Core Curriculum for
Ambulatory Care Nursing

Third Edition

Candia Baker Laughlin, MS, RN-BC

Editor

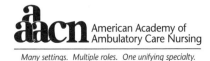

American Academy of
Ambulatory Care Nursing

Many settings. Multiple roles. One unifying specialty.

Core Curriculum for Ambulatory Care Nursing (3rd Edition)

Editor
Candia Baker Laughlin, MS, RN-BC

Managing Editor: Katie R. Brownlow, ELS
Editorial Assistant: Jamie Kalitz
Director of Editorial Services: Carol M. Ford
Layout Design & Production: Darin Peters
Director of Creative Design & Production: Jack M. Bryant

AAACN Executive Director: Cynthia Nowicki Hnatiuk, EdD, RN, CAE
AAACN Director of Association Services: Pat Reichart
AAACN Education Director: Rosemarie Marmion, MSN, RN-BC, NE-BC

Publication Management
Anthony J. Jannetti, Inc.
East Holly Avenue, Box 56, Pitman, NJ 08071-0056
856-256-2300; FAX 856-589-7463; www.ajj.com

THIRD EDITION
ISBN: 978-0-9846597-4-6

DISCLAIMER
The authors, reviewers, editors, and publishers of this book have made serious efforts to ensure that treatments, practices, and procedures are accurate and conform to standards accepted at the time of publication. Due to constant changes in information resulting from continuous research and clinical experience, reasonable differences in opinions among authorities, unique aspects of individual clinical situations, and the possibility of human error in preparing such a publication, the reader should exercise individual judgment when making a clinical decision, and if necessary, consult and compare information from other authorities, professionals, or sources.

SUGGESTED CITATION:
Laughlin, C.B. (Ed.). (2013). *Core curriculum for ambulatory care nursing* (3rd ed.). Pitman, NJ: American Academy of Ambulatory Care Nursing.

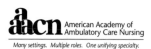

Many settings. Multiple roles. One unifying specialty.

East Holly Avenue/Box 56, Pitman, NJ 08071-0056
Phone: 800-262-AMBNURS (272-6877); Fax: 856-589-7463
Web site: www.aaacn.org; Email: aaacn@ajj.com

Contents

SECTION ONE – The Organizational/Systems Role of the Ambulatory Care Nurse

Contents

Foreword

The *Core Curriculum for Ambulatory Care Nursing* (3rd Edition) serves as an excellent resource for nurses, whether new to ambulatory care, seasoned in the specialty, or perhaps studying to sit for the ambulatory care certification exam.

Candia Baker Laughlin, MS, RN-BC, Editor of the *Core Curriculum*, served as President of AAACN from 2002–2003. Exactly ten years later, her clinical expertise, professional experience, and passion for the practice of ambulatory care nursing are strongly evident in this text. Laughlin, along with many chapter authors chosen for their ambulatory care practice expertise, have skillfully updated the *Core Curriculum* to include new content on topics such as nursing care of surgical patients in the ambulatory setting, telehealth nursing, integrative therapies, needs of high-risk patient populations, patient safety, and emerging clinical issues.

The design of the delivery of patient care in ambulatory care settings has changed since the *Core Curriculum* was last published in 2006. Change continues today. This redesign of the landscape of our health care environment is in large part due to the many initiatives of health care reform, such as accountable care organizations and patient-centered medical homes. Today, the specialty of ambulatory care nursing has more opportunity than ever before. New technology is emerging, and the role of the ambulatory care nurse is evolving, with the ultimate goal of improving patient outcomes. With this update, the *Core Curriculum* recognizes that as our specialty changes, so must our leadership and practice skills.

The AAACN Board of Directors and I would like to thank Editor Candia Baker Laughlin, as well as the many expert authors, editors, and reviewers who dedicated many hours to the *Core Curriculum*. We would also like to acknowledge two members of the Board of Directors — Linda Brixey, RN, and Nancy May, MSN, RN-BC — who reviewed the text on behalf of the Board. We have great respect for everyone who contributed in updating this edition, which covers a broad scope of topics on ambulatory care nursing.

The *Core Curriculum* is not only an excellent resource to advance practice and leadership skills, but it is also a valuable aid for those studying for ambulatory care nursing certification.

I hope you enjoy this magnificent contribution to the practice of ambulatory care nursing, where as nurses, we work in many settings and have multiple roles, but are part of one unifying specialty.

Suzanne N. Wells, MSN, RN
AAACN President, 2012–2013

Preface

The *Core Curriculum for Ambulatory Care Nursing* (3rd Edition) is a comprehensive reference intended to support the American Academy of Ambulatory Care Nursing's mission: "To advance the art and science of ambulatory care nursing." As the specialty of ambulatory care nursing has continued to grow in breadth and depth, the knowledge and skills required for practice and leadership in this arena do as well. No text can cover all the topics an ambulatory care nurse may need, nor provide the depth in any single topic. Additionally, the health care environment and science continue to rapidly change. However, this reference is written to address a very broad scope, and points the reader to additional resources to seek supplementary information or identify changes in the field.

This edition of the *Core Curriculum* has been organized and expanded to address the educational needs of nurses new to the specialty and those with experience, as well as to provide a review for those who seek specialty certification as an ambulatory care nurse. As the specialty has changed, so has the content of the American Nurses Credentialing Center's examination. The changes in the content and organization of this edition not only reflect the new knowledge, but also the content of the certification exam. Additionally, feedback and requests from readers of the second edition have been incorporated.

Features of the third edition include:

- New chapters addressing ambulatory nursing care of surgical patients and emerging concepts and practice models related to chronic illness care.
- Expanded content on telehealth nursing, patient safety, complementary and alternative therapies, the impact of health care reform, and the needs of special patient populations, such as the homeless or victims of abuse.
- The latest content on emerging clinical issues, which may be observed by nurses in almost any ambulatory care setting, such as autism spectrum disorder, common emergency conditions, and HIV/AIDS as a chronic condition.

Authors of each chapter or topic were selected for their expertise in the area, and other experts reviewed the content to ensure its accuracy and relevance. In recognition of the value of this continuing education activity, contact hours are offered following the study of each chapter (see p. xviii).

The Ambulatory Care Nursing Conceptual Framework, developed by a "think tank" of AAACN expert members in 1998 and revised in 2010, is the basis for the text's organization. The sections of the book reflect the framework's three roles identified for the ambulatory care nurse: organization/systems role, professional role, and clinical role. The core areas of knowledge and skills within each of those three roles are reflected in those sections of the text. The core knowledge and skill dimensions that are part of the clinical role are applied to patient populations served by ambulatory care nurses, and are defined as well, acutely ill, chronically ill, or terminally ill.

The content is presented in outline format for easy review and reference. Key terms that are defined in the text are also captured in the Glossary. Many Web resources, community agencies, and published references are identified throughout the text and at the end of chapters for further information.

The American Academy of Ambulatory Care Nursing and its association management firm, Anthony J. Jannetti, Inc., are commended for their vision and leadership in supporting the publication of the *Core Curriculum for Ambulatory Care Nursing*. It is fortunate that so many authors and reviewers provided a wealth of expertise from their diverse settings, backgrounds, and geographic locations across the United States and Canada. All these individuals have demonstrated tremendous commitment to advancing the art and science of ambulatory care nursing that is evident in the pages that follow.

Candia Baker Laughlin, MS, RN-BC
Editor

Contributors

Nancy M. Albert, PhD, CCNS, CHFN, CCRN, NE-BC
Director, Nursing Research & Innovation, and
  Clinical Nurse Specialist
Kaufman Center for Heart Failure
Cleveland Clinic
Cleveland, OH

Jennifer Allen, MSQSM, RN, CPAN
Nursing Transition Coordinator
Walter Reed National Military Medical Center
  Bethesda
Bethesda, MD

Diana Anderson, BSN, RN, CPN
Site Nurse, Ambulatory – Atlantic County
  Specialty Care Center
The Children's Hospital of Philadelphia Care
  Network
Pediatric and Adolescent Specialty Care
Mays Landing, NJ

Ida M. Androwich, PhD, RN-BC, FAAN
Professor and Director HSM
Loyola University Chicago
Chicago, IL

Marie Beisel, MSN, RN, CPHQ
Senior Project Manager
University of Michigan, Ambulatory Care Services
Ann Arbor, MI

Catherine M. Besthoff, RN, MHA, CPHQ
Director, Program Evaluation
North Shore – LIJ Health System
Krasnoff Quality Management Institute
Great Neck, NY

Mary Anne Bord-Hoffman, MN, RN-BC
Nurse Manager
VA Palo Alto Healthcare System, San Jose
  Community Based Outpatient Clinic
San Jose, CA

Kathy Bratcher, MS, RN
Director, Clinical Development and Training
Palo Alto Medical Foundation
Palo Alto, CA

Michelle Budzinski-Braunscheidel, BSN, RN
Team Leader, Pediatric Specialties
Cleveland Clinic
Cleveland, OH

Deborah Byrne-Barta, BSN, RN-BC, CPN
Site Nurse
The Children's Hospital of Philadelphia Care
  Network
Pediatric and Adolescent Specialty Care
Voorhees, NJ

Renée Y. Cecil, MSN, RN
Subspecialty Practice Nurse IV/Nurse
  Coordinator
The Children's Hospital of Philadelphia
Philadelphia, PA

Patricia D. Chambers, BHScN, RN
Manager
Alberta Health Services
Calgary, Alberta
Canada

Mark Cichocki, RN
HIV Nurse Educator
University of Michigan HIV/AIDS Treatment
  Program
Ann Arbor, MI

Debra Ann Clementino, MS, RN, JD
RN Case Manager, Hospice Home Care
Grace Hospice
Lansing, MI

Mary Elizabeth Davis, MSN, RN, CHPN, AOCNS
Clinical Nurse Specialist
Memorial Sloan Kettering Cancer Center
New York, NY

Pamela Del Monte, MS, RN-BC
Associate Chief Nurse/Ambulatory Care Service
Department of Veterans Affairs – DVAMC
Durham, NC

Contributors

Gail DeLuca, MS, FNP-BC
Assistant Professor
St. Xavier University
Chicago, IL

Eileen M. Esposito, DNP, RN-BC, CPHQ
Principal & Executive Consultant
Ambulatory Expert Solutions
Jerchio, NY

Kristene K. Grayem, MSN, CNP, RN
Director of Nursing, Clinical Systems & PI
Akron Children's Hospital
Akron, OH

Sheila A. Haas, PhD, RN, FAAN
Professor, Niehoff School of Nursing
Loyola University Chicago
Maywood, IL
Past President
American Academy of Ambulatory Care Nursing

Annette S. Hamlin, BSN, RN
Education Coordinator
Akron Children's Hospital
Akron, OH

Clare Hastings, PhD, RN, FAAN
Chief Nurse Officer
National Institutes of Health Clinical Center
Bethesda, MD
Past President
American Academy of Ambulatory Care Nursing

Jane Holloway, BSN, RN
Education Coordinator
Akron Children's Hospital
Akron, OH

Anne T. Jessie, MSN, RN
Senior Director of Ambulatory Nursing Practice
Carilion Clinic
Roanoke, VA

E. Mary Johnson, BSN, RN-BC, NE-BC
Patient Navigator
Center for Health Affairs
Cleveland, OH
Past President
American Academy of Ambulatory Care Nursing

Peggy Kaminsky, MSN, RN, CIC
Infection Prevention Manager
Kaiser Foundation Hospital Redwood City
Redwood City, CA

Roslyn C. Kelly, MSN, RN-BC, CDE
Managed Care Diabetes Nurse Educator
Veterans Affairs Maryland Health Care System
Baltimore, MD

Kathy Kesner, MS, RN, CNS
CNS Educator
University of Colorado Hospital
Aurora, CO

Margaret Ross Kraft, PhD, RN
Assistant Professor
Loyola University Chicago
Maywood, IL

Candia Baker Laughlin, MS, RN-BC
Director of Nursing, Ambulatory Care Services
University of Michigan Health System
Ann Arbor, MI
Past President
American Academy of Ambulatory Care Nursing

June Levine, MSN, RN
National Consultant Ambulatory Nursing
Ben Hudnall Memorial Trust
Kaiser Permanente
Oakland, CA

Patricia Lucarelli, MSN, RN-BC, CPNP, APN
Pediatric Nurse Practitioner
Jersey Shore University Medical Center
K. Hovnanian Children's Hospital
Neptune, NJ

Margaret Fisk Mastal, PhD, RN
Independent Consultant
Alexandria, VA
Past President
American Academy of Ambulatory Care Nursing

Wanda Mayo, BSN, RN, CPN
Case Manager
Amerigroup Corp
Grand Prairie, TX

Contributors

Jennifer Mills, LCDR, NC, USN, MSN, CNS-BC
Division Officer, General Internal Medicine
  Services
Walter Reed National Military Medical Center
Bethesda, MD

Barbara Pacca, BSN, RN, CPN, HTP
Field Nurse
Children's Hospital Home Care
King of Prussia, PA

Susan M. Paschke, MSN, RN-BC, NEA-BC
Chief Clinical & Quality Officer
VNA of Ohio
Cleveland, OH
President-Elect, 2012-2013
American Academy of Ambulatory Care Nursing

Joan M. Paté, MS, BSN, RN-BC
Legal Nurse Consultant
Sandia Medical-Legal Consultant, LLC
Rio Rancho, NM

CAPT Wanda C. Richards, MSM, MPA, BSN
Assistant Deputy Commander, BRAC and
  Nursing Integration
Walter Reed National Military Medical Center
Bethesda, MD

Sherry Smith, MSN, MBA, RN
Chief Consulting Officer
3CT, Call Center Consulting Team
Gilford, NH

Jane Westmoreland Swanson, PhD, RN, NEA-BC
Director, Geri and Richard Brawerman Nursing
  Institute
Cedars-Sinai
Los Angeles, CA
Past President
American Academy of Ambulatory Care Nursing

Deborah D. Tinker, MSN, RN, CENP
Director, Ambulatory Nursing
University of Wisconsin Hospital & Clinics
Madison, WI

Christina Watwood, MPH/MHA, BSN, RN
Operations Engineer
Vanderbilt University Medical Center
Nashville, TN

Sarah Jane Whalen-Espin, MSN, CCRN, RN-BC
Clinical Nurse Educator
The Villages VA Outpatient Clinic
NF/SG Veterans Health System
The Villages, FL

Carol Jo Wilson, PhD, FNP-BC
Dean and Professor
University of St. Francis
Joliet, IL

Reviewers

Jo Ann Appleyard, PhD, RN
Director, Undergraduate Program
Clinical Assistant Professor
University of Wisconsin – Milwaukee College of
    Nursing
Milwaukee, WI
Past President
American Academy of Ambulatory Care Nursing

Amy Bacon, BSN, RN, AE-C
Respiratory Care Nurse Educator
GlaxoSmithKline Pharmaceuticals
Houston, TX

Martha R. Baker, MS, RN, MA
Clinical Faculty
Kaiser Permanente
Denver, CO

Elizabeth Barnhart, FNP
Clinical Nursing Director
Tufts Medical Center
Boston, MA

Carole A. Becker, MS, RN
Clinical Content Analyst
Relay Health, A Division of McKesson
Scottsdale, AZ

Donna M. Carroll, BSN, RN-C
Staff Nurse Primary Care – Ambulatory Clinic
The VA Outpatient Clinic
The Villages, FL

Regina Conway-Phillips, PhD, RN
Assistant Professor
Loyola University Chicago
Marcella Niehoff School of Nursing
Chicago, IL
Past President
American Academy of Ambulatory Care Nursing

Debbie Dannemeyer, BSN, RN-BC, MAS
Ambulatory Practice Leader
Assistant Medical Group Administrator
Kaiser Permanente
Anaheim, CA

Linda Dilley, BSN, RN
Kelsey-Seybold Clinic
Sugar Land, TX

Renee Dursun, BSN, RN
Pediatric Nurse Care Coordinator – Telephone
    Triage
Shriners Hospital for Children
Chicago, IL

Marna K. Flaherty-Robb, MSN, RN, CNS
Chief Nursing Information Officer
University of Michigan Hospitals and Health
    System
Ann Arbor, MI

Ruth L. Fritskey, MSN, RN, AOCN
IRB Research Nurse
Cleveland Clinic
Cleveland, OH

Adina S. Gutstein, MSN, CRNP, FPCNA
Nurse Practitioner
Cardiovascular Medical Associates, PC
Philadelphia, PA

Linda Harden, BSN, MS, RN-BC
Chief Nursing Office
Henry Ford Medical Group
Detroit, MI

Cheedy Jaja, PhD, MPH, MN, RN
Assistant Professor of Nursing
College of Nursing
Georgia Health Sciences University
Augusta, GA

Barbara S. Kiernan, PhD, APRN, PNP-BC
Chair and Associate Professor, Biobehavioral
    Nursing
Georgeia Health Sciences University
Augusta, GA

Debra Kirkley, PhD, RN
Director, Professional Practice & Development
Group Health Cooperative
Seattle, WA

Reviewers

Robin J. Kruger, BSN, RNC-TNP
Clinical Instructor
Cleveland Clinic Nurse on Call
Cleveland, OH

Sharon Lanzetta, MSN, RN, BC
Unit Director, PACU, PTU, SOU
University of California Los Angeles (UCLA)
Los Angeles, CA

Aaron J. Loeb, MBA, MS, RN
Clinical Educator
Kelsey-Seybold Clinic
Houston, TX

Nancy May, MSN, RN-BC
Chief Nursing Officer – Ambulatory Practice
Scott and White Healthcare
Temple, TX

Caroline R. McKinnon, PhD(c), PMHCNS-BC
Clinical Instructor
Georgia Health Sciences University, College of
    Nursing
Augusta, GA

Phyllis J. Mesko, CPN, RN
Staff Nurse, PACU
Akron Children's Hospital
Akron, OH

Vannesia D. Morgan-Smith, MGA, RN, NE-BC
Administrative Manager of Patient Services
Children's National Medical Center
Washington, DC

Carol Ann Nash, BSN, RN
Hypertension Nurse Clinician
Mayo Clinic Division of Nephrology and
    Hypertension
Rochester, MN

Lori Musolf Neri, MSN, CRNP, CLS, FPCNA
DIrector, Center for Cardiac Risk Prevention
The Heart Care Group
Allentown, PA

Susan A. Olsson, BSN, RN-BC
Occupational Health Nurse
University of Michigan Health System
Ann Arbor, MI

Mary K. Parker, CNS
Division Officer, General Surgery Clinic
United States Navy
Bethesda, MD

Susan Peterson, RN
Nursing Supervisor, Gastroenterology
Kelsey-Seybold Clinic
Houston, TX

Rebecca Linn Pyle, MSN, RN, B-C
Director of Nursing, Digestive Health Institute
Children's Hospital Colorado
Aurora, CO
Past President
American Academy of Ambulatory Care Nursing

Sandra W. Reifsteck, MS Ed, RN, FACMPE
Director, Office of Development and Quality
    Outcomes
Institute for Healthcare Communication
New Haven, CT
Past President
American Academy of Ambulatory Care Nursing

Diane Resnick, RN-BC, MPA
Manager, Jane H. Booker Family Health Center
Jersey Shore University Medical Center, Meridian
    Health
Neptune, NJ

Michael H. Ross, MSN, RN, ACNS-BC
Clinical Nurse Specialist
Andersen Air Force Base Medical Clinic
United States Air Force
Andersen AFB
Guam

Carol Rutenberg, RN-BC, C-TNP, MNSc
President
Telephone Triage Consulting, Inc.
Hot Springs, AR

Reviewers

Pamela Sanford, MSN, RN-BC, CNS
Clinical Educator III
Scott and White Healthcare
Temple, TX

Paula Schipiour, MS, RN
Nursing Faculty
Robert Morris University
Chicago, IL

Matthew D. Schreiner, RN
Infectious Disease Clinic Nurse
Michigan State University
Kalamazoo Center for Medical Studies
Kalamazoo, MI

Dawn D. Smith, RN
RN Supervisor
Kelsey-Seybold Clinic
Sugar Land, TX

Deborah A. Smith, DNP, RN
Associate Professor
Georgia Health Sciences University
Augusta, GA

Rowena P. Stevens-Ross, BSN, MSN/MBA, RN
Certified Legal Nurse Consultant/Nurse
    Entrepreneur
Escondido, CA

Lisa Swerczek, BSN, RN
Coordinator
St. Louis Children's Hospital Answer Line
St. Louis, MO

Susan Trapp, BSN-BC, RN
Nurse Manager
UNMC Physicians
Bellevue, NE

Dana Tschannen, PhD, RN
Clinical Assistant Professor
University of Michigan, School of Nursing
Ann Arbor, MI

Dedria R. Tuck, BSN, RN, CPN
Clinical Team Leader, Family Medicine Residency
Carilion Clinic
Roanoke, VA

Mary Hines Vinson, DNP, RN-BC, CMPE
Associate Chief Nursing Officer, Ambulatory
    Nursing and Patient Care Services
Duke University Health System
Durham, NC

Catherine York, MSN, RN, CRNP
Nurse Practitioner, Cardiology
Heart Care Group
Allentown, PA

Acknowledgements

The authors who researched and wrote the 22 chapters in this publication are all experts in ambulatory care nursing, and it has been my privilege to work with each of them. Many had contributed similar content in earlier editions, and they carefully researched, updated, and revised it to support best practices in today's health care environment. I was also pleased to recruit some new authors, all of whom proved to be excellent and rose to the challenges of the scope and nature of this text. Additionally, I thank the content experts who reviewed every page, most of whom reviewed several chapters or sections of chapters. Writing and reviewing content for a textbook requires hard work and perseverance. I owe a debt of gratitude to each one of them for their responsiveness and commitment.

I want to express a special recognition to the memory of Tracey Offutt, BSN, RN, who passionately committed and began authoring content for this edition, but passed away unexpectedly. My sincere condolences continue to go to her husband, Jason Offutt, and the rest of her family.

I would also like to thank those individuals who supported the development of this third edition. I am immensely grateful to Jamie Kalitz, our Editorial Assistant, who provided her support and expertise in managing deadlines, tracking chapters, communicating with authors and reviewers, and reassuring me when I became anxious. I thank Katie R. Brownlow, ELS, our Managing Editor, for her guidance, encouragement, support, and superb editorial skill. I thank the AAACN Board of Directors for offering me this opportunity.

Finally, I want to thank those who provided me personal and professional mentorship, counsel, encouragement, and support. My wonderful husband, Harry, has provided tremendous support to make this project possible. My friend and AAACN partner, Cynthia Nowicki Hnatiuk, EdD, RN, CAE, who has recognized and encouraged my passion for AAACN for many years, persuaded me that I could do this again and declared that she was "counting on me." Finally and most importantly, I owe an immeasurable debt to my dear mother, Patricia Baker, who I lost during the course of the composition of this text. She has always been my role model as a person and as a nurse, and taught me to do what I care about and to care about what I do.

Candia Baker Laughlin, MS, RN-BC
Editor

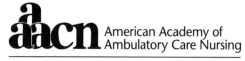
American Academy of Ambulatory Care Nursing

Many settings. Multiple roles. One unifying specialty.

The American Academy of Ambulatory Care Nursing is a welcoming, unifying community for registered nurses in all ambulatory care settings. This professional organization offers:

MISSION: Advance the art and science of ambulatory care nursing.

VISION: Professional registered nurses are the recognized leaders in ambulatory care environments. They are valued and rewarded as essential to quality health care.

- Connections with others in similar roles
- Help in advancing practice and leadership skills
- Advocacy that promotes greater appreciation for the specialty of ambulatory care nursing

CORE VALUES: Individually and collectively, our members are guided by our deep belief in:
- Responsible health care delivery for individuals, families, and communities
- Visionary and accountable leadership
- Productive partnerships, alliances, and collaborations
- Appreciation of diversity
- Continual advancement of professional ambulatory care nursing practice

STRATEGIC GOALS:
1. Serve Our Members – Enhance the professional growth and career advancement of our members.
2. Expand Our Influence – Expand the influence of AAACN and ambulatory care nurses to achieve a greater positive impact on the quality of ambulatory care.
3. Strengthen Our Core – Ensure a healthy organization committed to serving our members and expanding our influence.

MEMBERSHIP: Over 2,300 registered nurses who practice in varying ambulatory care settings such as hospital-based outpatient clinics/centers, solo/group medical practices, telehealth call centers, university hospitals, community hospitals, military and VA settings, managed care/HMOs/PPOs, colleges/educational institutions, patient homes, and free-standing facilities. Members are managers and supervisors, administrators and directors, staff nurses, care coordinators, educators, consultants, advanced practice nurses, and researchers.

MEMBERSHIP BENEFITS: Academy membership benefits include discounted rates to the AAACN National Preconference and Conference, offering multiple practice innovations, industry exhibits, and numerous networking opportunities. Other benefits include: distance learning programs, special member rates on publications and the fee to take the ANCC ambulatory care nursing certification exam, the bimonthly newsletter *(ViewPoint)*, subscription to **one** of three journals *(Nursing Economic$, MEDSURG Nursing,* or *Pediatric Nursing),* opportunity to join a special interest group (Leadership, Patient Education, Pediatrics, Staff Education, Telehealth Nursing Practice, Veterans Affairs, and Tri-Service Military), awards and scholarship programs, access to national experts and colleagues through the AAACN online membership directory, monthly E-newsletter, email discussion lists, Online Library, an Expert Panel, Web site (aaacn.org), and online Career Center.

AAACN PUBLICATIONS/EDUCATION RESOURCES:
- *Scope and Standards of Practice for Professional Ambulatory Care Nursing*
- *Ambulatory Care Nursing Certification Review Course Syllabus*
- *Ambulatory Care Nursing Certification Review Course DVD*
- *Ambulatory Care Nursing Orientation and Competency Assessment Guide*
- *Ambulatory Care Nursing Review Questions*
- *Core Curriculum for Ambulatory Care Nursing*

- *Scope and Standards of Practice for Professional Telehealth Nursing*
- *Telehealth Nursing Practice Core Course (TNPCC) DVD*
- *Telehealth Nursing Practice Essentials Textbook*

AAACN COURSES:
- Ambulatory Care Nursing Certification Review Course*
- Telehealth Nursing Practice Core Course (TNPCC)*

* Both courses can be presented at your location – call the National Office for details. Site licenses for multiple users are available. Courses are also available on DVD and in the Online Library at www.aaacn.org/library.

ANNUAL CONFERENCE:
AAACN provides cutting-edge information and education at its annual conference, usually held in the month of March, April, or May. Nurses from across the country, as well as international colleagues, come together to network, learn from each other, and share knowledge and skills. Renowned speakers in the field of ambulatory care present topics of current interest. An Exhibit Hall featuring the products and services of vendors serving the ambulatory care and telehealth community provides information and resources to attendees.

CERTIFICATION:
AAACN values the importance of certification and promotes achieving this level of competency through its educational products to prepare nurses to take the ambulatory care nursing certification examination. AAACN strongly encourages all telehealth nurses to become certified in ambulatory care nursing. Because telehealth nurses provide nursing care to patients who are in ambulatory settings, they must possess the knowledge and competencies to appropriately provide ambulatory care. Ambulatory certification is and will continue to be the gold standard credential for any nursing position within ambulatory care.

CORPORATE COLLABORATIONS:
Together, working with corporate colleagues, AAACN continues to advance the delivery of ambulatory care to patients. AAACN is open to alliances or collaborations with corporate industry to achieve mutual goals. Corporations are encouraged to contact the national office to suggest ways AAACN can work with them to advance the practice of ambulatory care nursing.

American Academy of Ambulatory Care Nursing
East Holly Avenue, Box 56, Pitman, NJ 08071-0056
Phone: 800-262-6877; Fax: 856-589-7463
Email: aaacn@ajj.com; Web site: www.aaacn.org

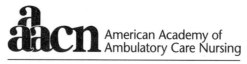

American Academy of
Ambulatory Care Nursing

Many settings. Multiple roles. One unifying specialty.

Position Statement: The Role of the Registered Nurse in Ambulatory Care

Background

Ambulatory care nursing is a unique realm of specialized nursing practice. Ambulatory nurses are leaders in their practice settings and across the continuum of care. They are uniquely qualified to influence organizational standards related to patient safety and care delivery in the outpatient setting. Ambulatory care nurses are knowledge workers who function in a multidisciplinary, collaborative practice environment, where they utilize critical thinking skills to interpret complex information and guide patients and families to health and well being (Swan, Conway-Phillips, & Griffin, 2006).

"Historically, the outpatient setting was the 'professional home' of physicians. They saw the majority of their patients in their offices and referred them for other services or levels of care, as needed. Registered nurses were few, as the system was physician driven. However, fiscal caps for hospital care and technological advances moved patients from inpatient venues into the ambulatory care setting. Patients required higher levels of care than in the traditional outpatient settings, and the ambulatory venue saw a growth in the number of professional nurses" (Mastal, 2010, p. 267).

The transition of health care from the inpatient to the outpatient setting has led to challenges with access to care and coordination of services, and has increased the complexity of care delivered outside hospital walls. This shift has dramatically increased the need for professional nursing services, as patients and their families require increased depth and breadth of care. Ambulatory RNs facilitate patient care services by managing and individualizing care for patients and their families, who increasingly require assistance navigating the complex health care system. In addition to the provision of complex procedural care, professional nursing services provide support with decision-making, patient education, and coordination of services.

"Many characteristics differentiate ambulatory care nursing from other specialty practices, including the settings, the characteristics of the patient encounters, and focus on groups, communities, and populations, as well as individual patients and their families" (Mastal, 2010, p. 267). The current ambulatory care setting is diverse and multifaceted, requiring nurses highly skilled in patient assessment and with the ability to implement a broad range of nursing interventions in a variety of settings. RNs in ambulatory care must possess strong clinical, education, and advocacy skills, and demonstrate the ability to manage care in complex organizational systems. Registered nurses are uniquely qualified, autonomous providers of patient/family-centered care that is ethical, evidence-based, safe, expert, innovative, healing, compassionate, and universally accessible.

Efforts to conserve financial and nursing resources, along with a lack of understanding of differing roles, has led many organizations to under-utilize RNs in ambulatory settings. The economic benefit of care delivered by RNs has been demonstrated by their impact on patient satisfaction, quality patient outcomes, patient safety, reduced adverse events, and reductions in hospital/emergency department admissions (Haas, 2008; Institute of Medicine, 2011; O'Connell, Johnson, Stallmeyer, & Cokingtin, 2001). The future of the American health care system depends upon our ability to utilize registered nurses to the maximum of their expertise, licensure, and certification.

Position Statement

It is the position of the American Academy of Ambulatory Care Nursing that:
- RNs enhance patient safety and the quality and effectiveness of care delivery and are thus essential and irreplaceable in the provision of patient care services in the ambulatory setting.
- RNs are responsible for the design, administration, and evaluation of professional nursing services within the organization in accordance

with the framework established by state nurse practice acts, nursing scope of practice, and organizational standards of care.

- RNs provide the leadership necessary for collaboration and coordination of services, which includes defining the appropriate skill mix and delegation of tasks among licensed and unlicensed health care workers.
- RNs are fully accountable in all ambulatory care settings for all nursing services and associated patient outcomes provided under their direction.

References

Haas, S.A. (2008). Resourcing evidence-based practice in ambulatory care nursing. *Nursing Economic$, 26*(5), 319-322.

Institute of Medicine. (2011). *The future of nursing: Leading change, advancing health.* Washington, DC: The National Academies Press.

Mastal, M.F. (2010). Ambulatory care nursing: Growth as a professional specialty. *Nursing Economics$, 28*(4), 267-269, 275.

O'Connell, J., Johnson, D., Stallmeyer, J., & Cokingtin, D. (2001). A satisfaction and return-on-investment study of a nurse triage service. *American Journal of Managed Care, 7*, 159-169.

Swan, B.A., Conway-Phillips, R., & Griffin, K.F. (2006). Demonstrating the value of the RN in ambulatory care. *Nursing Economic$, 24*(6), 315-322.

Additional Readings

American Academy of Ambulatory Care Nursing. (2006). *Core curriculum for ambulatory care nursing* (2nd ed). Pitman, NJ: Author.

American Academy of Ambulatory Care Nursing. (2010). *Scope and standards of practice for professional ambulatory care nursing.* Pitman, NJ: Author.

American Nurses Association. (2004). *Nursing: Scope and standards of practice.* Silver Spring, MD: Author.

American Nurses Association. (2005). *Principles for delegation.* Silver Spring, MD: Author.

Haas, S.A., Gold, C.R., & Androwich, I. (1997). Identifying issues in nursing workload. *ViewPoint, 19*(2), 8-9.

Hnatiuk, C. (2006). The economic value of nursing. *ViewPoint, 28*(4), 1, 15.

Lucarellli, P. (2008). Thinking outside the exam room: Accessing community resources for patients in ambulatory care settings. *Nursing Economic$, 26*(4), 273-275.

Price, M.J., & Parkerton, P.H. (2007). Care delivery challenges for nurses. *American Journal of Nursing, 107*(6), 60-64.

Swan, B.A., & Griffin, K.F. (2005). Measuring nursing workload in ambulatory care. *Nursing Economic$, 23*(5), 253-260.

Uppal, S., Jose, J., Banks, P., Mackay, E., & Coatesworth, A.P. (2004). Cost-effective analysis of conventional and nurse-led clinics for common otological procedures. *Journal of Laryngology and Otology, 118*(3), 189-192.

Vlasses, F.R., & Smeltzer, C.H. (2007). Toward a new future for healthcare and nursing practice. *Journal of Nursing Administration, 37*(9), 375-380.

**Approved by AAACN Board of Directors
December 2010**

This position statement is further supported by the AAACN Position Paper: *The Role of the Registered Nurse in Ambulatory Care.* Both documents may be accessed at www.aaacn.org.

American Academy of Ambulatory Care Nursing
East Holly Avenue, Box 56, Pitman, NJ 08071-0056
Phone: 800-262-6877; Fax: 856-589-7463
Email: aaacn@ajj.com; Web site: www.aaacn.org

CNE Evaluation Instructions

Core Curriculum for Ambulatory Care Nursing (3ʳᵈ Edition)

- Prior to beginning the learning activity, go to the Online Library www.aaacn.org/library and check the posted expiration date to be sure the CNE credit for this activity has not expired.

- To receive CNE credit for individual study after reading each chapter in this book, you must complete the corresponding evaluation in the Online Library. Contact hours for these activities are free to AAACN members.

- Visit **www.aaacn.org/library** and log in using your email address and password. (Use the same log in and password for your AAACN Web site account and Online Library account. First-time visitors will need to establish an account.)

- Click *Core Curriculum* under "Other CE Opportunities" in the navigation bar.

- Complete the online evaluation for the chapter(s) you have completed, and print your CNE certificate. Certificates are always available under "CNE Transcript" in the Online Library.

- Continuing nursing education (CNE) credit offered from this book is valid until the date posted in the Online Library.

Fees

AAACN Member: Free
Regular: $5 per chapter

These educational activities have been co-provided by Anthony J. Jannetti, Inc. and the American Academy of Ambulatory Care Nursing (AAACN).

Anthony J. Jannetti, Inc. is accredited as a provider of continuing nursing education by the American Nurses Association (ANCC) Credentialing Center's Commission on Accreditation.

AAACN is a provider approved by the California Board of Registered Nursing, provider number CEP 5366. Licensees in the state of California must retain the awarded certificate for four years after a CNE activity is completed.

These activities were reviewed and formatted for contact hour credit by Rosemarie Marmion, MSN, RN-BC, NE-BC, AAACN Education Director. Accreditation status does not imply endorsement by the provider or ANCC of any commercial product.

Potential Conflict of Interest Disclosures

Mary Elizabeth Davis: The author is a member of the Advisory Board of Genentech Patient and Nursing Education.

All other authors and reviewers reported no actual or potential conflict of interest in relation to the continuing nursing education activities.

The Organizational/Systems Role Of the Ambulatory Care Nurse

Chapter 1

Professional Ambulatory Care Nursing Practice

Margaret Fisk Mastal, PhD, RN

OBJECTIVES – *Study of the information in this chapter will enable the learner to:*

1. Discuss the historical evolution of ambulatory care nursing as a professional specialty.
2. Define ambulatory care nursing practice as a unique professional specialty.
3. Discuss the conceptual framework of ambulatory care nursing practice.
4. Discuss the scope and standards of practice for professional ambulatory care nursing practice.
5. Articulate the role of the registered nurse in ambulatory care.

KEY POINTS – *The major points in this chapter include:*

1. Ambulatory care nursing practice has evolved over the past four decades into a professional nursing specialty.
2. Ambulatory care nursing practice is a complex, multifaceted specialty that is both independent and collaborative as nurses partner with patients, caregivers, and other health care professionals to meet the health and illness needs of individuals, groups, communities, and populations.
3. The conceptual framework, or blueprint, for ambulatory care nursing practice is identified and defined in terms of three major interrelated concepts: patient, nurse, and environment.
4. The scope and standards of practice specify the circumstances that promote the effective management of increasingly complex nursing roles and specify the expectations of professional nursing practice in ambulatory care.
5. Professional registered nurses are essential and irreplaceable in the coordinated delivery of services in ambulatory settings, and bring economic benefits to ambulatory care by improving patient satisfaction, enhancing quality patient outcomes and patient safety, reducing the occurrence of adverse events, and diminishing hospital and emergency department admissions.

Modern professional ambulatory care nursing is a unique domain of nursing practice that focuses on health care for individuals, families, groups, communities, and populations. Ambulatory care nurses practice in settings distinctive from other nurses. They practice in primary and specialty care outpatient venues, non-acute surgical and diagnostic outpatient settings in the community, and via telehealth or electronic encounters with call centers, medical offices, or other outpatient settings. Usually, the patient initiates the contact with nurses and other health care providers in ambulatory care settings.

Patients in ambulatory care predominantly engage in self-care and self-managed health activities or receive care from family/significant others outside institutional settings. Nurses assist and influence patients and/or caregivers in making informed decisions about their self-care and health behaviors (Mastal, 2010).

Ambulatory care nursing is typified by registered nurses caring for high volumes of patients in short periods of time (usually less than 24 hours), often dealing with issues in each encounter that can be unknown and unpredictable. Ambulatory care nurses address, in partnership and collaboration with other health care professionals, patients' wellness, acute illness, chronic disease, disability, and end-of-life needs. As nurses, they are responsible for patient advocacy, coordination of nursing and other health services for continuity of care, implementation of nursing services, and applying evidence-based nursing knowledge to their practice.

I. Historical Evolution of Ambulatory Care Nursing Practice as a Professional Specialty

Ambulatory care nursing practice has evolved and experienced extensive changes over the past four decades. It has been a demanding and thought-provoking journey that has produced the highly specialized professional subspecialty it is today.

A. Historically, the outpatient setting was the "professional home" of physicians (Mastal, 2010).
   1. Physicians saw the majority of outpatients in their medical offices, referring them to other services or levels of care as needed.
   2. Registered nurses were few because the system was physician-driven.
B. Radical change during the latter quarter of the 20th century served as an impetus for patients to move from hospitals to outpatient settings for much of their care (Mastal, 2006).
   1. Diagnostic-related groups (DRGs) and other reimbursement changes for inpatient venues resulted in decreased lengths of stay and more outpatient surgeries.
   2. Technological advances were implemented that impacted care in all venues.
   3. Health promotion and disease prevention as priorities for quality living were acknowledged worldwide.
   4. Primary health care was defined as essential health care (World Health Organization [WHO], 1978).
   5. The Institute of Medicine (IOM) (1978) issued the first definition of primary care, conceptualized as personal health services – "accessible, comprehensive, coordinated, and continual care delivery by providers of personnel health services" (p. 5).
   6. Patients in outpatient settings required higher levels of care and the roles of nurses in ambulatory care expanded.
C. Formalization of ambulatory care nursing practice as a professional specialty.

1. Definition of ambulatory care nursing as a professional nursing specialty (American Nurses Association [ANA], 2003) required the following:
   a. Articulate the practice base.
   b. Provide for research and development of that base.
   c. Institute a system for nursing education.
   d. Establish the structures for delivering nursing services.
   e. Provide quality review mechanisms, including a code of ethics, standards of practice, and a system of credentialing.
   f. Evolve as a specialty nursing organization.
2. Visionary nurse leaders in ambulatory care settings leveraged collegial partnerships with physician groups, identifying the changing role of the nurse in outpatient settings.
3. The nurse leader group organized officially in 1979 and established the American Academy of Ambulatory Nursing Administration (AAANA), which:
   a. Established bylaws, recruited members.
   b. Began discussions with ANA.
   c. Conducted annual conferences.
   d. Developed and published the first edition of *Ambulatory Care Nursing Administration and Practice Standards* in 1987. Thereafter, standards have been updated every three years.
   e. Broadened focus beyond administration to all ambulatory care nursing and renamed the association the American Academy of Ambulatory Care Nursing (AAACN) in 1992.
   f. Recognized telehealth nursing as an expanding and integral aspect of ambulatory care nursing practice. Began to organize and formalize telephone nursing practice.

g. AAACN members partnered with ANA to publish the first monograph on the specialty, *Nursing in Ambulatory Care: The Future Is Here,* containing the first formal definition of ambulatory care nursing practice (AAACN/ANA, 1997).

h. Developed and published *Telephone Nursing Practice Administration and Practice Standards* (AAACN, 1997).

4. Isolation of the characteristics of professional nursing in ambulatory care.

a. Focus groups of experienced ambulatory care nurses identified the following characteristics of nursing practice in ambulatory care (Haas, 1998):
   (1) Nursing autonomy.
   (2) Patient advocacy.
   (3) Skillful, rapid assessment.
   (4) Holistic nursing care.
   (5) Client teaching.
   (6) Wellness and health promotion.
   (7) Coordination and continuity of care.
   (8) Long-term relationships with patients and families.
   (9) Telephone triage, consultation, follow-up, and surveillance.
   (10) Patient and family control as major caregivers, users of the health care systems, and decision-makers regarding compliance with care regimen.
   (11) Collaboration with other health care providers.
   (12) Case management.

b. First conceptual framework for ambulatory care nursing developed by an AAACN "expert member" think tank (Haas, 1998).
   (1) Identified two major concepts:
      (a) Patient – Defined in terms of persons who were healthy, acutely ill, chronically ill, and terminally ill.
      (b) Nurse – Defined in terms of three roles: Clinical, organizational/systems, and professional.

(2) Developed the first conceptual diagram depicting the two concepts and showing their relationship to each other.

5. Establishment of a credentialing process.
   a. Collaborated with the American Nurses Credentialing Center (ANCC) to delineate the core knowledge of the specialty for certification, building on the characteristics of ambulatory care nursing and the conceptual framework.
   b. Assisted ANCC to identify content experts for development of certification examination content.
   c. Developed study materials and a review course in addition to the standards, competencies, and telehealth nursing practice references.

II. Definition of Ambulatory Care Nursing Practice

The definition of ambulatory care nursing identifies the unique scope of practice and dimensions of practice that differentiate it from other nursing specialties.

A. Initial definitions of ambulatory care nursing identified by the following:
   1. Description of the practice setting.
   2. Description of the patients as those who were generally non-acute and were able to walk in for appointments.
   3. Length of care episodes were less than 24 hours in length (Haas, 2006).

B. Today's definition of ambulatory care nursing addresses:
   1. Patient populations served.
   2. Collaborative practice.
   3. Scope of practice and the defining characteristics/dimensions.
   4. Importance of quality in delivering nursing care and improved patient outcomes.
   5. Accountability for and autonomy in delivering ambulatory nursing care.

C. Definition of ambulatory care nursing practice.
   1. Professional ambulatory care nursing is a complex, multi-faceted specialty that encompasses independent and collaborative practice.

2. The comprehensive practice of ambulatory care nursing is built on a broad knowledge base of nursing and health sciences, and applies clinical expertise rooted in the nursing process.

3. Nurses use evidence-based information across a variety of outpatient health care settings to achieve and ensure patient safety and quality of care while improving patient outcomes.

4. Ambulatory care includes clinical, organizational, and professional activities engaged in by registered nurses with and for individuals, groups, and populations who seek assistance with improving health and/or seek care for health-related problems.

5. The ambulatory care registered nurse is accountable for the provision of nursing care in accordance with relevant federal requirements, state laws and nurse practice acts, regulatory standards, the standards of professional ambulatory care nursing practice, other relevant professional standards, and organizational policies (AAACN Task Force, 2011).

D. Defining characteristics – Differentiate ambulatory care nursing as a specialty distinct from other specialties and describe its major attributes.

1. Ambulatory nursing care requires critical reasoning and astute clinical judgment to expedite appropriate care and treatment, especially given that the patient may present with complex problems or potentially life-threatening conditions.

2 Ambulatory care registered nurses provide care across the lifespan to individuals, families, caregivers, groups, populations, and communities.

3. Ambulatory care nursing occurs across the continuum of care in a variety of settings that include (but are not limited to):
   a. Hospital-based outpatient clinics/centers.
   b. Solo and/or group medical practices.
   c. Ambulatory surgery and diagnostic procedure centers.
   d. Telehealth service environments.
   e. University and community hospital clinics.
   f. Military and Veterans Affairs settings.
   g. Nurse-managed clinics.
   h. Managed care organizations.
   i. Colleges and educational institutions.
   j. Freestanding community facilities.
   k. Care coordination organizations.
   l. Patients' homes.

4. Ambulatory care registered nurses interact with patients during face-to-face encounters or through a variety of telecommunication strategies, often establishing long-term relationships.

5. Telehealth nursing is an integral component of professional ambulatory care nursing that utilizes a variety of telecommunication technologies during encounters to assess, triage, provide nursing consultation, and perform follow-up and surveillance of patients' statuses and outcomes.

6. During each encounter, the ambulatory care registered nurse focuses on patient safety and the quality of nursing care by applying appropriate nursing interventions, such as:
   a. Identifying and clarifying patient needs.
   b. Performing nursing procedures.
   c. Conducting health education.
   d. Promoting patient advocacy.
   e. Coordinating nursing and other health services.
   f. Assisting the patient to navigate the health care system.
   g. Evaluating patient outcomes.

7. Nurse-patient encounters can occur once or as a series of occurrences, are usually less than 24 hours in length at any one time, and occur individually or in a group setting.

8. Ambulatory care registered nurses, acting as partners and advisors, assist and support patients and families to optimally manage their health care, respecting their culture and values, individual needs, health goals, and treatment preferences.

Figure 1-1.
Ambulatory Care Nursing Conceptual Framework Diagram

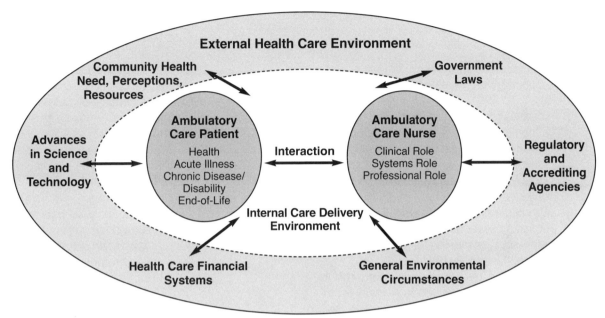

Source: AAACN, 2011b. Used with permission.

9. Ambulatory care registered nurses facilitate continuity of care using the nursing process, multidisciplinary collaboration, and coordination of appropriate health care services and community resources across the care continuum.

10. Ambulatory care registered nurses are knowledgeable about and provide leadership in the clinical and managerial operations of the organization.

11. Ambulatory care registered nurses design, administer, and evaluate nursing services within the organization in accord with relevant federal requirements, state laws and nurse practice acts, regulatory standards, relevant professional nursing standards, and institutional policies and procedures.

12. Ambulatory care registered nurses provide operational accountability for and coordination of nursing services, including the appropriate skill mix and delegation of roles and responsibilities for licensed and unlicensed nursing personnel.

13. Ambulatory care registered nurses apply the provisions of the American Nurses Association Code of Ethics for Nurses to their own professional obligations and for the patients entrusted to their care.

14. Ambulatory care registered nurses pursue lifelong learning that updates and expands their clinical, organizational, and professional roles and responsibilities (AAACN Task Force, 2011).

III. Ambulatory Care Nursing Conceptual Framework

The conceptual framework is a blueprint for the practice of ambulatory care nursing. It identifies the concepts that form the focus of the practice and provides a diagram of the relationship among the concepts (see Figure 1-1).

A. An ambulatory care nursing conceptual framework can assist in:

   1. Designing ambulatory care delivery models.

   2. Developing testing materials for competencies and certification.

3. Developing educational materials for ambulatory care nursing.
4. Developing orientation programs for ambulatory care nursing.
5. Providing a theoretical structure for research studies.

B. Initial conceptual framework for ambulatory care nursing was developed in 1998 (Haas, 1998).
   1. Created by a think tank leader group using a nominal group approach to delineate major areas of practice, knowledge, and skills.
   2. Identified and defined two major concepts: patient and nurse.
   3. Created a diagram that identified the relationship between the concepts.

C. Revision and expansion of the conceptual framework (Mastal, 2010).
   1. Developed by a Task Force of AAACN leaders; then submitted to AAACN members for review, editing, and final approval.
   2. Utilized and kept much of the work of the initial group who developed the first framework, especially as related to the concept of the nurse.
   3. Retained the concepts of "patient" and "nurse," but added a third concept – "environment."
      a. Patient – Includes the following assumptions:
         (1) Each patient is an individual, functioning holistically as a biological, psychosocial, and spiritual being.
         (2) Patients are the center of patient-nurse interactions, control decisions about their health care, have choices about interventions, and manage their health care between ambulatory care encounters.
         (3) The term *patient* refers to individuals, families, caregivers/support systems, groups, and populations that approach the health care system in a variety of situations and health states.

         (4) Patients usually live in the community, but may visit the ambulatory care setting from an institution (such as an assisted-living or group home) for a specific reason.
         (5) Health states are categorized as:
            (a) Wellness or health – Essentially healthy.
            (b) Acute illness – Ill, but usually healthy (may have sinusitis, appendicitis).
            (c) Chronic disease and/or disabled (such as diabetes, asthma, or heart disease).
               i. Individuals who are chronically ill can also have an acute exacerbation or an acute illness (for example, the individual with asthma can have an upper respiratory infection).
               ii. Individuals who are disabled can have a physical and/or a behavioral disability, as well as an acute illness, another chronic disease, or a secondary complication as a result of their disability.
            (d) End-of-life with terminal illness (such as cancer or end stage renal disease).
         (6) Ambulatory care nurses must be cognizant of all existing health states operating within the patient (Haas, 2006).
      b. Environment – Defines ambulatory nursing practice more clearly, setting it apart definitively from other professional nursing specialties (Mastal, 2010).
         (1) Shapes the nurse-patient relationship and interactions.
         (2) Encompasses organizational, social, economic, legal, and political factors within the organization and external to it.

(3) Conceptually, has two dimensions – Internal and external:

    (a) Internal environment – The care delivery environment:

        i. Where nurses practice.

        ii. Where patients access and receive care.

        iii. Dynamic and diverse with different types of settings.

    (b) External environment – Refers to both the geographic location of the specific health care organization and the contextual factors in the greater ambulatory environment:

        i. Community health needs, perceptions, and resources (e.g., rural and urban ambulatory care settings may address different patient needs and/or have different requirements and resources).

        ii. Federal and state laws relevant to health care and nursing practice.

        iii. General environmental circumstances (such as terrorist attacks, extreme weather conditions, and epidemics).

        iv. Health care financial systems and reimbursement regulations.

        v. Advances in science and technology related to health, diagnostics, communication, informatics, and other areas.

        vi. Regulatory and accrediting agencies' standards.

c. Concept of nursing – The scope of professional ambulatory care nursing is dynamic. It evolves continually in response to changing societal and organizational needs, directions, and preferences, as well as to the advancing and expanding knowledge base of ambulatory care nursing's theoretical and scientific domains (Mastal, 2010). The ambulatory care nurse functions in three major roles: Organizational, professional, and clinical (Haas, 2006).

(1) Ambulatory care nurses practice within the organization/system's role when they manage and coordinate resources and workflow in their setting. Organizational/system's role activities include:

    (a) Providing specialty practice and/or office support.

    (b) Managing health care fiscal matters (such as reimbursement and coding).

    (c) Collaborating with others.

    (d) Managing conflict.

    (e) Using informatics systems.

    (f) Addressing the contextual issues in the environment when providing care.

    (g) Ensuring care for the caregiver(s).

    (h) Managing priorities, delegating, and/or supervising.

    (i) Applying ambulatory care culture and cross-cultural competencies.

    (j) Practicing political and entrepreneurial skills.

    (k) Structuring customer-focused systems.

    (l) Adhering to workplace regulatory standards (such as the Equal Employment Opportunity Commission [EEOC] and the Occupational Safety and Health Administration [OSHA]).

    (m) Advocating for patients inter-organizationally and in the community.

    (n) Addressing legal issues.

    (o) Determining appropriate workload (Haas, 2006).

(2) Ambulatory care nurses practice within the professional role as they continuously practice according to standards, evaluate the outcomes of practice, and develop themselves and other staff. Professional role activities include:
  (a) Pursuing evidence-based practice.
  (b) Exercising leadership inquiry and utilizing research.
  (c) Participating in clinical quality improvement activities.
  (d) Developing staff.
  (e) Complying with regulatory requirements, managing risk and safety.
  (f) Caring for self holistically.
  (g) Applying the nursing code of ethics (Haas, 2006).

(3) Ambulatory care nurses practice in the clinical role when they provide care within each of the clinical specialty dimensions (Haas, 1998). Clinical nursing role activities apply to individuals, groups, and populations. They include:
  (a) Assessing, screening, and triaging patients in the setting, on the telephone, and/or electronically.
  (b) Providing health education for patients and caregivers.
  (c) Advocating for patients.
  (d) Managing health care across the continuum.
  (e) Practicing telehealth services.
  (f) Collaborating in resource identification and referral.
  (g) Conducting clinical procedures, independent, interdependent, and dependent.
  (h) Providing primary, secondary, and tertiary prevention.
  (i) Communicating and documenting nursing interventions.
  (j) Managing outcomes.
  (k) Developing and using nursing protocols.

  (l) Applying the nursing process in all encounters.

(4) Nursing responsibilities – Ambulatory care nurses are required to simultaneously address the concurrent needs of patients across the health-illness continuum. For example:
  (a) In the clinical role:
    i. Patient education dimension: The nurse understands that although chronically ill, patients still require wellness education.
    ii. Case management dimension: The nurse recognizes that cost effectiveness is maximized if case management protocols are implemented for chronically or terminally ill, and that case management protocols can also enhance recovery, prevent complications, and decrease costs in acute illnesses.
  (b) In the organizational role:
    i. Management dimension: The nurse understands that reimbursement for some interventions may differ if the patient is acutely ill versus well at the time of the encounter.
    ii. Care of the caregiver dimension: Although ambulatory nurses are attuned to caregivers of chronically or terminally ill patients, they also work with caregivers of acutely ill patients who need counseling or advice to see them through an exhausting acute illness.

(c) In the professional role:
   i. Evidence-based practice dimension: The nurse understands that protocols can be applied to health promotion for well populations, as well as treatment interventions for the chronically or terminally ill.
   ii. Staff development dimension: Ambulatory care nurses are responsive to needs of staff for development in areas of new therapies and pharmacologic agents for acute or chronically ill patients, but they are also aware of needs for staff development in the use of therapies and drugs for palliative care of the terminally ill (Haas, 2006).
(5) Major objectives of ambulatory care nursing have been identified:
   (a) Protect and promote health.
   (b) Minimize suffering.
   (c) Maximize patients' understanding during diagnostic and treatment phases.
   (d) Prevent illness and injury.
   (e) Apply appropriate nursing interventions to human responses in health, illness, disease, disability, and end-of-life situations.
   (f) Actively advocate for optimal health care for individuals, families, groups, communities, and populations (AAACN, 2010b).

IV. Scope and Standards of Practice for Professional Ambulatory Care Nursing

A. Purposes for use of the Scope and Standards of Practice for Ambulatory Care Nursing include:

1. Provide guidance for the structure and processes in delivery of ambulatory care nursing.
2. Serve as a guide for provision of quality patient care.
3. Facilitate professional nursing development.
4. Facilitate evaluation of professional nursing performance.
5. Stimulate participation in research and use of research findings.
6. Serve as a guide for quality management.
7. Serve as a guide for ethics and patient advocacy (Haas, 2006).

B. Scope of Ambulatory Care Nursing Practice.
1. In 2010, the first scope of practice statement was developed and became a part of the standards in the publication entitled, *Scope and Standards of Practice for Professional Ambulatory Care Nursing* (AAACN, 2010a).
2. "The scope of practice statement describes the *who, what, where, when, why,* and *how* of nursing practice. Each of these questions must be answered to provide a complete picture of the dynamic and complex practice of nursing and its evolving boundaries and membership" (ANA, 2010, p. 2). The AAACN (2010a) Scope of Practice statement includes:
   a. Definition of professional ambulatory care nursing.
   b. Conceptual framework of ambulatory care nursing.
   c. Evolution of modern ambulatory care and nursing practice.
   d. The ambulatory care practice environment (specialties and types of settings):
      (1) Primary care (internal medicine, pediatrics, family medicine, women's health, telehealth services).
      (2) Diagnostics and specialty care (medical specialties, surgical specialties, care management, ambulatory surgery, and diagnostic centers).

e. Science and art of ambulatory care nursing practice:
  (1) Science: The nursing process and analytical and critical thinking skills.
  (2) Art of practice: Based on respect for the dignity of others, compassionate caring, and dynamic processes, such as listening, mentoring, coaching, empathizing, teaching, culturally sensitive caring, accepting, providing presence, and resolving conflicts.
f. Nursing roles:
  (1) Advanced practice registered nurses (APRNs):
    (a) Types include certified registered nurse anesthetist (CRNA), certified nurse midwife (CNM,) clinical nurse specialist (CNS), nurse practitioner (NP).
    (b) In general, APRNs affiliate with physician groups as providers of health and medical care.
    (c) APRNs have acquired special clinical knowledge and skills, with many having master's and/or doctoral degrees.
    (d) APRNs are licensed and practice differently than registered nurses, with their scope of practice defined according to state practice acts.
  (2) Registered nurses:
    (a) Have completed an accredited diploma, associate degree, or baccalaureate nursing educational program.
    (b) Have successfully passed the national examination for nursing licensure.
    (c) Practice in clinical, educational, and management roles.
  (3) Licensed practical nurses (LPN) or licensed vocational nurses (LVN):
    (a) Scope of practice and supervision are defined by the state in which they practice.
    (4) Nursing staff are also usually composed of non-licensed staff (such as medical or nursing assistants and technicians who may function under the supervision of a registered nurse).
  g. Issues in ambulatory care nursing.
C. Standards of Professional Ambulatory Care Nursing – Standards establish the guidelines that promote the effective management and evaluation of increasingly complex ambulatory care nursing roles and responsibilities in a changing health care environment.
  1. The first set of *Nursing Administration and Practice Standards for Ambulatory Care* was published in 1987 and has been updated every three years.
  2. The first edition of the AAACN *Telephone Nursing Practice Administration and Practice Standards* was published in 1997. These standards are revised every three years and now use the title *Telehealth Nursing Practice Administration and Practice Standards.*
  3. Both sets of AAACN standards are the result of a collaborative effort of nurses from a diverse array of ambulatory settings in a variety of geographic locations.
  4. Ambulatory care nursing values are reflected in the AAACN standards. The values of AAACN as an organization (AAACN, 2010b) are:
    a. Responsible health care delivery for individuals, families, and communities.
    b. Visionary and accountable leadership.
    c. Productive partnerships, alliances, and collaborations.
    d. Appreciation of diversity.
    e. Continual advancement of professional ambulatory care nursing practice.
D. Definitions: Used as the common foundation in the development of standards.
  1. Standard – An authoritative statement developed and disseminated by a profes-

sional organization or governmental or regulatory agency by which the quality of practice, services, research, or education can be judged.

2. Patient – An individual who requests or receives nursing services. Also called client, consumer, member, or customer in many settings.

3. Family – Defined by the patient in his or her own terms and may include individuals related by blood or marriage, or in self-defined relationships. (This definition is intended to include the family in nursing care as appropriate. It is not intended as a legal definition of family.)

4. Nursing staff – Staff members who participate in delivering nursing care. These staff members are either registered nurses or are supervised by a registered nurse.

5. Health care team – Includes the patient, family, and other members of the health care system who are involved in the development and implementation and evaluation of the care plan.

6. Nursing services – Organized services delivered to groups of patients by nursing staff. Includes nursing care as well as services to support or facilitate direct care (such as referral and coordination of care).

7. Competency – Refers to the knowledge, skills, and behaviors identified as performance standards constituting the acceptable demonstration of ability in a role.

8. Evidence-based nursing practice – Process by which nurses make clinical decisions using the best available research evidence, their clinical expertise, and patient preferences in the context of available resources (Haas, 2006).

E. Components of each standard.
1. Standard statement.
2. Measurement criteria: Specific, measurable indicators that demonstrate compliance with the standard. Standards have two sets of criteria:
   a. Measurement criteria for all registered nurses in ambulatory care settings.
   b. Additional measurement criteria for nurse executives, administrators, and managers in ambulatory care settings.

F. Assumptions.
1. In addition to the *Scope and Standards of Practice for Professional Ambulatory Care Nursing,* registered nurses use nursing practice standards developed by professional nursing organizations, such as the American Nurses Association (ANA), Oncology Nursing Society (ONS), Association of periOperative Registered Nurses (AORN), and the Emergency Nurses Association (ENA), for care to specific patient populations.
2. Ambulatory care nurses also use clinical practice guidelines developed by federal agencies, such as the Agency for Research and Quality (AHRQ), to guide care for specific patient populations.

G. Ambulatory care nursing standards (AAACN, 2010a) include:
1. Standards of clinical practice:
   a. The six clinical practice standards address the science and art of nursing clinical practice in ambulatory care – The nursing process.
   b. The nursing process is a six-step rational, systematic method of planning, providing, and evaluating nursing care developed by Ida J. Orlando in the late 1950s as she observed nurses as they practiced. It has been refined by the profession over the intervening decades.
2. Standards of professional performance – The 10 professional performance standards for ambulatory care nursing identify a competent level of behavior in the organizational and professional dimensions of each ambulatory care nurse's specific role (see Tables 1-1 and 1-2). These behaviors include activities related to:
   a. Performance improvement.
   b. Education.
   c. Professional practice evaluation.
   d. Collegiality.
   e. Collaboration.

Table 1-1.
Standards of Practice for Professional Ambulatory Care Nursing

Standard 1 – Assessment

Ambulatory care registered nurses systematically collect focused data relating to health needs and concerns of a patient, group, or population.

Standard 2 – Nursing Diagnoses

Ambulatory care registered nurses analyze the assessment data to determine the diagnostic statements for health promotion, health maintenance, or health-related problems or issues.

Standard 3 – Outcomes Identification

Ambulatory care registered nurses identify expected outcomes in a plan of care individualized for a specific patient, group, or population.

Standard 4 – Planning

Ambulatory care registered nurses develop a plan that identifies strategies and alternatives to attain expected outcomes.

Standard 5 – Implementation

Ambulatory care registered nurses implement the identified plan.

Standard 5a – Coordination of Care

Ambulatory care registered nurses coordinate the delivery of care within the setting of practice and across health care settings.

Standard 5b – Health Teaching and Health Promotion

Ambulatory care registered nurses employ strategies that promote individual and community wellness.

Standard 6 – Evaluation

Ambulatory registered nurses evaluate progress toward the attainment of stated outcomes.

Standard 7 – Performance Improvement

Ambulatory care registered nurses enhance the quality and effectiveness of clinical practice, the organizational system, and professional nursing practice.

Standard 8 – Education

Ambulatory care registered nurses attain knowledge and competency that reflects current ambulatory care nursing practice.

Standard 9 – Professional Practice Evaluation

Ambulatory care registered nurses evaluate their own nursing practice in relation to professional practice standards and guidelines, relevant statutes, rules, regulations, and organizational position descriptions.

Standard 10 – Collegiality

Ambulatory care registered nurses positively interact with and contribute to the professional development of peers and colleagues.

Standard 11 – Collaboration

Ambulatory care registered nurses collaborate with patients, family members, caregivers, and other health professionals in the conduct of ambulatory care nursing practice.

Standard 12 – Ethics

Ambulatory care registered nurses apply the principles of professional codes of ethics that ensure individual rights in all areas of practice.

Standard 13 – Research

Ambulatory care registered nurses integrate relevant research findings into practice.

Standard 14 – Environment

Ambulatory care registered nurses actively engage in organizational initiatives that create and maintain an internal environment that is safe, hazard-free, ergonomically correct, confidential, and comfortable for patients, visitors, and staff.

Standard 15 – Resource Utilization

Ambulatory care registered nurses consider factors related to effectiveness, cost, and impact on practice and the organization in the planning and delivery of nursing and health care services in outpatient settings.

Standard 16 – Leadership

Ambulatory care registered nurses demonstrate leadership behaviors in practice settings, across the profession, and in the community.

Source: AAACN, 2010a. Used with permission.

Table 1-2.
Standards of Telehealth Nursing Practice

Standard 1 – Assessment

Telehealth registered nurses systematically collect comprehensive and focused data relating to health needs and concerns of a patient, group, or population.

Standard 2 – Nursing Diagnosis

Telehealth registered nurses analyze the assessment data to determine the diagnostic statements for health promotion, health maintenance, or health-related problems or issues.

Standard 3 – Outcomes Identification

Telehealth registered nurses identify expected outcomes in an individualized plan of care specific to the patient, group, or population.

Standard 4 – Planning

Telehealth registered nurses develop a plan that identifies strategies and alternatives to attain expected outcomes.

Standard 5 – Implementation

Telehealth registered nurses implement the identified plan of care to attain expected outcomes.

Standard 5a – Coordination of Care

Telehealth registered nurses coordinate the delivery of care within the practice setting and across health care settings.

Standard 5b – Health Teaching and Health Promotion

Telehealth registered nurses employ strategies that promote individual and community wellness.

Standard 5c – Consultation

Telehealth registered nurse leaders provide consultation to influence identified plans of care, enhance the ability of other professionals, and effect change.

Standard 6 – Evaluation

Telehealth registered nurses evaluate progress toward the attainment of stated outcomes.

Standard 7 – Ethics

Telehealth registered nurses apply the principles of professional codes of ethics that ensure individual rights in all areas of practice.

Standard 8 – Education

Telehealth registered nurses actively attain nursing knowledge and competency in order to reflect current nursing practice.

Standard 9 – Research and Evidence-Based Practice

Telehealth registered nurses incorporate relevant research findings into practice to maintain the standard of care within recognized best practice models, to promote continuous improvement, and to advance the practice of telehealth nursing.

Standard 10 – Performance Improvement

Telehealth registered nurses enhance the quality and effectiveness of telecommunication practices, the organizational systems, and professional telehealth nursing practice.

Standard 11 – Communication

Telehealth registered nurses communicate effectively using a variety of formats, tools, and technologies to build professional relationships and to deliver care across the continuum.

Standard 12 – Leadership

Telehealth registered nurses acquire and utilize leadership behaviors in practice settings, across the profession, and in the health care community at large.

Standard 13 – Collaboration

Telehealth registered nurses collaborate with patients, family members, caregivers, and other helath care professionals in the delivery of telehealth nursing practice.

Standard 14 – Professional Practice Evaluation

Telehealth registered nurses evaluate their own nursing practice in relation to patient outcomes; organizational policies, procedures, and job descriptions; nursing professional standards; and relevant governmental regulations and statutes.

Standard 15 – Resource Utilization

Telehealth registered nurses utilize appropriate resources to plan and provide telehealth services that are safe, effective, and financially responsible.

Standard 16 – Environment

Telehealth registered nurses perform work activities and care for patients in an internal environment that is safe, efficient, hazard-free, and ergonomically correct.

Source: AAACN, 2011b. Used with permission.

f. Ethics.

g. Research.

h. Environment.

i. Resource utilization.

j. Leadership.

V. Role of the Nurse in Ambulatory Care

A. Much of the health care formerly delivered in hospitals now occurs in ambulatory care settings. This shift has dramatically increased the need for professional nursing services as patients and families require increased depth and breadth of care interventions.

1. Registered nurse contributions to the care of patients in ambulatory settings.

   a. Facilitate patient safety and quality of care by managing, individualizing, and evaluating care for patients and families.

   b. Assist patients and families to navigate the complexities of the health care system.

   c. Participate in and/or conduct complex procedural care.

   d. Support patients in the decision-making process.

   e. Provide in-depth health education for patients, families, communities, and populations.

   f. Coordinate care across the health care continuum.

2. Economic benefit of care delivered by registered nurses as demonstrated by their impact on:

   a. Patient satisfaction.

   b. Quality patient outcomes.

   c. Patient safety.

   d. Reduced adverse events.

   e. Reductions in hospital and emergency department admissions (Haas, 2008; IOM, 2011; O'Connell, Johnson, Stallmeyer, & Cokington, 2001).

3. Position statement – Based on the above assumptions and data, AAACN issued the following position statement in 2011: "It is the position of the American Academy of Ambulatory Care Nursing that:

   a. "Registered nurses enhance patient safety and the quality and effectiveness of care delivery and are thus essential and irreplaceable in the provision of patient care services in the ambulatory setting."

   b. "Registered nurses are responsible for the design, administration, and evaluation of professional nursing services within the organization in accordance with the framework established by state nurse practice acts, nursing scope of practice, and organizational standards of care."

   c. "Registered nurses provide the leadership necessary for collaboration and coordination of services, which includes defining the appropriate skill mix and delegation of tasks among licensed and unlicensed nursing staff.

   d. "Registered nurses are fully accountable in all ambulatory care settings for all nursing services and associated patient outcomes" (AAACN, 2011a, p. 96).

References

American Academy of Ambulatory Care Nursing (AAACN). (1997). *Telephone nursing practice administration and practice standards.* Pitman, NJ: Author.

American Academy of Ambulatory Care Nursing (AAACN). (2010a). *Scope and standards of practice for professional ambulatory care nursing* (8th ed.). Pitman, NJ: Author.

American Academy of Ambulatory Care Nursing (AAACN). (2010b). *Strategic plan 2010.* Pitman, NJ: Author.

American Academy of Ambulatory Care Nursing (AAACN). (2011a). American Academy of Ambulatory Care Nursing position statement: The role of the registered nurse in ambulatory care. *Nursing Economic$, 29*(2), 96.

American Academy of Ambulatory Care Nursing (AAACN). (2011b). *Scope and standards of practice for professional telehealth nursing* (5th ed.). Pitman, NJ: Author.

American Academy of Ambulatory Care Nursing (AAACN)/ American Nurses Association (ANA). (1997). *Nursing in ambulatory care: The future is here.* Washington, DC: American Nurses Publishing.

American Academy of Ambulatory Care Nursing (AAACN) Task Force. (2011). *Definition of ambulatory care nursing.* Pitman, NJ: AAACN.

American Nurses Association (ANA). (2003). *Nursing's social policy statement* (2nd ed.). Silver Spring, MD: Author.

American Nurses Association (ANA). (2010). *Scope and standards of practice* (2nd ed.). Silver Spring, MD: Author.

Haas, S. (1998). Ambulatory care conceptual framework. *View-Point, 20*(3), 16-17.

Haas, S.A. (2006). Ambulatory care specialty nursing practice. In C.B. Laughlin (Ed.), *Core curriculum for ambulatory care nursing* (2nd ed., pp. 3-12). Pitman, NJ: American Academy of Ambulatory Care Nursing (AAACN).

Haas, S.A. (2008). Resourcing evidence-based practice in ambulatory care. *Nursing Economic$, 26*(5), 319-322.

Institute of Medicine (IOM). (1978). *Primary care in medicine. A manpower policy for primary healthcare: Report of a study.* Washington, DC: The National Academies Press.

Institute of Medicine (IOM). (2011). *The future of nursing: Leading change, advancing health.* Washington, DC: The National Academies Press.

Mastal, M.F. (2006). The context of ambulatory care nursing. In C.B. Laughlin (Ed.), *Core curriculum for ambulatory care nursing* (2nd ed., pp. 29-45). Pitman, NJ: American Academy of Ambulatory Care Nursing (AAACN).

Mastal, M. (2010). Ambulatory care nursing: Growth as a professional specialty. *Nursing Economic$, 28*(4), 267-269, 275.

O'Connell, J., Johnson, D., Stallmeyer, J., & Cokington, D. (2001). A satisfaction and return-on-investment study of a nurse triage service. *American Journal of Managed Care, 7*, 159-169.

World Health Organization (WHO). (1978). *Primary health care. Report of the international conference on primary health care.* Alma Ata, USSR, Geneva: Author.

Additional Readings

American Academy of Ambulatory Care Nursing (AAACN). (2010). *Ambulatory care nursing certification review course* (Revised syllabus). Pitman, NJ: Author.

Brixey, L. (Ed.) (2010). *Ambulatory care nursing orientation and competency assessment guide* (2nd ed.). Pitman, NJ: American Academy of Ambulatory Care Nursing (AAACN).

Espensen, M. (Ed.). (2009). *Telehealth nursing practice essentials.* Pitman, NJ: American Academy of Ambulatory Care Nursing (AAACN).

Haas, S.A., & Hackbarth, D.P. (1995). Dimensions of the staff nurse role in ambulatory care: Part II. *Nursing Economic$, 13*(3), 151-165.

Chapter 2

Ambulatory Care Nursing Practice Arena

Sheila A. Haas, PhD, RN, FAAN
Clare Hastings, PhD, RN, FAAN

OBJECTIVES – *Study of the information in this chapter will enable the learner to:*

1. Identify current trends in health care that impact ambulatory care nurses.
2. Describe ambulatory patient characteristics and differences between acute care and ambulatory care.
3. Discuss current practice settings and new delivery systems created by the 2010 Patient Protection and Affordable Care Act (PPACA).
4. Describe how to transition to ambulatory nursing practice.

KEY POINTS – *The major points in this chapter include:*

1. Opportunities and changes are occurring in the ambulatory care arena in response to the 2010 Patient Protection and Affordable Care Act (PPACA).
2. Ambulatory care practice arenas are varied and complex.
3. Nurses in ambulatory care have a variety of practice options.

Ambulatory care nurses practice in a diverse and changing environment. In the years since the first explicit descriptions of the domain of ambulatory nursing practice (Haas, Hackbarth, Kavanaugh, & Vlasses, 1995; Hackbarth, Haas, Kavanaugh, & Vlasses, 1995; Hastings, 1987; Verran, 1981), the scope and complexity of nursing practice in ambulatory care has broadened and increased. The pace of change intensified following passage of the Patient Protection and Affordable Care Act (PPACA) signed into law by President Obama in 2010. PPACA focused on health promotion and disease prevention, and provided increased access through insurance reform. Access to care for newly insured individuals would occur through ambulatory settings offering primary care. As health care increasingly moves out of the acute care hospital and into the community and home settings and focuses more on health promotion and disease prevention, nurses looking to ambulatory care as a practice setting continue to find a broad array of possible set-

tings, roles, and opportunities. It is important for nurses practicing in ambulatory care to be aware both of the diversity in roles and practice settings, as well as the common themes that are present across ambulatory practice settings.

This chapter will provide nurses in ambulatory care with an overview of the broad scope of ambulatory practice and clarify the common factors that occur in all ambulatory care settings. The differences between ambulatory and inpatient practice, as well as the often unexpected challenges faced by nurses transitioning from traditional inpatient roles to ambulatory care, will also be discussed. An understanding of the effect of the practice setting on nursing practice is important to enable nurses to effectively contribute to the health care team. Significant content in this chapter is abstracted with permission from the monograph *Nursing in Ambulatory Care: The Future Is Here* (American Academy of Ambulatory Care Nursing/American Nurses Association [AAACN/ANA], 1997).

I. **Current Trends in the Ambulatory Care Nursing Practice Arena**

The domain of ambulatory care nursing practice is defined as the overall scope of nursing practice in the ambulatory arena. It includes attributes of the environment in which practice occurs, patient requirements for care, and specific nursing role dimensions. The domain of ambulatory care nursing practice is being influenced by several major trends.

A. The movement of health care out of the hospital in an effort to enhance economics (i.e., to decrease costs).

1. Fueled by changes in insurance coverage for patients, reimbursement, and enhanced attention to wellness, health promotion, and disease prevention.

a. Over 30 years of diagnosis-related group (DRG)-based prospective payment for inpatient services have compressed hospital length of stay and pushed care into the ambulatory and home care settings.

b. Growth of population-based, capitated care has been an important feature of health care delivery response to prospective payment and reduced funding since the 1980s.

c. Mandates instituted by the 2010 PPACA have placed increased emphasis on wellness and preventive services, which are often provided in the ambulatory care setting.

d. Plans for implementing accountable care organizations (ACOs) as a component of health care reform have renewed incentives for preventing hospitalization and shifted economic risk for re-hospitalization to the provider of services.

e. Prevalence of 23-hour short-stay units has increased the use of outpatient observation or short-stay status as alternatives to an inpatient admission.

2. Changes accelerated by continued developments in technology have allowed more and more complex procedures to be managed in an ambulatory setting.

a. Minimally invasive surgical techniques and interventional radiology techniques that reduce morbidity and shorten recovery time.

b. Improved methods for short-term anesthesia that shorten recovery time.

c. Innovations in vascular access and intravenous pump technologies that allow patients to remain out of the hospital during long-term intravenous therapy.

d. Innovations in telemedicine and social networking, as well as access to smart technology that allows more complex monitoring to be provided remotely.

3. Early discharge creates the requirement for ambulatory follow-up, often in combination with home health visits.

a. Enhanced surgical techniques have shortened stays, but recovery still must be monitored, symptoms managed, drains removed, and wound healing assessed in ambulatory care.

b. Shortened hospital stays mean that pre- and post-intervention patient education and support must be done on an ambulatory basis.

c. Potential lack of reimbursement for readmissions creates a greater focus on assuring patient comprehension of health teaching and compliance with required health behavior and self monitoring.

4. Advances in the care of chronically ill patients.

a. A growing older adult population with multiple chronic illnesses requires care coordination for ongoing ambulatory treatment, assessment, monitoring, evaluation, and follow-up for chronic illness.

b. Ambulatory infusion and procedure centers are used as alternatives to inpatient care.

c. Outpatient invasive testing and treatment centers allow much of the ongoing care for severe chronic illness (such as hypertension, heart disease, asthma, cancer, and renal failure) to be provided in an ambulatory care setting.

d. Nurses are becoming involved in multidisciplinary disease management teams focused on the chronically ill.

B. Health care consumerism.

1. Consumer-driven health care (CDHC) is an approach that encourages consumer awareness, informed choice, and decision-making based on open, transparent, and credible information:

   a. Information includes availability, relevance, quality, and pricing of health care services, health care providers, and financing plans.

   b. CDHC empowers consumers to take greater control of and achieve greater satisfaction from their health care experience.

   c. Providers of health care offerings shall be considered "consumer-driven" if they are committed to publically releasing the information relevant to facilitating the consumer choice.

   d. Ambulatory care nurses are often the linchpin between consumers and the health care system.

2. Consumer expectations of quality and safety in health care are changing.

   a. Quality expectations are influenced by Institute of Medicine (IOM) (2001) findings:

      (1) Performance varies considerably within and across settings.

      (2) The health care system is fragmented, poorly organized, and does not make best use of resources.

      (3) Increase of chronic illness has had a major impact on the system.

      (4) System is confusing and too complex for consumers.

   b. IOM criteria for quality care (IOM, 2001, p. 67):

      (1) Care is safe – "We must avoid injuries to patients from the care that is intended to help them."

      (2) Care is effective – "We must provide services based on scientific knowledge to all who could benefit."

      (3) Care is patient-centered – "We must provide care that is respectful of and responsive to individual patient preferences, needs, and values, and ensure that patient values influence all clinical decisions."

      (4) Care is timely – "We must reduce waits and sometimes harmful delays for patients who receive care from nurses and other providers who give care."

      (5) Care is efficient – "We must avoid waste of equipment supplies, ideas, and energy."

      (6) Care is equitable – "We must provide care that does not vary in quality because of personal characteristics, such as gender, ethnicity, geographic location, and socio-economic status."

3. Health literacy has a recognized influence on patients' ability to access and collaborate with health care providers.

   a. Health literacy is the degree to which individuals have the capacity to obtain, process, and understand basic health information and services needed to make appropriate health decisions (U.S. Department of Health and Human Services [DHHS], n.d.). Health literacy is influenced by:

      (1) Knowledge and skills of lay and professional persons doing instructing.

      (2) Culture.

      (3) Context within which instruction occurs.

   b. Health literacy affects the ability to:

      (1) Navigate the health care system, including filling out complex forms.

      (2) Provide information, such as health history.

(3) Fully engage in self-care.

(4) Understand and appreciate concepts, such as risk.

c. Poor health literacy is linked to:

(1) Less frequent use of preventive services.

(2) Higher rates of hospitalization.

(3) Lack of knowledge regarding care for chronic conditions.

(4) Poorer health care status.

(5) Higher costs of health care.

(6) Stigma and shame.

C. Federal government expectations: *Healthy People 2020* (DHHS, 2012).

1. Healthy People 2020 mission:

a. Identify nationwide health improvement priorities.

b. Increase public awareness and understanding of determinants of health, disease, and disability, and the opportunities for progress.

c. Provide measurable objectives and goals that are applicable at the national, state, and local levels.

d. Engage multiple sectors to take actions to strengthen policies and improve practices that are driven by the best available evidence and knowledge.

e. Identify critical research, evaluation, and data collection needs.

2. Healthy People 2020 objectives:

a. Represent quantitative values to be achieved over the decade.

b. Are organized within identified topic areas.

c. Are managed by federal agencies.

d. Are supported by scientific evidence.

e. Address population disparities.

f. Are data-driven and prevention-oriented.

3. How to use Healthy People 2020 in the community.

a. Understand how health issues are changing in one's community over time.

b. Compare the health of one's community to that of other communities and the nation.

c. Use this information to talk with leaders in the area about the health issues that are important.

d. Sound the alarm when problems are getting worse or are not improving fast enough.

e. By getting involved, individuals can help make the United States a nation of healthy people living in healthier communities.

f. Healthy People 2020 lists specific objectives related to community health within the identified topic areas (DHHS, 2012).

D. Evolution of the nurse role as a result of the IOM reports *Crossing the Quality Chasm* (2001) and *The Future of Nursing* (2010) recommendations and key messages.

1. Quality and Safety Education in Nursing (QSEN) (Cronenwett et al., 2007).

2. QSEN competencies for education in pre-licensure programs in nursing and expected of all practicing nurses (QSEN, 2012):

a. *Patient-centered care* – "Recognize the patient or designee as the source of control and full partner in providing compassionate and coordinated care based on respect for patient's preferences, values, and needs."

b. *Quality* – "Use data to monitor the outcomes of care processes, and use improvement methods to design and test changes to continuously improve the quality and safety of health care systems."

c. *Teamwork and collaboration* – "Function effectively within nursing and inter-professional teams, fostering open communication, mutual respect, and shared decision-making to achieve quality care."

d. *Safety* – "Minimize risk of harm to patients and providers through both system effectiveness and individual performance."

e. *Evidence-based practice* – "Integrate best current evidence with clinical expertise and patient/family preferences and values for delivery of optimal health care."

f. *Informatics* – "Use information and technology to communicate, manage knowledge, mitigate error, and support decision-making."

3. *The Future of Nursing* report (IOM, 2010, p.1) recommendations and key messages:

   a. "Nurses should practice to the full extent of their education and training."

   b. "Nurses should achieve higher levels of education and training through an improved education system that promotes seamless academic progression."

   c. "Nurses should be full partners with physicians and other health care professionals in redesigning health care in the United States."

   d. "Effective workforce planning and policy-making require better data collection and information infrastructure."

II. Ambulatory Patient Characteristics

A. Ambulatory patients are not always "ambulatory."

   1. Patients may not walk in and walk out.

   2. Patient acuity varies from people who are healthy and being seen for health maintenance advice to patients who are acutely ill or chronically ill in crisis.

   3. Increasing numbers of patients have chronic illnesses managed at home with complex treatment regimens and medical equipment.

   4. Movement of elective surgeries to the ambulatory setting means patients have to be recovered after invasive procedures and anesthesia.

   5. Ambulatory sites may also provide service to patients who are actually inpatients at another facility.

   6. Ambulatory services are often delivered over the telephone or via the Internet.

B. Ambulatory patients are as diverse as inpatients in their clinical presentation. They may be:

   1. Acutely ill requiring triage and possible emergency care.

   2. Acutely ill requiring support, diagnosis, and treatment.

   3. Chronically ill with an acute exacerbation.

   4. Chronically ill requiring ongoing monitoring and assistance with self-management.

   5. In need of a clearly defined treatment or procedure, including recovery, monitoring, and discharge instructions.

   6. In need of education, reassurance, and support.

   7. In need of preventive services and self-care education.

C. Ambulatory patients are informed consumers.

   1. Media coverage and the availability of comparative quality of care data have created a skeptical and informed consumer group.

   2. Many people have access to the Internet; they come already knowing much about their condition, its prognosis, and current treatment.

   3. As health care adopts systematic assessment of patient satisfaction and public reporting of clinical outcomes, patients themselves have become more willing to come forward with complaints and provide feedback.

   4. Because of the growth in consumerism, nurses in ambulatory care are very likely to encounter situations in which patients question the rationale or quality of care.

D. Each patient has a constituency of family members and/or concerned others who may become involved with care and care decisions.

   1. Ambulatory care is community-based, often involving care that must be continued in the home between ambulatory visits.

   2. With the increase in early hospital discharge and self-managed chronic disease, it is necessary to involve others as caregivers in the home.

Table 2-1.
Differences Between Nursing Role in Ambulatory and Inpatient Settings

Aspect of Role	Inpatient Practice	Ambulatory Practice
Treatment episode	Inpatient admission	Visit or phone encounter
Observation mode	Direct and continuous	Episodic, often using patient as informant
Management of treatment plan	By nurse, with input from patient and family	By patient and family, with input from nurse
Primary intervention mode	Direct	Consultative
Organizational presence of nursing	Nurse-managed department	May or may not be formal structure for nursing
Workload variability and intensity	Determined by bed capacity and admission criteria	Theoretically determined by scheduling system; may also be affected by telephone volume

Source: Adapted from Hastings, 1987.

3. Involving family members or other significant individuals can enhance the effectiveness of patient education and increase the likelihood of adherence to the plan of care.

III. Comparison of Nursing Practice in Inpatient Acute Care and Ambulatory Care

Inpatient acute care is defined as hospital-based care in which patients are admitted overnight for diagnosis, treatment of an acute problem, or treatment of an acute exacerbation of a chronic problem. *Ambulatory care* is defined as outpatient care in which patients stay less than 24 hours and are discharged to their normal residential situation after care.

A. Summary of differences between the nursing role in ambulatory and inpatient settings (see Table 2-1).
   1. The key to the difference between nursing care in inpatient and ambulatory settings lies in differences in the underlying assumptions about the relationship between the patient and the nurse.
   2. Distinct differences exist in the level of accountability for care and control over the treatment plan assumed by both the patient and the nurse in the two settings.
   3. Although it is a requirement that RNs be present at all times in the inpatient setting to provide, supervise, or coordinate patient care, this requirement does not universally exist in ambulatory care.
   4. Differences in the focus of nursing practice in the two types of settings have led to different evolutions in the structure of care delivery and understanding of staffing requirements.
B. Patient contacts in the hospital setting.
   1. Patients are admitted to the hospital because they require nursing care. This fact is the basis for the requirement that all hospitalized patients be under the care of a registered nurse while they are admitted.
   2. Accountability for managing care is transferred to the nurse when the patient is admitted.
      a. This includes even those activities in which the patient was competent, such as medication administration.
      b. The nurse assumes total accountability for care and observation during admission.
C. Patient contacts in the ambulatory setting.
   1. Ambulatory visits usually initiated by the patient for the purpose of seeking medical care or following up from a previous visit.

2. Most prevalent site for ambulatory care is still the physician's office.
3. Between provider visits, patients are expected to manage their own self-care and treatments prescribed by the provider, and seek additional help, if needed.
4. Need for nursing in ambulatory care is not universal as it is in the hospital setting.
    a. Must define patients or groups of patients requiring nursing care provided or supervised by a registered nurse (RN).
    b. Must distinguish services provided or supervised by an RN from those provided by an advanced practice nurse, in collaboration with a team of independent providers, and also by medical assistants providing services that are delegated by and under the supervision of a physician.
    c. Must define level of care to be provided.
    d. No universal professional or regulatory standards exist on this issue.

D. Differences in the definition of treatment episode.
    1. Episode of care in acute care nursing is the hospital admission.
        a. Episode has defined beginning and end points (admission and discharge).
        b. Treatment period is continuous with an admission.
    2. Episode of care in ambulatory care is a visit or phone or electronic encounter.
        a. Treatment is episodic rather than continuous.
        b. Treatment period may include multiple episodes.
        c. Treatment period often has poorly defined beginning and end point.

E. Differences in observation mode and availability of patient.
    1. In acute care, the nurse has the opportunity to continuously observe the patient and collect assessment data.
        a. Variations in disease process and treatment effectiveness can be directly observed.

    b. Physical assessment can be used to corroborate patient-reported findings on an ongoing basis.
    2. In ambulatory care, opportunity for direct observation and physical assessment is minimal.
        a. The nurse must rely on the patient's report and description of symptoms, self-care, and results.
        b. The nurse must have a comprehensive understanding of the patient's condition and treatment to effectively probe for additional data.
        c. The nurse must often rely on the report of family members if the patient is unable to describe the situation.
        d. The assessment is compressed into a much shorter time frame.
        e. There are often gaps in critical information needed to make judgments about diagnosis and care.

F. Differences in management of the treatment plan.
    1. In acute care, control over implementation of the treatment plan resides primarily with the nurse, with the patient playing the role of active participant.
        a. Determining the approach.
        b. Timing of care.
        c. Modifications and adaptations to improve effectiveness or tolerance of treatment.
    2. In ambulatory care, control over implementation of the treatment plan resides primarily with the patient (and family), with the nurse serving in a consultative role.
        a. Approach is described, patient preferences assessed, and plan recommended during the visit or telehealth encounter, with possible demonstration or teach back by patient or family members.
        b. Timing is prescribed.
        c. Actual implementation occurs under the control of the patient when the nurse is not present.

d. Adaptations and modification are made by the patient, often not in consultation with health care providers.

e. Changes in health behavior or adherence are made by the patient, often without a detailed understanding of the rationale for treatment and implications of making changes.

G. Differences in nursing interventions.

1. Until recently, there was a clearly discernable difference in the types of interventions and locus of control over interventions between the hospital and ambulatory care nursing.

a. Historically, hospital-based care was initiated by the nurse, and related to monitoring, treatment, or self-care activities that the patient would be unable to perform.

b. Hospital-based interventions are often technologically complex and involve hands-on care.

c. In contrast, interventions by ambulatory care nurses historically tended to be patient-initiated, focused on health care advice, or instructing patients how to manage care at home or prepare for tests and procedures.

2. Recent changes in the health care system have blurred the boundaries of inpatient and outpatient care.

a. Patients with complex conditions and treatment regimens are being cared for in outpatient and day hospital settings.

b. There has been a dramatic growth in 23-hour short-stay units.

c. Complexity of ambulatory surgery has increased.

d. Increasingly, outpatients are being seen on inpatient units for evaluation and triage (e.g., oncology and labor and delivery).

e. This blurring will be accentuated with the implementation of ACOs and the assumption by the total organization of risks for poor outcomes or readmissions to the hospital.

H. Differences in the organizational position of nursing.

1. Traditionally, inpatient nurses:

a. Are part of an organized department of nursing and have a defined nurse executive with a voice at the governing body level.

b. Have regular continuing education opportunities.

c. Have detailed policies, procedures, and other resources.

d. Are required to document in an electronic health record.

2. Traditionally, ambulatory care nurses work within a variety of structures.

a. Often report to a non-nursing administrator.

b. May be hired directly by physicians in a group practice.

c. Except for large hospital-based or group practices, may not have a defined nursing administrative structure.

d. Even in the same organization, nurses in different ambulatory roles may have different reporting and supervisory relationships.

I. Differences in workload variability and intensity.

1. In acute care, the inpatient unit has a defined capacity that is based on bed size.

a. Although acuity and census may fluctuate, there is at least a theoretical limit to the number of patients for whom care is provided.

b. Unit admission and discharge criteria set a level of care, which predicts what types of patients may be seen.

2. In ambulatory care, workload is theoretically predicted by the appointment system.

a. Ambulatory care nurses know that the appointment system is easily bypassed by walk-ins and urgent visits.

b. No-show patients and resulting overbooking practices also add to problems predicting workload.

c. Workload is also projected based on telephone volumes, which may or may not be proportionate to appointments scheduled.

Figure 2-1.
Context for Ambulatory Care Nursing Practice

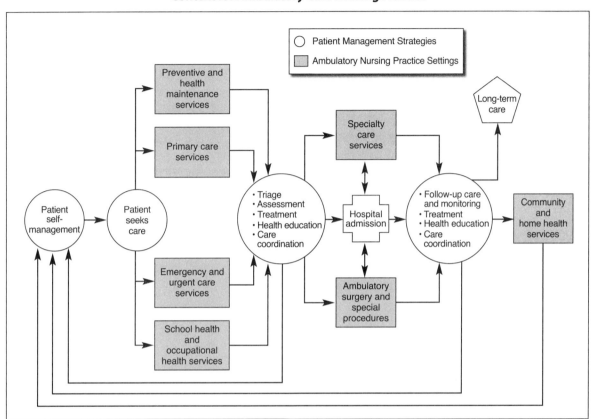

Source: Developed by Clare Hastings. Adapted from AAACN/ANA, 1997.

J. Impact of new accountability models for health care.
1. Impact of the Joint Commission Core Measures, Public Reporting (Hospital Compare), and Pay for Performance.
   a. Payment to acute care facilities dependent on outcomes that only become evident when the patient transitions to ambulatory care.
   b. Readmission and transitional care planning are an intense focus, with acute care facilities at risk for poor post-hospitalization outcomes (Boutwell et al., 2011; Mulder, Tzeng, & Vecchioni, 2012).
2. New roles for nurses in transitional care management.

a. Patient navigator roles (also called "pivot nurses") (Pedersen & Hack, 2010; Robinson-White, Conroy, Slavish, & Rosenzweig, 2010; Skrutkowski et al., 2008).
b. Transitional care models (Naylor et al., 2009) described further in Chapter 20, "Ambulatory Nursing Role in Chronic Illness Care."

IV. Current Practice Settings for Ambulatory Care Nurses
   Practice setting is defined as the type of organizational delivery system in which the nurse practices.
A. The context for ambulatory nursing practice.
   1. Nurses practice within a broad continuum of ambulatory care settings (see Figure 2-1).

2. The ambulatory health care system spans primary care, when the patient first seeks care, through acute care, chronic follow-up, and palliative care.
3. Nurses care for patients in every phase of preventive care, health maintenance, diagnosis, treatment, and follow-up as patients move in and out of acute care settings.

B. Ambulatory care nurses practice within several distinct organizational settings.
   1. Characteristics of the setting are determined by its organizational structure, its patient population, its financial and reimbursement structure, and the organization of its primary providers (usually physicians).
   2. Within each type of setting, there are also differences based on size, regional location, affiliation with a network or health system, and regional differences in health finance administration.
   3. Dimensions of clinical nursing practice are similar across settings; however, the frequency of performance of certain dimensions varies a great deal by setting (Haas et al., 1995).
   4. Major categories of practice setting include:
      a. University hospital outpatient departments.
      b. Community hospital outpatient departments.
      c. Solo and group medical practices.
      d. Health maintenance organization (HMO) clinics and services.
      e. Government health systems (federal, state, and local).
      f. Community and freestanding centers such as:
         (1) Occupational health centers.
         (2) School health clinics.
         (3) Shelters for the homeless.
         (4) Surgery/special procedure or infusion centers.
         (5) Urgent care centers.

C. University hospital outpatient departments.
   1. History and development.

   a. Teaching hospital outpatient clinics have been used since the early 1900s to provide teaching opportunities for medical students, residents, and other health care providers.
   b. Traditionally, care was provided free or at minimal charge to those primarily in the local community.
   c. Have also included specialty clinics based on the expertise of medical faculty members that pull referrals from a greater distance.
   2. Ambulatory nursing role.
      a. Nurses have been active collaborators in the development of teaching hospital clinics and programs.
      b. Nurses are often the only constant for patients receiving chronic illness care through cycles of rotating residents.
      c. Nurses in academic medical centers were among the first to begin to describe the role of the nurse in ambulatory care.
      d. Teaching hospital clinics are often the site for innovations in nursing care, including nurse-run clinics and other forms of collaborative practice.
      e. Because of the teaching focus, many teaching clinics have been plagued by long waits, poor access to urgent care, and difficulties obtaining medical records.
      f. Financial pressures and changing reimbursement have forced many academic medical centers to reorganize their teaching clinics, streamline operations, and improve patient support services or consider closing in the face of increasing costs and decreasing revenues.

D. Community hospital outpatient centers.
   1. History and development.
      a. Began as an outgrowth of the dispensary movement in the 1800s to serve the urban poor.
      b. As financial incentives and pressures changed, community hospital outpatient centers became more focused on

adjunctive services, such as ambulatory surgery and short-stay units.

c. Not financially or operationally competitive as a large source of primary care services.

2. Ambulatory nursing role.

a. Usually small programs with limited numbers of nursing staff.

b. Focus on the use of ancillary staff and use of RNs as working managers.

c. As more high-tech programs were implemented, use of RNs increased.

E. Medical group practices.

1. History and development.

a. Medical group practices are an outgrowth of the economic pressures on solo physician private practices.

b. Movement of patients out of the hospital and rapid growth of large multispecialty practices have increased the intensity of services provided in the medical group practice setting.

c. Many medical schools' faculties have formed group practices, providing reimbursement mechanisms and incentives that improve the financial status of the academic program.

2. Ambulatory care nursing role.

a. The nursing role is focused on facilitating the care of patients and the work of physicians.

b. The physician is usually the employer and often the supervisor of nurses.

c. Role components include triage and access management, managing and coordinating care, providing technical support for complex clinical procedures, and patient education.

F. Health maintenance organizations (HMOs).

1. History and development.

a. Since the 1970s, the number of prepaid comprehensive health plans that provide all services to members based on a fixed fee per month has grown.

b. This organizational structure created a whole new set of incentives and needs for care management.

c. Emphasis was to reduce the use of hospital days, and in general, this utilization stimulated development of processes to triage patients and directed them to a different level of care.

d. Incentives to reduce hospital utilization also led to a new focus on prevention and health maintenance.

2. Ambulatory care nursing role.

a. Extensive involvement in assessment and triage.

b. First sites to identify telephone triage as a specific nursing function.

c. Nurses are also involved in health maintenance activities, technical procedures (such as outpatient chemotherapy), and care management.

G. Federal health systems.

1. History and development.

a. Include federally mandated programs to serve specific populations.

(1) Department of Defense programs for active duty and retired military personnel.

(2) Department of Veterans Affairs programs for those with previous military service.

(3) U.S. Public Health Service programs, including Native American Health Service hospitals, clinics, and community health centers for underserved populations.

b. Systems represent large networks of organizations operating on a fixed budget.

c. Until recently, most services were provided free of charge to members of enrolled populations.

2. Ambulatory care nursing role.

a. Nursing practice supported by a longstanding tradition of well-trained unlicensed assistive personnel (Navy corpsmen and Army medics).

b. The nursing role has developed rapidly in recent years, involving nurses in health assessment and promotion/disease prevention, patient education, and the provision of complex procedures in the outpatient setting.

c. Federal health systems have been sites for development of innovative models and approaches to nurses providing primary ambulatory care services and the patient-centered medical home model of care (see description below and Chapter 20, "Ambulatory Nursing Role in Chronic Illness Care").

H. Community and freestanding centers.
1. Program types include:
   a. Surgery centers.
   b. Diagnostic centers.
   c. Local health departments.
   d. Free and grant-supported experimental clinics.
   e. College health centers.
   f. Occupational health offices in large employers.
   g. Retail clinics, such as those within chain drug stores.
2. Ambulatory care nursing role.
   a. Many centers small in size and scope.
   b. Nurses assume multiple roles.
   c. Many such sites have been experimental sites for piloting nurse-run clinics.

V. **New Delivery Systems Created by the 2010 Patient Protection and Affordable Care Act (PPACA)**
A. Patient-centered medical home – A model of care that includes personal physicians, whole-person orientation, coordinated and integrated care, and evidence-based medicine (Rosenthal, 2008).
1. Companion and complementary to ACOs or building blocks of ACOs.
2. Eligibility for care coordination and performance bonuses in patient-centered medical homes could include implementation of model care management processes for chronic care patients such as:
   a. Disease registries.
   b. Open access scheduling.
   c. Patient self-management programs (Wagner et al., 2001).

d. Linkage of electronic health records to specialty referral physicians and hospital.
e. Availability of nurse practitioners, physician assistants, dieticians, and pharmacists.
f. Lists of board-certified specialists used by the primary care practice.
g. Agreement to make performance data publically available.
3. New opportunities for ambulatory care nurses:
   a. Care coordination requires or allows nurses to:
      (1) Know patients well, and plan and coordinate care with the goal of delivering the *right care* at the *right time* in the *most efficient* way possible.
      (2) Work under established evidence-based practice (EBP) care management protocols.
      (3) Lead or participate in development and refinement of EBP protocols.
      (4) Collaborate on development of process and outcome indicators for EBP protocols.
      (5) Monitor (assessment and evaluation) current status of patients, often using telehealth modalities.
      (6) Make adjustments to treatment plan within specified EBP protocol parameters.
      (7) Collaborate and communicate with health team regarding patient status and needs.
      (8) Document all patient encounters in the electronic health record.
      (9) Refer patients who are out of alignment with outcome parameters to physican/advanced practice nurse.
      (10) Maintain a long-term supportive relationship with patients and families.
      (11) Act as a resource and advocate for patients and families.

(12) Collaborate on measurement of patient and family outcomes of care.

b. Telehealth.

c. Management roles in ambulatory care.

d. Advanced practice roles:

(1) Build on documented effectiveness of advanced practice nurses in primary care and disease management.

(2) Serve as primary care providers and full partners in the interdisciplinary team in the patient-centered medical home.

(3) Develop wellness and prevention plans for patients.

B. Accountable care organization (ACO) – A provider group, including at least primary care physicians, specialists, and hospitals, that accepts responsibility for the cost and quality of care delivered to a specific population of patients cared for by the group's clinicians (Inglehart, 2011; Shields, Patel, Manning, & Sacks, 2011; Shortell, Casalino, & Fisher, 2010).

1. The goal of the ACO is to deliver coordinated, efficient, and effective care.

2. ACOs that achieve quality and cost targets should benefit from financial gains.

3. Payment should be based on quality rather than quantity of care.

4. To enhance quality and cost-effectiveness, an ACO needs to be able to:

a. Care for patients across the continuum of care in different institutional settings and in the home.

b. Plan prospectively for budget and resource needs.

c. Effectively use evidence-based protocols and comparative effectiveness research.

d. Develop and support comprehensive, valid, and reliable measurement of its performance.

5. Initiatives to enhance quality and safety within ACOs.

a. Use of comparative effectiveness, research, and analysis.

b. Collaborative inter-professional teamwork.

c. Development and use of evidence-based guidelines.

d. Coordination of care across settings, including the patient-centered medical home.

e. Efficient communication across settings and with patients in the community.

f. Efficient, reliable, and valid data collection at point of care.

6. New opportunities for ambulatory care nurses.

a. RNs can be leaders, facilitators, and/or participants in all ACO quality and safety initiatives.

b. Potential for enhanced use of major role dimensions by ambulatory RNs:

(1) Advocacy.

(2) Telehealth.

(3) Patient education.

(4) Care coordination and transitional care.

(5) Community outreach (Haas et al., 1995).

VI. Transitioning into Ambulatory Care Nursing

A. Reasons nurses are making the transition to ambulatory care.

1. Increased emphasis on ambulatory care as a care delivery site.

2. Expansion of complex services offered in ambulatory care, with resulting needs for nursing support.

3. Nurses seeking alternative practice settings to the hospital.

a. Opportunities for greater professional autonomy.

b. Opportunities for increased collaboration with physicians.

c. Scheduling and lifestyle advantages.

d. Expectations that ambulatory care will provide a low-stress work environment.

B. Transition challenges.

1. Change in locus of control.

a. Experience of diminished control.

      (1) Over the general treatment regimen.

      (2) Over the timing and method of implementation.

      (3) Especially noticed by nurses transitioning from critical care.

  b. Combined with general sensory overload.

      (1) Large numbers of patients arriving for care.

      (2) Large numbers of providers.

  c. Lack of a shift start and end, with resulting requirement that the nurse stays to see to the needs of all patients in the setting.

  d. Changes in expected workload.

  e. Difficulty planning time and controlling pace of work.

2. Changes in data available.

  a. Requirement that clinical decisions be made with less than usual amount of data.

  b. Unavailability of continuous observation that allows the nurse to pick up subtle changes in the patient's condition.

  c. Reliance on new methods of assessment and integration of information.

      (1) Nuances of patient self-reporting.

      (2) Rapid observation and synthesis, combined with probing and assessment skills.

3. Changes in scope of services provided.

  a. May not be able or required to meet all assessed needs at a given visit.

      (1) May use referral or recommendation as opposed to direct intervention.

      (2) May create conflict in a newly transitioned nurse used to meeting the total needs of each patient.

  b. May apply health assessment standards based on inpatient experience.

      (1) Not appropriate for ambulatory visits.

      (2) This practice creates an unnecessary burden on both the nurse and the patient.

      (3) Critical transition task is to learn how to assess only the essential data for purpose of the visit and the patient's need.

  c. Scope of services may vary substantially from visit to visit.

      (1) For one visit, the nurse may briefly review the patient record and assign the patient to an unlicensed staff member.

      (2) For another visit, the nurse may do a complete assessment, and provide education and counseling or direct care.

  d. Important that population assessment be done.

      (1) Establish overall needs for nursing care within the population.

      (2) Identify major visit types and level of nursing care required for each.

      (3) Establish a process by which patients may gain access to the nurse as needed.

4. Changes in collaborative relationships.

  a. Relationships among health team members change; depending upon the task or challenge at hand, the nurse may be a team member or a team leader.

  b. Focus of nursing care shifts:

      (1) Away from the medical plan of care and implementing that plan.

      (2) Toward a more consultative role with patients, families, and physicians.

  c. The nurse is seen more as the coordinator and manager of care and less as direct implementer.

      (1) Creates opportunities for collaborative practice with physicians.

      (2) Identified by nurses practicing in ambulatory care as a valued aspect of the role.

  d. The nurse becomes a conduit between the physician directing care and the patient/family managing care at home.

e. Collaborative practice models and effective team function are critical and require excellent communication and negotiation skills (Kamimura, Schneider, Lee, Crawford, & Friese, 2012; Sinsky, Sinsky, Althaus, Tranel, & Thiltgen, 2010).

f. Requires demonstration of key competencies to be accepted as a colleague in patient management by physicians.

(1) Clinical competence.

(2) Confidence in decision-making.

(3) Ability to communicate effectively.

5. Diversity in practice assignments.

a. Often a shock for nurses transitioning from single specialty inpatient units.

b. Due to the episodic nature of care, some specialty programs may meet only once or twice per week.

c. The nurse may be assigned in multiple locations to fill out the week.

d. Requires broad competency to manage care for diverse groups of patients.

e. For experienced ambulatory nurses, this variability is the "spice" in their roles.

f. For the new nurse, it may seem like chaos.

C. Strategies to support a successful transition.

1. Nurses transitioning to ambulatory care need full orientation to the setting and the practice styles for each area assigned.

2. Although clinical competency is not usually the major issue, the new nurse will need assistance adapting practice approaches to the new setting.

3. Attention should be paid to signs that the new staff member is becoming overwhelmed with multiple demands.

References

American Academy of Ambulatory Care Nursing (AAACN)/ American Nurses Association (ANA). (1997). *Nursing in ambulatory care: The future is here*. Washington, DC: American Nurses Publishing.

Boutwell, A.E., Johnson, M.B., Rutherford, P., Watson, S.R., Vecchioni, N., Auerbach, B.S., & Wagner, C. (2011). An early look at a four-state initiative to reduce avoidable hospital readmissions. *Health Affairs (Millwood), 30*(7), 1272-1280.

Cronenwett, L., Sherwood, G., Barnsteiner, J., Disch, J., Johnson, J., Mitchell, P., ... Warren, J. (2007). Quality and safety education for nurses. *Nursing Outlook, 55*(3), 122-131.

Haas, S.A., Hackbarth, D.P., Kavanaugh, J.A., & Vlasses, E. (1995). Dimensions of the staff nurse role in ambulatory care. Part II: Comparison of role dimensions in four ambulatory settings. *Nursing Economic$, 13*(3), 152-165.

Hackbarth, D.S., Haas, S., Kavanaugh, J.A., & Vlasses, E. (1995). Dimensions of the staff nurse role in ambulatory care. Part I: Methodology and analysis of data on current staff nurse practice. *Nursing Economic$, 13*(2), 89-98.

Hastings, C. (1987). Classification issues in ambulatory care nursing. *Journal of Ambulatory Care Management, 10*(3), 50-64.

Inglehart, J.K. (2011). Assessing an ACO prototype – Medicare's physician group practice demonstration. *New England Journal of Medicine, 364*(30), 198-200.

Institute of Medicine (IOM). (2001). *Crossing the quality chasm*. Washington, DC: The National Academies Press.

Institute of Medicine (IOM). (2010). *The future of nursing: Leading change, advancing health*. Washington, DC: The National Academies Press.

Kamimura, A., Schneider, K., Lee, C.S., Crawford, S.D., & Friese, C.R. (2012). Practice environments of nurses in ambulatory oncology settings: A thematic analysis. *Cancer Nursing, 35*(1), E1-E7.

Mulder, B.J., Tzeng, H.M., & Vecchioni, N.D. (2012). Preventing avoidable rehospitalizations by understanding the characteristics of 'frequent fliers.' *Journal of Nursing Care Quality, 27*(1), 77-82.

Naylor, M.D., Feldman, P.H., Keating, S., Koren, M.J., Kurtzman, E.T., Maccoy, M.C., & Krakauer, R. (2009). Translating research into practice: Transitional care for older adults. *Journal of Evaluation in Clinical Practice, 15*(6), 1164-1170.

Pedersen, A., & Hack, T.F. (2010). Pilots of oncology health care: A concept analysis of the patient navigator role. *Oncology Nursing Forum, 37*(1), 55-60.

Quality and Safety Education for Nurses (QSEN). (2012). *Competency KSAs (pre-licensure)*. Retrieved from http://www. qsen.org/ksas_prelicensure.php

Robinson-White, S., Conroy, B., Slavish, K.H., & Rosenzweig, M. (2010). Patient navigation in breast cancer: A systematic review. *Cancer Nursing, 33*(2), 127-140.

Rosenthal, T.C. (2008). The medical home: Growing evidence to support a new approach to primary care. *The Journal of the American Board of Family Medicine, 21*(5), 427-440.

Shields, M.C., Patel, P.H., Manning, M., & Sacks, L. (2011). A model for integrating independent physicians into accountable care organizations. *Health Affairs (Millwood), 30*(1), 161-172.

Shortell, S.M., Casalino, L.P., & Fisher, E.S. (2010). How the center for Medicare and Medicaid innovation should test accountable care organizations. *Health Affairs (Millwood), 29*(7), 1293-1298.

Sinsky, C.A., Sinsky, T.A., Althaus, D., Tranel, J., & Thiltgen, M. (2010). Practice profile. 'Core teams': Nurse-physician partnerships provide patient-centered care at an Iowa practice. *Health Affairs (Millwood), 29*(5), 966-968.

Skrutkowski, M., Saucier, A., Eades, M., Swidzinski, M., Ritchie, J., Marchionni, C., & Ladouceur, M. (2008). Impact of a pivot nurse in oncology on patients with lung or breast cancer: Symptom distress, fatigue, quality of life, and use of healthcare resources. *Oncology Nursing Forum, 35*(6), 948-954.

U.S. Department of Health and Human Services (DHHS). (2012). *Healthy people 2020 – Home.* Retrieved from http://www.healthypeople.gov/2020/default.aspx

U.S. Department of Health and Human Services (DHHS). (n.d.). *Quick guide to health literacy.* Retrieved from http://www.health.gov/communication/literacy/quickguide/resources.htm

Verran, J. (1981). Delineation of ambulatory care nursing practice. *Journal of Ambulatory Care Management, 4*(2), 1-13.

Wagner, E.H., Glasgow, R., Davis, C., Bonomi, A., Provost, L., McCulloch, D. ... Sixta, C. (2001). Quality improvement in chronic illness care: A collaborative approach. *Journal on Quality Improvement, 27*(2), 63-80.

Additional Readings

Baghi, H., Panniers, T.L., & Smolenski, M.C. (2007). Description of practice as an ambulatory care nurse: Psychometric properties of a practice-analysis survey. *Journal of Nursing Measurement, 15*(1), 62-76.

Haas, S. (1998). Ambulatory care nursing conceptual framework. *ViewPoint, 20*(3), 16-17.

Institute of Medicine (IOM). (1999). *To err is human.* Washington, DC: The National Academies Press.

Moore-Higgs, G.J., Watkins-Bruner, D., Balmer, L., Johnson-Doneski, J., Komarny, P., Mautner, B., & Velji, K. (2003). The role of licensed nursing personnel in radiation oncology part B: Integrating the ambulatory care nursing conceptual framework. *Oncology Nursing Forum, 30*(1), 59-64.

Streeter, B.L. (2007). A clinical advancement program for registered nurses with an outpatient focus. *Gastroenterology Nursing, 30*(3), 195-200.

Chapter 3

Ambulatory Care Operations

Susan M. Paschke, MSN, RN-BC, NEA-BC

OBJECTIVES – *Study of the information in this chapter will enable the learner to:*

1. Describe the members of the ambulatory care team and the role of the professional nurse as team member, team leader, and care coordinator.
2. Compare and contrast appropriate delegation and supervision skills necessary for the professional ambulatory care nurse.
3. Discuss strategies to determine staffing requirements and skill mix in ambulatory care settings.
4. Evaluate the patient care environment regarding safety, security, hazards, and risks to patients and staff.

KEY POINTS – *The major points in this chapter include:*

1. The patient is a pivotal member of the ambulatory health care team; in addition, the team is composed of the patient's family and/or significant others and the group of health care professionals who provide care and services.
2. The professional nurse follows the standards of delegation and maintains responsibility and accountability for tasks that are delegated to other members of the health care team.
3. Nurses in ambulatory care settings are accountable for evaluating the patient care environment and developing safety and infection control plans and process improvement initiatives to ensure a safe and efficient environment for care.
4. Staffing in ambulatory care presents unique challenges – no formula, tool, or methodology is applicable across the variety of ambulatory care settings.
5. Management of equipment and supplies using the "just in time" rather than the "just in case" philosophy is essential for efficient use of space.

A mbulatory care operations are those recurring activities and processes involved in the day-to-day business of ambulatory care. The quality of care provided to patients is dependent on the integrity of caregivers and care delivery systems, as well as environmental supports that provide the infrastructure to the ambulatory setting. Members of the health care team are responsible for providing quality care based on their professional expertise, scope of practice, and skills. Determining and providing the appropriate number and type of personnel can have a direct effect on the ability to meet patient requirements for care and the desired quality outcomes. The total patient experience is also impacted by the processes for patient access and scheduling, workflow and facility design, resource and environmental management and attention to the safety and security of patients and staff, and the handling of various emergency situations.

I. The Ambulatory Health Care Team

Generally, the patient initiates contact with the ambulatory care system to meet his or her concerns regarding wellness or health care needs (American Academy of Ambulatory Care Nursing [AAACN], 2010). Thus, the patient is a pivotal member of the ambulatory health care team; the team is additionally composed of the patient's family or significant others in partnership with a group of health care professionals who provide care and services in an ambulatory setting. These health care professionals collaborate to ensure multidisciplinary assessments and treatment plans that focus on continuity of care and coordination of resources to meet patient needs.

A. Members of the ambulatory care team include:
   1. Registered nurses (RNs).
   2. Advanced practice registered nurses (APRNs).
      a. Nurse practitioners (NPs).
      b. Clinical nurse specialists (CNSs).
      c. Certified nurse midwives (CNMs).
      d. Certified registered nurse anesthetists (CRNAs).
   3. Physicians (MDs, DOs).
   4. Physician assistants (PAs).
   5. Licensed practical nurses or licensed vocational nurses (LPN/LVNs).
   6. Unlicensed assistive personnel (UAPs).
      a. Medical assistants (MAs).
      b. Nursing assistants or patient care assistants (NAs or PCAs).
   7. Clerical and secretarial support personnel.
   8. Professionals and non-professionals from other disciplines, such as pharmacy, therapies (respiratory, speech, occupational, or physical), social work, nutrition, behavioral health, home care.

B. Primary care.
   1. The primary care team consists of a care provider aligned with a group of other health care practitioners responsible for the comprehensive care of a single or group of patients and serving as the point of access to the health care system. The team coordinates access to other levels of care as necessary.
   2. Roles of the team.
      a. *Physicians/APRNs/PAs* – Providers of care responsible for the delivery and management of patient care.
      b. *Social workers* – Provide psychosocial assessments, ongoing counseling, and treatment; serve as consultants to the team for psychosocial issues.
      c. *Dietitians* – Perform nutritional screening and/or assessment; develop, implement, and educate the patient and family regarding nutrition therapy plans.
      d. *Pharmacists* – Educate patients about medications, including expected outcomes, side effects, precautions, interactions, and reactions.
      e. *Behavioral health* – Serve as mental health resources to assist with assessment and treatment of patient conditions.
      f. *Therapists (respiratory, physical, occupational, speech)* – Treat a variety of patient conditions and educate patients regarding ongoing care at home.
      g. *Clerical support* – Register patients, schedule appointments, contact patients, retrieve medical records and other pertinent information to enable providers to deliver care.
      h. *Clinical support/nursing services personnel (RNs, LPN/LVNs, UAPs).*

C. Nurses in ambulatory care settings play an integral role as members of the primary or specialty care team.
   1. RNs provide direct care to patients, as well as coordinate care to ensure continuity and appropriateness of care.
   2. Nurses have the ability to perform many roles of other health care team members in the event that these team members are not available, such as nutrition education, medication education, psychosocial support, and clerical duties.
   3. Roles specific to the professional registered nurse include:
      a. Telephone triage/advice/screening.
         (1) Use of formalized triage protocols for specific complaints to determine the most appropriate course of action.
            (a) Immediate intervention – Emergency department or urgent care.
            (b) Intervention within 24 hours.
            (c) Routine appointment.
            (d) Education and support to provide self-care or family member care at home.

    (2) Patients with multiple complaints, a complex medical history, or poor historians may not be appropriately managed with protocols based on symptoms.

    (3) Assessment, judgment, and critical thinking skills are necessary for this role.

b. Direct care and treatment of patients.

    (1) Scheduled patients.

    (2) Triage and care of walk-in patients.

    (3) Management of urgent or emergent situations.

c. Referrals to other members of the health care team or to community services, such as home care, hospice, assisted living, or nursing homes.

d. Case management – "The collaborative process that assesses, plans, implements, coordinates, monitors, and evaluates options and services to meet an individual's health needs through communication and use of available resources to promote quality, cost-effective outcomes" (Marquis & Huston, 2009, p. 216).

    (1) The professional registered nurse possesses the appropriate knowledge, judgment, and skill to coordinate the care of the patient across the continuum of care (AAACN, 2010).

    (2) Not every patient requires case management.

e. Supervision of LPN/LVNs and UAPs – Includes monitoring, evaluation, education, and delegation of appropriate tasks to appropriate and competent individuals.

f. Patient advocacy – See Chapter 8, "Patient Advocacy and Use of Community Resources."

g. Health and wellness education – Teaching the patient and family to safely care for themselves outside of and between visits to the health care setting.

    (1) Includes assessment of the patient's readiness to learn; physical, emotional, or cultural barriers to learning; preference for method of learning; and the patient's response to the educational session (The Joint Commission, 2010).

    (2) Includes information on disease, treatments, medications, self-care management, lifestyle risk factors, and community resources. Pre- and post-education evaluation and teach back provide assessment of learning.

    (3) Focuses on health promotion and disease prevention for both individual and groups.

    (4) Includes health promotion information regarding food and nutrition, smoking cessation, drug and alcohol consumption, exercise and physical activity, and home, vehicle, and environmental safety – Based on objectives set forth in *Healthy People 2020* (U.S. Department of Health and Human Services, 2010).

    (5) Educates in congruence with nursing theory. See Chapter 16, "Patient Education and Counseling."

    (6) Evaluates the need for end-of-life planning – Educates patients about their rights to plan for medical care and provides information regarding advance directives (e.g., living wills, durable power of attorney for health care, and treatment preferences, such as palliative and/or hospice care).

h. Quality/performance improvement.

    (1) Identification of quality or performance improvement opportunities is the responsibility of all members of the health care team.

    (2) Patient outcomes are key indicators of quality care.

D. Scope of practice – Defines the procedures, actions, and processes permitted for a licensed individual and is limited to that which the law allows for specific education and experience, and specific demonstrated competency.

1. RNs, LPN/LVNs, APRNs – The scope of practice for each level of nursing care is determined by the nurse practice act of the state where the individual is licensed to practice.

2. PAs – The scope of practice for physician assistants is determined by the delegatory decisions made by the supervising physician in accordance with state laws and regulations set forth by the state medical board.

3. MAs – The scope of practice for medical assistants is regulated by the state medical board because medical assistants must work under a licensed person's direct supervision when performing clinical duties delegated by the licensee.

   a. May perform administrative, clerical, or clinical tasks.

   b. Must possess appropriate educational and/or on-the-job training and demonstrate competence prior to tasks being delegated.

   c. May take exam to become certified (CMA) or registered (RMA).

E. Competence.

1. Competence is defined as the ability to demonstrate the technical, interpersonal, and/or clinical skills necessary to perform the responsibilities of the job.

2. Assessment of competence may require actual demonstration of skills.

3. Frequency of competence assessment is dependent upon the skill, behavior, or activity being assessed.

   a. Initial competency verification – Completed during orientation of new nursing staff.

   b. Annual competency verification – Annual assessment of skills and techniques. High-risk or low-volume activities may require more frequent assessment.

II. Delegation and Supervision

According to the Joint Statement on Delegation by the American Nurses Association (ANA) and National Council of State Boards of Nursing (NCSBN) (2006), delegation is the process for a nurse to direct another person to perform nursing tasks and activities while maintaining responsibility and accountability for the tasks. The professional registered nurse uses delegation to ensure that routine tasks are performed by others, thereby allowing the nurse to handle complex problems or those that require a higher level of knowledge, skill, or expertise.

A. Delegation is a learned skill and improves with practice (Marquis & Huston, 2009).

B. Common mistakes in delegation include:

1. Under-delegating due to:

   a. Lack of trust in others to perform the task.

   b. Fear of resentment from subordinates.

   c. Lack of experience in delegation.

2. Over-delegating due to:

   a. Insecurity in performance of the task.

   b. Continually relying on exceptionally competent employees – May lead to burnout and decreased productivity.

3. Improper delegation.

   a. Delegation to the wrong person, at the wrong time, for the wrong reason (Huston, 2007).

   b. Delegation of tasks beyond the capability of the individual.

   c. Delegation of decision-making without adequate information.

C. Delegation to unlicensed assistive personnel (UAPs).

1. Definition of UAP – Individuals who are trained to function in an assistive role to the licensed registered nurse in the provision of patient/client care activities as delegated by the nurse (ANA & NCSBN, 2006).

2. UAPs can perform tasks and non-nursing functions, enabling the professional registered nurse to perform nursing functions and activities.

3. Delegation of tasks can increase the liability of the professional registered nurse if done improperly. Delegation principles include:
   a. The RN may delegate elements of care, but may not delegate the nursing process itself.
   b. The RN has the duty to answer for personal actions relating to the nursing process.
   c. The RN takes into account the knowledge and skills of any individual to whom the RN may delegate elements of care.
   d. The decision of whether or not to delegate or assign is based upon the RN's judgment concerning the condition of the patient, the competence of all members of the nursing team, and the degree of supervision that will be required of the RN if a task is delegated.
   e. The RN delegates only those tasks for which she or he believes the other health care worker has the knowledge and skill to perform, taking into consideration training, cultural competence experience, and facility/agency policies and procedures.
   f. The RN uses critical thinking and professional judgment when following *The Five Rights of Delegation:*
      (1) Right task.
      (2) Right circumstances.
      (3) Right person.
      (4) Right directions and communication.
      (5) Right supervision and evaluation.
   g. RNs monitor organizational policies, procedures, and position descriptions to ensure there is no violation of the nurse practice act (ANA & NCSBN, 2006).
D. Delegation algorithm (Johnson, 1995) – Series of questions to assist with appropriate delegation to UAPs:
   1. Is the task within the scope of nursing practice? If no, the task cannot be performed or delegated by the professional nurse.
   2. Does the task require nursing knowledge, skill, or independent judgment? If yes, the task cannot be delegated.
   3. Is the task within the level of educational preparation and demonstrated competence of the individual to whom it is to be delegated? If no, the task cannot be delegated.
   4. Is the professional nurse available to supervise? If no, the task cannot be delegated.
   5. Is the patient's condition such that someone other than a professional nurse can perform the task? If no, the task cannot be delegated.
   6. Does the task involve initial assessment, analysis, development of a plan of care, or evaluation of patient progress? If yes, the task cannot be delegated.
E. Supervision – The provision of guidance and oversight of a delegated nursing task (ANA & NCSBN, 2006).
   1. Supervision is a role expectation of all professional nurses.
   2. Supervision requires development of the following skills:
      a. Ability to direct and guide other professionals, LPN/LVNs, and UAPs.
      b. Effective communication, direction, monitoring, and evaluation of the progress and completion of the task.
      c. Evaluation of patient outcomes.
      d. Evaluation of staff satisfaction.
   3. Strategies for effective supervision of unlicensed assistive personnel (UAPs).
      a. Know the individual, education level and training, the role expectations, and level of competence.
      b. Allocate time for oversight of the work of the UAP – Allows for observation of and timely feedback regarding performance.
      c. Use open, respectful, and constructive communication regarding the task and the performance.
      d. Adhere to patient care and work performance standards for self and others.

4. Role of nurse manager or nurse executive regarding the supervisory role of the professional nurse is to:
   a. Support the professional nurse in the role of supervisor.
   b. Assure appropriate training and skill development in supervision to meet job requirements. Provide remedial training as necessary.
   c. Assess job satisfaction and promote retention in the supervisory role.

III. Determining Staffing and Skill Mix in Ambulatory Care

A. Definitions.
   1. *Staffing* – The process of determining and providing the appropriate number and mix of nursing personnel to meet the requirements for patient care and desired outcomes.
   2. *Skill mix* – The various types of nursing staff by job classification necessary to care for the patient population being served (Dunham-Taylor & Pinczuk, 2006).
   3. *Workload* – Refers to the amount and difficulty associated with providing patient care and related activities in a specified period of time.
   4. *Staffing ratio* – The ratio of nurses or nursing personnel to providers (a licensed practitioner, such as a physician or NP).

B. Factors influencing staffing.
   1. Process of care delivery.
      a. Volume and types of services provided.
      b. Complexity of patients.
      c. Number of providers and practice styles.
      d. Use of midlevel providers.
      e. Available space and patient flow.
      f. Number and types of nursing personnel available, including UAPs.
      g. Availability of consult and support services.
      h. Presence of medical residents, students, or other trainees.
   2. Types of patient encounters.
      a. Scheduled vs. unscheduled.
      b. New vs. established/follow-up visits.
      c. Office visit vs. procedure.
      d. Urgent or emergent situation.
      e. Direct physical care or treatment vs. education or counseling.
      f. In-person vs. telephone or other telecommunication device contact.
      g. Special needs populations (e.g., geriatric, pediatric, sight or hearing impaired).
   3. Provider requirements for assistance.
      a. Prior to visit.
      b. During visit.
      c. Following visit.
      d. Telephone support – Phone care, prescription refills.

C. Staffing models in ambulatory care.
   1. Goal of staffing model is to increase efficiency and maintain needed flexibility.
   2. No models are available for use across all ambulatory care settings due to multitude of settings and wide variety of patients.
   3. No accurate patient acuity or classification systems are currently available for ambulatory care for general application.

IV. Practice and Office Support

The quality of patient care provided in any ambulatory setting is as dependent upon the environmental supports as it is on the skills and abilities of providers. Patient scheduling and access, workflow and resource management, environmental safety, and emergency preparedness are important factors in the daily operations of ambulatory care settings and play a key role in patient and staff satisfaction.

A. Patient scheduling and access – In the past, patient visits were arranged according to a pre-set schedule of appointment time frames with the intent of reducing wait times for patients and providers. Variations in scheduling now allow for group appointments, wave appointments, and sometimes, no appointments. Efficient scheduling enhances utilization of nursing and support staff, space, and ancillary services, and allows for appropriate preparation and gathering of necessary information prior to the visit. The degree to which the scheduling plan or system functions effectively can impact the smooth flow of patients into and out of the ambulatory setting and is a key driver of patient satisfaction.

1. Access and scheduling.
   a. *Access* – Defined as the extent to which a facility or service is available according to an individual's need or desire.
   b. Pre-scheduled appointment times (appointments made in advance, which may limit availability for same-day appointments) vs. open or advanced access (which typically facilitates available same-day appointments any time of day).
   c. Scheduled appointments vs. walk-in appointments.
   d. Centralized scheduling of appointments vs. decentralized scheduling.
2. Appointment types.
   a. Set time (patients scheduled every 15 minutes for the hour) vs. block time (all patients for the hour scheduled at the same time and taken first come, first served).
   b. Fixed time increments (appointments scheduled every 15 minutes) vs. varied time increments (appointments scheduled for different amounts of time based on condition or presumed need).
   c. Individual (single patient per time slot) vs. group (several patients with same or similar conditions scheduled together).
3. Visit types.
   a. New patient vs. established patient.
   b. Provider referral vs. patient self-referral.
   c. Primary care vs. specialty care.
4. Other variables.
   a. Provider variables.
      (1) Type of provider.
         (a) Primary care vs. specialty care.
         (b) Nurse practitioner vs. physician assistant vs. physician.
         (c) Procedure nurse vs. patient education nurse.
      (2) Provider traits.
         (a) Experienced vs. beginning practitioner.
         (b) On-time vs. chronically late.
         (c) Support needed: None, some, or much.
         (d) Availability: Requirements for meetings, teaching, research, or administrative duties.
   b. Patient variables.
      (1) Nature of problem.
         (a) Urgent vs. non-urgent.
         (b) New patient/new problem vs. existing problem.
         (c) Established patient/new problem vs. existing problem.
         (d) Acute vs. chronic illness/disease.
      (2) Special needs.
         (a) Interpreter required: Foreign language, American Sign Language (ASL).
         (b) Physical limitations: Non-ambulating or difficulty ambulating, sight or hearing impaired.
         (c) Acutely ill.
   c. Support variables.
      (1) Staffing.
         (a) Number of staff and ratio of staff to providers.
         (b) Skill mix – Types of staff, such as RN, LPN or LVN, MA, PCA, technician.
      (2) Space.
         (a) Number of exam rooms per provider.
         (b) Appropriate room types: Exam, treatment, procedure, observation, recovery, infusion.
   d. Business variables.
      (1) Intake/customer service representatives.
      (2) Insurance verification/pre-authorization.
      (3) Special equipment availability.

(4) Available information: Medical records/reports.

(5) Computerized systems for integration of schedules with patient medical records, registration, billing, sequencing of appointments.

(6) Policies/procedures for reminder calls to patients, late arrivals, no shows, or cancellations.

B. Layout and design issues – The design of an ambulatory care facility can enhance or impede the flow of patients and daily operations. Standardization and planning in the design and set-up of the workspace supports maximum flexibility of room utilization and puts supplies and equipment in closer proximity to patients and staff, thereby enhancing productivity and efficiency. All facilities must comply with the *Americans with Disabilities Act* of 1990 and the regulations for ambulatory health care facilities identified by the Facilities Guidelines Institute, Inc. (FGI, 2010). Consideration should be given to:

1. Provision for privacy for patients in all areas, including appropriate levels of acoustical and visual privacy.

2. Private, confidential areas for registration, insurance authorization, financial discussions, and payment transactions.

3. Waiting area sized to accommodate patients and those who accompany them – Safe and appropriate areas for children, elderly, bariatric patients.

4. Separate areas for those with suspected communicable illnesses.

5. Security protection in certain areas – Video cameras, panic buttons, safety glass enclosures, lock-down capabilities.

6. Easily accessible and sufficient number of ADA-compliant public restrooms.

7. Identified areas for mobile phone use and internet accessibility.

C. Environmental management – Appropriate management plans assure a safe, accessible, and functional environment of care. Ambulatory care settings present special challenges due to patient mix, the nature of undiagnosed conditions, and the movement of patients through multiple areas of the ambulatory care environment (Association for Professionals in Infection Control and Epidemiology, Inc [APIC], 2009). Ambulatory care nurses have accountability for evaluation of patient care environments and the subsequent development of safety and infection control plans, ongoing monitoring, and implementation of process improvements related to patients and staff (The Joint Commission, 2010).

1. Safety.

a. Factors affecting patient safety.

(1) Physical disability.

(2) Altered mental status/impaired judgment.

(3) Effects of medications.

(4) Fall risk – Assessment and identification of high-risk patients.

(5) Appropriate furnishings and equipment for population served:

(a) Children – Appropriately sized furniture, safe toys, electrical outlet covers.

(b) Elderly – Non-movable chairs, safety rails.

(c) Bariatric – Oversized chairs, scales, wheelchairs, radiology equipment for obese patients.

(d) Specialty specific:

i. Rehabilitation patients – Wheelchair/other assistive device accessibility.

ii. Orthopedic patients – Higher seating.

iii. Immuno-compromised – High-efficiency particulate arresting (HEPA) air filtration.

b. Factors affecting staff safety.

(1) Availability of personal protective equipment – Appropriately sized gloves, masks, goggles, face shields, gowns, aprons, respiratory protection.

(2) Ergonomically appropriate work stations and furniture – Height-adjustable chairs, keyboard wrist protectors, non-glare computer screens.

(3) Safe patient handling equipment – Patient transfer and lift devices, powered examination and procedure tables.

(4) Safe handling of hazardous materials/waste.

    (a) Accessible material safety data sheets (MSDS) for all hazardous materials.

    (b) Appropriate storage facilities.

    (c) Spill kits/exposure protocols/ emergency procedures/appropriate sharps containers.

    (d) Safe and appropriate disposal process.

2. Security.

  a. Control access.

    (1) Staff identification system – Secured staff-only access areas.

    (2) Procedure areas with specialized equipment.

    (3) Secured areas for prescription pads, needles, syringes, medications, controlled substances.

  b. Security situations/emergencies.

    (1) Aggressive/escalating patient behavior.

    (2) Suspicious persons/activity.

    (3) Suicide risk.

    (4) Persons in possession of weapons.

    (5) Bomb threats.

    (6) Threats to staff or patients.

3. Medical emergencies.

  a. Maintain staff competence.

    (1) Recognition of acute changes in patient condition.

    (2) Certification in basic life support (BLS)/cardiopulmonary resuscitation (CPR).

    (3) Provision of first aid.

    (4) Knowledge of urgent/emergent procedures.

  b. Provide appropriate equipment.

    (1) Age-appropriate for patients served.

(2) Preventive maintenance and equipment checks to assure continual state of readiness.

  c. Documentation/risk management.

    (1) Document event and outcome in patient medical record.

    (2) Provide hand-off communication to assure continuity of patient care.

    (3) Incident reporting for process improvement and risk management.

4. Infection control.

  a. Recognize health exposure risks and presence of infection.

    (1) Symptoms of infection, such as suspicious-looking or -smelling wound drainage, diarrhea, or respiratory secretions.

    (2) Airborne diseases (including chicken pox, measles, tuberculosis, influenza, SARS, Avian influenza, and other foreign, emerging, or potentially re-emerging disease, such as smallpox).

    (3) Exposure to high-risk body fluids through needlesticks, splash to mucous membranes (eyes, nose, mouth), or contact with non-intact skin.

    (4) Identify reportable diseases as regulated by local, state, and federal health agencies – Maintain current list.

      (a) Ensure mechanisms exist for timely reporting.

      (b) Educate staff regarding who can/is required to report.

      (c) Document in patient/employee medical records.

  b. Provide staff orientation/ongoing education relating to general infection control principles and site-specific procedures, including annual competency assessment regarding revisions in infection control requirements.

    (1) Disease transmission.

    (2) Standard and enhanced precautions.

(3) Respiratory hygiene.

(4) Employee safety related to exposure.

c. Prevent transmission through:

(1) Hand hygiene compliance (Centers for Disease Control and Prevention [CDC], 2002).

(2) Use of personal protective equipment (required by OSHA) – Avoid direct contact with blood, respiratory or excretory secretions, wound drainage, aerosols, or contaminated articles or patient belongings.

(3) Use of immunizations for staff as recommended by CDC and institutional policy.

(4) Use of standard precautions with all patients.

(5) Adherence to post-exposure procedures – Administer first aid, follow prophylaxis procedures and monitoring per CDC recommendations.

(6) Use appropriate containers to hold contaminated items for transport, disposal, or reprocessing, such as covered metal containers.

d. Surveillance.

(1) Tracking and trending of infections – More challenging in ambulatory settings due to intermittent visits.

(2) Appropriate patient follow-up to prevent transmission to other patients, health care workers, family, and friends.

(3) Assure follow-up on laboratory results reporting (such as wound, urine, throat, and genital cultures).

(4) Develop ongoing quality monitoring and performance improvement program based on results of surveillance activities.

5. Disinfection and sterilization.

a. Definitions.

(1) *Disinfection* – A process that destroys many or all pathogenic microorganisms, except bacterial spores, on inanimate objects usually by use of liquid chemical or wet pasteurization (Rutala, Weber, & The Healthcare Infection Control Practices Advisory Committee [HICPAC], 2008).

(a) High-level disinfection – Kills all microorganisms, except large numbers of bacterial spores, with appropriate solution for determined exposure time (such as 2% glutaraldehyde for 20 minutes).

(b) Low-level disinfection – Kills most vegetative bacteria, some fungi, and some viruses in a shorter period of time (less than 10 minutes).

(2) *Sterilization* – Process that destroys or eliminates all forms of microbial life and is carried out in health care facilities by physical or chemical methods, such as pressurized steam (autoclave), dry heat, ethylene oxide gas, hydrogen peroxide gas plasma, and liquid chemicals (Rutala, Weber, & HICPAC, 2008).

(3) *Cleaning or decontamination* – The removal of visible soil (organic and inorganic material) from objects or surfaces accomplished manually or mechanically using water with detergents or enzymatic products (Rutala, Weber, & HICPAC, 2008).

b. Requirements – Must provide a consistent standard of care for all patients.

(1) *Critical items* – Must be *sterilized.*

(a) Items that enter sterile tissue or the vascular system.

(b) Include surgical instruments, catheters, implants, and ultrasound probes that enter sterile body cavities.

(2) *Semi-critical items* – Must use *high-level disinfection,* at least (could be sterilized, but not required).

(a) Items that contact mucous membranes or non-intact skin.

(b) Include respiratory and anesthesia equipment, some endoscopes, laryngoscope blades, cystoscopes, esophageal and anorectal manometry probes and catheters, and diaphragm fitting rings.

(3) *Non-critical items* – Must be *cleaned* or *decontaminated,* at least – Considered *low level disinfection* (could use high-level disinfection or sterilization, but not required).

(a) Items that contact intact skin, but not mucous membranes.

(b) Include BP cuffs, crutches, bedpans, bedside commodes, and environmental items.

c. Examination rooms.

(1) Clean examination rooms between patients, including removal of soiled linen and equipment, cleaning soiled surfaces, and changing table paper.

(2) Clean examination tables, counter tops, treatment carts, and floors daily.

(3) Disinfect patient care equipment between patients.

(4) After a patient with an airborne transmitted illness, close the room for the prescribed amount of time based on the number of air exchanges required and disinfect the room prior to reuse.

d. Equipment and supplies.

(1) Separate clean and soiled supplies and linen.

(2) Discard disposable equipment after single use into designated waste receptacles.

(3) Discard syringes, needles, glass vials, and all sharps into appropriate sharps containers; use needleless technology whenever possible.

(4) Follow manufacturer's instructions for reprocessing/high-level disinfecting procedures for endoscopic equipment and accessories.

6. Refrigerators and freezers.

a. Separate storage for medication, food, and specimens.

b. Monitor temperature daily and record manually or via electronic data capture (NB: with Vaccines for Children, CDC requires twice daily temperature monitoring with a recordable/traceable thermometer).

c. Maintain temperature within acceptable range – Implement immediate actions if temperature is out of range.

d. Clean and/or defrost at regular intervals.

D. Management of equipment and supplies. To function efficiently, a process for procuring and maintaining medical equipment and supplies is necessary. The process will include the safe and effective use of equipment, staff education, and competency assessment relating to the equipment, and a cost-effective method for purchasing equipment and supplies.

1. Selection of equipment and supplies.

a. Purchasing specifications.

b. Shared pricing contracts to assure lowest possible cost.

c. Service/maintenance contracts and warranties.

d. Availability of "loaner" equipment and expedited delivery of supplies.

2. Inventory management.

a. "Just in time" vs. "just in case" philosophy – Limit inventory to what is needed at present to preserve financial investment – Avoids "stockpiling."

(1) Agreement on standardization of items.

(2) Increased frequency of ordering/purchasing.

(3) Designated "par levels" based on usual usage patterns – Tracking and trending.

b. Preventive maintenance/service.

        (1) Initial inspection of all powered medical equipment for compliance with appropriate specifications prior to initial use.

        (2) Routine scheduled inspections that adhere to manufacturer's recommendations for frequency of evaluation of equipment – Ensures appropriate functioning and readiness for use when needed.

        (3) Staff responsible for checking all critical alarms for audibility and correct functioning.

        (4) Availability of back-up equipment, such as battery-operated for use in emergency conditions.

   c. Safe Medical Device Act – 1990.

        (1) Federal legislation designed to inform the FDA of any medical product that caused or is suspected to have caused serious illness, injury, or death in a patient or employee.

        (2) Leads to investigation of the product and determination of level of risk for continued use – Products may be suggested for limited uses or be taken out of service based on FDA rulings.

E. Emergency preparedness.

  1. Identify specific procedures in response to internal and external disasters (such as fire, explosion, earthquake, hurricane, tornado, flooding, terrorism).

  2. Define facility's role in community-wide disaster response.

  3. Provide staff orientation and ongoing education.

    a. Role and responsibility during emergency/disaster.

    b. Skills required for response.

    c. Competency assessment at least annually.

    d. Scheduled drills to practice and test procedures.

    e. Evaluation of response and performance.

  4. Establish communication plans and back-up systems for use during disasters/emergencies.

  5. Develop plans to obtain supplies and equipment during disasters/emergencies.

  6. Develop primary and alternative evacuation plans, including access to transport equipment if needed.

  7. Establish plans for utilities disruption/failure.

    a. Which patient care activities can continue and which need to be stopped for patient and staff safety?

    b. Alternative sources for essential utilities (emergency power, telecommunications, water, steam).

    c. Emergency procedures for system failures.

    d. Location of emergency shut-off controls for medical gases, water, and power, and procedure to be used.

    e. Process for repair services.

  8. Develop business recovery plan – How and when to resume business "as usual."

References

American Academy of Ambulatory Care Nursing (AAACN). (2010). *Scope and standards of practice for professional ambulatory care nursing* (8th ed.). Pitman, NJ: Author.

American Nurses Association (ANA) & National Council of State Boards of Nursing (NCSBN). (2006). *Joint statement on delegation*. Washington, DC: Author.

Association for Professionals in Infection Control and Epidemiology, Inc. (APIC). (2009). *APIC text of infection control and epidemiology* (3rd ed.). Washington, DC: Author.

Centers for Disease Control and Prevention (CDC). (2002). Guideline for hand hygiene in health care settings. *Morbidity and Mortality Weekly Report (MMWR), 51*(RR-16), 1-56.

Dunham-Taylor, J., & Pinczuk, J.Z. (2006). *Health care financial management for nurse managers: Merging the heart with the dollar.* Sudbury, MA: Jones & Bartlett Publishers.

Facilities Guidelines Institute, Inc. (FGI). (2010). *Guidelines for design and construction of healthcare facilities.* Retrieved from http://www.fgiguidelines.org

Huston, C.J. (2007). 10 tips for successful delegation. *Journal of Nursing Management, 39*(3), 54-56.

Johnson, E.M. (1995). Assistive personnel in ambulatory care. *ViewPoint, 17*(3), 1.

Joint Commission, The. (2010). *Comprehensive accreditation manual for hospitals.* Oakbrook Terrace, IL: Author.

Marquis, B.L., & Huston, C.J. (2009). *Leadership roles and management functions in nursing: Theory and application* (6th ed.). Philadelphia: Lippincott, Williams & Wilkins.

Rutala, W.A., Weber, D.J., & The Healthcare Infection Control Practices Advisory Committee (HICPAC). (2008). *Guideline for disinfection and sterilization in healthcare facilities.* Atlanta: Centers for Disease Control and Prevention.

U.S. Department of Health and Human Services (DHHS). (2010). *Healthy people 2020.* Washington, DC: Author.

Additional Readings

Potter, P., DeShields, T., & Kuhrik, M. (2010). Delegation practices between registered nurses and nursing assistive personnel. *Journal of Nursing Management, 18*(2), 157-165.

Reed, P.G., & Shearer, N.C. (2009). *Perspectives on nursing theory* (5th ed.). Philadelphia: Lippincott, Williams & Wilkins.

Rose, K.D., Ross, J.S., & Horwitz, L.I. (2011). Advanced access scheduling outcomes: A systematic review. *Archives of Internal Medicine, 171*(13), 1150-1159.

Roussel, L., & Swansburg, R.C. (2009). *Management and leadership for nurse adminstrators* (5th ed.). Sudbury, MA: Jones & Bartlett Publishers.

U.S. Food and Drug Administration (FDA). (2010). *How to report problems with products regulated by FDA.* Retrieved from http://www.fds.gov/AboutFDA/ContactFDA/ReportaProblem/default.html

Chapter 4

Health Care Fiscal Management

Anne T. Jessie, MSN, RN

OBJECTIVES – *Study of the information in this chapter will enable the learner to:*

1. Describe how care delivery and payment models impact daily operations and budgetary planning and management.
2. Recognize common revenue sources.
3. Apply knowledge of managed care financial principles in daily practice, as well as mechanisms to ensure quality and appropriate care.
4. Describe common coding systems.
5. Gain an understanding of the business of health care and its relationship to the budgeting process.
6. Identify the need to understand how health care reform impacts fiscal management in ambulatory care.

KEY POINTS – *The major points in this chapter include:*

1. Ambulatory care nurses have significant opportunities to impact health care costs related to hospital admission and readmission through chronic disease management and care coordination, promoting preventive health activities, and managing care transitions across the continuum of care.
2. Managed care and health care reform present new opportunities for ambulatory care nurses to improve quality outcomes.
3. Nurses can contribute to the financial health of organizations by applying knowledge of health care financial management, program planning, and budget management.
4. Participating in care coordination and managing transitions in care are critical areas where ambulatory care nurses can assist in controlling health care costs and improve patient outcomes.

The magnitude of public expenditures for health care within the United States has escalated to a level requiring thoughtful, purposeful, and actionable steps toward health care reform. The government's role in financing and regulating health care has significantly increased with the passage of the Patient Protection and Affordable Care Act (PPACA) (Democratic Policy and Communications Committee [DPCC], 2010). As a result of the constantly changing landscape of health care and legislative environments, ambulatory care nurses must develop an understanding of the concepts of health care economics within the context of health care reform. Decisions made by nurses not only affect the financial viability of the organizations for which they work, but may directly affect the financial well-being of their patients.

Ambulatory care registered nurses take a holistic approach when planning and delivering patient care and managing resources. The ambulatory care nurse considers "factors related to the availability of resources, effectiveness, efficiency, cost and benefits, and impact on ambulatory care clinical practice and the organization" (American Academy of Ambulatory Care Nursing [AAACN], 2010, p. 37). Ambulatory care nurses employ cost-effective interventions to maximize wellness and prevent illness, as well as manage acute and chronic diseases (AAACN, 2010). In addition, the nurse educates and advocates for the patient and caregiver to make informed decisions regarding the costs, risks, and benefits of health care services.

In this chapter, the ambulatory care nurse will be provided with a basic knowledge of health care finance, which will allow for knowledgeable and active participation in providing cost-effective patient care services. The reader will acquire knowledge of commonly used financial terms and acronyms applicable in the work setting. Basic financial concepts will be defined, such as revenue stream, cost accounting, cost benefit analysis, managed care concepts, and coding and reimbursement mechanisms. Additionally, the role of the nurse in accountable care organizations (ACOs), patient-centered medical homes (PCMHs), and transitions in care will be described.

The nurse's awareness of how clinical behaviors impact the cost of health care services is essential in the ambulatory care environment. Failure to understand and apply clinical guidelines and decision pathways may result in otherwise avoidable emergency department visits, hospitalizations, and other costly tests and interventions. The ambulatory care nurse's specific role in the continuum of care focuses on the integration of the plan of care, measurement of outcomes, the provision of patient education, and the assurance of timely and appropriate access to care. These activities result in lower costs, higher quality, and continuous improvements in care management and care delivery.

I. **Quality, Costs, and Financing**
A. Dunham-Taylor and Pinczuk (2006) described the importance of linking patient values and expectations with achieving quality and financial accountability. Attention must be paid to what patients value. "Value is determined by the three elements of cost, quality, and service" (Dunham-Taylor & Pinczuk, 2006, p. 32).
    1. Cost is driven by available resources.
    2. Quality is linked to safety and outcomes.
    3. Service refers to the timing and type of care provided.
B. Involving the patient in determining what care will be provided within the context of cost contributes to compliance with the treatment plan and directly impacts patient satisfaction and desired patient outcomes.

C. The goals for health care put forth by the Institute of Medicine (IOM, 2001) suggest that health care professionals should become more attuned to the patient's perspective. The goals are for health care to be safe, effective, patient-centered, timely, efficient, and equitable (IOM, 2001).
D. Aligning payment policies with quality improvement is a necessary component of health care reform.
E. However, most providers receive payments from a variety of payers with a mix of incentive and rewards programs, and inconsistent expectations can inhibit quality improvement.

II. **Financial Environment of Health Care Organizations**
A health care organization providing health services will be financially viable if it receives revenues from services provided in an amount equal to or greater than the dollars expended to provide the services. Patient service revenue represents the amount that results from the provision of patient care services. Additional sources of revenue may include government payments at the local, state, or federal level for services such as educational programs and research or foundation grants.
A. Fees are the method of charging patients or payers for services rendered during an episode of care.
    1. Fees are determined starting with the basic costs required to provide a service.
    2. Defining service units and identifying direct and indirect costs are necessary prior to establishing fees.
    3. Nurses need to adopt and utilize a standard set of definitions for cost information to be interpreted consistently and communicated effectively (see Table 4-1).
B. The total costs of running an ambulatory practice can be categorized into fixed, variable, and mixed costs (see Table 4-2).
C. To cover all costs, practices must generate more revenue on patient visits and procedures than the costs incurred by the delivery of care.
    1. *Net income* is defined as revenue, less expense, after all expenses are paid.

Table 4-1.
Service Units and Direct and Indirect Costs

Cost Measurement	Definition	Examples
Service unit	A basic measure of a product or service being provided by an organization.	In ambulatory care, individual patient encounters, such as office visits, procedures, or nurse-only visits.
Direct costs	Costs of resources for providing a specific service directly related to the delivery of patient care.	Nursing salaries, supplies, medications.
Indirect costs	Costs within a service unit that are not incurred for direct patient care.	Clerical support staff, rent, laundry, housekeeping, utilities.

Source: Adapted from Finkler, Kovner, & Jones, 2007.

Table 4-2.
Fixed and Variable Costs

Costs	Definition	Examples
Relevant range	Normal range for an expected activity for a cost center.	Anticipated number of patient office visits monthly or yearly.
Fixed costs	Costs that are fixed in the context of a relevant range. Cost does not change with a change in visit volumes.	Manager salary, rent, minimum staff, and support staff requirements.
Variable costs	Costs that vary with changes in volumes of service units.	Medications, supplies, direct staffing beyond minimum, overtime.
Mixed costs	Costs that include both fixed or variable costs.	*Utilities:* Minimum costs are fixed, but may vary based on weather extremes or need for periodic extended hours. *Staffing:* Minimum level is fixed, with variation related to volume.

Source: Adapted from Finkler, Kovner, & Jones, 2007.

2. Additional factors in net income are insurance contractual adjustments and non-collectable bad debt.
3. Fees must be set to determine net income.
4. Net income needs to be determined for the following:
   a. Developing plans for new programs.
   b. Funding capital expenses (such as information technology systems or building projects).
   c. Contributing to retained earnings for operations in future years.
   d. Paying out profits or dividends to shareholders in a for-profit health care entity.
D. Revenue is the total amount of income received or that is entitled to be received based on services rendered or goods provided. Net patient revenue is the amount of revenue that an organization is legally allowed to collect (Finkler, Kovner, & Jones, 2007).
   1. The rapidly changing health care environment and a payer's focus on controlling costs can directly affect an organization's revenue stream or their sources and amounts of revenue.

2. Medicare, Medicaid, and other insurance types have coverage limits and payment levels that change frequently and can significantly affect the revenue stream.
3. A charge or fee for a service often does not reflect the actual amount collected. The actual amount received is commonly referred to as the *collectible*.
4. Bad debt occurs when an insurer, an employer, or a patient does not pay a bill.
5. A fee may be set based on the usual, customary, and reasonable (UCR) amount.
   a. *Usual* refers to the amount normally charged for a given health care service.
   b. *Customary* is based on the percentile of aggregated fees charged in a given geographic area for the same service.
   c. *Reasonable* is defined as the lowest customary charge by a physician for a service or the prevailing charge by a group of physicians in an area for a particular service.
6. Discounts are often negotiated by health care organizations to secure a contract with another organization. This provides some assurance of business volume. An example is a number of physical examinations performed by a nurse practitioner for a particular company according to a sole provider agreement.

III. Health Care Payers

Payers are individuals, employers, insurance companies, or government agencies that directly pay for health care services (Dunham-Taylor & Pinczuk, 2006).
A. Payment methods include:
   1. Fee-for-service: Reimbursement method in which payment is made for each service or item provided. This method can contribute to encouraging a doctor or organization to provide more medical care by paying for each service provided. Examples include use of advanced imaging, such as MRI or CT scan, without screening with diagnostic X-ray first or ordering laboratory screening, which may not be indicated by history and clinical findings.

2. Managed care: Prepayment or capitated reimbursement, as described below.
3. Employer-provided insurance: The employing organization offers health plan choices or provides an employer-funded plan where the company bears the risk. The organization contracts with third-party administrators to manage the plan.
4. In addition to insurance payment, health care fees may include the following:
   a. Private pay: Individual pays the total cost for health care services received.
   b. Out-of-pocket expense: Money paid by an individual for health care services received that are not covered by insurance or other third-party sources. Could be 100% for services that are not covered by the plan (e.g., plastic surgery), the portion that is not paid by the patient's insurance plan, or the full payment for a service not pre-approved by the insurer.
   c. Co-payment: Dollar amount paid by an individual for a specific service defined in the insurance plan each time a health service is used.
   d. Deductibles: Amount an insured individual must pay before insurance covers costs. For example, an individual may have a $200 deductible for hospitalization before the payer will reimburse for the remainder of the hospital stay.
B. Types of health insurance programs available in the United States are described in Table 4-3.

IV. Managed Care Concepts

Finkler and colleagues (2007) described managed care as a system that combines financing and care delivery through comprehensive benefits delivered by selected providers with financial incentives for enrolled members to use these providers. The goals of managed care are quality, cost-effectiveness, and accessibility of health care. It is a coordinated system of health care that achieves outcomes (reduced utilization and improved population health) through preventive care, case management, and the provision of medically necessary, appropriate care.

Table 4-3.
Types of Health Payment Plans

Key Terms	Insurance Type	Service Provided
Governments fund or provide health plans (federal, state, local).	Medicare	Coverage for hospital expenses (Part A) and physician services (Part B) for individuals over age 65 or other individuals who meet qualifying criteria.
	Medicaid	Plan jointly funded by state and federal governments to cover indigent populations and is managed by the state providing the coverage.
	TriCare	A federal program covering families of active duty military personnel, retired military personnel, and their spouses and dependents. Previously known as Civilian Health and Medical Program of the United States (CHAMPUS).
	Indian Health Service	Federal program for community health center programs for defined populations.
	Prisons	Other: Limited state and local health care coverage programs focused on at-risk populations and are needs-based.
Private insurance: Includes commercial indemnity and managed care plans. Individual or employer chooses insurance (e.g., Aetna, Blue Cross/Blue Shield).	Commercial indemnity plans	Insurer contracts to pay for care received up to a fixed amount per episode of care. Example: In an 80/20-indemnity plan, the insurer pays 80% and the insured is responsible for 20% (or remainder) of the fee.
	Managed care plans	Example: The insurer may offer health maintenance organization plans (HMOs), preferred provider organization plans (PPOs), or point-of-service plans (POS) (these will be described under *Managed Care Concepts* later in this chapter).

A. Prepaid health insurance: A fixed amount paid to the contracted provider of care each month for each enrollee for specific services defined by the health care plan.

B. Capitation: A managed care approach that pays providers a flat fee per patient regardless of the care that the patient consumes.
   1. The provider is responsible for delivering or coordinating the delivery of all services required under the conditions of the provider contract.

   2. An example is a plan that pays a per-member-per-month (PMPM) amount to a physician group to provide primary care services for each patient in the plan.

C. Managed care is a system that places the primary care provider at the point of entry to acquire health care services.
   1. Care managers are designated to authorize the provision of services and have the responsibility for overseeing utilization of services.

Table 4-4.
Types of Managed Care Plans

Managed Care Plan	Definition
Preferred Provider Organization (PPO)	Program in which contracts exist between providers and the health care plan. Providers agree to provide care for negotiated set rates. Set prices are usually less than current prevailing rates. The plan provides financial incentives for patients to utilize in-network providers through decreased out-of-pocket expense.
Point of Service (POS)	Organization offers members either in-network, HMO-type coverage with low co-insurance and deductibles but with limited choice, or out-of-network choices at higher rates (Finkler et al., 2007).
Health Maintenance Organization (HMO)	An organized system that accepts responsibility to provide or deliver an agreed-upon set of basic and supplemental health maintenance and treatment services to an enrolled group of persons. The group is reimbursed through a predetermined fixed periodic prepayment made by, or on behalf of, each person or family unit enrolled.
	The provider is encouraged to provide appropriate medical care in exchange for higher premiums, but assumes risk of not being paid if predefined quality outcomes are not met.
	In some HMO plans, primary care physicians (PCPs) are used as gatekeepers who manage all aspects of care, authorizing referrals to other providers. They are often paid panel management fees with incentives for providing comprehensive services within their own practice.
	HMOs can have open access, allowing for self referrals without PCP authorization if in-network.
Independent Practice Association (IPA)	Members include individual and group practice physicians that contract with an HMO to provide services for a negotiated fee. Physicians provide services to one or more HMOs, but also treat other patients not covered by HMOs (Dunham-Taylor & Pinczuk, 2006).
Physician Hospital Organization (PHO)	Entity formed by a hospital and group of physicians to obtain payer contracts and achieve market objectives. Physicians maintain ownership of their practices and agree to accept managed care patients based on their agreement with the physician hospital organization (PHO). The PHO is governed by both the physicians and the hospital, and serves jointly as a negotiating and contracting unit (Finkler et al., 2007).
Medicare Managed Care	Reimbursement is paid on a capitated, per-member basis each month instead of fee-for-service. Fees are based on average adjusted per capita cost historically paid in a given geographic region for Medicare-eligible enrollees.
Medicaid Managed Care	Programs are new with a focus on patient care coordination and cost management.

2. The goal of care management is to direct patients to the most cost-effective services, and indicate which providers are included in the plan and how the payment will be made.

3. Efforts to reduce duplication of services and control costs create new professional demands on ambulatory care nurses, emphasizing efficient resource allocation, coordinated care planning, and managing care transitions, with a focus on quality outcomes.

D. Managed care may be provided through a variety of kinds of plans (see Table 4-4).

E. ACOs are a type of managed care system created by health care reform and composed of a group of providers of medical care services that share in risks and rewards of providing quality care at a fixed reimbursement rate. This is further described later in this chapter.

Table 4-5.
Care Delivery Programs

Method of Care Delivery	Example
Disease management	The use of standardized, evidence-based care plans to manage patients with specific chronic medical conditions to ensure that best practice is employed to manage patient care processes.
Health promotion	Education of patients on illness prevention and wellness by engaging patients in self-care activities that improve individual health and well-being.
Case management/ care coordination	Population-based management of panels of patients over time that are at risk for co-morbidities, re-hospitalizations, or adverse outcomes. Focus is on maximizing control of chronic disease and facilitating early detection and prevention of disease exacerbations. Ambulatory care nurses often coordinate the transition of care across the care continuum.

F. Mechanisms to ensure quality and appropriateness of managed care plans:
1. Health Plan Employer Data and Information Set (HEDIS®).
   a. National Committee for Quality Assurance's (NCQA) measures of managed care plans on important indicators of quality, access, patient satisfaction, membership, utilization, finance, and descriptive information on health plan management and activities (Finkler et al., 2007).
   b. Measures allow for comparisons of various managed care plans against performance targets and allow for employers to choose not to enter into contractual agreements if targets are not met.
2. Precertification or prior authorization.
   a. Process of obtaining authorization or certification from a health care plan for hospital admissions, referrals, procedures, or tests.
   b. Precertification or authorization from a payer allows for review of clinical appropriateness of the service and helps ensure the service is cost-effective.
   c. Ambulatory care nurses assist in obtaining precertification and approval for medications and expensive procedures.

3. Concurrent review: Utilization review of costly cases is often performed to ensure hospitalized patients are being managed most efficiently relative to length of stay and discharge planning needs.
4. Case management: A method for managing the provision of health care to members/patients with catastrophic or high-cost medical conditions. The focus is on coordinating the care to improve the continuity and quality of care, as well as lower costs.
5. Care delivery programs: Ambulatory care nurses facilitate the provision of care to the right patient, in the right setting, providing the right care, by the right provider, at the right time. Care delivery systems can contribute positively to the efficient, cost-effective provision of care (see Table 4-5).

V. **Centers for Medicare and Medicaid Services (CMS)**
A. The Centers for Medicare and Medicaid Services (CMS), formerly called Health Care Financing Administration (HCFA), within the U.S. Department of Health and Human Services, determines the standard rules and reporting mechanisms for heath care services.
1. To control the rising costs fueled by fee-for-service payments, in 1983, HCFA implemented fixed payments for defined hospital services and related lengths of stay and costs of care called diagnosis-related groups (DRGs).

a. DRGs were intended to positively impact hospital operational efficiencies and contribute to maintaining financial stability and improved quality of care.

b. Hospitalized patients are placed into specific groups based on their principle diagnosis, surgical procedure, age, complications, and comorbidities.

c. Payment for each patient in a specific group is the same; fees are predetermined, fixed, and independent of the actual cost of the care incurred in treating the patient (Finkler et al., 2007).

d. Advances in technology and reduced payments from HCFA/CMS have had significant effects on hospital lengths of stay, resulting in lesser costs assigned to DRGs.

e. DRGs have fostered a shift of care from inpatient settings to ambulatory care due to a decrease in hospital reimbursement.

f. Ambulatory care nurses have a significant opportunity to affect the cost of an inpatient admission, a case, an encounter, or service through care coordination and managing transitions in care.

B. Resource-based relative value scale (RBRVS) is used by CMS to determine payment to physicians for the services rendered to Medicare patients.

1. A weighted procedure method known as a relative value unit (RVU) established by HCFA/CMS is used to approximate the work done by physicians based on knowledge and skills required.

2. The RVU includes three elements: Values for the physician work, the practice expense, and the malpractice expense for the delivery of the service.

3. Regional pricing is considered by HCFA/CMS when reimbursement rates are set for a particular service.

VI. Coding

Coding is a standard method used to report patient care services provided to private or government health plans to receive payment.

A. Health Care Common Procedure Coding System (HCPCS): Uniform method established by HCFA/CMS for providers and medical suppliers to report professional services, procedures, supplies, and medications to health plans.

1. HCPCS provides a common language for communicating services provided and ensures valid profiles for fee schedules.

2. The system supports education and research in health care services by allowing for local, regional, and national data comparisons.

3. There are two levels of HCPCS codes:

a. HCPCS Level 1: The *Physicians' Current Procedural Terminology* (CPT), CPT 2011: An internationally recognized coding system, published by the American Medical Association (2011), for reporting medical services and procedures. Codes representing services provided by nurses are also described, but individual payers determine if nurses are eligible providers or if the service is covered.

(1) Evaluation and Management (E&M): Category of CPT codes that represent non-procedural provider encounters (such as an office visit for an earache, blood pressure monitoring, or a comprehensive medical examination).

(2) CPT 99211: An E&M code for a minimal office visit for an established patient not requiring a physician. It is the only code that a nurse can bill independent of a physician encounter.

b. HCPCS Level II: Alphanumeric codes created for supplies and drugs not listed in CPTI (such as ambulance services, durable medical equipment, and drugs).

B. ICD-9: *International Classification of Diseases, 9th Revision, Clinical Modification* (ICD-9-CM): An internationally recognized system for the purposes of indexing morbidity and mortality internationally; also used in the U.S. for coding patients' conditions for billing (U.S. National Center for Health Statistics, 2010).
   1. CMS requires the use of ICD-9-CM codes on claims submitted by health care providers.
   2. The numerical code must represent an accurate translation of the diagnostic statement or terminology documented by the provider and may be a sign, symptom, or condition.
   3. Coders are individuals who may be employed by health care organizations to provide an accurate picture of the patient's condition using numerical codes to translate the physician's documentation into billable services.
   4. Electronic coding systems: Electronic systems (computers) translate physician on-line documentation in clinical information systems into billable service codes.

C. ICD-10: *International Classification of Diseases, 10th Edition, Clinical Modification Procedure Coding System* (ICD-10-CM/PCS): New classification system that collects more detailed clinical information to reflect advancements in clinical medicine (CMS, 2010). Replacing ICD-9 to provide greater detail to describe patients' medical conditions, procedures, and hospital services.
   1. ICD-10-CM: Diagnosis classification developed by the Centers for Disease Control and Prevention. Uses 3–7 alpha or numeric digits.
   2. ICD-10-PCS: Procedure classification system developed by CMS for use in inpatient settings only. Uses 7 alpha or numeric digits.

D. Documentation: Describing the reason for a patient's encounter. Must appear on a source document.
   1. Source documents include any documentation of a patient encounter.

   2. Encounter forms, emergency reports, billing forms, and patient records are examples of source documents that may vary from facility to facility.

E. Compliance: The provider of health care services must follow standard coding guidelines and be prepared to provide documentation that the service provided matches the service billed. Failure to do so could result in allegations of fraud and significant monetary fines, and may result in loss of licenses by hospitals or professionals.

F. Ambulatory patient groups (APGs): Patient classification system designed in 1997 to explain amount and type of resource used in ambulatory care visits in hospital outpatient departments; forerunner to the more commonly used ambulatory payment classifications (APCs).

G. APCs were adopted in 2000 by CMS for outpatient prospective payment in hospital outpatient departments and ambulatory surgery centers. Kongvstedt (2004) described APCs as similar to DRGs for hospitals.
   1. APCs are based on procedures rather than diagnoses.
   2. APCs provide for severity adjustment.
   3. More than one code may be billed if more than one procedure is performed; however, additional charges are discounted.

VII. Resource Management

Organizations are responsible for effectively managing resources, people, capital, equipment, and supplies. Ambulatory care nurses have an active role in planning for and allocating all resources, and have direct impact on resource utilization and controlling expenses.

A. Non-labor resource management: Management of office and medical-surgical supplies, linen, pharmaceuticals, and durable medical equipment that affects unit costs. Nurses manage and influence daily operational costs using the following methods:
   1. Inventory management to identify the minimum volume of supplies needed using par levels.

2. Selection of the least expensive supply alternative that satisfies quality standards through product evaluation.
3. Tracking and trending use of supplies.
4. Use of budget variance reports.
5. Utilizing supply invoices to match items requested with supplies received.

B. Labor resource management: Managing numbers and levels of staff and the hours they are paid typically has greater cost implications than non-labor resource management.
1. Practice efficiency is facilitated by staffing for the right level of care and volume.
2. Ambulatory practice nurse leaders determine the staffing mix required for services and assign work based on staff education, training, competence, scope, and licensure.
3. Staffing needs are also based on the volume and type of procedures performed, anticipated acuity of patients to be seen, number of scheduled office encounters, and predicted scheduling and telephone management needs.

VIII. Financial Planning

Planning is an essential role of financial management and is typically carried out via the budgeting process. Some institutions plan using projections of financial targets for margin improvement. Financial and nurse managers both contribute and share detailed financial information to plan for organizational growth, expansion of services, and maintenance or improvement of financial stability. Planning from all departments is coordinated and aggregated to define the organization's overall financial plan (Finkler et al., 2007). A financial plan provides a framework in which health care organizations can plan for and manage processes, quantify predicted expenses, and manage costs, as well as specify action steps necessary to attain an organization's goal and objectives.

A. Margin projection planning utilizes the gross margin (the difference between revenue and cost of services) and marginal cost (the additional cost related to a change in activity) to guide revenue planning.

1. Margin projections consider volume-driven increases in variable costs and additional fixed costs.
2. Marginal utility refers to the additional benefit or utility gained from the purchase of one more unit or added service.
3. Marginal cost analysis is the process used to evaluate current services provided to guide decisions to change the volume or type of services offered based on marginal costs – the cost of treating one patient (if fixed costs are static, an increase in patient volume may actually cost less).

B. Improvement plans are based on an analysis that looks for opportunities to increase efficiency and quality, while decreasing waste.

C. Budgeting is a logical way for a health care organization to plan for and manage its processes.
1. Strategic, longer-term plans drive operational or shorter-term budget cycles.
2. Budgets consider the following information to formulate organizational goals: Historical performance, projected number of visits, number of encounters, number of patients in a physician's panel, projected capitated fees, salary and non-salary dollar expenses, and overtime rates.
   a. Historical performance combined with expansion of existing services and planned new services allow one to forecast anticipated revenues and associated expenses.
   b. Goals are described using statements that define what is to be achieved, specific objectives to be measured, and the time frame for completion.
   c. Benefits of budget planning: Promotes effective decision-making, considers alternatives, specifies major assumptions (e.g., fee increases, inflation), and uses financial and statistical indicators that monitor operations and productivity.

D. Strategic plan: Plan that typically spans three to five years and is used to drive operational goals and short-term budget cycles. Strategic plans have the following elements (Finkler et al., 2007):

1. Mission.
2. Long-term goals.
3. Competitive strategy.
4. Policies.
5. Needed resources key assumptions.

E. Financial reports: Statements that convey information about an organization's financial condition and the results of activities for a defined period of time.
   1. Items typically reported in ambulatory care and other health care agencies include:
      a. Productivity indicators, such as relative value units per full-time equivalent (FTE) or visits per worked hours.
      b. Anticipated vs. actual volume of office encounters or surgical procedures.
      c. Anticipated versus actual expenses.
      d. Projected verses actual revenue.
   2. Ambulatory nurses might also receive a variety of other reports that assist with tracking processes, such as:
      a. Reports of referrals to specialty departments.
      b. Ambulatory encounters completed.
      c. Procedures billed.
   3. Variance reports can be used to demonstrate differences between actual results compared to the plans.

F. Programming: Financial planning for programs is a component of the overall strategic planning process and focuses on costs and benefits associated with specific programs (Finkler et al., 2007).
   1. Existing programs may be considered for expansion, downsizing, or elimination. New programs may also be planned.
   2. Programs can assist organizations with meeting stated goals and objectives.
   3. The following tools can assist in defining and developing programs:
      a. Feasibility study – Includes market analysis, patient interest surveys, facility requirements, local duplication, or absence of like programs.
      b. Cost-benefit analysis – A formal financial analysis that determines the cost of the program and projected revenues, as well as identifies and quan-

tifies program benefits. Assumptions are included regarding expenses and revenue based on projected volumes. Analysis is usually completed before starting a new program or service and may be included in the feasibility study.

G. Types of budgets: Capital and operational budgets are most commonly used in health care planning.
   1. Capital budgets plan for the acquisition of investments outside of operational planning that will be used by the organization beyond the year in which they are acquired (Finkler et al., 2007). Capital budgets are estimated and designed with input from individual departments and typically include high-dollar items that will be paid for over several years, such as acquisition or renovation of buildings, new and replacement equipment, and new information technology.
   2. Operating budget: Plan for the day-to-day operating activity statistics, revenue, and expenses for an organization and are prepared for one year.
      a. Statistical or activity budget – Measures of workload or activity for each operational area.
      b. Expense budget – Projection of expected costs related to specific programs or departments and based upon their anticipated volume of activity (such as payroll and supplies) (see Table 4-1).
         (1) Direct expenses – Specifically identifiable as aligned to a specific program.
         (2) Indirect costs – Spread across multiple programs proportionate to their size and activity, such as building and equipment depreciation, and bad debt estimates.
      c. Revenue budget – Projection of specific revenues related to programs or departments based on projected volumes in the statistical budget.

H. Managerial accounting: A process used by financial managers in which they collect and report information on revenues and expenses of a specific department or program and are responsible for aggregate department budgets into the larger organizational strategic plan.

I. Analysis: An analysis of financial plans that includes reporting, trending, and tracking results.
1. Factors that are critical to the continued provision of a service or program are defined by management.
2. Organizations identify key performance indicators that assist with a balanced approach to planning and forecasting, and measure organizational performance against a plan.
3. Balanced scorecards are used for strategic management purposes as a way to examine internal performance typically in four areas:
   a. Customer service (patient satisfaction).
   b. Financial perspective (activity, expense, cost, and revenue data).
   c. Internal processes.
   d. Learning and growth (Finkler et al. 2007).

IX. Financial Implications of Health Care Reform

The patient-centered medical home (PCMH) is the leading model proposed for health care redesign because it aligns with provisions in the Patient Protection and Affordable Care Act (PPACA) (2010) to address cost, quality, and workforce shortfalls.

A. There is early evidence that PCMH efforts related to care management programs have resulted in significant savings in Medicaid populations; it has been shown that it is cheaper to prevent or closely manage disease than it is to pay for complications (Carver & Jessie, 2011).
B. Despite the demonstrated value of the PCMH model of care in improving patient outcomes, the current fee-for-service payment structure does not consistently reimburse for services delivered by non-physicians or for care that is outside of an office visit or procedure.
C. Health care reform initiatives, such as ACOs, are positioned to sustain the PCMH model by

rewarding systems for improved outcomes (see Chapter 2, "Ambulatory Care Nursing Practice Arena"). Core characteristics of ACOs:
1. Provider-led organizations.
2. A strong primary care base that is accountable for costs across the continuum of care.
3. Payments are linked to quality that reduce overall costs.
4. Reliable performance measurement that supports quality improvement and demonstrates that savings are realized through improvements in care (McClellan, McKethan, Lewis, Roski, & Fisher, 2010).

D. Ambulatory care nurses are positioned to close the gap between coverage and access, coordinating increasingly complex care for a wide range of patients, while maintaining efficiency, quality, and safety; and enabling the full economic value of their contributions (IOM, 2011).

References

American Academy of Ambulatory Care Nursing. (2010). *Scope and standards of practice for professional ambulatory care nursing* (8th ed.). Pitman, NJ: Author.

American Medical Association (AMA). (2011). *Physicians' current procedural terminology, CPT 2011* (standard ed.). Chicago: Author.

Carver, M.C., & Jessie, A. (2011). Patient-centered care in a medical home. *The Online Journal of Issues in Nursing, 16*(2). Retrieved from http://www.nursingworld.org/MainMenuCategories/ANAMarketplace/ANAPeriodicals/OJIN/TableofContents/Vol-16-2011/No2-May-2011/Patient-Centered-Care-in-a-Medical-Home.html

Centers for Medicare and Medicaid Services (CMS). (2010). *ICD-10-CM/PCS: An introduction.* Retrieved from http://www.cms.gov/ICD10

Democratic Policy and Communications Committee (DPCC). (2010). *Patient Protection and Affordable Care Act (PPACA).* Retrieved from http://www.dpc.senate.gov/health reformbill/health bill04.pdf

Dunham-Taylor, J., & Pinczuk, J.Z. (2006). *Health care financial management: Merging the heart with the dollar.* Boston: Jones & Bartlett Publishers.

Finkler, S.A., Kovner, C.T., & Jones, C.B. (2007). *Financial management for nursing managers and executives.* St. Louis, MO: Saunders Elsevier.

Institute of Medicine (IOM). (2001). *Crossing the quality chasm: A new health system for the 21st century.* Washington, DC: The National Academies Press.

Institute of Medicine (IOM). (2011). *The future of nursing: Leading change, advancing health.* Washington, DC: The National Academies Press.

Kongvstedt, P. (2004). *Managed care: What it is and how it works* (2nd ed.). Boston: Jones & Bartlett Publishers.

McClellan, M., McKethan, A., Lewis, J., Roski, J., & Fisher, E.S. (2010). A national strategy to put accountable care into practice. *Health Affairs, 29*(5), 982-990.

U.S. National Center for Health Statistics. (2010). *International classification of diseases, 9ᵗʰ revision, clinical modification* (6ᵗʰ ed.). Hyattsville, MD: Author.

Additional Readings

D'Angelo, L. (2006). Health care fiscal management. In C. Laughlin (Ed.), *Core curriculum for ambulatory care nursing* (2ⁿᵈ ed., pp. 73-83). Pitman, NJ: American Academy of Ambulatory Care Nursing (AAACN).

Griffin, K.A., & Swann, B.A. (2006). Linking nursing workload and performance indicators in ambulatory care. *Nursing Economic$, 24*(1), 41-44.

Swann, B.A., Haas, S.A., & Chow, M. (2010). Ambulatory care registered nurse performance measurement. *Nursing Economic$, 28*(5), 337-339, 342.

Unruh, L. (2008). Nurse staffing and patient, nurse, and financial outcomes. *American Journal of Nursing, 108*(1), 62-69.

Chapter 5

Informatics

Ida M. Androwich, PhD, RN-BC, FAAN
Margaret Ross Kraft, PhD, RN

OBJECTIVES – *Study of the information in this chapter will enable the learner to:*

1. Define the concept of nursing informatics as it applies to ambulatory care nursing.
2. Discuss the benefits and requirements for an electronic health patient record (EHR).
3. Define the application of "meaningful use" (MU) criteria.
4. Identify criteria for evaluating technology for use in the ambulatory setting.
5. Describe the role of standardized languages, particularly focusing on the Nursing Minimum Data Set (NMDS) nursing elements (diagnosis, intervention, outcome, and intensity).
6. Describe the potential of clinical decision support systems (CDSS) and evidence-based practice (EBP) to manage performance outcomes and enhance clinical care.
7. Discuss current issues relating to privacy and confidentiality of medical record information.

KEY POINTS – *The major points in this chapter include:*

1. Nurses are surrounded with an overwhelming increase in technological capabilities.
2. It is essential for ambulatory care nurses to be familiar with a wide range of health care information technology applications and to be informed users of health information technology.
3. Nursing informatics applications are in all areas of nursing: clinical practice, administration, education, and research.
4. Nurses are uniquely positioned to define requirements, develop, implement, and evaluate applications that support patient-centered care and care-coordination.
5. Because of the power and potential of automated, computer-based documentation, the translation of nursing documentation from the paper record to the electronic record involves more than merely translating what was done on paper to the computer.
6. An ideal information technology is one that is consistent with and supports the workflow of the clinician.
7. An information system must be capable of providing information to a provider at the point of care to assist in decision-making about the present encounter, as well as able to capture data and information that can be aggregated to inform future encounters.
8. Nurses have an important role in the promotion of the development and use of personal health records (PHRs).
9. The Office of the National Coordinator for Health Information Technology (n.d.) has been established to provide standards that ensure that meaningful use (MU) of information is a national goal.
10. The computer has virtually unlimited storage and great information processing capability, whereas man has limited storage and memory, but much experience, knowledge, intuition, and judgment. Nurses must build on both the strengths of man and the computer (Weed, 1997).

Nurses have long demonstrated the ability to accept and incorporate new technology into their professional practice. David Brailer, the National Health Information Technology Coordinator calls nurses "early adopters" and states that their input is essential to the realization of the nation's health information goals (Taylor, 2005). Consequently, it is essential for ambulatory care nurses to understand nursing informatics and be informed users of information technology. Nurses are surrounded with an overwhelming increase in technological capabilities.

Technology, the practical application of science, can be classified as either information-oriented or therapeutic in use. Therapeutic technologies in the ambulatory care setting could include laser and cryosurgery, pharmacotherapeutics, and magnetic resonance imaging (MRI), as well as various electronic monitoring devices. Information technologies can be classified as either information-producing or information-managing. The electronic health record (EHR) is information-oriented. Other information technologies include Web-based information retrieval and storage, telehealth delivery modes for patient education, and clinical decision support systems that automate care processes. Teich and Wrinn (2000) described information systems of the future in which review of results, electronic records, referral processing, secure messaging, order entry for prescriptions and tests, and decision support systems were possible. The development and use of these systems will affect role elements of the nurse in ambulatory care settings. With many of the coordination of care activities that would normally belong to the registered nurse becoming automated, how will the ambulatory care registered nurse of the 21st century reshape the role? Kerfoot (2000) identified a technical intelligence quotient as a survival skill for nurses in the new millennium. She defined technical intelligence quotient as not merely being aware of how a specific technology works, but as understanding the relationships among the technology, the users, and the affected systems and how they interact to produce outcomes.

This chapter focuses on developing a basic understanding of information technology applications and the issues associated with using technology to meet patient needs and enhance health care delivery in the ambulatory care setting. Today more than ever, every nurse practicing in ambulatory settings must be familiar with a range of health care information technology applications. Ambulatory care nurses also need to understand how to best use informatics and information technology to improve the quality of patient care and support professional practice. There is also a need to leverage information available through technology to evaluate potential risks to patients, patient populations, and the practice environment.

I. **Definition of Nursing Informatics and Applications**

A. *Nursing informatics* is defined by the American Nurses Association (ANA, 2006b) as "a specialty that integrates nursing science, computer science, and information science to manage and communicate data, information, and knowledge in nursing practice" (p. 46).

B. A conceptual basis for the understanding of information technology was developed by Graves and Corcoran (1989).

1. Information is derived from data (basic facts or observations) organized in such a manner as to have meaning to the user.

2. Knowledge is an evaluation or recognition of something with familiarity that is gained through experience that can put the information to use.

C. Over the past two decades, professional nursing has recognized the importance of informatics in the health care arena.

1. Automated systems in health care have existed for over 35 years (Saba & McCormick, 2012) and were initially developed to meet the financial need for reimbursement. As early as the 1980s, nurses recognized that relevant patient information obtained using information technology could provide support for patient care decisions, operations, education, and research.

2. Information systems deal with data that have been structured and named and can be counted. That which is nameless can-

Figure 5-1.
Role of Knowledge in Care Process and Information Systems

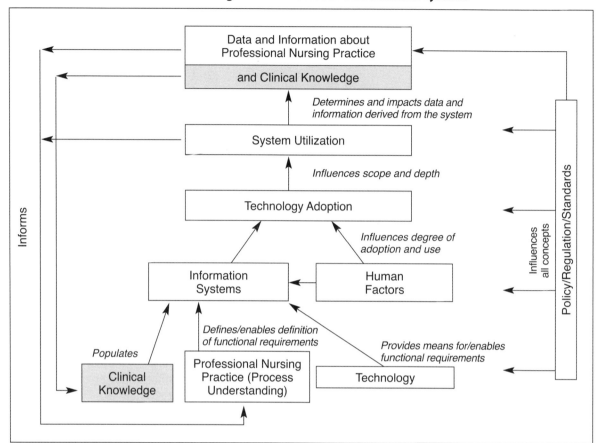

Source: Androwich et al., 2003. © American Nurses Association. Used with permission.

not be counted, and consequently, has no impact. What is named incorrectly or incompletely, when counted, leads to irrelevant information, prohibiting practical use or a sensible interpretation.

3. Information systems that support nursing practice require the incorporation of clinical knowledge/clinical content (see Figure 5-1). Such systems must be capable of both providing information to a clinician at the point of care to assist in decision-making about the present encounter, as well as providing data and information that can be aggregated to inform future encounters.

4. Nursing informatics applications are in all areas of nursing: Clinical practice, administration, education, and research.
    a. Nursing practice activities in ambulatory care that are supported by computers include:
        (1) Generating patient-focused work lists.
        (2) Incorporating evidence-based content at the point of care to support decisions.
        (3) Transmitting orders to ancillary departments.

(4) Scheduling procedures.

(5) Retrieving test results.

(6) Charting medications and treatments.

(7) Changing the plan of care.

(8) Documenting discharge or after visit summaries.

(9) Monitoring device documentation.

(10) Providing decision support and best practice advice, including reminders and alerts.

(11) Using computerized educational applications for patients and families.

b. Nursing administration information system applications are designed to meet the following ambulatory care data needs (Saba & McCormick, 2012):

(1) Allocating of resources (staffing and scheduling, patient classification, acuity, inventory, patient billing, budgeting and payroll, nursing intensity, claims processing, and referrals).

(2) Ensuring that practice standards are established and implemented (quality assurance/outcomes management, regulatory reporting, consumer surveys, evidence-based practice).

(3) Evaluating care delivery models (personnel files, risk pooling, costing nursing care, case mix).

(4) Collaborating and planning (forecasting and planning, preventive maintenance, unit activity reports, utilization review, shift summary reports, census).

(5) Planning, organizing, implementing, and controlling the care of individuals and populations (computer-based patient records, poison control, allergy and drug reactions, incident reports, communication networks, training and education).

c. Nursing education applications in ambulatory care include:

(1) Using computer-assisted instruction for patient education.

(2) Developing simulation learning scenarios.

(3) Using computer-adaptive testing for competency assessment.

(4) Distance learning for continuing staff education.

(5) Accessing Internet resources.

(6) Computerized tracking of competencies.

d. Nursing research in ambulatory care is supported by information technology including:

(1) Conducting computerized literature searches.

(2) Supporting complex statistical analysis of data.

(3) Developing standardized language documentation strategies.

(4) Using population-based decision support.

5. Nurses who have information science and computer science expertise combined with health care expertise are uniquely positioned to assume leadership roles in translating the information needs of caregivers to those designing the actual systems to capture patient care data.

6. All nurses need to be able to translate the data/information provided by existing systems and to evaluate it to promote improved patient care.

II. The Computerized Patient Record/Electronic Health Record

The computerized patient record (CPR), or the electronic health record (EHR) as it is now called, is an "electronic patient record that resides in a system specifically designed to support users by providing accessibility to complete and accurate data, alerts, reminders, clinical decision support systems, links to medical knowledge, and other aids" (Institute of Medicine [IOM], 1991, p. 6).

A. Uses of an EHR (adapted from IOM CPR Report, 1991).

1. Documentation of services provided.
2. Promotion of continuity of care (serves as a communication tool).
3. Description of diseases and causes (supports diagnostic work).
4. Support for decision-making about the diagnosis and treatment of patients.
5. Facilitation of care in accordance with clinical practice guidelines.
6. Generation of reminders (e.g., preventive or health maintenance action needed).
7. Allocation of resources and assess workload.
8. Analysis of trends and develop forecasts.

B. Requirements of an EHR (adapted from IOM CPR Report, 1991).
1. Record content.
   a. Uniform core data elements.
   b. Standardized coding systems and formats.
   c. Common data dictionary.
   d. Information on outcomes of care and functional status.
2. Record format: Integrated record with all providers, disciplines, and sites of care included.
3. System performance standards.
   a. Rapid retrieval.
   b. 24-hour access.
   c. Easy data input.
   d. Available at convenient places.
4. Linkages.
   a. With other information systems (such as laboratory, radiology, and pharmacy).
   b. With relevant literature.
   c. With other institutional databases and registries.
   d. Electronic transfer of billing information.
5. Intelligence.
   a. Decision support.
   b. Clinician reminders.
   c. Customizable alert or alarm systems (for example, for allergies and drug interactions).
6. Reporting capabilities.
   a. Standard clinical reports.
   b. Customized reports.
   c. Derived documents (e.g., insurance forms and mandated reports).
   d. Trend reports and graphics.
7. Control and access: Safeguards against violations of confidentiality and unauthorized use.
8. Training and implementation.
   a. Effective user training required for system use.
   b. Graduated implementation possible.
C. Because of the power and potential of automated, computer-based documentation, the translation of nursing documentation from the paper record to the electronic record involves more than merely translating what was done on paper to the computer.

III. Evaluation of Information Systems

Evaluating computer technology, particularly software, for use in ambulatory care settings is an important role of the nurse leader.

A. A major reason for dissatisfaction with software applications is unmet expectations on the part of the user. This often occurs because the ability to communicate between the domain expert in the problem domain (the nurse in the clinical area) and the domain expert in the solution domain (the programmer) is inadequate.
B. A number of questions that should be addressed before purchasing any software include:
1. How much flexibility is in the software? Is it possible to customize?
2. Can the software be modified if situations change?
3. What type of technical support and training are available? How much will they cost?
4. Will this software interface with other existing software? What will it take in terms of programming to build interfaces? Is the software compatible with existing hardware?
5. What is the plan for upgrades? How much will they cost?

6. Is the system equipped with adequate back-up? Adequate security (sign-on codes or passwords)?
7. Is the system user-friendly? This entails screen design, commands, menus, and navigation throughout the program. For example, can screens be skipped for a simple entry, or does the program require a lock-step, screen-by-screen approach? Can the user go back and edit one data element without redoing the entire entry?
8. What industry standards does the software meet? For example, Health Language 7 (HL7) is the accepted standard for messaging in health care.

C. The development of "meaningful use" incentives by the Office of the National Coordinator for Health Information Technology and the Centers for Medicare and Medicaid (CMS) programs provides financial incentives for the use of a certified EHR in a meaningful manner. Such applications can include the use of this EHR technology to electronically exchange health information to improve the quality of care and to submit clinical quality and other care measures to accrediting agencies.
1. Meaningful use includes an organization's ability to use health care information technology to improve the quality of care and inform clinical decisions at the point of care.
2. Meaningful use criteria is being phased in between 2011 and 2015.
3. Phase I of the meaningful use process is the development of a baseline for electronic data capture and information sharing.
4. Phase II and III will be based on the development of future rules.
5. Benefits of meaningful use beyond financial incentives include reduction in errors, availability of records and data, reminders and alerts, clinical decision support, and e-prescribing/refill automation.

IV. **Nursing Minimum Data Set in Ambulatory Care**
A. The concept of the nursing minimum data set (NMDS) was developed as a way to ensure that all data important to the practice of nursing was collected in a standardized manner in every encounter, across all settings. The NMDS includes 16 data elements that would be collected by all nurses, for all patient encounters, across all settings (Werley & Lang, 1988).
1. Patient elements.
   a. Age.
   b. Gender.
   c. Unique patient identifier: May be medical record number, Social Security number, or another unique means of patient identification.
   d. Payment mechanism: Insurance coverage or reimbursement information.
   e. Medical diagnosis: Typically coded in ICD-9 coding.
   f. Disposition: Refers to discharge status, not as relevant to ambulatory care setting; useful information for ambulatory care would include living arrangements (e.g., lives alone).
2. Facility.
   a. Facility identifier: Facility type or provider code.
   b. Dates of care: In ambulatory care, pertains to encounter date.
   c. Unique provider identification: This is new for nursing to have a unique provider number, and automated or computerized documentation is often the sign-on ID.
3. Nursing care provided.
   a. Nursing diagnosis.
   b. Nursing intervention.
   c. Nursing outcome.
   d. Nursing intensity.
B. Although not widely implemented in practice, the NMDS is viewed as a goal that would allow for aggregation and comparison of nursing practice across settings.

C. The NMDS is designed so that a comparison of patient-centered data can be made in order to evaluate the effectiveness of nursing interventions across practice settings, across specialties, across specialty settings, and geographic boundaries.

D. The NMDS data elements have many elements in common with the *Uniform Hospital Discharge Data Set* (UHDDS) and the *Uniform Ambulatory Care Discharge Data Set* (UACDDS).

E. The UACDDS is similar to UHDDS, but is based on a patient encounter, not on an admission. Currently, there is no standard for these data, although the importance of establishing a core set of ambulatory care data is widely recognized. Ideally, information such as living arrangements of patient, patient's support systems, medications, and the patient's ability to manage activities of daily living, should be collected on each patient.

V. Standardized Languages

"If you cannot name it, you cannot teach it, research it, practice it, finance it, or put it into public policy." — Norma Lang, PhD, RN, FAAN (1998)

A. Unified, not necessarily uniform, languages are necessary to document and use the nursing elements in the NMDS (diagnosis, intervention, outcomes, and intensity) or other large datasets.

B. To support the use of multiple vocabularies and classification schemes, the American Nurses Association (ANA) formed a committee to set criteria for an accepted nursing language and to approve languages meeting the criteria.

C. The ANA Committee on Nursing Practice Information Infrastructure (CNPII), formerly the Steering Committee on Databases to Support Nursing Practice, proposes policy and program initiatives regarding nursing classification schemes, uniform nursing data sets, and the inclusion of nursing data elements in national databases.

D. The CNPII recommended that the profession work toward the development of a unified nursing language system that would allow linking or mapping of similar terms while retaining the integrity and purpose of each specific scheme/vocabulary. This unified system would facilitate development, analysis, and use of nursing data sets.

E. The CNPII also developed specific criteria for vocabularies to be eligible for recognition. These criteria include:
1. Clinical usefulness for making diagnostic, intervention, and/or outcome decisions.
2. Explicit rationale going beyond an application or synthesis/adaptation of vocabularies/classification schemes currently recognized by ANA.
3. Precise definitions in clear and unambiguous terms.
4. Reliability of the vocabulary terms.
5. Validated as useful for clinical purposes.

F. As of January 2006, a number of languages were deemed to have met these criteria and have been approved by the ANA. They include the following:
1. North American Nursing Diagnosis Association's (NANDA) nomenclature for nursing diagnosis.
2. Nursing Interventions Classification (NIC), developed by a team at the University of Iowa led by Joanne McCloskey-Dochterman and Gloria Bulechek, is a taxonomy for classifying nursing interventions.
3. Clinical Care Classification (CCC) (formerly Home Health Care Classification [HHCC]), Saba's Georgetown System for Patient Problems, Interventions, and Outcomes.
4. Omaha (the Omaha VNA's system for problems, interventions, and outcomes).
5. Nursing Outcomes Classification (NOC) developed by a team led by Marion Johnson, Meridean Maas, and Sue Moorhead at the University of Iowa.
6. Nursing Management Minimum Data Set (NMMDS).
7. Perioperative Nursing Data Set (PNDS) developed by the Association of periOperative Registered Nurses.
8. Systematic Nomenclature for Medicine-Reference Terminology (SNOMED-CT®) (College of American Pathologists).

9. Nursing Minimum Data Set (NMDS) (described earlier in this chapter).
10. International Classification for Nursing Practice (ICNP®) (International Council of Nurses [ICN].
11. Logical Observation Identifiers Names and Codes (LOINC®) – There has been recent work on understanding the selection of a nursing terminology (Anderson, Keenan, & Jones, 2009). This article looked at the use of different terminologies and discussed how commonly used each of the various languages is in research. Alternatively, contact information about the individual terminologies is available on the ANA (2006a) Web site (http://www.nursing world.org/npii/terminologies.htm).

G. Standardized languages can be used for:
1. Outcomes data collection, retrieval, analysis.
2. Decisions about care management.
3. Quality management and improvement.
4. Decision support.
5. Statistical and epidemiologic reporting (vital statistics, tumor registries).
6. Administrative applications (billing, cost data).

H. In conclusion:
1. Vocabulary is an urgent issue in nursing and nursing informatics.
2. Vocabulary is central to the integration of patient care data and research.
3. Standardized vocabularies support date retrieval and benchmarking.

VI. Documentation Strategies

A. Health professionals document care for many reasons:
1. To communicate care provided to all providers.
2. To provide continuity of care; to ensure a historical, narrative record of an episode or episodes of care and the patient's responses to treatment.
3. To document care provided or not provided for legal reasons.
4. To facilitate reimbursement (Turley, 1996).

B. In general, there are two approaches to automated nursing documentation – The established nursing process approach and the newer interdisciplinary critical pathway/protocols approach.
1. The nursing process approach is based on the traditional paper forms used by nurses. This format addresses multiple functions.
   a. Nursing admission assessment.
   b. Discharge instructions via menu lists.
   c. Specific data documentation such as vital signs, weights, and intake and output measurements.
   d. Provision of standardized care plans for nurses to be individualized for patients.
   e. Documentation of nursing care in the progress note format.
   f. Documentation of medication administration via medication administration records (MARs).
2. The critical pathway/protocols approach, an approach particularly popular with the rise of managed care, is an interdisciplinary approach to documentation and is based on use of critical pathways or protocols to structure documentation.
   a. The provider selects one or more critical pathways for the patient.
   b. Standard physician or other clinician order sets are included in pathway and are automatically processed.
   c. The system is capable of tracking variances from anticipated care (critical pathway) and is able to aggregate variance information for analysis by provider.
   d. The above approach provides a feedback loop, and the information is used to improve care and client outcomes.
3. Research has demonstrated that electronic documentation has the ability to improve patient care and that practices with EHRs have better outcomes (Cebul, Love, Jain, & Herbert, 2011).
4. With the advent of new and emerging models of care, such as medical homes, care coordination, and accountable care organizations (ACOs), it is essential that ambulatory care organizations have the

ability to document nursing care in electronic record systems.

5. With the help of health IT, health care providers will have:

    a. "Accurate and complete information about a patient's health. That way they can give the best possible care, whether during a routine visit or a medical emergency."

    b. "The ability to better coordinate the care they give. This is especially important if a patient has a serious medical condition."

    c. "A way to securely share information with patients and their family caregivers over the Internet for patients who opt for this convenience. This means patients and their families can more fully take part in decisions about their health care."

    d. "Information to help doctors diagnose health problems sooner, reduce medical errors, and provide safer care at lower costs" (Office of the National Coordinator for Health Information Technology, 2011).

VII. Decision Support Systems (DSS)

Nurse leaders are constantly challenged to keep up with the rapidly growing and constantly changing information base relevant to practice. Computers can assist in this process by bringing necessary information to the nurse in forms that will leverage the information-seeking and decision-making processes. These systems provide decision support in the form of bringing evidence, expertise, and scarce resources to the provider at the point of care. Nurse leaders must use all available evidence to increase the probability of "doing the right thing." In the future, institutions will be successful in delivering quality care to the extent that they have comparable, reliable, relevant data for cost, utilization, and outcome studies; for guideline development; for performance management; and for identification of best practices (Androwich & Kraft, 2012).

A. An automated decision support system provides an ambulatory nurse with a tool that enhances the nurse's ability to make effective and timely decisions in semistructured and uncertain situations.

B. Structure of any decision support system includes:

    1. Some type of user interface that facilitates or triggers inquiries.

    2. A knowledge base (database) containing expert information organized to promote decision-making.

    3. An inference engine with analytic models that can generate alternative solutions.

C. An example of how a decision support system might operate in a clinical setting is the scheduling of immunizations.

    1. The system would ask for input of the child's date of birth, weight, immunization history, and other pertinent facts.

    2. The database would use the information provided to compare with accepted practice standards contained in the knowledge base.

    3. The algorithm in the inference engine would then be used to provide a recommendation for the next immunization to be scheduled.

D. Characteristics of a decision support system include:

    1. Ability to organize and interpret large amounts of data.

    2. Standardized decision-making criteria.

    3. Provision of expert level assistance to novice.

    4. Allowance for capturing (extracting and documenting) knowledge of experts.

E. A goal is to develop an intelligent health care system – A learning organization that promotes a culture of knowledge and empowerment among its members.

F. The trend in ambulatory patient care is to organize care around targeted patient populations (e.g., high cost or high volume). Care planning relies upon identification of best practice models from the literature that derives recommendations from large population studies.

G. ACOs and the implementation of "meaningful use" will require collection and reporting of these data and are progressively going to attach rewards/incentives and penalties to clinicians and organizations for meeting these data.

H. Population-based decision support is one form of a decision support system. In these situations, data from a number of patients are aggregated and used to provide information to support patient care for individual patients.

1. These systems are essential for disaster preparedness to enable the early detection of trends via syndromic surveillance, as well as providing resource management and decision support in actual disasters (O'Carroll, Yasnoff, Ward, Ripp, & Martin, 2003).

2. The term *syndromic surveillance* applies to surveillance using health-related data (typically symptom clusters) that precede a given diagnosis and signal a sufficient probability of a number of cases or a potential population outbreak that would warrant further response.

3. Though historically the syndromic surveillance has been used to target the investigation of potential cases, public health officials are increasingly exploring the usefulness of syndromic surveillance methods in detecting outbreaks associated with bioterrorism (Haas & Androwich, 2011).

I. Evidence-based practice is the integration of the best research evidence with clinical experience to facilitate clinical decision-making (Sackett, Strauss, Richardson, Rosenberg, & Haynes, 2000). This same principle can be used in planning care for patient populations. Evidence-based nursing sources of evidence include:

1. Computerized literature databases, such as the Cumulative Index of Nursing and Allied Health Literature (CINAHL) (www.cinahl.com) and the National Library of Medicine's (NLM) Medline (www.nlm.gov).

2. Online, published, systematic evidence reviews, such as The Cochrane Collaboration (www.cochrane.org), the Agency for Healthcare Research and Quality (AHRQ) (www.ahrq.gov), Zynx Health (www.zynx.com) for interdisciplinary plans of care, and CINAHL's Clinical Innovations Database (CCID) (www.cinahl.com).

J. The goal of evidence-based practice (see Chapter 11, "Evidence-Based Practice and Performance Improvement") for ambulatory care nurses is to determine the best care options, answer clinical questions, and identify areas for care improvement.

VIII. Telehealth Issues

A. *Telehealth* can be defined as the use of modem telecommunications and information technology to provide health care to individuals at a distance and to transmit information to provide care (Hebda & Czar, 2009) (see Chapter 9, "Telehealth Nursing").

B. Information quality – Few generally accepted standards are available for providers and consumers to use to evaluate the quality of information offered on the Internet.

C. The "AAACN metric" is one method that can be used by ambulatory nurses to evaluate information for use and to teach patients how to be savvy information consumers (Androwich, 1999).

1. **A**ccuracy – How valid and reliable does this information seem? Is it consistent with "mainstream" knowledge or is it apparent that it is evidence-based?

2. **A**uthorship – What is expertise and credibility of author(s)? Does the author of the information have a commercial interest in the product referenced? If so, is the commercial relationship explicit? What organization(s) is the author or site associated with? Are they credible?

3. **A**ttribution – Is the information referenced? Are the citations reliable, and do they include experts and trusted sources in the content area?

4. **C**urrency – How current is the information? When was the information posted?

5. **N**ursing Practice Relevance – Is this important to my patients? Is it a POEM? (**Pa**tient-**O**riented **E**vidence that **M**atters – Matters because it will require and inform practice change.)

D. The overall soundness of a source is evaluated based on the above criteria.

IX. Privacy and Confidentiality/Standards/Accreditation

A. The Health Insurance Portability and Accountability Act of 1996 (HIPAA) provides safeguards for patient health care data (U.S. Department of Health and Human Services, 2003). At minimum, this means that measures are in place to protect against:
1. Unauthorized access and harm to patient care data (system security).
2. Accidental or intentional disclosure to unauthorized persons or unauthorized data alteration (data security).
3. Transmission of sensitive information to unauthorized recipients (data confidentiality).
4. Lack of consistency and accuracy of data stored in data-based systems (data integrity).

B. At the federal level, the National Committee on Vital and Health Statistics (NCVHS, 2012) has been charged by Congress with providing recommendations related to the nature, characteristics, quality, and degree of security needed for various types of data elements. NCVHS deals with all issues that pertain to:
1. National health information infrastructure (NHII).
2. Population health data.
3. Data quality.
4. Standards and security.
5. Privacy and confidentiality.
6. Interoperability (the ability to share data and information electronically).
7. Recommendations for personal health records.

C. The Joint Commission (2012) has standards that relate to information and the use of information in patient care in ambulatory care settings. Some of these involve:
1. Measures that protect information confidentiality, security, and integrity (user access, retrieval of information without compromising security or confidentiality, written policies controlling patient records, and guarding records and information).
2. Uniform definitions and methods for data capture to facilitate data comparison within and among health care organizations.
3. Education on principles of information management and training for system use.
4. Accurate and timely transmission of information (24-hour availability, minimal delay of order implementation, pharmacy system designed to minimize errors, and quick turnaround of test results).
5. Integration of clinical and nonclinical systems.
6. Client-specific data information: System collects and reports individual data and information that can be used to support practice, aid research, and support decision-making.
7. Aggregation of data/information, which informs care and improves operations performance.
8. Knowledge-based information – Literature is available in print or electronic form.
9. System provides useful comparative data/information.

X. Emerging Issues in Ambulatory Health Care Informatics

A. ACOs – Hospitals, groups of doctors, and other health care providers who work together to deliver coordinated, high-quality care to the Medicare patients they serve.
1. This model of health service delivery offers doctors and hospitals financial incentives to provide high quality care to Medicare beneficiaries while keeping costs down.
2. ACO participation is voluntary and began in 2012.
3. Coordination of care helps ensure that patients get the right care at the right time, avoiding unnecessary duplication of services and preventing medical errors.

B. Personal health record (PHR) – A lifelong resource of health information owned and managed by the individual. The PHR is separate from and does not replace the legal medical record. Ideally, it will contain information from the individual and providers in an electronic format.

1. This record is owned by the individual, who also determines how information is shared with providers, caregivers, and family.
2. Integration of PHRs with EHRs of providers allows data and secure communication to be shared between a consumer and his or her health care team.
3. PHR use helps individuals to be more successful in pursuit of their own health, encourages patient engagement in their own health care, and can bridge the information gap between individuals and health care providers.
4. PHRs are a tool nurses can use to have a better informed and motivated patient/client acting on behalf of better health with an enhanced patient compliance.
5. Ambulatory care nurses can promote the development and use of PHRs and help patients identify the data elements important to such a record.

C. Interactive Voice Response Technology (IVRT) – Integrates computers and telephone technology with speech recognition and automation to allow a computer to detect voice and touch tones using a normal phone call.
1. The IVRT system can respond with prerecorded or dynamically generated audio to direct callers how to proceed through a menu. IVRT systems can be used to control almost any function that can be broken down into a series of simple menu choices.
2. Ambulatory care applications of IVRT include appointment scheduling and reminders, as well as post-appointment/procedure follow-up.
3. IVRT allows for a referral to a human resource when needed.
4. IVRT is shown to improve client satisfaction while controlling communication costs.

D. Major nursing issues that are driving or need to drive increased focus and attention on informatics:
1. The "patient story" should serve as the basis of EHR summary screens.
2. New roles for ambulatory care nurses involve personal health records, IVRT, care coordination, and patient education.

3. Standardized national tools are needed related to patient self-care management, family caregiver assessment, continuity of care documentation and transfer forms to support safe and effective care coordination for transitions.
4. Significant progress in medication safety is crucial.

E. The impact of social media on changing ambulatory care nursing practice presents opportunities and issues.

References

American Nurses Association (ANA). (2006a). *ANA recognized terminologies that support nursing practice.* Retrieved from http://www.nursingworld.org/npii/terminologies.htm

American Nurses Association (ANA). (2006b). *The scope of practice for nursing informatics.* Washington, DC: Author.

Anderson, C., Keenan, G., & Jones, J. (2009). Using bibliometrics to support your selection of a nursing terminology set. *CIN: Computers, Informatics, Nursing, 27*(2), 82-90.

Androwich, I. (1999). Evidence-based practice: Harvesting the evidence. *Chart, 96*(2), 5.

Androwich, I.M., Bickford, C.J., Button, P.S., Hunter, K.M., Murphy, J., & Sensmeier, J. (2003). *Clinical information systems: A framework for reaching the vision.* Washington, DC: American Nurses Publishing.

Androwich, I.M., & Kraft, M. (2012). Incorporating evidence: Use of computer-based clinical decision support systems for health care professionals. In V. Saba, & K. McCormick (Eds.), *Essentials of sursing informatics* (pp. 167-179). New York: McGraw-Hill.

Cebul, D., Love, T., Jain, A., & Herbert, C. (2011). Electronic health records and quality of diabetes care. *New England Journal of Medicine, 365*, 825-833.

Graves, J., & Corcoran, S. (1989). The study of nursing informatics. *Image, 21*(4), 227-231.

Haas, S., & Androwich, I. (2011). Ambulatory care nursing: Challenges for the 21st century. In P.S. Cowen, & S. Moorhead (Eds.), *Current issues in nursing* (8th ed., pp. 177-190). Philadelphia: Mosby.

Hebda, T., & Czar, P. (2009). *Handbook of informatics for nurses and healthcare professionals* (4th ed.). Upper Saddle River, NJ: Prentice Hall.

Institute of Medicine (IOM). (1991). *The computer-based patient record: An essential technology for health care.* Washington, DC: The National Academies Press.

Joint Commission, The. (2012). *Standards for ambulatory care.* Oakbrook Terrace, IL: Author.

Kerfoot, K. (2000). TIQ (Technical IQ): A survival skill for the new millennium. *Nursing Economic$, 18*(1), 29-31.

Lang, N. (1998, March 25-28). *Language, classification, and data: A powerbase for clinical practice: If you cannot name it...* Paper presented at the 23rd Annual Conference for American Academy of Ambulatory Care Nursing. Atlanta, GA.

National Committee on Vital and Health Statistics (NCVHS). (2012). *Home page.* Retrieved from http://www.ncvhs.hhs.gov/

O'Carroll, P., Yasnoff, W., Ward, M.E., Ripp, L., & Martin, E. (Eds.). (2003). *Public health informatics and information systems.* New York: Springer-Verlag, Inc.

Office of the National Coordinator for Health Information Technology. (2011). *Home page.* Retrieved from http://healthit.hhs.gov/

Saba, V., & McCormick, K. (Eds.). (2012). *Essentials of nursing informatics.* New York: McGraw-Hill.

Sackett, D.L., Strauss, S.E., Richardson, W.S., Rosenberg, W.M.C., & Haynes, R.B. (2000). *Evidence-based medicine: How to practice and teach EBM.* London: Churchill Livingston.

Taylor, N. (2005). National health IT coordinator applauds nurses as early adopters. *Nursing Management, 36*(10), 2-6.

Teich, J., & Wrinn, M. (2000). Clinical decision support systems come of age. *MD Computing, 17*(1), 43-46.

Turley, J. (1996). Toward a model of nursing informatics. *Journal of Nursing Scholarship, 28*(1), 309-313.

U.S. Department of Health and Human Services. (2003). *Office of Civil Rights (OCR) summary of the HIPAA privacy rule.* Retrieved from http://www.hhs.gov/ocr/privacy/hipaa/understanding/summary/index.html

Weed, L. (1997). New connections between medical knowledge and patient care. *British Medical Journal, 315*(7102), 231-235.

Werley, H., & Lang, N. (Eds.). (1988). *Identification of the nursing minimum data set.* New York: Springer.

Chapter 6

Legal Aspects of Ambulatory Care Nursing

Joan M. Paté, MS, BSN, RN-BC
Debra Ann Clementino, MS, RN, JD

OBJECTIVES – *Study of the information in this chapter will enable the learner to:*

1. Discuss the regulation of nursing practice.
2. Identify the legal problems for and liability issues related to nursing assessment and critical thinking skills in the ambulatory setting.
3. Describe the various laws related to patient rights.
4. Describe the purpose of clinical documentation and record retention requirements.
5. Describe negligence and sources of professional liability.
6. Identify the circumstances under which information must be reported to legal authorities and others.
7. Discuss the purpose and implications of the fraud and abuse laws.
8. Explain workplace regulatory compliance issues.

KEY POINTS – *The major points in this chapter include:*

1. Health care is governed by laws from many sources.
2. Nursing practice is regulated by state "Practice Acts."
3. Several legal problems may arise resulting from nursing assessment and analysis.
4. Patients have rights reflected in the Patient Self Determination Act, HIPAA, EMTALA, state regulations for consent and advanced directives, and other statutes and case law.
5. Laws require complete and accurate documentation of health care services.
6. Nurses are legally responsible for their own actions and for reporting incompetent or otherwise inappropriate behavior of other professionals.
7. Nurses are required to comply with workplace regulations, such as those from EEOC and ADA.

The purpose of this chapter is to provide nurses with a basic understanding of some of the many legal issues that arise regularly in the practice of nursing, and particularly, in ambulatory care settings. It is important to note that the laws and regulations that affect nursing differ significantly from state to state, and policies designed to facilitate compliance vary across institutions. It is critical for every ambulatory care nurse to become familiar with the specific state laws, including the state nurse practice act, as well as institutional policies and procedures that may apply to his or her practice and use them as sources of legal decision-making.

I. General Overview

The law, defined broadly, is a group of rules and standards developed by legislatures, administrative agencies, and courts that govern the conduct of individuals and institutions within a community. The practice of health care is governed by federal, state, and in some cases, local laws. Health care providers enter into contracts or adopt institutional policies and procedures that serve as additional standards with which they are expected to comply and against which their conduct or practice is measured.

A. Sources of law.
1. Constitutions (federal, state).
2. Statutes or codes.
   a. Federal laws.
      (1) Usually passed by Congress and signed by the President.
      (2) Compiled into the United States code.
   b. State laws.
      (1) Usually passed by state legislatures and signed by governors, or enacted by popular vote through referenda or voter initiatives.
      (2) Compiled into various state codes.
      (3) Vary from state to state.
3. Regulations.
   a. Rules promulgated by federal agencies (such as the U.S. Department of Health and Human Services [DHHS] or the Securities and Exchange Commission [SEC]) and state agencies (such as state health departments and insurance commissioners).
   b. Supplemented by formal and informal agency guidance.
      (1) Written interpretive guidelines that describe how agencies enforce the law.
      (2) User manuals and program memoranda.
      (3) Congressional testimony by agency representatives.
      (4) Other official communications.
4. Judicial and administrative agency action.
   a. Court decisions and court orders issued as a result of criminal enforcement or civil litigation (rules or standards developed by courts over time are referred to as "common law").
   b. Administrative agency decisions and orders issued in connection with disputes among private parties or arising from agency enforcement of regulations.
5. Contracts.
   a. Legal agreements among two or more parties.
   b. May be enforced by courts, or in some cases, through private arbitration proceedings.

B. Types of law.
1. Criminal law.
   a. Defined by statute; supplemented by regulations; interpreted by judges.
   b. Violation may be punished by fines and/or imprisonment, depending on the seriousness of the offense.
   c. Sources of investigation and enforcement.
      (1) Federal agencies (such as the U.S. Department of Justice, U.S. Food & Drug Administration).
      (2) State agencies (such as the attorney general, state police).
      (3) Local authorities.
   d. Examples of conduct that may violate criminal laws.
      (1) Practice of nursing without a license.
      (2) Illegal prescription or use of controlled substances; drug diversion.
      (3) Fraud.
      (4) Assisted suicide.
      (5) Failure to report child or elder abuse, or neglect.
2. Civil law.
   a. Defined by statute, regulation, and common law; interpreted by administrative agencies and judges.
   b. Violation can be punished by fines, civil penalties, damages, or other sanctions, including suspension or revocation of licensure.
   c. Sources of enforcement.
      (1) Federal agencies (e.g., DHHS).
      (2) State agencies (e.g., state health departments or insurance commissioners).
      (3) Private parties (e.g., patients harmed by negligent care; employees hurt by discriminatory practices or violation of workplace safety rules).
   d. Examples of conduct that may be the subject of civil disputes.

(1) Malpractice/professional negligence or misconduct.
(2) Violation of legal or ethical standards protecting patient rights (some patient rights laws, such as Health Insurance Portability and Accountability Act [HIPAA], may be enforced criminally depending on the circumstances).
(3) Improper claims or reimbursement.
(4) Breach of contract.

II. Regulation of Nursing Practice

The practice of medicine, nursing, and other health professions is defined and regulated at the state level by a combination of laws and regulations usually referred to as "Practice Acts."

A. Nurse practice acts.
1. Each state enacts and administers its own laws and regulations.
   a. Rules (laws) vary from state to state.
   b. Rules are reviewed and updated periodically to reflect changes in nursing practice.
   c. The National Council of State Boards of Nursing (NCSBN, 2011) developed a Model Nursing Practice Act, intended to guide boards of nursing in considering revisions to State Nurse Practice Acts and Nursing Administrative Rules.
      (1) Models are a way to promote a common understanding of what constitutes the practice of nursing across the nation.
      (2) The NCSBN Model Nursing Practice Act is updated as nursing and policy evolve.
2. Usually enforced by oversight boards (e.g., "Board of Nursing") created under the acts.
   a. Members are designated in different ways depending on the state (may be chosen by public officials or professional societies, or designated automatically based on office/affiliation/location).
   b. Responsible for investigating complaints and concerns raised by patients, colleagues, others, and for disciplining unprofessional, unethical, and incompetent individuals.
   c. Types of discipline issues include nursing practice, boundary violations, chemical dependency, abuse, fraud, and positive criminal background checks.
   d. Involved at varying levels in health professional recovery programs for nurses and other licensed individuals with mental health or chemical dependency/problems.
3. Often supplemented by general requirements in broader "occupational codes" that apply to all health professionals.

B. Guiding principles of nursing regulation (via nurse practice acts).
1. Protect the public from unsafe nursing practice or practitioners.
2. Regulate the competence of all practitioners by the board of nursing; define the practice of nursing and establish the scope and standards of practice.
3. Require due process and ethical decision-making for practitioners.
4. Promote competent practice by qualified professionals; protect the title of "nurse" from improper use by unqualified individuals.
5. Establish education, training, and administrative requirements for licensure/relicensure.
6. Respond in a timely manner to the evolving marketplace and health care environment, such that the scope of practice has clarity and is consistent with the community needs for nursing care.
7. Use evidence-based standards of practice for advances in technology, demographic and social research.

C. Nursing practice across state lines.
1. Situations.
   a. Physical practice in multiple locations (e.g., in two cities that straddle a state border on opposite sides, or in multiple locations as a traveling nurse).

b. Telephone or Internet-based triage or case management, in which patients in multiple states may seek health care information and advice.

c. Telehealth services through which patients are assessed and even treated remotely using high-tech devices (such as computerized stethoscopes, otoscopes, and ophthalmoscopes), as well as equipment that images, digitizes, and transmits radiology studies.

2. Many states prohibit and even criminalize the practice of nursing without a current local license.

a. State boards, which have the responsibility for protecting patients who live in their states, generally take the position that the practice of nursing occurs wherever the patient is located at the time of service.

b. Requirements for licensure vary. In some cases, it may be necessary to hold separate licenses in multiple states. Some states have created alternative processes.

(1) Some states permit the practice of nursing by "endorsement," which requires nurses to submit their licenses and other information to the local board for approval, a cumbersome and expensive process, particularly for RNs, who practice in many states.

(2) Some states adhere to a "mutual recognition model," such as the Nurse Licensure Compact (NLC).

3. Nurse Licensure Compact.

a. Enacted in 24 of 50 states, with 6 states in pending legislation in 2012.

b. Features of nurse licensure compact.

(1) Allow nurses to practice across state lines, physically or electronically, unless one is under discipline or a monitoring agreement that restricts interstate practice. Nurses are licensed where they live (the "home state").

(2) A nurse who practices in states other than the home state (called "remote states") under a compact must comply with the laws and regulations of each state.

(3) Discipline in a remote state does not necessarily result in discipline in the home state, but information is shared across jurisdictions, and discipline in one state may lead at least to investigation in others.

(4) Advanced practice registered nurses (APRNs) are not included in the NLC. APRNs must apply in each state in which they practice. Exemption: Federal facilities.

c. Most states that have adopted the NLC have adopted a version that applies only to RNs and LPNs/LVNs.

d. The APRN Compact offers states the mechanism for mutually recognizing APRN licenses/authority to practice. This step is significant for increasing access and accessibility to qualified APRNs.

e. As of 2011, only three states (Iowa, Utah, and Texas) have agreed to mutually recognize the APRN Compact and have passed laws authorizing joining the APRN Compact. No date has been set for implementation of the APRN Compact.

4. The law is still in flux, and rules are changing constantly; it is important for nurses to check on the rules of any state in which they plan to practice, whether by physical presence or remotely (a good source of information is www.ncsbn.org/nlc).

D. Delegation of authority.

1. Some states allow licensed practitioners to delegate their authority to perform certain services to other licensed or unlicensed practitioners.

2. Where this occurs, a physician (for example) may delegate clinical tasks not usually within the scope of a nurse's practice to a nurse or other individual who has appropriate education, experience, and expertise.

a. Delegation usually must be recorded in writing.
b. The delegating health professional (the physician, in this example) remains ultimately responsible for the service.
3. A delegating nurse is responsible for individualized assessment of the patient, situational circumstances, and ascertaining delegatee competence before delegating a task (NCSBN, 1995).
   a. The nursing process (such as assessment, planning) cannot be delegated.
   b. Supervision, monitoring, evaluation, and follow-up by the RN are crucial components of delegation to another.
   c. Critical elements of delegation decisions include:
      (1) Qualifications of the delegatee.
      (2) Nature of the nurse's authority, as established by the law in the state of practice.
      (3) The nurse's personal competence in the area of nursing relevant to the task being delegated.
4. Definition of delegation.
   a. A skill requiring clinical judgment and final accountability of client care.
   b. State nurse practice acts determine what level of licensed nurse is authorized to delegate.
   c. Five rights of delegation (NCSBN, 1995).
      (1) Right task.
      (2) Right circumstance.
      (3) Right person.
      (4) Right direction/communication.
      (5) Right supervision/evaluation.
5. Common delegation errors.
   a. Under-delegating.
   b. Over-delegating.
   c. Improper delegating.
E. Credentialing and privileging.
   1. Credentialing.
      a. Review and verification of credentials (education, training, licensure, certification, experience) of nurses. Most states required a criminal background check prior to granting licensure (NCSBN, 2011).
      b. This is the process that gives a nurse the authority to practice in an institution.
      c. Credentialing occurs upon employment, and in most cases, at designated intervals, often on a 2-year cycle.
      d. Credentialing is part of The Joint Commission oversight (Smolenski, 2005).
      e. Depending on the institution, credentialing may occur through standard clinical credentialing processes used for medical staff credentialing or through equivalent human resources processes.
      f. Additional requirements in credentialing are needed for APRNs, such as an active collaborative practice agreement; such requirements must be on record with the employer prior to credentialing (Phillips, 2009).
         (1) Collaborative agreements describe the relationship between an advanced practice nurse, such as a nurse practitioner, and a collaborating physician who allows the nurse practitioner to practice independently within the agreed guidelines.
         (2) Once the collaborative agreement is obtained, the credentialing process proceeds; re-credentialing and renewal of the collaborative agreement is required at least every two years.
   2. Privileging.
      a. Among nurses, applies to nurse practitioners, midwives, and nurse anesthetists only (mid-level provider).
      b. Process by which a hospital governing body grants permission for the APRN to provide specific aspects of patient care. Examples of privileges are admitting, prescribing, and performing procedures (Hittle, 2010).

c. Nurse practitioners and midwives should also seek credentialing by health insurance providers (Medicare, Medicaid, insurance organizations). Credentialing by these payer groups allows the nurse practitioner to bill for care provided and to receive reimbursement (Hittle, 2010).

3. Peer review.

a. The process of reviewing and assessing the clinical competence and conduct of health professionals on an ongoing basis.

b. An integral part of quality assessment and improvement processes, whereby nurses systematically assess, monitor, and make judgments about the quality of nursing care provided by peers as measured against professional standards of practice (Haag-Heitman, 2009).

c. Should occur regularly and on an ad hoc basis in response to adverse events or concerns, but also in support of specific initiatives of quality and safety.

d. Overcoming barriers to peer review can be accomplished using an adapted version of SBAR (Situation-Background-Assessment-Recommendation) named SBIR. Components of SBIR Include:

(1) State the *Situation*.

(2) Describe the *Behavior*.

(3) State the *Impact* on the RN team, patient, or family.

(4) Make a *Recommendation* for change in the behavior or practice, and choose a solution (Haag-Heitman, 2009).

4. Confidentiality of credentialing and peer review information.

a. The process of credentialing and peer review is privileged in most states – Third parties have no right (or very limited rights) to access it.

b. The federal Patient Safety and Quality Improvement Act of 2005, P.L. 109-41, provides additional federal protection for some peer review and quality improvement activities.

c. To protect the peer review privilege, information about the process should always be maintained confidentially and not be voluntarily disclosed to third parties (except the institution's agents and representatives) or to anyone without a need to know.

III. Ambulatory Nursing Practice and Related Liability Issues

Health care is increasingly practiced by telephone, over the Internet, and through other non-traditional media, rather than in-person. Health care facilities, managed care organizations, individual physician practices, and other organizations regularly hire nurses to triage incoming calls and dispense general health care advice. Telehealth nursing practices and legal issues related to this area will be discussed in Chapter 9 ("Telehealth Nursing"). In the following section, a variety of medical-legal issues that relate to the practice of ambulatory nursing will be discussed.

A. General rules for verbal orders (orders given by providers and executed by registered nurses).

1. May be for medication, treatment, tests, intervention, or other patient care.

2. Should be limited to urgent situations in which immediate written or electronic communication is not feasible; should not be used frequently or as common practice for the convenience of providers.

3. The National Patient Safety Goals (The Joint Commission, 2011) identify the risk of miscommunication of information when verbal orders are utilized and have been effective in reducing the use of verbal orders.

4. Documentation guidelines for the nurse receiving the verbal order.

a. Write legibly.

b. Include date and time.

c. Include any information relevant to the order, including patient name, relevant history, information documenting the need for and appropriateness of ordered treatment or service, etc.

d. Include a note on how the order was received (e.g., "t.o." for "telephone order" or "v.o." for "verbal order" given in person).

e. Have the order authenticated in writing or electronically by the ordering provider very shortly after the order is executed, usually no later than the next encounter with the patient or within 48 hours, whichever is sooner (medical staff bylaws generally state when a verbal order must be authenticated).

(1) If the ordering provider is unavailable, the covering physician may countersign.

(2) Medicare regulations prohibit a nurse practitioner or physician's assistant from authenticating a physician's verbal order.

5. Managing risk in the receipt of verbal orders.

a. Ask any relevant questions.

b. Read the content of the order back to the ordering provider before hanging up.

c. Reduce the order to writing immediately and sign the order.

d. Ensure that the ordering (or covering) physician has countersigned the order within the prescribed time frame.

e. A nurse may refuse to take a verbal order if he or she feels uncomfortable doing so.

B. Boundary violations.

1. Boundary violations or crossings are an occupational hazard in nursing and the health care profession (Holder & Schenthal, 2007).

2. Boundary violations occur when a nurse fails to adhere to a therapeutic relationship, such as having a "favorite" patient and arranging the care of others around this favorite.

3. Boundary issues may begin as harmless incidents, such as believing that the nurse is the only person who can provide adequate care to a particular patient.

4. Examples of boundary violations/issues include:

a. Giving out one's telephone number or socializing with patients after discharge or in non-working hours.

b. Sexual conduct with a patient.

c. Accepting loans or valuable gifts, borrowing anything from patients.

d. Picking up groceries for a homebound patient.

e. Social contact with former patients or their relatives, especially in the case of a minor.

5. NCSBN (2005) identifies five guiding principles to help nurses differentiate between what is a therapeutic relationship and what is not one:

a. Respect human dignity.

b. Avoid personal gratification at the patient's expense.

c. Do not interfere with a patient's personal relationships.

d. Promote patient autonomy and self-determination.

e. Promote a fiduciary relationship (one that's based on trust).

C. Hand-off communication (Crane, 2010).

1. Defined as the transition from one health care provider to another or from one setting to another.

2. Root cause of adverse sentinel events in up to 70% of reports compiled by The Joint Commission. Needed follow-up care slips through the cracks or vital information is not shared in a timely fashion (Crane, 2010).

3. Some type of written communication method is recommended, such as SBAR, to ensure vital signs, presenting complaints, allergies, and medications are communicated to receiving facility or provider.

D. Reporting of incompetent/inappropriate behavior of colleagues (Messinger, 2009).

1. In most states, it is mandatory to report violations of ethical practice (such as HIPAA violation), boundaries, or nursing practice (such as patient abandonment) to the state board of nursing.

2. Any lawsuit involving a licensed nurse found negligent must be reported to the state board of nursing.

E. Impaired critical thinking.
   1. Absence of critical thinking may lead to incorrect conclusions or failure to take timely action when needed.
   2. Critical thinking is both an action and a process. The process of critical thinking employs multiple steps that include an ongoing evaluation by the registered nurse. When critical thinking is absent, errors in patient treatment and management may occur.
   3. Types of errors in critical thinking include (Iyer & Levin, 2007, pp. 13-15):
      a. Drawing incorrect parallels between two cases — This may occur when the nurse is thinking about a case and may be influenced by a recent experience. Example: A nurse is assigned two patients with back pain. The first patient fell down some stairs and has compression fractures in her back with pain. The second patient with back pain has no history of trauma. This patient's pain may be minimized by the nurse when this patient's pain may actually indicate spinal cord decompression or a dissecting aortic aneurysm, both conditions that require prompt assessment and intervention.
      b. Making a premature diagnosis – Not considering all available information.
      c. Over-reliance on the findings of others – Not taking the time to investigate abnormal findings as found or reported by ancillary staff.
      d. Failing to recognize the significance of abnormal findings or values, such as a decreased pulse in a patient receiving morphine.
      e. Over-reliance on protocols – Protocols are helpful guidelines in many situations; however, they should not replace situations that require critical thinking and timely action.
      f. Over-confidence in one's abilities and experience can also increase the likelihood of an error when the nursing process is not used correctly.
      g. Caring for patients with similar names may result in errors in medication administration and treatment.
F. Ambulatory nursing liability (Paté, 2010) requires the nurse to conduct:
   1. Accurate assessment and re-assessment utilizing the nursing process.
   2. Critical analysis of data, with timely intervention for abnormal or worrisome symptoms.
   3. Specific areas of risk and requisite nursing actions are indicated (see Table 6-1).

IV. **Patient Self Determination: Informed Consent**

Informed consent is the process by which a patient is provided relevant information about a proposed test, treatment, or procedure and given the opportunity to ask questions and receive understandable answers, resulting in a voluntary decision to either proceed or not to proceed with the test, treatment, or procedure.
A. Legal basis: Patient Self Determination Act and state laws, which may vary.
   1. Competent adult patients are legally entitled to accept or decline recommended medical tests or treatments.
   2. Provision of care without informed consent may be professionally unethical, create professional liability, and in egregious cases, be viewed as civil or criminal battery.
   3. Limited exceptions are recognized in most states and include:
      a. Emergency treatment.
      b. Involuntary commitment for psychiatric evaluation and treatment.
      c. Testing of patients for serious communicable diseases after possible transmission (e.g., accidental blood exposure).
   4. Duty to obtain informed consent.
      a. Rests with the primary provider.
      b. If the provider is a physician, the physician may delegate the process of obtaining informed consent to a nurse.

Table 6-1.
Safeguards Against Legal Problems Resulting from Nursing Assessment and Analysis

Area of Risk	Appropriate Action
Collection of data (vital sign measurements)	• Understand abnormal vs. normal data. • Age-specific differences and co-morbidity influences. • Post normal data measures in intake areas.
Unscheduled patient visits (walk-ins)	• Develop a policy for unscheduled visits; RN assesses and determines level of urgency and hand-off.
Scope of nursing practice	• Understanding of limitations. • Differences between the RN and LPN scope of practice (e.g., LPN collects data, cannot make an assessment).
Patient safety: Fall and pain risk assessments	• Patients are assessed at the entry to the clinic for pain level (numeric, Wong-Baker) and risk for falls. Intervention taken when at-risk for fall, such as wheelchair, patient escort.
Reassessment after treatment or medication administration	• Policies in place for patient reassessment at a specific interval (e.g., 15 minutes) after treatment. Generally, a pain scale is used or symptoms of an allergic reaction are assessed for injections.
Medication errors	• Pre-assess for history of problems with injections, the medication prescribed; instruct the patient on the safety precautions needed after medication administration. • Use of 5 rights.
Documentation accuracy	• Timely, accurate documentation. • Use a charting method that uses "cues" to elicit responses. EMR – Templates or smart phrases commonly used in nursing interventions. • Frequent chart reviews for accuracy.
Resuscitation readiness (procedures and equipment) education	• Frequent mock codes/drills in clinic. • Use case scenarios for continuing education. • CNE focused on unit, patient population.

Source: Paté, 2010. Used with permission.

B. Informed consent is obtained if the patient received the following information and opportunities:
1. Nature of the treatment.
2. Benefits or outcome anticipated.
3. Possible risks involved and the probability of each risk, if ascertainable.
4. Alternatives to treatment.
5. Consequences associated with declining treatment.
6. Opportunity to raise questions and be provided with understandable answers.
7. Opportunity to make a voluntary decision, which is free of undue influence.

C. Disclosure issues prior to informed consent.
1. State courts have held that a primary provider must disclose his or her own HIV/AIDS status to patients before performing any invasive test or treatment.
2. State laws may require disclosure of various conflicts of interest or financial relationships with providers to whom a patient may be referred.

D. Documentation of informed consent.
1. Both a verbal and written consent are legally effective.
2. When obtained verbally, consent should be documented in the medical record.

3. Written informed consent may be required in some cases, including high-risk procedures, HIV/AIDS testing, and genetic testing.

4. Good documentation of informed consent, particularly when signed by the patient (or surrogate), may help reduce professional liability exposure.

E. Legal competency to consent: Minors.
   1. The age of "majority" (when a person is considered an adult) is determined by state law and may range between the ages of 18 and 21.
   2. In general, a minor (a person who has not attained the age of majority) may not consent to his or her own health care unless:
      a. Legally emancipated (e.g., declared independent of parents by court order).
      b. Otherwise recognized to have the capacity to make adult decisions (common examples include adolescents who are married or who are on active duty in the Armed Forces).
   3. Many state laws include exceptions to facilitate a minor's access to sensitive services including care for:
      a. Pregnancy/prenatal care; birth control.
      b. Mental health.
      c. Substance abuse.
      d. Serious communicable diseases, such as HIV/AIDS and other sexually transmitted diseases (STDs).
   4. Generally, a parent, person acting *in loco parentis* (in the place of the parents), or legal guardian must consent to health care services in any other circumstances.

F. Legal competency to consent: Adults.
   1. An adult patient is usually presumed to be competent unless a court decides otherwise.
   2. A person may be incompetent if he or she lacks the ability or capacity to understand the information presented during the informed consent process.
   3. A person may be legally incompetent for the following reasons:
      a. Mental retardation.
      b. Dementia.
      c. Brain damage.
      d. Stroke.
      e. Unconsciousness.

G. Although state law varies, if the patient is legally incompetent, the following persons may provide consent:
   1. A parent of a minor.
   2. A legal guardian of the incompetent person.
   3. A person appointed in a living will or a durable power of attorney.
   4. Anyone standing in *loco parentis* (in the place of the parents) for a minor.
   5. Patient's next of kin.

H. Although state law varies, an emancipated minor, living independently from parents and self-supporting, may provide consent for him or herself.

I. Although state law varies, a minor seeking treatment for drug abuse, sexually transmitted infections, pregnancy, and prevention of pregnancy may provide consent for him or herself.

V. Patient Self Determination: Advance Directives

A. Most states recognize one or more forms of advance directives, which allow competent adults to make certain kinds of health care decisions in advance of an acute (such as a car accident) or chronic (e.g., dementia or stroke) incapacity, thus ensuring their wishes are respected even if they are unable to communicate them directly.

B. Types of advance directives:
   1. Living will – Written statement describing the kind of care the patient does and does not want; it is usually very specific regarding different types of available treatments, including ventilator, dialysis, nutrition, and hydration.
   2. Durable power of attorney for health care – Document naming another individual, usually a relative or close friend (sometimes referred to as a patient advocate), as the person empowered to make health care decisions on the patient's behalf if/when the patient becomes incompetent.

3. Do not resuscitate (DNR) order instructing medical personnel to refrain from using heroic measures to save a life after cardiopulmonary failure.

C. Typically, advance directives must be in writing, voluntarily signed by the patient while competent, and witnessed or notarized.

VI. Patient Transfer Issues (Emergency Medical Treatment and Active Labor Act – EMTALA)

In 1986, Congress passed the Emergency Medical Treatment and Active Labor Act (EMTALA) to ensure patient access to emergency services regardless of ability to pay. EMTALA and similar state laws around the country (also known as "anti-dumping" statutes) help ensure timely public access to emergency treatment and safe delivery of newborns.

A. Application.
1. Law applies to hospitals with emergency departments that participate in the Medicare program. Medicare participating hospitals without dedicated emergency departments have more limited requirements.
2. Law protects all patients, regardless of Medicare status, insurance coverage, or ability to pay, who:
   a. Present to emergency departments requesting emergency examinations or treatment.
   b. Appear for unscheduled visits to ambulatory units (such as psychiatry or labor and delivery) of the hospital that regularly provide emergency care.
   c. Appear on hospital property or in a hospital-owned ambulance.
3. Law includes protections for providers who refuse to authorize a transfer of an unstable patient and for hospital employees who report violations.

B. An emergency medical condition covered by EMTALA is a medical condition manifesting itself by acute symptoms of sufficient severity (including severe pain) such that the absence of immediate medical attention could be reasonably expected to result in:

1. Placing the health of the patient (or in the case of a pregnant woman, the health of the woman or her unborn child) in serious jeopardy.
2. Serious impairment to bodily functions.
3. Serious dysfunction of any bodily organ or part.

C. Active labor is considered an emergency medical condition. Any woman who presents with contractions is considered to be in potentially active labor and must be given an appropriate medical screening examination.

D. Requirements when a patient presents to the emergency department.
1. Hospital must provide an appropriate medical screening examination (MSE) and relevant ancillary services to determine whether an emergency medical condition exists.
2. If the hospital determines the individual has an emergency medical condition, the hospital must do one of the following:
   a. Provide further examination and stabilizing treatment as necessary to stabilize the condition.
   b. If reasonably unable to do so (such as lack of expertise), arrange for the transfer of the patient to an appropriate facility.
3. Hospital may not delay MSE or stabilizing treatment to inquire about insurance or payment status.
4. Transfer rules.
   a. Transferring hospital must provide the necessary medical treatment within its means to minimize the risk to the health of the patient.
   b. Transferring hospital must provide the patient's relevant medical records to the receiving hospital.
   c. Transfer must be performed by competent staff and with appropriate medical supplies.
   d. Hospital may not transfer an unstable patient unless:
      (1) Patient requests the transfer in writing after being informed of the hospital's obligations and risks of the transfer.

(2) Physician or other qualified medical personnel certifies that the benefits of care to be received at the receiving facility outweigh the risk to the patient of undergoing transfer.

    e. The receiving hospital must accept the patient if it has specialized capabilities or facilities necessary to treat the patient and sufficient capacity to do so.

  5. The patient may refuse to accept treatment or transfer, but the hospital must attempt to document such refusal.

E. EMTALA imposes numerous additional administrative requirements impacting institutional policies and procedures, and imposes stiff penalties for non-compliance.

F. Advanced practice nurses and EMTALA.

  1. EMTALA generally recognizes the role of "qualified medical professionals" (QMPs) (including APRNs) in delivering health care.

  2. Current regulations and interpretive guidance generally allow a QMP (e.g., a nurse midwife) to conduct a medical screening examination.

  3. For a woman having contractions, a physician (rather than the QMP) must certify false labor to determine that no medical emergency exists (e.g., that the patient is not in active labor).

G. Legislation in 2002 authorized the waiver of sanctions for EMTALA violations during a public health emergency.

H. After Hurricane Katrina, the Centers for Medicare and Medicaid Services (CMS), which enforces EMTALA, authorized the waiver of sanctions on hospitals located in national emergency area if the hospital redirected or relocated a patient to another location to receive a MSE. Specific circumstances for application of the waiver apply within a limited time period.

I. EMTALA was further modified during the 2009-2010 H1N1 influenza pandemic providing guidance for managing extraordinary emergency department surges using two approaches: Options requiring a waiver and those not requiring a waiver.

VII. HIPAA and Other Patient Rights

Protection of patient privacy is a central ethical obligation of health care practitioners. State laws, accreditation requirements, and professional ethical standards require nurses and other health care providers to take steps to protect patient privacy and other patient rights. These privacy protections include protecting confidentiality of protected health information, notifying patients of provider privacy practices, and ensuring patients access to their personal health information (PHI).

A. HIPAA.

  1. Federal law establishes a "floor" for privacy protection through the Health Insurance Portability and Accountability Act of 1996 and implementing privacy and security regulations (together, referred to as HIPAA).

  2. HIPAA applies to all health plans, health care clearinghouses, and those health care providers (including nurses) who bill electronically for their services.

  3. HIPAA basics.

    a. Patients have a right to control their PHI.

    b. Patients must "authorize" use or disclosure of their PHI in limited situations.

    c. Patients have a right to revoke a prior authorization.

    d. Exceptions to the authorization requirement include:

      (1) Use of PHI for patient care (treatment), claims and payment, and core health care operations.

      (2) Mandatory public health disclosures, such as:

        (a) Abuse, neglect, domestic violence.

        (b) HIV/AIDS diagnosis.

        (c) Cancer diagnosis.

        (d) Immunization.

      (3) De-identification of PHI for later use.

      (4) Certain uses and disclosures for research activities.

      (5) Disclosures required by law (such

as in response to a court order or a law enforcement agency demand).

    (6) Disclosure to coroners, medical examiners, and funeral directors.

    (7) Disclosure to organ banks or entities facilitating organ donation.

  e. Special protections apply to psychotherapy notes (process notes created by mental health professionals and separated from the regular medical record).

  f. Patients have other rights, including the right to notice of privacy practices, the right to access their records, the right to request special confidentiality protections, the right to amend inaccurate records, and the right to information about disclosures made without their authorization.

4. State laws also regulate use and disclosure of PHI. In addition to general protections that may be more restrictive than HIPAA, many state laws grant special protection to PHI about:

  a. STDs or serious communicable diseases, such as HIV/AIDS.

  b. Tests or diseases that may create employment or insurance risks for patients, such as genetics testing or cancer diagnoses.

  c. Mental health or substance abuse diagnosis and treatment.

5. Health Care Integrity and Protection Data Bank.

  a. Contains information related to HIPAA violations and subsequent adverse actions against providers and entities.

  b. Data bank information is only disclosed to federal and state government agencies, health plans, and self-requests for disclosure.

B. Other patient rights (vary by state and institution):

1. Consideration, respect for individual dignity.

2. Non-discrimination.

3. Adequate, appropriate care.

4. Access to PHI about the condition, plan of care, chances of recovery, and responsible providers.

5. Adequate and appropriate pain and symptom management.

6. Clear communications in a language and manner understandable to the patient.

7. Refusal of treatment.

8. Involvement in own care and decisions where feasible.

9. Freedom from physical and emotional abuse.

10. Freedom from physical and chemical restraints except in very limited circumstances authorized by law, accreditation standards, and institutional policies.

11. Making complaints or grievances.

12. Refusal to participate in experimental treatments or procedures.

13. Receipt of financial information (bill, sources of financial assistance).

14. Information about rights and responsibilities.

VIII. Abandonment

Patient abandonment occurs when the professional relationship between a health care provider (HCP) and patient is terminated abruptly and without the patient's consent. A provider (RN, APN, MD)-patient relationship is established when a patient seeks health care services and the practitioner agrees to provide them. There are limitations on a practitioner's ability to refuse to provide services. In emergency situations, for example, the provider's agreement may not be necessary. Moreover, a practitioner may not generally discriminate against patients based on statutory or contractually protected classifications (such as sex, race, religion, national origin, or insurance status).

A patient may terminate his or her relationship with a provider (including an APRN) at any time. The provider, however, has legal and ethical obligations to facilitate continuity of care and avoid harm caused by prematurely terminating a relationship.

A. Provider's responsibilities when a patient terminates.

  1. If further treatment is needed, inform the patient of the risks of termination of care.

2. Refer the patient to an alternative provider, if requested.
3. Provide copies of patient records to the new provider to facilitate continuity of care.
4. Document the fact that the patient requested termination of the relationship, preferably on a form signed by the patient, or, if not feasible, then in a written verification letter sent to the patient.
5. If a patient is instructed to follow up, but fails to show up for appointments or call, reasonable attempts should be made to contact the patient and provide the information listed above.

B. Circumstances under which a provider may terminate.
1. Provider becomes unavailable to provide further treatment due to relocation, illness, injury, or disability.
2. Patient is disruptive or refuses to cooperate with treatment plans.
   a. Termination is not automatic.
   b. To avoid an abandonment claim, attempt a behavioral contract and document instances of noncompliance before terminating the relationship.
3. Reasons for establishing the relationship have been resolved.
   a. Example: A pregnant patient delivers. After post-partum checkup, the provider has no obligation to provide ongoing gynecological services or to provide maternity care for a subsequent pregnancy.
   b. Instructions should be provided to the patient for any additional necessary follow-up care.
4. The provider has inadequate credentials or scope of practice to address patient's needs. (Example: A primary care nurse practitioner is unable to provide a needed surgical intervention).
5. The patient is unwilling or unable to pay for further treatment (except when EMTALA applies – see above).

C. Nursing abandonment.

1. Occurs after a nurse has accepted responsibility for an assignment within a scheduled shift.
2. When a nurse fails to give reasonable notice to an employer of the intent to terminate the employer/employee relationship or contract leading to serious impairment of the delivery of professional care to patients (Morales, 2011).
3. "Examples of nursing abandonment situations are:
   a. Leaving the unit for lunch during a scheduled shift without transferring assignment to another nurse.
   b. Inappropriate transfer to lesser skilled personnel.
   c. Failing to respond to a patient's call for help.
   d. Failure to triage a patient's severity and situations with simultaneous needs" (Morales, 2011, p. 1).
4. Acceptable situations for refusal of assignments are:
   a. Refusal to accept responsibility for patient assignment after giving reasonable notice to employer/agent.
   b. Refusal based on a lack of competence to carry out assignment.
   c. Refusal to work a double shift or additional work hours beyond posted work schedule when proper notification has been given.
5. State board of nursing notification.
   a. Mandatory reporting of an unsafe patient care/situation by supervisor/manager.
   b. Any person may report an unsafe situation to the board of nursing.

D. The nurse-patient relationship and minimizing liability include:
1. When the nurse accepts responsibility for providing nursing care based upon a written or oral report of patient needs.
2. The relationship ends when that responsibility has been transferred to another nurse, along with appropriate communication regarding the patient's needs.

E. The provider's (such as an APRN's) responsibility when terminating the relationship is to minimize liability.
1. Notify the patient in writing by certified mail/return receipt requested.
2. Give the reason(s) for the withdrawal of care.
3. Identify a qualified substitute or an organization where qualified substitutes may be found. If the relationship is being terminated because specialized care is required, refer the patient to a provider of the specialized service.
4. Provide the patient with sufficient time to find an alternative provider.
5. Offer to be available to the patient for a specified period (typically no less than 30 days) to avoid a gap in services before a relationship is established with the alternative provider.
6. Inform the patient that treatment will be provided in an emergency until a new provider is found.
7. Offer to transfer medical records.
F. Interruptions in service.
1. The provider may be temporarily unavailable due to vacation, meetings, or illness.
   a. Replacement should be arranged, if feasible.
   b. The patient should be informed of alternatives.
2. Two patients may require care at the same time.
   a. The provider must prioritize each patient's needs.
   b. One patient must not be abandoned entirely to attend to another.
G. Home health care settings.
1. Home nursing services may be discontinued when:
   a. Source of payment no longer exists.
   b. Environment is unsafe for the home health nurse visits.
   c. The physician orders care to be terminated when no longer medically necessary.
2. If home health services are discontinued, documentation should generally include:

a. Written notice to the patient and physician.
b. Alternative measures taken to prevent endangerment to the patient, such as identification of alternative and accessible community resources.
H. Penalties for abandonment.
1. Malpractice liability (or in some states, potentially other theories of liability, such as breach of contract).
2. Licensing sanctions (e.g., Board of Nursing).

IX. Legal Aspects of Clinical Documentation

Complete and accurate documentation of health care services is required by federal and state law, accreditation requirements, professional standards, and industry practice. The quality of documentation may affect the outcome of a professional liability case. The care one takes in documenting nursing assessments and interventions could prove the standard of care was met and establish one's credibility with a jury (Austin, 2011). Nurses, like other health care practitioners, may be held liable for inappropriate treatment as a result of inadequate documentation.

A. The purpose of the medical record:
1. Provide the most credible evidence or legal proof that the care given to the patient met the legal standard of care.
2. Serve as a communication tool for health care providers that tells the "patient's story," while he or she is receiving care at a facility or clinic.
3. Provide attorney's information to help analyze the merits of a malpractice claim and as a defense to claims of negligence or intentional misconduct.
4. Implement quality improvement initiatives.
5. Review of services and needs for utilization review to determine the appropriate level of care and to obtain third-party reimbursement.
B. Elements of good documentation (applicable laws, accreditation, institutional policies, and licensing standards may require more or different elements depending on the circumstances).

1. Patient's symptoms, using the patient's words in "quotation marks."
   a. This action is particularly recommended when those quotes contain highly significant information.
   b. Exact quotes contain a high degree of credibility and may clearly describe the patient's concern or condition.
2. Objective observations.
3. Identification and analysis of any patient problems.
4. Nursing actions taken (e.g., treatment plan, procedures performed, drugs prescribed or administered).
5. Patient's response to medication, treatment, and/or intervention.
6. Signature, date, and time of every entry.
   a. Entries are signed with at least first initial, followed by last name, and then the clinician's status, such as RN or LPN.
   b. Gives the reader of the medical record a better understanding of what occurred during the shift or encounter and who provided the care.
   c. Assists concurrent and subsequent caregivers to better understand what care has been given, when, and by whom.
   d. Compliance to this element of charting is critical to an attorney when he or she evaluates the medical record to construct a case and develop a time line of events.
C. Characteristics of good documentation:
   1. Factual.
   2. Objective – Void of personal opinions or observations unrelated to the care of the patient.
   3. Accurate.
   4. Appropriate – Reflects the nursing process.
   5. Consistent.
   6. Timely.
   7. Complete – In a large organization, records generally should not be maintained in decentralized shadow files accessible only by the nurse or team within that unit.

D. Guidelines for charting in the medical record (Iyer & Levin, 2007):
   1. In paper documentation, always use ink, never erasable media. Most institutions have moved to the exclusive use of blue or black ink with paper medical records.
   2. Use neat and legible handwriting.
   3. Use correct spelling and grammar.
   4. Use only authorized abbreviations and avoid abbreviations prohibited by law, accreditation standards, or institutional policy.
      a. Use of incorrect abbreviations may lead to medical errors, and as such, many health care institutions have banned the use of dangerous and/or misleading abbreviations (Iyer & Levin, 2007).
      b. Unapproved abbreviations often enter the organization when new employees are hired. Covering this requirement during unit orientation may preclude unauthorized use.
   5. Recording in military time (e.g., 1530) eliminates much confusion about the time of day.
   6. Never erase or delete an entry unless required by law.
      a. If an error occurs, draw a line through the error so that the entry is still readable. Write "error" above it with your initials.
      b. For electronic documents, do not destroy the only electronic record. If it is inaccurate, flag it, archive it, or find some other way to notify the user that it is not to be relied upon.
   7. Always use the appropriate form.
   8. Documenting omitted care or medications. Agency policies specify this procedure.
      a. In a paper record, document on each line without leaving spaces between entries.
      b. Document an omission as a new entry.
      c. Avoid adding to a previously written entry.
   9. Making inappropriate comments – Avoid accusations and finger pointing, especially following an adverse event or patient injury (Iyer & Levin, 2007). Common situations in

nursing negligence cases that give rise to finger pointing by another include:

   a. The patient has been injured.

   b. The patient could have been injured.

   c. Physician's orders have not been carried out, and the nurse is trying to cover him or herself.

10. Patient allergies.

   a. Facility policy usually defines how allergy information is documented.

   b. Allergies to medications must be documented for every clinic visit.

   c. Electronic medical records may have a warning system to flag an order that is contrary to a known allergy and/or change the color of the allergy listed (such as red) to bring attention to the medication allergy.

E. Electronic medical records and documents.

1. Congress, federal agencies, and many states have adopted laws and issued regulations permitting health care providers to create and maintain documents solely in electronic form.

2. Examples.

   a. Electronic Signatures in Global and National Commerce Act (eSIGN) – A federal law.

   b. Uniform Electronic Transactions Act (UETA) – A model law adopted by many states.

   c. Food and Drug Administration, 21 C.F.R. Part 11 (regulations on use of electronic signatures and records).

3. Specific EMR/EHR federal regulations.

   a. 1974 – Privacy Act.

   b. 1986 – Electronic Communications Privacy Act (use of fax machines).

   c. 1990 – ADA.

   d. 1996 – HIPAA Privacy Rule.

   e. 2004 – National HIT Office.

   f. 2009 – HITECH.

4. Laws have specific requirements regarding security of record-keeping systems and authentication of users and user signatures.

5. Minimum security measures should always be enforced, including:

   a. Avoid maintaining medical records on personal computers or devices that may be susceptible to tampering, intrusion, or theft.

   b. Back up files regularly.

   c. Maintain up-to-date anti-virus and anti-spyware applications on the computer used.

   d. Never share a user identification code, password, or other access code with anyone.

   e. Report any equipment theft, potential intrusion, or improper password use promptly to institutional officials, or if one is unaffiliated with an institution, to local law enforcement personnel.

6. Potential quality gaps with EMR/EHR (Rhysnburger, 2011).

   a. Order errors or lack of provider signature.

   b. Delays in diagnosis or treatment may be apparent in the documentation.

   c. Documentation does not demonstrate compliance to standard of care.

   d. Documentation may demonstrate out-of-scope practices.

   e. Treatment/time gaps stand out in documentation.

   f. Documentation demonstrates medication order errors.

   g. Metadata (a large synthesis of related information) may invalidate stated or written documentation.

   h. Nearly impossible to recreate exactly what a clinician saw at a given time.

   i. Time sequence of EMR review and actions difficult to place in chronological order because information is housed in multiple areas.

   j. Use of "smart phrases" (list of common areas of documentation) may cue the nurse to include all elements of documentation required for a treatment or intervention. (Example of a smart phrase is: ***splint applied to ***site. Neurovascular checks reveal palpable pulse, pink extremity. One fills in the starred areas and personalizes the phrase for each patient.)

7. Safeguards to limit liability (Rhysnburger, 2011).
   a. Documentation of clinical findings.
      (1) Document accurately.
      (2) Document completely.
      (3) Document thought process (e.g., the nursing process).
   b. Computerized order entry.
      (1) Ensure that document and orders are placed in the correct medical record.
      (2) Ensure all orders are "signed" prior to closing records; otherwise it is a "pended" or incomplete chart.
      (3) Orders must be written *prior* to implementation; otherwise seen as a compliance "red flag" and is an unauthorized order. This means the nurse does not have an active order to carry out. He or she has increased legal liability because of acting independently, and payment may be denied.
   c. Diagnostics – Labs/imaging.
      (1) Follow-up tests not ordered or performed in a timely manner.
      (2) Documentation of MD/staff review with appropriate action taken.
      (3) Timely notification of patient for abnormal test results.
   d. Clinical decision support tools.
      (1) Adequate training on tools.
      (2) Appropriate use of tool; documentation of rationale for not using tool.
      (3) Adequate supportive clinical documentation.
   e. Messaging.
      (1) Avoid routing errors.
      (2) Avoid overuse of auto-text responses (e.g., failure to individualize documentation).
      (3) Avoid HIPAA violations (e.g., documentation of providing PHI to someone other than patient).
      (4) Attention to scope of practice issues (e.g., right person performing the task).

F. Document retention and destruction.
   1. All types of legal rules and precedents govern the retention and destruction of medical and administrative records of health care providers and institutions, including:
      a. Privacy laws.
      b. Tax laws.
      c. Food and drug laws (including laws regulating clinical research).
      d. Rules of evidence.
      e. Court or administrative decisions.
   2. Rule of thumb for health care records.
      a. Retain for at least six years.
      b. Many laws, regulations, institutional policies, and contract requirements demand even longer periods, especially related to the care of children.
      c. Minors' health care records should be retained at least six years or until age 21, whichever is longer. Records for a minor who never becomes competent (e.g., due to mental status) may need to be retained for life.
   3. Contracts may call for return or destruction of records, but laws, regulations, and institutional policies may demand otherwise.
   4. Institutional policies may require destruction of records after a certain amount of time has elapsed to address storage capacity, security, and other problems.
   5. Never destroy documents when on notice of a claim or lawsuit to which the documents are relevant.
      a. The court may draw a negative inference against the former holder of the record and assume the documents would have been supportive of the other party's case.
      b. Depending on how egregious inappropriate destruction may be, the court may hold the person who destroyed the records in contempt and may assess significant penalties.
   6. Re-creation of the EMR/EHR may result in a fragmented image of the actual record (Rhysnburger, 2011).
      a. Metadata are discoverable and must be produced when requested.

Figure 6-1.
Professional Liability/Malpractice Claim

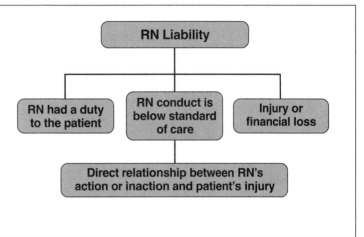

Source: Paté, 2010. Used with permission.

b. Use only trained legal records clerks to respond to records production requests.

X. Professional Liability/Malpractice

Nurses are responsible and may be held personally liable for their own actions, and in many circumstances, have a legal and ethical obligation to report incompetent nursing practice.

A. Professional negligence defined (four elements) (see Figure 6-1).
  1. A duty of care is owed to the patient.
     a. Requires that the nurse had established a relationship with the patient. Depending on the circumstances, relationships may be established inadvertently (e.g., when a stranger seeks health care advice during a social gathering).
     b. Duty is defined by reference to what a "reasonably prudent ambulatory care nurse would have done under similar circumstances in the United States" (Paté, 2010).
  2. The nurse breached that duty.
     a. His or her actions deviated from the standard of care.

b. Examples of breach of a duty of care:
  (1) Failure to use sterile technique during a dressing change.
  (2) Failure to follow an established medical protocol or guideline.
  (3) Practice beyond scope of the individual's education and experience (even if within the Scope of Practice Act).
  (4) Failure to disclose, such as failure to report an adverse reaction to the administration of a drug or failure to report an error.
  (5) Failure to ensure continued assessment or observation of an acutely ill individual, such as not re-assessing vital signs on a patient with elevated pulse, blood pressure, or temperature.
  3. The patient suffered damages, such as:
     a. Physical injury.
     b. Psychological injury.
     c. Financial loss.
  4. The nurse's breach of duty of care "proximately" caused the patient's damages.
     a. There is a reasonably direct relationship between the nurse's action or inaction and the patient's injury.

b. "But for" the nurse's action or inaction, the patient would not have been harmed.

B. Sources of claims and litigation.
 1. Poor or unexpectedly adverse outcomes.
 2. Most do not result in litigation.
    a. According to at least one older study conducted by the Secretary's Commission on Medical Malpractice (Health, Education, and Welfare), more than half of claims were based on minor or emotional issues, not major adverse events, such as death or disability (Atchison et al., 2001).
    b. Relationship between provider and patient is often more important than actual outcome of treatment (Hickson, Clayton, Githens, & Sloan, 1992; Hickson et al., 1994).
 3. Some reasons that patients file lawsuits include:
    a. Significant injury requiring future medical and other costs.
    b. Need for answers.
    c. Perceived rude or unsympathetic providers.
    d. Poor communication resulting in unreasonable expectations on the part of the patient.
 4. Specific issues include:
    a. Inadequate or inappropriate assessment or re-assessment.
    b. Inadequate informed consent process and documentation (such as failure to fully disclose risks and alternatives to proposed treatment). Note: The patient's consent to treat that is signed when a patient seeks medical care does not cover invasive procedures, such as suturing a laceration or performing minor procedures.
    c. Failure to observe and communicate changes in patient's condition.
    d. Failure of a nurse to question potentially inappropriate or dangerous orders.
    e. Medication administration errors.
    f. Inadequate or incomplete documentation of services provided.
    g. Non-compliance with the standard of care. The standard of care is defined as the care a reasonably prudent nurse would do in a similar situation in the United States. When a registered nurse is asked, "Is your care of Mr. Doe within the standard of care in 2010?" The registered nurse must know the applicable nursing standards for that specialty or area of practice at the time of the injury or illness. Within the ambulatory/clinic/outpatient setting, the *Scope and Standards of Practice for Professional Ambulatory Care Nursing* (AAACN, 2010) would apply.
    h. Ethical violations, including violation of patient privacy.
    i. Failure to ensure patient safety, such as identifying those at risk for falls and implementing safeguards.
 5. New nurse managers – Questions to ask risk management (Cohen, Cox, Klitch, & Webb, 2004).
    a. What types of liability issues have been identified in my clinic(s) in the past two years?
    b. How did the management staff address those issues? Were the actions successful?
    c. Are there any lawsuits pending in my clinic(s) that I need to be aware of?
    d. How does this department want to be notified when liability issues are identified in my clinic(s)?
    e. What are the most prominent types of legal action taken against this organization?
    f. What actions/plans have worked best to deter lawsuits in this organization?
    g. What type of training or continuing education does the risk management department provide for learning more about how liability issues are handled?

XI. Other Regulations Impacting Ambulatory Nursing Practice: Reporting Mandates, Fraud and Abuse (Whistle Blowing), and EEOC

A. Reporting mandates.

Federal and state laws and institutional policies require nurses and others to report incompetent, unethical, unprofessional, and other inappropriate behavior, as well as disciplinary actions undertaken to address such conduct and successful malpractice claims.

1. Federally required reporting.
   a. Adverse professional review actions and professional liability payments.
      (1) Reportable events include:
         (a) Suspension or revocation of licensure.
         (b) Limitation, restriction, suspension, or revocation of clinical credentials through credentialing or peer review activities related to professional competence or conduct, including incompetent clinical care or unethical conduct.
         (c) Malpractice payments.
      (2) Mandatory reporting for physicians.
      (3) Permissive reporting for nurses.
   b. Health care fraud.
2. State law-required reporting.
   a. Reporting requirements generally apply both to licensed facilities employing health care practitioners and to licensed practitioners themselves.
   b. Reportable events related directly to health care professionals may include:
      (1) Adverse professional review actions, and in some cases, professional liability payments.
         (a) Usually mandatory for all licensed practitioners.
         (b) Reports may trigger licensing board investigations.
      (2) Incompetent practice or practice outside the scope of a license.
      (3) Substance abuse and controlled substance violations.
      (4) Mental impairment.
      (5) Privacy breaches and other unethical conduct.
      (6) Fee-splitting, kickbacks, and other potentially abusive activities.
      (7) Criminal convictions.
   c. Failure to report a reportable event may, in and of itself, trigger adverse licensure action.
3. Public health reporting.
   a. Federal and state law includes mandates for reporting information that may impact the public health.
   b. Examples of required public health reporting.
      (1) Serious communicable diseases.
      (2) Cancer diagnoses.
      (3) Abuse, neglect, or domestic violence.
      (4) Gunshot wounds or other evidence of violent criminal activity.
      (5) Defective devices.

B. Fraud and abuse (whistleblowing).

Many federal and state laws have been enacted to protect the government and taxpayers from unscrupulous contractors and patients from incentives to provide unnecessary and sometimes dangerous health care services (or fail to provide necessary services). A few of these laws are:

1. False Claims Acts.
   a. Federal law originally enacted in the 1800s to combat defense procurement abuses in the Civil War era.
   b. Prohibits any entity from making a "false claim" to a government entity to induce undeserved payment. Applies even if the government suffers no actual damages.
   c. Private citizens may sue on behalf of the government, even if the government does not want to pursue the case.
   d. Law includes whistleblower protection provisions designed to encourage reporting of abusive organizations and individuals.

2. Prohibitions on kickbacks and referrals.
   a. Laws and regulations prohibit the solicitation, receipt, or offer of a payment of a kickback, bribe, or other type of payment, whether cash or in-kind, in return for referring a patient for an item or service for which payment may be made under a federal health care program (Medicare, TRICARE).
   b. Federal anti-self referral law ("Stark") applies only to referrals made by physicians to certain designated health care services in which they or their immediate family members have a financial interest.
   c. Many states have adopted equivalent schemes to offer additional protection to Medicaid programs.
   d. Kickbacks or referrals may sometimes result in false claims.
3. If one has financial relationships with referral sources or is a source of referrals to another health care provider, he or she should check with legal counsel to make sure those relationships comply with the fraud and abuse laws.
4. Other offenses.
   a. Government has many other ways to prosecute misconduct.
   b. Examples include health care fraud, mail fraud, wire fraud, and false statements.

C. Workplace issues: EEOC.
   Nurses and nurse managers are required to comply with regulations providing for equal opportunity and safety in the workplace. The Equal Employment Opportunity Commission (EEOC) is a federal agency that issues and enforces regulations concerning workplace discrimination.
   1. Responsible for enforcement of various anti-discrimination laws:
      a. Civil Rights Act: Prohibits employment discrimination based on race, color, religion, sex, or national origin.
      b. Equal Pay Act: Requires equal pay for men and women doing substantially similar jobs.
      c. Age Discrimination in Employment Act: Prohibits discrimination based on age of employees who are 40 years of age or older.
      d. Americans with Disabilities Act:
         (1) Provides equal opportunity rights to disabled citizens.
         (2) Deals with equal opportunity in employment, access to state and local government agencies, public accommodations, transportation, and telecommunications.
         (3) Applies to state and local government and all employers with 15 or more employees.
         (4) Defines a disabled person as someone who has a substantial physical or mental impairment that significantly limits a major life activity.
   2. Establishes rules for receiving and acting on complaints, including:
      a. Jurisdiction.
         (1) Except for Equal Pay Act violations, most violations of anti-discrimination laws must be filed with EEOC before going to court.
         (2) Failure to file with EEOC may result in loss of legal rights.
      b. Time limits.
         (1) General rule: Complaints must be filed within 180 days of an alleged violation.
         (2) Time limit may be extended to 300 days if the discrimination is covered by state or local anti-discrimination laws.
      c. Process.
         (1) EEOC investigates the complaint to determine whether the facts seem to support a violation of the law. Follow-up may occur when the case is not clear-cut.
         (2) EEOC may act as a mediator if charging party and employer both agree.

(3) If mediation is not pursued or is unsuccessful, EEOC may dismiss the charge.

    (a) EEOC may file a lawsuit on behalf of the employee.

    (b) EEOC may issue a "right to sue" letter that allows the employee to file a lawsuit within 90 days.

3. Remedies to discrimination, after a finding of discrimination by a court, may include:

    a. Accommodation of the employee, as needed.

    b. Hiring, promotion, or reinstatement.

    c. Payment of money damages, including back pay or front pay necessary to make the victim "whole" (place the victim in the position he or she would have had if not for the discrimination).

    d. Payment of attorneys' fees, expert witness fees, and court costs.

    e. Payment of punitive damages if the employer acted with malice or reckless indifference (not available against employers that are federal, state, or local governments).

    f. Other corrective action.

References

American Academy of Ambulatory Care Nursing (AAACN). (2010). *Scope and standards of practice for professional ambulatory care nursing* (8th ed.). Pitman, NJ: Author.

Atchison, D., Dabelstein, L., Kuhn, A.M., Murphy, R., Thomas, J., West, S.J., & Youngberg, B.J. (2001). *Nursing-legal survival: A risk management guide for nursing.* Oak Brook, IL: University Health System Consortium.

Austin, S. (2011). Stay out of court with proper documentation. *Nursing 2011, 41*(4), 24-29.

Cohen, S., Cox, S.H., Klitch, B.A., & Webb, S.K. (2004). *Core skills for nurse managers: A training tool kit.* Marble Head, MA: HCPro, Inc.

Crane, M.E. (2010). *Avoiding malpractice risks in the patient handoff.* Retrieved from http://www.medscape.com/BusinessofMedicine

Haag-Heitman, B. (2009). *Froedtert Hospital hosts Magnet™ workshop on peer review.* Retrieved from www.nursecredentialing.org/Magnet/MagnetEvents/RecognitionWorkshops.aspx

Hickson, G.B., Clayton, E.W., Entman, S.S., Miller, C.S., Githens, P.B., Whetten-Goldstein, K., & Sloan, F.A. (1994). Obstetricians' prior malpractice experience and patients' satisfaction with care. *Journal of the American Medical Association, 272*(20), 1583-1587.

Hickson, G.B., Clayton, E.W., Githens, P.B., & Sloan, F.A. (1992). Factors that prompted families to file medical malpractice claims following perinatal injuries. *Journal of the American Medical Association, 267*(10), 1359-1363.

Hittle, K. (2010). Understanding certification, licensure, and credentialing: Credentialing and privileging. *Journal of Pediatric Health Care, 24*(3), 203-206.

Holder, K.V., & Schenthal, S.J. (2007). Watch your step: Nursing and professional boundaries. *Nursing Management, 38*(2), 24-29.

Iyer, P.W., & Levin, B.J. (2007). *Nursing malpractice* (3rd ed.). Tucson, AZ: Lawyers and Judges Publishing.

Joint Commission, The. (2011). *National patient safety goals.* Retrieved from http://www.jointcommission.org/assets/1/6/2011_NPSGs_HAP.pdf

Messinger, M. (2009). Staying off the slippery slope: Knowing and maintaining professional boundaries in your nursing practice. *Nursing News & Views: Official Publication of the New Mexico Board of Nursing, 4*(4), 19-21.

Morales, K. (2011). *Patient abandonment.* Retrieved from http://www.nursetogether.com/Career/Career-Article/itemid/1829.aspx

National Council of State Boards of Nursing (NCSBN). (1995). *Concepts and decision-making process: National Council position paper on delegation.* Retrieved from http://www.ncsbn.org/regulation/nursingpractice.

National Council of State Boards of Nursing (NCSBN). (2005). *Working with others: A position paper.* Retrieved from http://www.ncsbn.org/regulation/nursingpractice

National Council of State Boards of Nursing (NCSBN). (2010). *Nurse Licensure Compact (NLC): Fact sheet for licensees and nursing students.* Retrieved from http://www.ncsbn.org/nlc/index.asp

National Council of State Boards of Nursing (NCSBN). (2011). *Model Nursing Practice Act and Model Nursing Administrative Rules.* Retrieved from http://www.ncsbn.org/regulation/nursingpractice.

Paté, J.M. (2010, May). *Pitfalls and pearls in ambulatory nursing: Are you practicing safely?* Presentation at the 35th Annual Conference for American Academy of Ambulatory Care Nursing. Las Vegas, NV.

Phillips, S.J. (2009). Despite legal issues, APNs are still standing strong. *The Nurse Practitioner, 34*(1), 19-41.

Rhysnburger, J. (2011, May). *Avoiding legal pitfalls when using electronic medical records.* Presentation at the 36th Annual Conference for American Academy of Ambulatory Care Nursing. San Antonio, TX.

Smolenski, M.G. (2005). Credentialing, certification, and competence: Issues for new and seasoned nurse practitioners. *Journal of the American Academy of Nursing Practitioner, 17*(5), 201-204.

Additional Readings

Alfaro-Lefevre, R. (1995). *Critical thinking in nursing: A practical approach.* Philadelphia: W.B. Saunders Company.

Andrews, M., Goldberg, K., & Kaplan, H. (1996). *Nurse's legal handbook* (3rd ed.). Springhouse, PA: Springhouse.

Carroll, R. (2006). *Risk management handbook for health care organizations.* San Francisco: Jossey-Bass.

Cartwright-Vanzant, R. (2011). Standard of care. *Journal of Legal Nurse Consulting, 22*(1), 14-18.

"Delegation as a management function." (2011). *Nursing Management*. Retrieved from http://currentnursing.com/nursing_management/delegation.html

Guido, G.W. (2005). *Legal and ethical issues in nursing*. Upper Saddle River, NJ: Prentice Hall.

Hauser, B.R. (1996). *Women's legal guide* (1st ed.). Golden, CO: Fulcrum.

National Council of State Boards of Nursing (NCSBN). (2011a). *Advanced Practice Registered Nurse Compact*. Retrieved from http://www.ncsbn.org/regulation/nursingpractice

National Council of State Boards of Nursing (NCSBN). (2011b). *Guiding principles of nursing regulation*. Retrieved from http://www.ncsbn.org/regulation/nursingpractice

Peternelj-Taylor, C. (2002). Professional boundaries: A matter of therapeutic integrity. *Journal of Psychosocial Nursing & Mental Health Services, 40*(4), 22-29.

Reid, A.J. (2001). *Law all nurses should know*. Retrieved from http://www.continuingeducation.com/nursing/lawstoknow/index.html

Walker, R. (2011). Legal file: Elements of negligence and malpractice. *The Nurse Practitioner: The American Journal of Primary Health Care, 36*(5), 9-11.

Chapter 7

Patient Safety and Regulatory Standards In Ambulatory Care

Kathy Bratcher, MS, RN
Peggy Kaminsky, MSN, RN, CIC
Deborah D. Tinker, MSN, RN, CENP

OBJECTIVES – *Study of the information in this chapter will enable the learner to:*

1. Discuss the evolution of a culture of safety as it relates to health care.
2. Describe the resources and key elements available to help an organization evaluate and improve its culture of safety.
3. Identify methods to improve the safety of medication administration in ambulatory care.
4. Define strategies to reduce the risk of health care-associated infections.
5. Describe health care regulatory and accrediting agencies.
6. Identify National Patient Safety Goals applicable to ambulatory care practice.

KEY POINTS – *The major points in this chapter include:*

1. Consumer groups, health care benefit providers, patient safety advocacy organizations, and regulatory agencies emphasize the importance of pursuing the highest standards of care for patient safety, partially in response to publications about medical errors.
2. Ambulatory care nurses working in a variety of settings are responsible for a continuous quality improvement approach to assure the prevention of errors and the promotion of patient safety.
3. Current trends support a non-punitive approach to health care error reduction with a "just culture" rather than a "culture of blame" focus.
4. Safe management of medications and prevention and control of infections are key to a robust patient safety program in ambulatory care.
5. Government agencies hold health care institutions accountable for safety and quality of the environment and of care.
6. Several regulating agencies oversee that health care institutions adhere to standards and requirements of safety and quality.

*P*atient safety has been defined as the prevention of health care errors and the elimination or mitigation of patient injury caused by health care errors (National Patient Safety Foundation, n.d.), health care that consistently does the right thing at the right time for the right person (U.S. Department of Veterans Affairs, 2011), and a discipline in the health care professions that applies safety science methods toward the goal of achieving a trustworthy system of health care delivery (Emanuel et al., 2008). The body of science supporting patient safety is fairly young and changing rapidly.

The concept of an organizational culture is focused on safety developed in response to the Chernobyl nuclear disaster in 1986. After investigating the incident, the International Atomic Energy Agency (IAEA) cited a "poor safety culture" as a contributing factor in the incident, and subsequent nuclear safety reports stressed the importance of a *safety culture* in preventing errors (International Nuclear Safety Advisory Group, 1999). In 1994, Dr. Lucian L. Leape applied the term to health care organizations in the article, "Error in Medicine" (Leape, 1994). But the catalyst for the current increased interest in patient safety was the publication of three Institute of Medicine (IOM) reports: *To Err Is Human* (2000), *Crossing the Quality Chasm* (2001), and *Keeping Patients Safe* (2003). In response to these publications, consumer groups, health care benefit providers, patient safety advocacy organizations, and regulatory agencies began to emphasize the importance of pursuing the highest standards of care for patient safety. Ambulatory care nurses working in a variety of settings are responsible for participating in activities to assure the prevention of errors and to promote patient safety.

I. A Safety Culture

A. Institute of Medicine (IOM) reports.
   1. IOM is an independent, non-profit organization that works to provide unbiased and authoritative advice to decision-makers and the public to improve health.
   2. *To Err Is Human* (IOM, 2000) drew public attention to errors in health care.
      a. Focuses on preventable errors that occur in the health care environment.
      b. Is credited with enlightening the public regarding the existence and prevalence of medical error.
      c. Discusses how reporting systems affect patient safety endeavors.
   3. *Crossing the Quality Chasm* (IOM, 2001) detailed steps health care should take to correct the preventable errors in health care systems.
   4. *Keeping Patients Safe* (IOM, 2003) reported on the effects of the work environment on error.
      a. Specifically addresses the work environment of nurses.
      b. Describes the critical role nurses play in keeping patients safe.
   5. *The Future of Nursing: Leading Change, Advancing Health* (IOM, 2010) details four key messages to nurses of the future, including the message that nursing must play an important role on the health care team.
B. A commitment to safety is key for an organization wishing to establish a "culture of safety." The components of a safety culture vary among researchers. The Agency for Healthcare Research and Quality (AHRQ) states that a culture of safety must contain these key components:
   1. Acknowledgment of the high-risk nature of an organization's activities and the determination to achieve consistently safe operations.
   2. A blame-free environment where individuals are able to report errors or near misses without fear of reprimand or punishment.
   3. Encouragement of collaboration across ranks and disciplines to seek solutions to patient safety problems.
   4. Organizational commitment of resources to address safety concerns (AHRQ, 2005).
C. A culture of safety survey helps an organization assess its organizational or departmental safety culture and track changes over time. Validated surveys can be developed internally or are available from the following organizations:
   1. AHRQ.
   2. Institute for Safe Medication Practices (ISMP).
D. Improvement depends on learning from errors and near misses, which in turn relies on reporting. In October 1997, Dr. Lucian L. Leape explained in a presentation to the United States Congress, "The single greatest impediment to error prevention in the medical industry is that we punish people for making mistakes."
   1. A "culture of blame" discourages reporting and learning from errors by blaming individuals for human errors.
   2. Health care has traditionally supported a culture of blame that has led to underreporting of errors.
   3. A non-punitive systems approach to safety allows more open reporting of incidents and near misses, providing a learning opportunity for the organization.
   4. A "just culture" focuses on identifying and addressing systems issues that lead individuals to engage in unsafe behaviors, while maintaining individual accountability, establishing zero tolerance for reckless behavior (Marx, 2009).

E. Tools available for organizations adopting a non-punitive system include:
    1. James Reason's (1997) Unsafe Acts Algorithm used in the implementation of a Fair and Just Culture (available through the Institute for Healthcare Improvement).
    2. David Marx's (2009) Just Culture algorithm (available at JustCulture.org and through AHRQ).
F. Multiple organizations have contributed to the enhancement of patient safety and the development of strategies to create successful patient safety cultures.
    1. National Patient Safety Foundation (NPSF) (www.npsf.org).
        a. Founded in 1997 as a not-for-profit research and education organization.
        b. Utilizes a collaborative approach to patient safety awareness and activities.
        c. Involves patients and their families as partners.
        d. Supports a culture of safety without blame.
    2. Institute for Healthcare Improvement (IHI) (www.ihi.org).
        a. Not-for profit-organization founded in 1991 in response to the IOM report, *Crossing the Quality Chasm.*
        b. IHI shares best practices and improvement knowledge through tools and partnerships with health care organizations around the world.
        c. Mission: Improving health care.
            (1) IHI (2012) aims to "improve the lives of patients, the health of communities, and the joy of the health care workforce" by focusing on the following goals:
                (a) Safety.
                (b) Effectiveness.
                (c) Patient-centeredness.
                (d) Timeliness.
                (e) Efficiency.
                (f) Equity.
    3. AHRQ (www.ahrq.gov).
        a. Mission is to improve the quality, safety, efficiency, and cost-effectiveness of health care.

b. Focus and strategic goals:
    (1) The goal of AHRQ research is measurable improvements in health care, gauged in terms of improved quality of life and patient outcomes, lives saved, and value.
    (2) The agency's overall focus is:
        (a) Safety and quality: Reduce the risk of harm by promoting delivery of the best possible health care.
        (b) Effectiveness: Improve health care outcomes by encouraging the use of evidence to make informed health care decisions.
        (c) Efficiency: Transform research into practice to facilitate wider access to effective health care services and reduce unnecessary costs.
c. Programs include *AHRQ Patient Safety Network* (PS Net), a professional informational source for patient safety literature, news, and other resources.
    4. VA National Center for Patient Safety (NCPS) (www.patientsafety.gov).
        a. Established in 1999 by the U.S. Department of Veterans Affairs to develop and nurture a culture of safety throughout the Veterans Health Administration.
        b. Goal is the nationwide reduction and prevention of inadvertent harm to patients as a result of their care.
        c. Components of NCPS include a patient safety awards program, the mandate that all VA contracts include patient-safety performance requirements, and an adverse event reporting system.
    5. Institute for Safe Medication Practices (ISMP) (www.ismp.org/about/mission.asp).
        a. The mission is to advance patient safety by preventing medication errors.
        b. ISMP engages in the following activities:

(1) Collect and analyze reports of medication-related hazardous conditions.

(2) Disseminate timely medication safety information, risk-reduction tools, and error-prevention strategies.

(3) Educate the health care community and consumers about safe medication practices.

(4) Collaborate with other patient safety organizations, educational institutions, governmental agencies, and other health care stakeholders.

(5) Advocate the adoption of safe medication standards.

(6) Conduct research to provide evidence-based safe medication practices.

II. Health Care-Associated Infections: Infection Prevention and Control

A. The basic principles of infection prevention and control will apply to any setting, yet ambulatory care poses some specific challenges due to the patient mix, central waiting rooms, increasing patient acuity, and increases in invasive procedures and services provided in the outpatient setting.

B. The Centers for Disease Control and Prevention (CDC) and the Healthcare Infection Control Practices Advisory Committee (HICPAC) summarized the basic components of an infection control program in ambulatory care in the report *Guide to Infection Prevention in Outpatient Settings: Minimum Expectations for Safe Care* (CDC, 2011).

C. The basic goals of an organization's infection control program are to protect the patient, protect health care workers and others in the health care environment, and to do these in a cost effective manner (Jennings, Friedman, & Wideman, 2005).

D. In the 1980s, the development of "universal precautions" for handling blood and blood products was focused upon protecting the health care worker from bloodborne pathogen exposure.

1. "Standard precautions" were subsequently developed to include other body fluids.

2. Additional components were incorporated to protect patients by ensuring that health care personnel do not carry infectious agents to patients on their hands or via equipment used during patient care.

E. Surveillance.

1. Infection control surveillance is undertaken to:

a. Decrease infection rates and ultimately reduce morbidity, mortality, and cost.

b. Reduce community-acquired infection rates through prevention strategies, including immunization, patient education, and compliance with mandatory reporting.

c. Identify potential clusters or outbreaks.

d. Educate health care personnel regarding risks relevant to their practice.

e. Evaluate and improve infection prevention strategies.

f. Comply with regulatory and accreditation requirements and standards.

2. A surveillance plan will identify indicators, define how and who to collect the data, and describe how the process will be evaluated for effectiveness.

F. Monitoring and reporting health care-associated infections (HAIs).

1. CDC describes Standard Precautions as the minimum infection prevention practices that apply to all patient care, regardless of suspected or confirmed infection status of the patient, in any setting where health care is delivered (Siegel, Rhinehart, Jackson, Chiarello, & The Healthcare Infection Control Practices Advisory Committee, 2007).

2. Standard precautions include:

a. Hand hygiene.

(1) Hand hygiene is essential to reduce the risk of spreading infections in ambulatory care settings.

(2) CDC (2002) and the World Health Organization (WHO) (2009) have both published guidelines and resources for effective hand hygiene programs.

(3) Alcohol-based hand rubs are effective against a broad spectrum of pathogens, and can increase compliance with recommended hand hygiene practices by requiring less time, irritating hands less, and facilitating hand hygiene at the site of patient care.

(4) Soap and water should be used for hand hygiene when hands are visibly soiled (e.g., dirt, blood, body fluids), or after caring for patients with known or suspected infectious diarrhea (e.g., *Clostridium difficile*, norovirus). Rubbing of hands with lather should continue for 20 seconds.

(5) Indications for hand hygiene include before and after touching a patient, before performing a clean or aseptic procedure, after an exposure to blood or body fluids, and after removing gloves.

b. Use of personal protective equipment (PPE) (such as gloves, gowns, masks, respirators, goggles, and face shields).

(1) Intended to protect the wearer from exposure to or contact with infectious agents.

(2) Gloves are worn for potential contact with blood, body fluids, mucus membranes, non-intact skin, or contaminated equipment.

(3) A cover gown is worn to protect skin and clothing where contact with blood or body fluids is anticipated.

(4) Mask, goggles, or a face shield is worn to protect mucus membranes during procedures expected to spray or splash body fluids.

(5) A surgical mask is worn when placing a catheter or injecting into the subdural or epidural space.

c. Safe injection practices.

(1) Practices reduce the risk of infection transmission during the preparation and administration of parenteral medications.

(2) The investigation of four large outbreaks of hepatitis B virus and hepatitis C virus among patients in ambulatory care facilities in the United States from 2000–2002 identified a need to define and reinforce safe injection practices (CDC, 2003).

(3) Complete guidance on safe injection practices can be found in the CDC's *Guideline for Isolation Precautions: Preventing Transmission of Infectious Agents in Healthcare Settings* (Siegel et al., 2007).

d. Safe handling of potentially contaminated equipment or surfaces in the patient environment.

(1) Equipment or items in the patient environment likely to have been contaminated with infectious body fluids must be handled in a manner to prevent transmission of infectious agents.

(2) Personnel should wear gloves for direct contact with potentially contaminated items or surfaces.

(3) Heavily soiled equipment should be contained for transport to another area for cleaning.

(4) Reusable equipment must be properly cleaned and disinfected or sterilized before use on another patient. Items must be cleaned before disinfection or sterilization can occur.

e. Respiratory hygiene/cough etiquette.

(1) Refers to the concept of containing respiratory secretions at the point of origin.

(2) In the clinic setting, patients may be asked to cough into tissues that are placed in the trash after use, followed by hand hygiene.

(3) Patients may be given facemasks to contain secretions.

(4) Supplies for respiratory hygiene and signs directing patients in their use should be placed throughout the outpatient setting.

(5) Patients with respiratory symptoms should be directed to identify themselves to health care personnel so they can be segregated as soon as possible.

III. Regulatory Requirements

A. Health care regulatory and accrediting agencies monitor health care practitioners and facilities, provide information about industry changes, promote safety, and ensure legal compliance and quality services.

1. Federal, state, and local regulatory agencies often establish rules and regulations for the health care industry, and their oversight is mandatory. Some agencies, such as those for accreditation, involve voluntary participation, but are important because they provide rankings or certification of quality.

2. Expectations may vary according to the organization or the particular area within the field.

3. Some ambulatory settings are part of a hospital system and are seen as hospitals for applicable standards; some ambulatory sites are independent and would follow ambulatory standards.

B. Federal and state regulations.

1. Nurse practice acts.

   a. State agencies are empowered by state legislation to enforce the nurse practice act in each state.

   b. The acts vary from state to state.

   c. Nurses must be knowledgeable and follow the regulations outlined in their state's nurse practice act, which defines the scope of practices for nurses.

   d. Most states have an online resource for more details from the respective state's board of nursing.

2. Government and the provision of health services.

   a. The U.S. Department of Health and Human Services (DHHS) is the United States government's principal agency for protecting the health of all Americans and providing essential human services, especially for those who are least able to help themselves. (http://www.hhs.gov/about/). Agencies within DHHS include:

      (1) Administration for Children and Families (ACF).

      (2) Administration on Aging (AoA).

      (3) Agency for Healthcare Research and Quality (AHRQ).

      (4) Agency for Toxic Substances and Disease Registry (ATSDR).

      (5) Centers for Disease Control and Prevention (CDC).

      (6) Centers for Medicare & Medicaid Services (CMS).

      (7) Food and Drug Administration (FDA).

      (8) Health Resources and Services Administration (HRSA).

      (9) Indian Health Service (IHS).

      (10) National Institutes of Health (NIH).

      (11) Program Support Center (PSC).

      (12) Substance Abuse and Mental Health Services Administration (SAMHSA).

   b. CMS administers the Medicare program and works in partnership with the states to administer Medicaid, the State Children's Health Insurance Program (SCHIP), and health insurance portability standards.

      (1) Medicare is a social insurance program for people age 65 and older and for some disabled people under 65 years of age.

(2) The Medicaid program rules and resources vary from state to state and from group to group, but are generally limited to coverage for pregnant women, children and adolescents, and individuals who are elderly, blind, or disabled.

(3) The CMS Conditions of Participation (COPs) are part of the Code of Federal Regulations (http://www.access.gpo.gov/nara/cfr/waisidx_04/42cfr482_04.html). Sections of the Conditions of Participation include (but are not limited to):

   (a) Patients' rights.

   (b) Quality assessment and performance improvement.

   (c) Nursing services.

   (d) Medical record services.

   (e) Pharmaceutical services.

   (f) Laboratory services.

   (g) Food and dietetic services.

   (h) Utilization review.

   (i) Physical environment.

   (j) Infection control.

c. The FDA is responsible for the oversight of drugs, medical devices, vaccines, blood products, and biologics; establishing rules for testing; clinical trials; and approval of new products. The FDA monitors safety, medical errors, and adverse reactions to treatment, and alerts the health care industry of risks associated with treatments.

d. The Occupational Safety & Health Administration (OSHA) is the enforcement arm of the Occupational Safety and Health Act, signed into law in 1970.

(1) OSHA sets workplace safety and health standards, and inspects workplaces for compliance with those standards. The employer has responsibilities, as does the employee. Below are the responsibilities of the employer. Detailed information is available on the OSHA Web site (http://osha.gov).

(2) Employers have certain responsibilities under the Occupational Safety and Health Act of 1970. The following list is a summary of the most important ones.

   (a) Provide a workplace free from serious recognized hazards and comply with standards, rules, and regulations issued under OSHA.

   (b) Examine workplace conditions to make sure they conform to applicable OSHA standards.

   (c) Make sure employees have and use safe tools and equipment, and properly maintain this equipment.

   (d) Use color codes, posters, labels, or signs to warn employees of potential hazards.

   (e) Establish or update operating procedures and communicate them so that employees follow safety and health requirements.

   (f) Provide medical examinations and training of employees when required by OSHA standards.

   (g) Post the OSHA poster (or the state-plan equivalent) at a prominent location within the workplace, informing employees of their rights and responsibilities.

   (h) Report any fatal accident or one that results in the hospitalization of three or more employees to the nearest OSHA office within eight hours.

   (i) Keep records of work-related injuries and illnesses. (Note: Employers with 10 or fewer employees and employers in certain low-hazard industries are exempt from this requirement.)

(j) Provide employees, former employees, and their representatives access to the Log of Work-Related Injuries and Illnesses (OSHA Form 300).

(k) Provide access to employee medical records and exposure records to employees or their authorized representatives.

(l) Provide the OSHA compliance officer the names of authorized employee representatives who may be asked to accompany the compliance officer during an inspection.

(m) Do not discriminate against employees who exercise their rights under the Act.

(n) Post OSHA citations at or near the work area involved. Each citation must remain posted until the violation has been corrected, or for three working days, whichever is longer. Post abatement verification documents or tags.

(o) Correct cited violations by the deadline set in the OSHA citation and submit required abatement verification documentation.

IV. Accreditation Agencies

A. The Joint Commission, previously the Joint Commission on Accreditation of Healthcare Organizations (JCAHO) (www.jointcommission.org).

1. The Joint Commission's mission is to continuously improve health care for the public by evaluating health care organizations and inspiring them to excel in providing safe and effective care of the highest quality and value.

2. Quality standards were first adopted between 1979 and 1981. Since then, standards have been regularly modified and performance improvement language has been integrated, as well as standards and elements of performance to improve organization-wide patient safety and quality of care processes.

3. The Joint Commission evaluates and accredits more than 19,000 health care organizations and programs in the United States. These organizations represent a variety of settings, including:
   a. Ambulatory health care.
   b. Behavioral health care.
   c. Critical access hospital.
   d. Home care.
   e. Hospital.
   f. Laboratory.
   g. Long-term care.

4. Accreditation standards are evaluated by survey on a three-year cycle, but in mid-cycle, the organization also assesses its own compliance in the Periodic Performance Review (PPR).

5. The following are general chapters that contain elements of performance; chapters may vary according to setting:
   a. Environment of care (EC).
   b. Emergency management (EM).
   c. Human resources (HR).
   d. Infection prevention and control (IC).
   e. Information management (IM).
   f. Leadership (LD).
   g. Medical staff (MS).
   h. Medication management (MM).
   i. National Patient Safety Goals (NPSGs).
   j. Nursing (NR).
   k. Provision of care, treatment, and services (PC).
   l. Performance improvement (PI).
   m. Rights and responsibilities of the individual (RI).
   n. Waived testing (RIEC).

6. National Patient Safety Goals (The Joint Commission, 2011) are a series of specific actions that organizations accredited by The Joint Commission are required to meet with the purpose of preventing medical errors and improving processes for patient safety.

a. National Patient Safety Goals are reviewed, refined, or modified, and published each year, and are a critical component of The Joint Commission's overall standards of safe, high-quality care.

b. Many are derived from the root causes of reported serious events, called sentinel events.

c. Accredited organizations are evaluated for continuous compliance with the elements of performance associated with the National Patient Safety Goals.

d. The current goals are available online (The Joint Commission, 2011). The topic areas for the 2011 National Patient Safety Goals include:
   (1) Identify patients correctly.
   (2) Use medicines safely.
   (3) Maintain and communicate patient medicines.
   (4) Prevent infection.
   (5) Prevent mistakes in surgery.

7. The Joint Commission's Disease-Specific Care Certification Program is designed to evaluate clinical programs across the continuum of care. Organizations accredited by The Joint Commission may seek certification for many chronic diseases or conditions. A list of certified programs includes (but is not limited to):
   a. Acute coronary syndrome.
   b. Alzheimer's disease.
   c. Asthma (pediatric).
   d. Brain injury rehabilitation.
   e. Breast cancer.
   f. Cardiac rehabilitation.
   g. Chemical dependency.

8. The Joint Commission has developed an advanced level of certification in five clinical areas. These programs must meet the requirements for Disease-Specific Care Certification plus additional, clinically specific requirements and expectations.

9. Certification by The Joint Commission is required by CMS for hospitals seeking reimbursement for lung volume reduction surgery and ventricular assist devices.

10. The Joint Commission Nursing Advisory Council was established to counsel The Joint Commission on present and evolving nursing-related issues that are affecting health care quality and patient safety. The council provides input to The Joint Commission on initiatives that affect the nursing profession.

B. National Committee for Quality Assurance (NCQA) (www.ncqa.org).

1. Works in partnership with managed care organizations, health care purchasers, state regulators, and consumers to develop standards and performance measures that effectively evaluate the structure and functions of medical and quality management systems in managed care organizations.

2. Healthcare Effectiveness Data and Information Set (HEDIS®) is a tool used by more than 90% of America's health plans to measure performance on important dimensions of care and service. These measures include goals specific to adults and children.

3. Many health plans report HEDIS data to employers and consumer groups, and use their results to make improvements in their quality of care and service or select the best health plan for their needs.

4. Consumers can access comprehensive HEDIS data through the State of Health Care Quality report, a comprehensive look at the performance of the nation's health care system.

5. The HEDIS Measures are divided into 5 areas:
   a. Effectiveness of care.
   b. Access/availability of care.
   c. Satisfaction with the experience of care.
   d. Use of services.
   e. Cost of care.

6. Patient-Centered Medical Home – NCQA's initial Physician Practice Connections® – Patient-Centered Medical Home™ (PPC-PCMH) (2008) program reflects the input of the American College of Physicians, American Academy of Family Physicians, American Academy of Pediatrics, Ameri-

can Osteopathic Association, and others in the revision of Physician Practice Connections to assess whether physician practices are functioning as medical homes.

C. Other accrediting agencies (non-exclusive list).
1. American Osteopathic Association (AOA): Osteopathic hospitals.
2. Community Health Accreditation Program, Inc. (CHAP), a subsidiary of the National League of Nursing: Home care and community health organizations.
3. Accreditation Commission for Health Care, Inc. (ACHC): Home care services.
4. The Accreditation Association for Ambulatory Health Care (AAAHC): A private, non-profit agency that offers voluntary, peer-based review of the quality of health care services of ambulatory health organizations, including ambulatory and surgery centers, managed care organizations, as well as Indian and student health centers, among others (AAAHC, 2012). AAAHC offers a program for accreditation for those organizations seeking Medical Home certification.

D. Additional resources.
1. Publicly reported quality data on the Web.
   a. HealthGrades (www.healthgrades.com).
   b. Hospital Compare (www.hospitalcompare.hhs.gov).
   c. Joint Commission Quality Check (http://www.jointcommission.org).
   d. The Leapfrog Group (www.leapfroggroup.org).
   e. 2012 Accreditation Handbook for Ambulatory Health Care designed for ambulatory care organizations seeking AAAHC accreditation.
   f. HEDIS 2011 Volume 2 – A resource for anyone involved in collecting, calculating, or submitting data.
   g. HEDIS 2011 Volume 3 – Complete instructions for administering all the survey-based HEDIS Measures, including surveys from the Consumer Assessment of Healthcare Providers.

2. Recommendation for the components of an infection prevention program can be found from the CDC.
   a. Immunization of Healthcare Workers, 1997.
   b. Guidelines for Preventing the Transmission of *Mycobacterium tuberculosis* in Health-Care Settings, 2005.
   c. Hand Hygiene in Healthcare Settings, 2002.
   d. Sharps Safety for Healthcare Settings.
   e. Guideline for Isolation Precautions: Preventing Transmission of Infectious Agents in Healthcare Settings, 2007.
   f. Guide to Infection Prevention in Outpatient Settings: Minimum Expectations for Safe Care.

References

Accreditation Association for Ambulatory Health Care (AAAHC). (2012). *About AAAHC.* Retrieved from http://www.aaahc.org/en/about

Agency for Healthcare Research and Quality (AHRQ). (2005). *AHRQ patient safety network (PSNet).* Retrieved from http://psnet.ahrq.gov/primer.aspx?primerID=5

Centers for Disease Control and Prevention (CDC). (2002). *Guideline for hand hygiene in health-care settings.* Retrieved from http://www.cdc.gov/mmwr/preview/mmwrhtml/rr5116a1.htm

Centers for Disease Control and Prevention (CDC). (2003). Transmission of hepatitis B and C viruses in outpatient settings — New York, Oklahoma, and Nebraska, 2000-2002. *MMWR Morbidity and Mortality Weekly Report, 52*(38), 901-906.

Centers for Disease Control and Prevention (CDC). (2011). *Guide to infection prevention in outpatient settings: Minimum expectations for safe care.* Retrieved from http://www.cdc.gov/HAI/pdfs/guidelines/Ambulatory-Care-04-2011.pdf

Emanuel, L., Berwick, D., Conway, J., Combes, J., Hatlie, M., Leape, L., ... Walton, M. (2008). *What exactly is patient safety?* Retrieved from http://www.ahrq.gov/downloads/pub/advances2/vol1/Advances-Emanuel-Berwick_110.pdf

Institute for Healthcare Improvement (IHI). (2012). *Vision and values.* Retrieved from http://www.ihi.org/about/Pages/IHIVisionAndValues.aspx

Institute of Medicine (IOM). (2000). *To err is human: Building a safer health system.* Washington, DC: The National Academies Press.

Institute of Medicine (IOM). (2001). *Crossing the quality chasm: A new health system for the 21st century.* Washington, DC: The National Academies Press.

Institute of Medicine (IOM). (2003). *Keeping patients safe: Transforming the environment for nurses.* Washington, DC: The National Academies Press.

Institute of Medicine (IOM). (2010). *The future of nursing: Leading change, advancing health.* Washington, DC: The National Academies Press.

International Nuclear Safety Advisory Group. (1999). *Basic safety principles for nuclear power plants.* Retrieved from http://www-pub.iaea.org/MTCD/publications/PDF/P082_scr.pdf

Jennings, J.A., Friedman, C., & Wideman, J.M. (2005). Ambulatory care. In *APIC text of infection control and epidemiology* (2nd ed., pp. 50-1-50-9). Washington, DC: Association for Professionals in Infection Control and Epidemiology.

Joint Commission, The. (2011). *National Patient Safety Goals.* Retrieved from http://www.jcrinc.com/National-Patient-Safety-Goals/

Leape, L.L. (1994). Error in medicine. *Journal of the American Medical Association, 272*(23), 1851-1857.

Leape, L.L. (1997, October 12). *Testimony.* United States Congress, House Committee on Veterans' Affairs.

Marx, D. (2009). *Patient safety and the just culture.* Retrieved from http://www.myvbch.org/documents/MarxPresentation.pdf

National Committee for Quality Assurance (NCQA). (2008). *Standards and guidelines for Physician Practice Connections® – Patient-Centered Medical Home™ (PPC-PCMH).* Washington, DC: Author.

National Patient Safety Foundation. (n.d.). *Mission and vision.* Retrieved from http://www.npsf.org/about-us/mission-and-vision/

Reason, J. (1997). *Managing the risks of organizational acidents.* Hampshire, England: Ashgate Publishing Limited.

Siegel, J.D., Rhinehart, E., Jackson, M., Chiarello, L., & The Healthcare Infection Control Practices Advisory Committee. (2007). *Guideline for isolation precautions: Preventing transmission of infectious agents in healthcare settings.* Retrieved from http://www.cdc.gov/hicpac/pdf/isolation/isolation2007.pdf

U.S. Department of Veterans Affairs. (2011). *Patient safety: Get involved!* Retrieved from http://www.patientsafety.gov/patients.html

World Health Organization (WHO). (2009). *WHO guidelines on hand hygiene in health care.* Retrieved from http://whqlibdoc.who.int/publications/2009/9789241597906_eng.pdf

Additional Readings

Agency for Healthcare Research and Quality (AHRQ). (2010, September). *At a glance.* AHRQ Publication No. 09-P003. Rockville, MD: Author.

Flin, R., Mearns, K., O'Connor, P., & Bryden, R. (2000). Measuring safety climate: Identifying the common features. *Safety Science, 34,* 177-192.

Langley, G.L., Nolan, K.M., Nolan, T.W., Norman, C.L., & Provost, L.P. (2009). *The improvement guide: A practical approach to enhancing organizational performance.* San Francisco: Jossey-Bass Publishers.

Leape, L.L. (2009). Errors in medicine. *Clinica Chimica Acta, 404*(1), 2-5.

Chapter 8

Patient Advocacy and Use of Community Resources

E. Mary Johnson, BSN, RN-BC, NE-BC

OBJECTIVES – *Study of the information in this chapter will enable the learner to:*

1. Describe the context of ethical concepts and advocacy behavior in nursing practice.
2. Discuss applications of health promotion and planning for care delivery for differing health status of population groups (such as well, acutely ill, chronically ill, and terminally ill patients).
3. Discuss the changing landscape of health care delivery in the 21st century, including vulnerable patient populations (such as homeless persons, abuse victims, and immigrants).
4. Describe features of customer-focused care in ambulatory health care.

KEY POINTS – *The major points in this chapter include:*

1. Advocacy is a core concept in professional nursing, historically and in contemporary times.
2. Ethical principles and advocacy behaviors are connected concepts and values that direct the actions of individuals, decisions of management groups, and the mission and values of health care systems.
3. Pending health care reform will require increased engagement and knowledge for ambulatory nurses to successfully help patients and families become partners in their health care decisions and outcomes of care.
4. Partnerships with community resources will become increasingly more important in helping support and promote continuity of care of everyone, including vulnerable and high-risk populations.

In recent years, nurses have come to recognize and better understand that the current health care delivery system has changed direction, including preventive care models focused on improving the health status of the patient populations they serve and treat on a daily basis. A greater awareness of influential forces that underlie health care and its societal context has been emerging in the course of the first decade of this new century. These emerging changes pose difficult challenges, but they are not insurmountable (American Nurses Association [ANA], 2010).

Virtually all nurses understand and support the concept of advocacy for improved health care to all populations. Ambulatory nurses recognize that decisions made at multiple levels ultimately affect the lives of their patients and all citizens – at the institutional level where nurses are employed, at the community level where they live, and at the state and federal legislative levels of this country. They also recognize that advocacy begins at the grass roots level of ambulatory practice and extends into the community.

Nurses are aware that patients and their families can feel quite vulnerable when illness is diagnosed and outcomes are uncertain. This is often combined with a limited view and understanding of how the health care delivery system actually functions. This delivery system can be difficult to navigate (e.g., testing sequencing, pre-op testing requirements, repeat authorizations necessary for some treatment or procedure plans, referrals to multiple specialties). While the explosion of technology has made increased knowledge about specific diseases and possibilities for treatment available, it has also contributed to the confusion about what is the "right" course of treatment for the individual seeking health care. For example, credible and reliable health care sources provide conflicting guidelines for screening mammography for women, and multiple treatment modalities and options are available for diagnosed prostate cancer care. These and other examples offer opportunities in which ambulatory nurses can advocate for patients, providing education that respects and empowers individual decisions about health care. Nurses are in the unique position of understanding both the language of medicine and the clinical practice model of health care delivery. It is the combination of these two key processes that provides a strong base for patient advocacy, and it is precisely those same processes that often create confusion and anxiety on the part of the patients and families.

The relationship between the patient and the health care team has been described as fiduciary, meaning a relationship built on a public confidence involving trust. This trust is translated by the public (patients) to mean that the health care team will act in the best interest of the patient. It is within this trust and commitment as a profession that nursing frames decision-making and advocacy behaviors in response to the needs of patients and families. The accepted principles of biomedical ethics include the concept that professionals must possess the knowledge, skill, and diligence to uphold the moral and legal standards of due care. Understanding how the nursing profession performs this role through ethical decision-making and advocacy behaviors is fundamental to the nursing practice in ambulatory care (Johnson, 2000). Ambulatory nurses are required to have a sound personal and professional ethical code (American Academy of Ambulatory Care Nursing [AAACN], 2010).

Ethical and advocacy principles are connected through a framework of accepted concepts and actions to be taken by individuals and/or professional organizations. The mission of AAACN is to "advance the art and science of ambulatory care nursing" (AAACN, 2011b). A significant contribution toward meeting this mission is the publishing and

timely revisions of the AAACN (2010) *Scope and Standards of Practice for Professional Ambulatory Care Nursing*. This publication delineates the scope and standards for professional ambulatory practice, as well as defining the conceptual framework of ambulatory nursing practice (AAACN, 2010). Within this document, standards include specific reference to role knowledge and skill dimension of advocacy for all patient populations (standards guide ethical practice and patient advocacy) (AAACN, 2010). Philosophically and organizationally, these public documents are congruent with nursing's commitment as a profession.

Current practice has seen ambulatory nurses' advocacy role expand and evolve into a role that is better described as that of a "patient navigator" in health care systems. While acknowledging the increasing complexity and uncertainty of how health care delivery systems function, this type of role and service will take on increased importance and will best be performed by ambulatory care nurses. Ideally, this role combines engaging and educating the patient/family, accessing internal care resources, and partnering with available community services to provide coordination and continuity of care for patients and families. In addition to appropriate access to care, reasonable cost of care delivery and high quality of care are features of customer-focused care in the ambulatory health care setting.

I. Historical and Professional Context of Patient Advocacy

A. According to Virginia Henderson (1961), the definition of nursing is "to assist the individual, sick or well, in the performance of those activities contributing to health or its recovery (or to a peaceful death) that he would perform unaided if he had the necessary strength, will, or knowledge, and to do this in such a way as to help him gain independence as rapidly as possible" (p. 42).

B. The nursing profession is:
1. An essential part of society.
2. Dynamic and reflects the changing nature of societal need.
3. "Owned by society" in the sense that a "profession acquires recognition, relevance, and even meaning in terms of its re-

lationship to that society, its culture and institutions, and its other members" (Henderson, 1961, p. 2).

4. Fundamentally respectful of the inherent worth, dignity, and human right of every individual (ANA, 2010).

C. Authority for the practice of nursing is based upon:
  1. A social contract that acknowledges professional rights and responsibilities, as well as mechanisms for public accountability (ANA, 2001).
    a. Specific, concise statement of moral obligations and duties of everyone who enters nursing.
    b. Non-negotiable ethical standard.
    c. Expression of nursing's understanding of its commitment to society (Fowler, 2010).
  2. Specific state nurse practice acts.
  3. Accepted standards of practice.
  4. Relevant federal and state laws and regulatory standards.
  5. Organizational policies (AAACN, 2011a).

D. People seek the services of nurses:
  1. To assist with improving health and/or seek care for health-related problems (AAACN, 2011a).
  2. To obtain information, education, and treatment related to health and illness.
  3. To identify both short- and long-term health outcomes and goals.
  4. To act as advocates for individuals dealing with barriers encountered in obtaining health care (ANA, 2001).

E. Performance of an advocacy role in ambulatory is exercised through:
  1. Understanding customer-focused care features.
    a. Encounters are initiated by patient.
    b. The patient's expectation of the system is to provide quality care at a reasonable cost.
    c. Care providers are accountable.
  2. Providing access to care.
  3. Providing ongoing assessment and evaluation of patient.
  4. Collaborating and participating in coordination of care.

5. Educating and valuing informed decision-making by the patient, such as through educating the patient about the range of options of care (e.g., for prostate cancer – watchful waiting, radiation, surgery, drug therapy, or combination of interventions).
6. Supporting mechanisms that assist in measuring patient satisfaction and responding appropriately to these data.
7. Participating in risk management programs and initiatives at all levels of practice.
    a. Accountability.
    b. Transparency.
8. Moral courage of the individual nurse (Lachman, 2010).

F. AAACN's *Scope and Standards of Practice for Professional Ambulatory Care Nursing* (2010) includes measurement criteria that state nursing staff members will:
  1. Actively engage in identifying and resolving the ethical concerns of patients, colleagues, or systems.
  2. Advocate for informed decision-making by the patient/family or legally designated representative.
    a. Ensure that patients have opportunities to voice opinions regarding care and services received, and have these issues reviewed and resolved without fear of recrimination.
    b. Educate and support patients in developing skills for self-efficacy.

G. AAACN's *Definition of Professional Ambulatory Care Nursing* (2011a) includes:
  1. Promoting patient advocacy.
  2. Acting as partners and advisors, and assisting and supporting patients and families to optimally manage their health care.

H. The relationship between a nurse and patient involves full and active participation of the patient and the nurse in the plan of care, and occurs within the context of the values and beliefs of the patient and the nurse. The same values and assumptions apply when the recipient of nursing is a family or community (ANA, 2010).

I. The ethical principle of autonomy reinforces this partnership based on trust and respect. This core principle represents the foundation of professional nurses' practice.

II. Linkage of Advocacy, Ethics, Nursing Ethics, and Risk Management

A. Advocacy – Public support for or recommendation of a particular cause of policy (Dictionary.com, 2012); act or process of advocating or supporting (a cause or proposal) on behalf of another (Steinmetz, 1997). The AAACN conceptual framework defines advocacy as compassion, caring, emotional support that is culturally competent and relevant to the patient's age (AAACN, 2010).

B. Ethics – A branch of philosophy dealing with the values related to human conduct, with respect to the rightness or wrongness of certain actions, and to the goodness and badness of the motives and ends of such actions; a set of moral principles or values, the principles of conduct governing an individual or a group (Steinmetz, 1997).

C. Nursing ethics – Involves choosing between two or more options, none of which may be totally desirable, to guide actions within the nurse's scope of practice (Gold, 2006).

D. Risk management – An organization-wide program to identify risks, control occurrences, prevent damage, and control legal liability. It is a process whereby risks to the institution are evaluated and controlled (Velianoff & Hobbs, 2000).
   1. Universal Protocol, "Do Not Use" List of Abbreviations, Patient Satisfaction, Electronic Medical Record, and the National Patient Safety Goals (NPSGs) by the Joint Commission (2011) correspond to risk management practices within organizations.
   2. Shared governance councils can offer an opportunity for identifying issues, reducing risk, and promoting patient advocacy at the unit level.

E. The linkage of ethics and advocacy principles for ambulatory nursing practice is in recognizing (understanding) that ethics provides a conceptual framework and advocacy provides opportunity for appropriate actions (behaviors) in implementing decisions made on behalf of patients.

1. A complex balance of learned principles and rules (justice, respect for autonomy) and learned professional values and virtues (health, well-being, and independence) exists (Fowler, 2010).
2. "Moral courage" is an essential skill required of nurses. Moral courage involves the individual's capacity to overcome fear and stand up for his or her core values and ethical obligations. Acting morally requires knowledge of professional ethical obligations (Lachman, 2010).
3. Organizational advocacy is identified through risk management activities combined with leadership actions that seek to support improving organizational performance (IOP) initiatives that are focused on quality outcomes, patient safety, and safe working environment.

III. Present Context of Patient Advocacy
The present day social-political environment of the health care system presents challenges on many fronts that require advocacy for patient/family.

A. Scientific advancement in medicine in past decade.
   1. Potential availability and application of advancements. Examples include:
      a. Human genome project leading to identifying specific treatment options for individuals.
      b. Improved transplantation options.
      c. Research protocols.
      d. Microscopic endoscopy applications.
      e. Virtual clinics.
      f. Expanded laproscopic and robotic surgery.
      g. eMedicine, such as the program at Cleveland Clinic in which second opinion is done without seeing the actual patient, based on specific data points collected by ambulatory nurses and reviewed by expert physician staff.

B. Allocation and rationing of medical advancements can occur as a result of:
   1. Geographic location.
   2. Cost containment pressure.
   3. Provider(s)' expertise and competence.

4. Provider(s)' satisfaction with reimbursement available for care provided by the patient's coverage plan.
5. Political/legislative mandates, such as individual state's decisions about type of services to be provided to their residents if they are paying under Medicaid (e.g., not providing abortion, not paying for selected drugs due to cost, or other expensive treatments).
6. Institutional decision(s) that consider cost/benefit analysis about specific therapies and experimental procedures investing in new program development. Incorporated within this analysis needs to be a process for adjudicating leadership decisions when different insurance plans deny or limit certain care to patients, or when transferring care to differing institution would be more appropriate.

C. Financial issues.
1. Governmental initiatives/decisions.
   a. Medicare/Medicaid programs: Promotion of managed care systems to elderly and poverty-level populations. The traditional Medicare program is a modified fee-for-service base. Payment amounts are limited, but access to providers is not.
   b. Omnibus Reconciliation Bill of 2010 (COBRA): Offers premium assistance to cover workers involuntarily terminated (in response to high unemployment in the country at that time) (Maximus, Inc., 2011).
   c. Corporate compliance: The health care industry continues to develop and implement systematic processes for measuring adherence to internal and external indicators of standards of care and regulatory bodies. Institutional oversight for measuring and improving processes is required (such as insurance plan criteria, research activities, billing practices).
   d. Pay-for-performance measures: Reimbursement structures based on outcomes (such as pressure sores,

hospital readmission rates, absence of never events). These measures are progressively increasing the demand for access to ambulatory care services (see Chapter 2, "The Ambulatory Care Practice Arena," and Chapter 4, "Health Care Fiscal Management").
   (1) Established goals for individual or institutional performance being rewarded (financial and/or other incentives).
   (2) Preventive care for Medicaid population receiving increased payments.
   (3) Medicare payments to include selected preventive services (e.g., Welcome to Medicare preventive visit) (Haas, 2011a).
   (4) Accountable care organizations (ACOs), patient-centered medical homes (PCMHs), electronic medical records (EMRs), meaningful use.

D. Private sector insurers.
1. Fee-for-service market is experiencing higher individual cost; this type of insurance plan has allowed for more choices by individuals about health care options. Represents a decreasing percentage of health care insurance product offering in the current environment.
2. Proliferation of managed care insurance products, which have become increasingly more standard throughout the country, including high-risk Medicare and Medicaid HMO plans.
   a. Failure of these ventures has also occurred, resulting in decreased access for Medicare and Medicaid populations.
   b. HMOs' decision-making/approval processes can create a moral dilemma for health care providers. Differing managed care plan offerings exist, and the decision about what is offered is generally the employer's choice. These plans often outline a decision-making process about when and what testing

and consulting services may be implemented. These protocols are designed using algorithms (associated with specific symptoms/disease management guidelines). Appeal processes exist for challenged or denied services.

E. Business sector issues.

1. Budget constraints exist for health care dollar.

   a. Increased co-pays, putting coverage at risk.

   b. Institutions' evaluation and decisions about insurance plans options offered to employees are based on shared risk and responsibility. Increasingly, employers are offering case management for "at risk" employees with selected diagnoses (such as diabetes, asthma, hypertension).

   c. Employers' hiring decisions may include an assessment of health status of potential candidates (such as history of smoking, morbid obesity).

   d. Employers are offering preventive/ wellness-focused programs for employees/ families, often partnering with available community resources (such as Weight Watchers®, Silver Sneakers®, and smoking cessation programs).

   e. Employees may decide to delay seeking health care due to fear, cost, or access, putting health at risk.

   f. Demand for quality outcomes of insured employees requires health care agency accountability for care.

   g. Operational challenges, including redesign of ambulatory care operations practice patterns, result from of the expansion of safety initiatives and the compressed length of stay (LOS) in hospital environments.

F. Political response to today's health care market focuses on recognizing and providing solutions involving:

1. Evaluating eligibility criteria and securing long-term funding of Medicare/Medicaid programs and the Patient Protection and Affordable Care Act (PPACA) (Haas, 2011b).

2. Evaluating programs for effectiveness and efficiencies, including:

   a. Defining clinical outcomes.

   b. Application of professional practice guidelines.

   c. Ensuring ongoing, documented performance improvement processes and measurement. For example, failure, mode, and effects (FME) process encourages a proactive review of new services/program before implementing (organized worry).

3. Understand the focus of PPACA.

   a. Health insurance reform.

   b. Health promotion, wellness, and quality health care.

   c. Enhancing access to safe, quality health care (Haas, 2011b).

4. Recognition of the aging U.S. population, demographics, and effect on health care systems.

5. Providing solutions involving Patient's Bill of Rights – Patient/family has the right to have complaints reviewed (The Joint Commission, 2010).

6. Responding to the rising number of uninsured and underinsured Americans (approximately 49.9 million uninsured, 50 million underinsured in 2010) (DeNavas-Walt, Proctor, & Smith, 2011; Robert Wood Johnson Foundation, 2009).

7. Concern by the American population about inability of U.S. to afford health care reform (Haas, 2011b).

G. Performance improvement is required on an ongoing basis.

1. Evaluation begins with patient rights/ responsibilities (autonomy).

2. Balance between cost and quality of care delivered (justice).

3. Nursing identification of and participation in the evaluation of performance improvement activities.

4. External review and regulatory agencies.

5. Internal review systems, including risk management program(s), are integrated into improving organizational performance (The Joint Commission, 2010) (see Chapter 7, "Patient Safety and Regulatory Standards in Ambulatory Care," and Chapter 11, "Evidence-Based Practice and Performance Improvement").

IV. **Implementing Advocacy for Patients/Families**

Advocating for patients and their families is most effective when linked to education about both health/disease management and the health care system itself.

A. Empowerment of the patient and family to make informed decisions.
1. Until early 1990s, health care providers often encouraged patients to have symptoms evaluated through an office visit. This system did little to affirm and reassure the decision-making of patients and families, often promoting a sense of vulnerability on the part of patients/families.
2. Education and understanding of nurses about health care reform initiatives under PPACA is important to their ability to assist patients/families.
3. In 1992, the American Hospital Association stated in *A Patient's Bill of Rights* that effective health care requires collaboration between patients and physicians and other health care professionals, moving toward partnership between providers and patients/families.
4. This shift recognizes the reality of care being episodic in nature and typically provided by patient and/or family between encounters with the health care system.
   a. Requires education of patients/families to evaluate and manage illnesses through a combination of self-care, telephone management, and office visits.
   b. Requires education of patient/family to support their ability to assimilate, interpret, and evaluate information for decision-making, such as through "Speak Up" initiatives and "smart patient" (The Joint Commission, 2010).
   c. Recommends providing access through Internet technology to information to enhance the patient's/family's understanding of basic disease process(es) and treatment options (Sennett, 2000). The Internet can also provide incorrect health information that can influence patient decision-making and outcomes of care.

B. Clinical operations must be designed to safely respond to new program offerings and be appropriately monitored.
1. Creating clinical operations focused on specific patient population with specific diagnosis to provide comprehensive care to meet needs (such as bariatric clinics, spine centers, stroke programs).
2. Offering flexible hours for delivery of services (for example, primary care and specialty care clinics open seven days per week, independent advanced practice nurse practices, onsite health care offered by employers 24/7).

C. Nurses' role in advocacy behaviors is based on:
1. Assessment of patient status (well, acutely ill, chronically ill, or terminally ill).
2. Needs, including increased awareness of abuse issues, domestic violence, elder, and child.
3. NPSGs (The Joint Commission, 2011).
4. Reassessment, recognition, decision-making, and organizational systems are available to provide care are essential elements of nursing assessment.

D. Advocacy skills required include:
1. Expert clinical assessment skills – Recognizing different types of health promotion.
2. Critical thinking and analysis to formulate a plan of care with patients.
   a. Understanding disease processes, disease management, health literacy, family dynamics, and organizational and community resources.
   b. Understanding basic survival skills in disease management.

c. Understanding of scope of practice as defined by the state board of nursing rules and regulations of professional practice.

d. Recognized rules and regulations of aligned health care providers who contribute to patient care services (e.g., state pharmacy boards, medical boards).

3. Recognition and appropriate response to changes in system(s) that create risk to patient/family or staff.

4. Ability to provide operational accountability for continuity and coordination of services (AAACN, 2011a).

5. Expert intervention skills.

a. Assisting patients and families with lifestyle skills: Current adaptation to health challenges.

b. Health promotion: Proactive, holistic approach to lifestyle.
(1) Primary prevention: Wellness promotion.
(2) Secondary prevention (early detection, diagnosis, and treatment).
(3) Tertiary prevention, recovery and rehabilitation, and specific measures to minimize disability and increase function (see Chapter 17, "Care of the Well Client").

6. Continued learning about implications of health care reform (such as Health Care and You [www.healthcareandyou.org], Commonwealth Fund [www.commonwealthfund.org/Health-Reform.aspx], *How Health Care Reform Really Works* [video from Ellen-Marie Whelan, Center for American Progress]) (Haas, 2011b).

7. Operational accountability for continuity and coordination of services.

a. Communications skills to partner with patients/families/health care team.

b. Knowledge of systems to coordinate care across service lines/institutions/community to provide continuity.
(1) Increased outreach efforts within the community (e.g., free mammography screening, influenza vaccine immunization at schools and churches).
(2) Health fairs offering screening/education, retail malls offering exercise opportunities, and kiosk education to individuals.
(3) Creation of primary/urgent care clinics in pharmacies/retail stores, with advanced practice nurses as primary providers.
(4) Federal programs that support local community outreach (such as Homeless Emergency and Rapid Transition to Housing [HEARTH] Act) that coordinate and provide services for vulnerable populations (such as homeless individuals, abuse victims, individuals with mental illness, individuals with AIDS). Programs are designed to provide basic wrap-around services at the local level, and have required reporting of data and progress at specific intervals to state and federal agencies (Homeless Management Information Systems [HMIS]).

8. Awareness and sensitivity of the fiscal impact of care decisions.

E. Nurse plays central role in working with patients/families to assure they receive:
1. Right access.
2. Right provider.
3. Right time frame.
4. Right level of care.

F. Patient satisfaction measurement is a subjective data collection that responds to the perception of care delivered, understanding that perception is reality to the patient.
1. Measurement indicators and processes.
a. Patient survey feedback in a timely fashion at provider level, unit level, and institutional level.
b. Accreditation agencies review findings and institutional response to these findings.

c. Third party payers' evaluations of care provided direct contracting with specific health care institutions to provide selected services for their insured members – Identified "centers of excellence" based on outcomes data (such as Lowe's Cardiac Surgery nationwide program contracted to Cleveland Clinic).

2. Complaint resolution process. Service recovery programs that resolve issues when the patient expresses concern/complaints. Units/institutions need to create an atmosphere of objectivity and specific processes for this to happen – Recognizing own values and biases of health care personnel.

3. Performance improvement activities at the unit level improving processes based upon patient feedback (such as improving access and wait times).

4. Employee engagement and workplace satisfaction evaluation.

G. Techniques for promoting advocacy and positive patient relations.

1. Acknowledge individuality and autonomy.
2. Acknowledge issues and responsibilities.
3. Be aware of verbal and non-verbal behaviors.
4. Provide and support service recovery programs (proactive approach to problem identification and resolution).
   a. Formal Ombudsman program.
   b. Service recovery programs.
   c. Patient service navigators – Liaison to patient/family during health care delivery process.
   d. Institutional Web site aimed at educating the public about nursing's professional role and responsibilities involving patient care.

V. Future Advocacy Opportunities for Nurses in Ambulatory Care

A. Challenge to advocate related to:
1. Increasing complexity of presenting patients.
2. Awareness of vulnerable populations, such as:

a. Homeless persons.
b. Minorities.
c. Addicted persons.
d. Immigrants.
e. Women and children in impoverished conditions.
f. Mentally ill persons.
g. Returning military.
h. Victims of domestic violence, elder abuse, or child abuse.
i. Unemployed.

B. Evolving community partnership(s) to identify, understand, and coordinate resources for specific vulnerable populations (such as Explorys [www.explorysmedical.com], Northeast Ohio Patient Navigation Collaborative [NEOPNC], Cuyahoga Health Access Partnership [CHAP] [http://cuyahogahealthaccess.org]).

C. Leadership behaviors that create and support opportunities for nurses to collaborate in helping to resolve issues and offer solutions in matters involving patient complaints, performance improvement results, risk management initiatives, and specific program changes.

1. Initiate specific operational decision-making (e.g., unit level includes evaluation of current services provided and the ability to add additional new program development, and modify or delete certain aspects of processes).

2. Express voice in health care resources/allocation (such as evaluation of appropriate equipment, space, personnel, and systems to meet changing practice).

3. Partner in learning from other professions.
   a. Identify centers of excellence with quality outcomes.
   b. Apply appropriate adaptation of results for specific environments and populations. For example:
      (1) The Institute of Medicine (IOM) (2011a) blueprint for relieving pain in America.
      (2) National Alliance to End Homelessness (2012).

4. Learn from other professional experience (e.g., a review of literature and reports, such as *The Checklist Manifesto*, a book

by Atul Gauande [2011] on preventing mistakes in the OR setting; writings about patient-centered medical homes [PCMHs] and accountable care organizations [ACOs]; IOM reports on health care delivery system in America).

5. Assist patients/families to understand their rights and responsibilities in participating in the health care system (e.g., build trusting partnerships, make choices available and understand).

6. Assure shared responsibility between the patient/family and health care team.
   a. Everyone has a role in making health care safe, including doctors, health care executives, nurses, and health care technicians.
   b. Health care organizations across the country are working to make health care safe. As a patient, one can make care safer by being an active, involved, and informed member of the health care team.
   c. Awareness of The Joint Commission's intent regarding patient responsibility (The Joint Commission, 2010).

D. Leadership coordination – Skills necessary to organize and manage an undertaking while moving forward on agreed goals. Ambulatory care nurses can apply these skills in their work setting and the community to benefit patients.
   1. Understanding community resources regarding disaster planning, first responders, importance of self-management by patients/families beginning with basic needs (food, housing, medications).
   2. Consider process for integrating the Patient Self-Determination Act of 1991 (Rouse, 1991) (see Chapter 6, "Legal Aspects of Ambulatory Care Nursing").
   3. Identify ambulatory patients requiring an acute care inpatient episode and begin discharge planning in ambulatory setting prior to admission (e.g., crutch walking for patients with joint replacements, teaching patient/family infusion services, specific medication regimens [such as warfarin], durable medical equipment that may be re-

quired in plan of care following certain procedures).
   4. Promote increased communications, using various technologies, between and across ambulatory/acute care/home care/rehab/hospice settings to improve the continuity of care for patients/families.
      a. Meet periodically with providers to promote understanding and updates of systems to establish processes that help ensure safe, effective patient care.
      b. Ensure flow of written communication regarding the plan of care, utilizing available technology, and electronic medical record compatibility.
      c. Establish hand-off communication processes.

VI. **External Environment and Resources**
A. Community education/involvement in promoting understanding of how to live a healthy lifestyle.
   1. Local school systems and colleges.
      a. Support nutritional school lunch programs.
      b. Promote physical exercise (e.g., Let's Move [www.letsmove.gov).
      c. Introduce preventive health measures in curriculum.
      d. U.S. Department of Agriculture changes in school for improved healthier meals program.
   2. Advocacy groups to address specific public health concerns. National fast food chains have introduced "healthy choices" on their menus in the past few years. In spite of efforts by advocacy groups to address the issue of good nutrition, food marketing to youth continues to contribute to childhood obesity (Harris, Pomeranz, Lobstein, & Brownell, 2009).
B. Advocacy resources.
   1. Internet resources for advocacy in ambulatory care.
      a. Patient Advocate Foundation (www.patientadvocate.org).
      b. Institute of Medicine (www.iom.edu).

c. Howard P. Freeman Patient Navigation Institute (www.hpfreemanpni.org).
d. Everybody Needs a Nurse (www.everybodyneedsanurse.com).
e. State insurance departments (www.healthguideusa.org).
f. Centers for Medicare and Medicaid Services (CMS) (www.cms.gov).
g. American Hospital Association-Society for Healthcare Consumer Advocacy (www.shca-aha.org).

2. Professional organizations/societies.
   a. American Nurses Association – Health Care Reform (www.nursingworld.org/MainMenuCategories/Healthcare Policy/Health-Care-Law.aspx).
   b. Consumer's guide to health reform.
   c. HealthCare.gov: Insurance Finder tool (http://finder.healthcare.gov).
   d. American Association of Retired Persons (AARP) (http://www.aarp.org).

3. Church community, including parish nursing programs, where available.

4. Professional organizations/political activism.
   a. Professional organizations support the nurse's ability to advocate.
      (1) Create standards of care to benefit patients.
      (2) Create and/or support "white paper" statements on specific issues.
      (3) Provide ongoing education for nurses.
      (4) Publish journals and texts to support care of patients.
   b. Professional organizations advocate directly.
      (1) Support lobbying efforts aimed at improving health care (for example, www.cohcaonline.org).
      (2) Propose and support public policy related to health care changes.
   c. Collaborate, participate, and support think tank efforts focused on helping to design, improve, and overhaul the current health care system.

(1) *The Future of Nursing: Leading Change, Advancing Health* (IOM, 2011b).
(2) Health Commentary (www.healthcommentary.org).
(3) AAACN initiative to participate and engage in health care reform (www.aaacn.org/HCReform).

5. Create business opportunities.
   a. Intermediary between patients and insurance company.
   b. Expanding roles within health care organizations in quality management, and evaluating and monitoring compliance indicators of quality as they relate to patient safety and outcomes.
   c. Independent consultants: Based on recognized expertise (such as redesign, accreditation process, clinical medical information system design [MISD] systems, research, and risk management/quality measurement, patient navigators).

References

American Academy of Ambulatory Care Nursing (AAACN). (2010). *Scope and standards of practice for professional ambulatory care nursing* (8th ed.). Pitman, NJ: Author.

American Academy of Ambulatory Care Nursing (AAACN). (2011a). *Definition of professional ambulatory care nursing.* Retrieved from http://www.aaacn.org/aboutaaacn/Ambulatory_Care_Nursing_Defined/AmbulatoryCareNursingDefinition.pdf

American Academy of Ambulatory Care Nursing (AAACN). (2011b). *Mission statement.* Retrieved from http://www.aaacn.org

American Hospital Association (AHA). (1992). *A patient's bill of rights.* Retrieved from http://www.patienttalk.info/AHA-Patient_Bill_of_Rights.htm

American Nurses Association (ANA). (2001). *Code of ethics for nurses with interpretive statements.* Washington, DC: American Nursing Press.

American Nurses Association (ANA). (2010). *The nurse's role in ethics and human rights: Protecting and promoting individual worth, dignity, and human rights in practice settings.* Retrieved from http://gm6.nursingworld.org/MainMenuCategories/Policy-Advocacy/Positions-and-Resolutions/ANAPositionStatements/Position-Statements-Alphabetically/Nursess-Role-in-Ethics-and-Human-Rights.pdf

DeNavas-Walt, C., Proctor, B.D., & Smith, J.C. (2011). *Income, poverty, and health insurance coverage in the United States: 2010.* Retrieved from http://www.census.gov/prod/2011pubs/p60-239.pdf

Dictionary.com. (2012). *Advocacy.* Retrieved from http://dictionary.reference.com/browse/advocacy

Fowler, M. (2010, May 19-20). *Standard VI: Ethics in ambulatory care: The moral milieu of the AAACN ethics standard/"ethical practices" and the ambulatory nurse.* Presentation at the 3rd Annual Ambulatory Nursing Symposium. Pasadena, CA.

Gauande, A. (2011). *The checklist manifesto: How to get things right.* New York: Picador.

Gold, C. (2006). Ethics. In C.B. Laughlin (Ed.), *Core curriculum for ambulatory care nursing* (2nd ed., pp. 183-188). Pitman, NJ: American Academy of Ambulatory Care Nursing.

Haas, S. (2011a). Ambulatory nurse leaders: Developing opportunities for patient-focused care navigation. *ViewVoint, 33*(4), 11.

Haas, S. (2011b). The new health care reform law: What patients need to know. *ViewPoint, 33*(1), 7-8.

Harris, J.L., Pomeranz, J.L., Lobstein, T., & Brownell, K.D. (2009). A crisis in the marketplace: How food marketing contributes to childhood obesity and what can be done. *Annual Review of Public Health, 30*, 211-225.

Henderson, V. (1961). *Basic principles of nursing care.* London: International Council of Nursing.

Institute of Medicine (IOM). (2011a). *Relieving pain in America: A blueprint for transforming prevention, care, education, and research.* Retrieved from http://iom.edu/Reports/2011/Relieving-Pain-in-America-A-Blueprint-for-Transforming-Prevention-Care-Education-Research.aspx

Institute of Medicine (IOM). (2011b). *The future of nursing: Leading change, advancing health.* Washington, DC: The National Academies Press.

Johnson, E.M. (2000). Advocating for patients. *ViewPoint, 22*(4), 1, 6-7.

Joint Commission, The. (2010). *2010 hospital accreditation standards (HAS) intent.* Oakbrook Terrace, IL: Author.

Joint Commission, The. (2011). *National patient safety goals.* Retrieved from http://www.jcrinc.com/National-Patient-Safety-Goals/

Lachman, V. (2010). Do-not-resuscitate orders: Nurses' role requires moral courage. *MEDSURG Nursing, 19*(4), 249-251, 236.

Maximus, Inc. (2011). *COBRA – Continuation coverage assistance appeals project.* Retrieved from http://www.continuationcoverage.net

National Alliance to End Homelessness. (2012). *Policy.* Retrieved from http://www.endhomelessness.org/section/policy

Robert Wood Johnson Foundation. (2009). *At the brink: Trends in America's uninsured – A state-by-state analysis.* Retrieved from http://www.rwjf.org/files/research/20090324ctuw.pdf

Rouse, F. (1991). Patients, providers and PDSA: Patient Self-Determination Act. *Hastings Center Report, 21*(5), S2-S3.

Sennett, C. (2000). Ambulatory care in the new millennium: The role of consumer information. *Quality Management in Health Care, 8*(2), 82-87.

Steinmetz, S. (Ed.). (1997). *Random House Webster's unabridged dictionary* (2nd ed.). New York: Random House.

Velianoff, G.D., & Hobbs, G.R. (2000). *Quality improvement and risk management.* Philadelphia: W.B. Saunders.

Additional Readings

Haas, S. (1998). Ambulatory care nursing conceptual framework. *ViewPoint, 20*(3), 16-17.

Haas, S. (2011a). Evolving informed understanding of the health care reform law. *ViewPoint, 33*(5), 7, 13.

Haas, S. (2011b). Health care reform law at one year: What ambulatory care nurses and patients need to know. *ViewPoint, 33*(3), 6-7.

Haas, S. (2011c). Understanding "value driving elements" of ACOs and PCHMs. *ViewPoint, 33*(6), 8-9.

Huber, D.L. (2010). *Leadership and nursing care management* (4th ed.). Maryland Heights, MO: Saunders.

Mastal, M.F. (2006). The context of ambulatory care nursing. In C.B. Laughlin (Ed.), *Core curriculum for ambulatory care nursing* (2nd ed., pp. 29-45), Pitman, NJ: American Academy of Ambulatory Care Nursing.

Savage, T. (1999). Ethics, the outpatient pediatric nurse and managed care. *Pediatric Nursing, 25*(2), 197-207.

Wilson, C.J., & De Luca, G. (2006). Care of the well patient: Screening and preventive care. In C.B. Laughlin (Ed.), *Core curriculum for ambulatory care nursing* (2nd ed., pp. 267-285). Pitman, NJ: American Academy of Ambulatory Care Nursing.

Chapter 9

Telehealth Nursing

Sherry Smith, MSN, MBA, RN

OBJECTIVES – *Study of the information in this chapter will enable the learner to:*

1. Define telehealth nursing practice.
2. Discuss the scope of telehealth nursing practice, its purpose, and its role within ambulatory care nursing.
3. Describe the core dimensions fundamental to telehealth nursing practice.
4. Discuss the use of decision support tools for assessment and care management.
5. Describe the professional competencies of telehealth nursing practice.
6. Identify risk management strategies that support the safe practice of telehealth nursing.

KEY POINTS – *The major points in this chapter include:*

1. Telecommunication technology in health care includes telephones (including telephony), computer, the Internet, interactive video, and teleconferencing.
2. A relationship is created between the consumer and the nurse with each telehealth encounter, and the nurse has a duty to provide safe and effective care.
3. Telehealth nursing follows the nursing process with emphasis on assessment and communication skills.

This chapter will describe telehealth nursing and its support of improved access, quality, and cost-efficiency of health care delivery, regardless of whether the setting is a centralized call center, decentralized ambulatory practice setting, or remote from home. Consumers seek assistance in making health care decisions, finding answers to their health care questions, learning more about self-management of specific conditions, and receiving emotional support. Proactive contact with consumers by telehealth nurses supports health management, health promotion, and transitional care strategies. Telehealth nursing practice supports the endeavors of the Institute of Medicine (IOM), which is partnering with the Robert Wood Johnson Foundation to investigate transformational improvements in the practice of nursing in the re-formed health care system (IOM, 2008). Today, telehealth nursing practice is recognized as a nursing subspecialty by the American Academy of Ambulatory Care Nursing (AAACN) and the American Nurses Association (ANA) (AAACN, 2010a, 2010b).

I. **Telehealth Nursing Practice Defined**
A. Definitions approved and adopted by the Telehealth Nursing Practice Special Interest Group (AAACN, 2011).
   1. *Telehealth:* The delivery, management, and coordination of health services that integrate electronic information and telecommunications technologies to increase access, improve outcomes, and contain or reduce costs of health care (AAACN, 2011). *Telehealth* is used as an umbrella term to describe the wide range of services delivered across distances by all health-related disciplines.

2. *Telehealth nursing:* The delivery, management, and coordination of care and services provided via telecommunications technology within the domain of nursing. Telehealth nursing is a subset of telehealth, encompassing all types of nursing care and services delivered across distances. *Telehealth nursing* is a broad term encompassing practices that incorporate a vast array of telecommunications technologies (e.g., telephone, fax, electronic mail, Internet, video monitoring, and interactive video) to remove time and distance barriers for the delivery of nursing care.

3. *Telephone nursing:* All care and services within the scope of nursing practice that are delivered over the telephone. A component of telehealth nursing practice restricted to the telephone.

4. *Telephone triage:* An interactive process between nurse and client that occurs over the telephone and involves identifying the nature and urgency of client health care needs and determining the appropriate disposition. A component of telephone nursing practice that focuses on assessment and prioritization and referral to the appropriate level of care.

B. Evolution of telehealth nursing practice.

1. The word *triage* originated from the French word "trier," which means to pick or sort. It was used by the French military to designate where wounded soldiers would be sent. Later, the U.S. military used the term to identify a sorting station for wounded soldiers, which would then be transported to secondary facilities (Newberry, 2003).

2. An often-repeated story identifies the first telehealth interaction occurring during a telephone call by Alexander Graham Bell. He was calling for Mr. Watson, his assistant, to come and help him with an injury to his hand.

3. In the last half of the 1970s, as managed care models emerged, health maintenance organizations (HMOs) began using telephone triage and advice services as a "gatekeeping" effort to control patients' access to care.

4. In the early 1980s, hospital marketing departments began providing physician and service referral, class registration, and consumer health education, along with triage and advice services to attract and retain market share.

5. The proliferation of managed care organizations further expanded telehealth services to address:
   a. Demand management.
   b. Recertification and referral authorization.
   c. Customer services providing information and assistance regarding benefits, eligibility, and assistance with provider relations.
   d. Member services, including enrollment, health risk appraisals, and primary care provider selection.

6. Increased incidence of chronic illness, rising health care costs, and increased emphasis on the delivery of quality health care have influenced the development of services that incorporate telehealth nursing as a care delivery strategy.
   a. Disease management.
   b. Care management, including transitional care.
   c. Case management.
   d. Clinical prevention services.

7. The role of the telehealth nurse will continue to expand as health care reform measures are implemented. The care coordination/care management/case management roles will become critical to the reduction of readmissions and emergency department visits in emerging integrated care environments (IOM, 2011).
   a. Care transitions.
   b. Post-discharge follow-up.
   c. Improved access to ambulatory care services.

II. Scope of Practice for Telehealth Nursing Practice

State boards of nursing define the scope of nursing practice for each state. It is important for registered nurses to be familiar with the Nurse Practice Act and the rules and regulations in the practice of nursing in their state of residence. A scope of practice statement describes the who, what, where, when, why, and how of nursing practice (ANA, 2010).

A. Experienced registered nurses deliver telehealth nursing care in all settings of ambulatory care as well as in formal call center programs. They utilize their knowledge and apply the nursing process to meet the actual or potential health needs of patients. They are supported by telecommunication technology and decision support tools to provide care 24/7.

B. The purpose of telehealth nursing practice.
1. Improve access to health care for individuals, groups, and specific patient populations at risk.
2. Improve the quality of health care outcomes through patient-centered, collaborative care.
3. Improve the cost efficiency of care delivery by meeting the needs of patients with timely and appropriate resources.

III. Standards of Telehealth Nursing Practice

Standards are authoritative statements used by the nursing profession to describe the responsibilities for which its practitioners are accountable. Standards reflect the values and priorities of the profession. They provide direction for professional nursing practice and a framework for the evaluation of this practice. Standards of professional nursing practice describe a competent level of nursing practice and professional performance common to all registered nurses (ANA, 2010).

A. Standards relevant to telehealth nursing.
1. Legal standards.
   a. State nurse practice acts.
   b. The rules and regulations for the practice of nursing.
2. Professional standards pertaining to telehealth nursing practice.
   a. Developed by accrediting professional organizations and applied to general or specialty practice.
   b. *Scope and Standards of Practice for Professional Telehealth Nursing* was first published in 1997 by AAACN. Standards were reviewed and broadened, and the publication was renamed to its current title in 2001 to reflect the advancement of practice. The standards were last revised and published in 2011.
   c. General standards applicable to telephone nursing: American Association of Office Nurses (AAON), *Office Nursing Practice Standards for Quality Care of Patients* (Jones, 2004).
   d. Position statement applicable for telephone nursing: Emergency Nurses Association (ENA), *Position Statement Telephone Advice*, developed in 1991, most recently revised in 2010 (ENA, 2010).
   e. Position statement applicable for telehealth nursing: National Association of School Nurses (NASN), *Position Statement: The Use of Telehealth Technology in the Practice of School Nursing* (NASN, 2010).
3. Regulatory standards.
   a. Developed by local and state health departments and federal agencies, such as the Americans with Disabilities Act (ADA) and Occupational Safety and Health Administration (OSHA).
   b. Developed by national organizations such as:
      (1) The Joint Commission (2011) *2011 Comprehensive Accreditation Manual for Standards for Ambulatory Care.*
      (2) American Accreditation Healthcare Commission/URAC (2008) has developed *Health Call Center Accreditation Standards* for organizations that provide clinical triage and health information services.

4. Organizational standards.
   a. Define performance expectations for the telehealth practice nurse within the organizational structure.
   b. Organizational standards include:
      (1) Policies and procedures.
      (2) Position descriptions.
      (3) Performance standards.
      (4) Standards of care.
      (5) Decision support tools.

IV. Core Dimensions Fundamental to Telehealth Nursing Practice

While core dimensions provide a basis for all nursing practice, telehealth nursing has its own unique dimensions that set it apart from other nursing subspecialties. The most notable difference in telehealth nursing practice is not being in the physical presence of the patient. This results in adaptation of the nursing process, with increased emphasis on assessment and communication skills.

A. Dimensions of telehealth nursing practice.
   1. Systematically assesses patient needs using decision support tools, critical thinking, and clinical judgment.
   2. Builds rapport and trust quickly to assess patient's/caller's needs and to determine urgency in time-limited encounters.
   3. Applies relevant communication techniques utilizing telecommunication devices to interact and educate patients. All interactions use plain language to improve the health literacy of consumer served.
   4. Facilitates collaboration for the planning of care with patients, their support systems, and providers of health care.
   5. Documents the telecommunication interaction.
   6. Utilizes telecommunication technology to provide patient care.
   7. Demonstrates knowledge of legal issues specific to telehealth nursing practice.
   8. Evaluates outcomes of telehealth practice using quality measurements.
   9. Maintains confidentiality of telehealth encounters.

B. The nursing process in telehealth nursing practice – The nursing process consists of inter-

Figure 9-1.
Model of Telehealth Nursing Practice

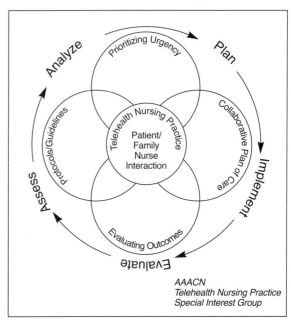

AAACN
Telehealth Nursing Practice
Special Interest Group

Source: AAACN, 2009. Used with permission.
© American Academy of Ambulatory Care Nursing.

related steps that provide the blueprint for consistent care delivery in all patient settings, including telehealth. AAACN has developed a model that illustrates the interactive, circular relationship of the nursing process for telehealth nursing practice (see Figure 9-1). The core reflects the interaction between the nurse and the patient/caregiver. The nurse prioritizes the urgency of the situation based on assessment data, utilizes decision support tools, and collaborates with other health care professionals and the patient/caregiver to develop a plan of care, implement appropriate interventions, and evaluate the outcome (AAACN, 2009).

1. Assessment – Data collection.
   a. The reason for the call or patient's chief complaint.
   b. Medical history – Confirming diagnosed health care problems, allergies, prescribed and over-the-counter medications, and alternative therapies.

c. History of symptoms and associated symptoms.

d. Focused assessment of the patient's actual or potential health needs.

2. Analyze and plan – Continually analyze the data gathered to develop an effective plan of care.

a. Use decision support tools to prioritize the triage category (such as emergent, urgent, non-urgent).

b. Reference other resources as appropriate and/or collaborate with others.

c. Determine the disposition of the patient based on acuity of symptoms (e.g., 9-1-1, emergency department, walk-in clinic, or self-care) and nursing diagnosis.

3. Implementation – Putting the plan into action.

a. Define plan that is patient-centered.

b. Carry out interventions that are in control of the nurse (such as transferring calls to 9-1-1, scheduling of provider appointment).

(1) Facilitate follow-up care and coordinate resources (such as referrals).

(2) Provide information and education (such as instructing about home care measures for symptoms).

c. Intervention carried out by the patient/caregiver. Nurse utilizes communication/counseling skills that induce actions to achieve desired outcomes.

d. Documentation of nursing process.

4. Evaluation – Achievement of expected outcome.

a. Patient's understanding, acceptance, and implementation of the plan of care, including when to call back for further intervention.

b. Follow-up actions and plans of the nurse.

c. Analyze/re-evaluate effectiveness of each step of the nursing process.

V. Telehealth Assessment

Registered nurses do not medically diagnose, but assess patients and make critical decisions regarding appropriate care. Assessing patients in most practice settings involves face-to-face interactions in which the nurse is able to use all sensory input (auditory, visual, olfactory, and tactile), along with both verbal and non-verbal communication. The assessment of patients using telecommunication devices is unique because the locus of assessment changes. Additionally, the nurse must be sensitive to verbal and emotional cues communicated through speech as well as the presence of background sound (AAACN, 2009).

A. The locus of assessment shifts to the patient/caregiver.

1. The nurse must guide the patient in assessing symptoms.

a. The nurse needs to listen, interpret, and direct the patient during the assessment process.

b. The patient is an active partner in the assessment and is the primary assessor (for example, the patient must actively determine the site of pain and describe the location to the nurse).

c. There must be clear delineation between the patient being an active participant in assessment and the patient self-diagnosing.

2. The locus of assessment may not be with the patient, but with the caller/caregiver who is with the patient.

a. The caregiver becomes the eyes and ears for the nurse.

b. The nurse directs the caregiver to describe what he or she observes.

B. The locus of care is not physically with the nurse. The patient/caregiver carries out interventions appropriate for the assessed needs.

C. The telecommunication encounter is time-limited.

1. The communication must be focused upon moving the caller to the next best step or level of intervention.

2. The nurse must focus on the most important needs of the encounter.

Figure 9-2.
Telehealth Nursing Communication Model

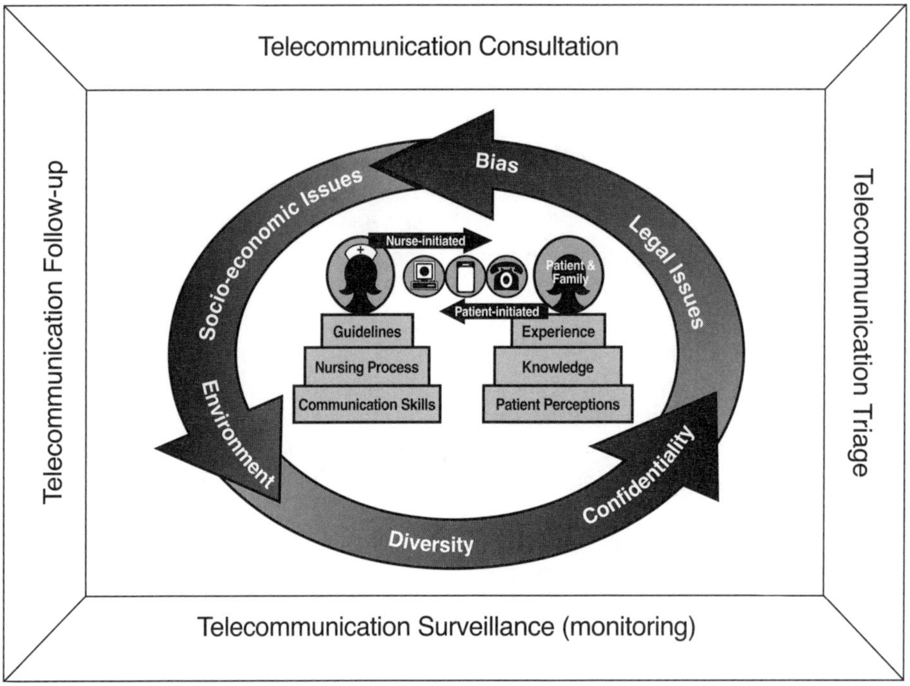

Source: AAACN, 2009. Used with permission.
© American Academy of Ambulatory Care Nursing.

3. Extensive needs of a caller/patient may indicate that an in-person assessment is required.

VI. Telehealth Communication

The key to the telehealth assessment is the interaction with the patient or caregiver. The nurse must develop a partnership to initiate interactive health care management. Interactions are brief, with communication techniques focusing on obtaining detailed information without the use of tactile or visual senses (see Figure 9-2).

A. The nurse directs the caller to examine self or the patient.
   1. The caller uses techniques provided by the nurse.
   2. The nurse interprets the caller's description of symptoms, location, and appearance.
B. The nurse must establish trust immediately to elicit accurate information.

1. Identifies self to caller with name and title.
2. Identifies the patient by name, and if the patient is not the caller, the relationship to the caller.
3. Identifies the patient's relationship to the provider (e.g., established patient or new patient).
C. The nurse demonstrates expert communication skills.
   1. Uses plain language in all communications to improve health literacy of populations served.
   2. Uses open-ended and close-ended questions appropriately.
   3. Uses active listening techniques.
   4. Verifies the reason for the call from the patient's/caller's perspective and identifies preferences.
   5. Identifies any hidden agendas for the call (such as exploring why the caller is really

calling and what the caller expects to achieve/obtain from the interaction).

6. Clarifies the caller's statements to understand his or her descriptions.
   a. Directs the caller to clarify location of symptoms by instructing to point to the area and describe in relation to well-known anatomical part (e.g., the "belly button").
   b. Asks the caller to quantify and qualify symptoms by using pain scales, common sizes (such as pea size, quarter size).
7. Utilizes terminology consistent with the patient's/caller's level of comprehension.
8. Utilizes counseling skills, such as motivational interviewing or positive reframing to support self-management behaviors.

D. The nurse manages multiple presentations or co-morbidity of symptoms.
   1. Hearing the caller describe multiple symptoms.
   2. Identifying primary symptoms and secondary symptoms.
   3. Sorting and prioritizing these symptoms.
   4. Discouraging caller's self-diagnosis and/or bias toward treatment.

E. The nurse maintains confidentiality of interactions.
   1. Patient interactions take place in a private environment away from other patients, visitors, and inappropriate personnel.
   2. Disclosure statements are signed by patients before information is provided to family members or others. Care of minor children or incompetent adults is handled according to legal statutes and institutional policy (see Chapter 8, "Legal Aspects of Ambulatory Care Nursing").
   3. Records of calls are safeguarded against breach in confidentiality and in accordance with HIPAA.

VII. Decision Support Tools

A decision support tool is a plan or guide for the assessment and management of an actual or potential health problem(s) for individuals, groups, or at-risk populations to reduce the risk of omissions and increase the predictability of desired outcomes. Decision support tools support but do not replace the use of the nursing process and critical thinking skills used by the telehealth nurse to meet the unique needs of a patient and his or her preferences, given the situation and available resources. *Protocols, guidelines, algorithms,* and *care pathways* are some terms used as descriptors for decision support tools.

A. Desirable attributes of evidence-based guidelines (IOM, 2011).
   1. *Validity* – Result in desired health and cost management outcomes.
   2. *Reliability* – Given like or similar clinical presentation, other clinicians concur with the content and process.
   3. *Applicability* – Explicitly describes the population to which they apply.
   4. *Flexibility* – Identifies specific clinical cautions for patient populations.
   5. *Clarity* – Unambiguous language and precise definitions of terms.
   6. *Multi-disciplinary input* – Participation by representatives of key affected groups in the development and review.
   7. *Scheduled review* – Defined review cycle.
   8. *Documentation* – Citation of references, assumptions, procedures, and analytic methods must be documented and described.

B. Purpose and benefits of using decision support tools for assessment, triage, and care management of patients.
   1. Provide safe, effective, appropriate care and disposition for the actual or potential health needs of individuals, groups, or patient populations.
   2. Provide standardization of care to achieve desired outcomes.
   3. Improve efficiency of assessment process.
   4. Decrease omissions or harmful practices.
   5. Facilitate the ease, efficiency, and retrievability of appropriate documentation.
   6. Support evidence-based interventions.
   7. Reduce liability risk.
   8. Meet accreditation standards.
   9. Enhance evaluation of performance.

10. Provide data repository for the study of telehealth nursing practice.

C. Content and structure of decision support tools.
1. Symptom-based or condition-specific. Not intended to medically diagnose, but to evaluate acuity of symptoms and facilitate appropriate care to improve health outcomes.
2. Description of the scope of guideline subject, defining what it does and does not include.
3. Overview or background information, discussing pertinent clinical indicators, risk factors, and assessment parameters for the subject.
4. Sequenced assessment questions to determine clinical needs and urgency of symptoms. Organized in groupings designating acuity level (e.g., emergent, urgent, non-urgent, self-care).
5. Clinical alerts that define or clarify the assessment parameters to increase reliability. Clinical alerts also include pertinent clinical information, such as age-specific risk factors, unusual presentations, or clinical rationale to support clinical judgment.
6. Self-care measures that provide detailed information on first aid or self-care to manage or resolve symptoms.
7. Defined directions for the patients/callers regarding "watchful waiting" or warning signs that describe symptoms to watch for and stated time frames for seeking care if these symptoms occur, worsen, or do not improve.
8. Disposition information describing the appropriate site, provider, and time frame of care, for example:
   a. *Emergent* – Call 9-1-1 or go to emergency department immediately.
   b. *Urgent* – Seek medical care within the next 4–6 hours.
   c. *Non-urgent* – Ranging from seek medical care within 24 hours to home/self-care.
9. Reference list citing sources used to develop the guideline.

D. Common ambulatory care situations utilizing guidelines.
1. Telephone triage, counseling, and education programs.
2. Case management and disease management services; may include use of home monitoring devices (Park, 2006).
3. Crises lines for suicide prevention, child abuse, poison control, and others.
4. Hotlines or support lines for HIV/AIDS, substance abuse, and others.
5. Ambulatory procedures and examinations (such as ocular examinations, auditory evaluation, glucose tolerance testing).
6. Anticipatory guidance counseling sessions.
7. Perioperative care.
8. Post-hospitalization follow-up.

E. Perceived disadvantages of using guidelines for assessment, triaging, and care of patients in a telehealth situation.
1. For professional registered nurse.
   a. May influence the nurse to focus on single condition or symptom. The presence of co-morbidity increases complexity of nursing intervention.
   b. Requires in-depth training and experience to become proficient.
   c. Patient interaction is more structured than an impromptu interaction.
2. For physician/provider.
   a. Perceived loss of control for each patient's plan of care.
   b. Conflict in allowing professional registered nurse empowerment in assessment and triage decisions.
3. For administration.
   a. Concern of guidelines being expensive to develop, maintain, or purchase.
   b. Concern of risk management issues if guidelines are not strictly followed by all nurses.

VIII. Professional Competencies

Defined competencies for telehealth nursing practice identify the behaviors and outcomes specific to providing efficient, effective, evidence-based care (AAACN, 2011). Competencies should be measurable and include:

A. Professional knowledge – A minimum of 3–5 years of applicable clinical nursing experience is the industry average/standard before employment in a telehealth nursing position (AAACN, 2009). However, individual organizations decide number of years of relevant experience based on services provided telephonically. Competencies include:

1. Call processing: Manages clinical calls using the nursing process.
2. Assessment: Demonstrates critical thinking skills in assessing covert and overt parameters relevant to the needs of the caller.
3. Age-specific competencies: Provides care consistent with the functional requirements of the person's developmental age.
4. Cultural awareness: Provides culturally sensitive care to diverse populations.
5. Interventions and outcomes: Uses clinical judgment and effective interventions to enhance patient/client outcomes.

B. Interpersonal skills.

1. Trust relationship: Establishes a trust relationship to elicit accurate patient/caller information.
2. Communication skills:
   a. Uses effective interpersonal communication skills to engage in, develop, and disengage in a therapeutic interaction.
   b. Uses plain language in communications with consumers to address health literacy issues.
   c. Uses communication skills to facilitate collaboration, such as negotiation, conflict resolution, and group decision-making.
3. Counseling skills: Utilizes counseling skills to facilitate patient self-management behaviors, such as motivational interviewing and positive reframing.
4. Customer service: Applies customer service skills when interacting with a caller.

C. Technical skills.

1. Telecommunication technologies: Adapts to equipment and demonstrates efficient use of technology devices to perform role.
2. Software programs: Understands, selects, and uses relevant software programs appropriately.
3. Care management and analysis: Uses selected program decision support tools to address caller/patient needs to identify actual and potential health risks.

D. Documentation of telehealth encounters: Documents telecommunications encounters that reflect care specific to the actual or potential health needs of the caller/patient. This may include call recording as well (Vinson, McCallum, Thornlow, & Champagne, 2011).

E. Personal and professional development: Accepts personal responsibility for maintaining and improving the knowledge and skills necessary to assess, triage, and manage patients.

1. Core education is included in the *Telehealth Nursing Practice Essentials* (AAACN, 2009).
2. Researching and defining practice as further concepts in medical and nursing management are developed, including personal health management, disease management, quality management, and outcome management.
3. Remaining abreast of telehealth changes and recommending improvements for practice.
4. Advancing telehealth nursing by demonstrating professional clinical knowledge, critical thinking, participating in quality improvement, and utilizing research related to clinical practice.

F. Resource management: Internal and external resource utilization. Locates and utilizes appropriate resources to meet the needs of caller/patient.

G. Practice and administrative issues: Practices in accordance with an ethical, legal, and organizational framework that ensures the caller's/patient's interest and well-being are met (AAACN, 2011).

IX. **Risk Management and Quality Improvement Strategies for Telehealth Nursing Practice**

With the initiation of each telehealth encounter, a relationship is created between the consumer and

Table 9-1.
Safeguards Against Legal Problems Resulting from Telephone Triage

- Use medically approved protocols to establish a standard of care. Do not deviate from the protocols unless changes are in writing and approved by the appropriate medical authority.

- Document the call and advice provided. For example, if a suit is filed 3 years later claiming the nurse did not advise the mother appropriately, the nurse's position is much more defensible if the documentation shows that protocols were followed and appropriate advice was given.

- Provide callers with an option to call back or seek medical attention sooner if they do not agree with the advice, if the condition persists or worsens, or if new symptoms develop.

- Develop a mechanism to regularly review documentation and advice for consistency, accuracy, and quality.

- Orient and train staff in telephone triage protocols, policies and procedures, phone encounter techniques, dealing with difficult calls, and documentation.

- Measure outcomes. Conduct regular consumer satisfaction surveys. Follow up promptly on problems and quality issues.

- Establish a positive helping relationship at the outset of the call. The average call lasts approximately 6 minutes. The effectiveness of this short encounter is often dependent on skillful communication. The initial contact can often make or break the caller's confidence and satisfaction with the telephone interaction.

- Encourage the caller to briefly describe the problem and its duration, onset, and location; past medical history; medications; and allergies. Be sure to obtain the age of the person with the problem.

- Use terminology the caller can understand. Avoid medical jargon as much as possible.

- Listen carefully to the caller and avoid jumping to conclusions. Callers may mask their real concern for fear of embarrassment, particularly regarding sensitive issues such as sexually transmitted infections or mental health problems.

- Try to talk to the person with the problem, directly if possible. Direct communication is usually more reliable and inclusive than secondhand information.

- Thoroughly assess the problem before determining an action plan. The caller may underplay the symptoms and want reassurance that the problem is insignificant.

- Pay attention to the degree of anxiety and concern expressed by the caller. Remember the telephone nurse is at a disadvantage and cannot see or touch the person. If the caller is emphatic that the person is ill even though protocols may recommend home care measures or observation while waiting for an appointment, encourage the caller to seek medical attention sooner. It is better to be overly cautious than to miss a serious condition.

- Attend conferences, workshops, and continuing education offerings to establish competency in communication skills, assessment, and telephone triage to reduce the risk of medical-legal problems.

Source: Briggs, 1997. Used with permission from the author.

the nurse, and the nurse has a duty to provide safe and effective care. It is expected that the nurse will provide a level of care that would be given by a reasonable, prudent nurse under the same or similar circumstances. Published professional standards, such as the *Scope and Standards of Practice for Professional Telehealth Nursing* (AAACN, 2011), define the responsibilities for which its practitioners are accountable. There are inherent risks with all clinical practice, and in a highly litigious environment, it is important to consider proactive strategies to reduce risk and to minimize potential liability associated with telehealth practice (see Table 9-1).

A. Program planning needed to meet quality standards.
   1. Define program mission and goals.
   2. Define roles and responsibilities consistent with state practice acts and professional standards.
   3. Develop policies and procedures specific to telehealth services to promote standardization that include, but are not limited to:
      a. Management of emergencies or at-risk situations (such as potential suicide, violence and abuse, childbirth, any basic life support situation, calls from minors, and reportable conditions).

b. Call management processes (such as maintaining confidentiality, dealing with anonymous callers or those refusing to provide information, time frame for returning calls/delay of care, inability to contact patient/caller, second- or third-party calls, dealing with non-compliant callers or repeat callers, and access to emergency medical services).

c. Knowledge and appropriate use of approved guidelines, including how to manage callers with multiple symptoms, overriding dispositions, and presenting symptoms not covered in a guideline.

4. Assignment of a medical director or panel of physicians to review guidelines and policies and procedures, serve as a resource for clinical issues, and participate in outcome management and quality improvement processes.

5. If providing telehealth across state lines, consult legal counsel to ensure compliance with applicable state laws (Waters, 2005) (see Chapter 8, "Legal Aspects of Ambulatory Care Nursing").

B. Documentation of telehealth encounters – Thorough and accurate documentation of telehealth encounters communicates relevant patient data to other health care providers to promote continuity of care and aid collaboration. Documentation supports reimbursement for care provided and/or helps define the value of telehealth services. It is also utilized by professional disciplines and accrediting agencies to judge the quality of care delivered. Complete documentation is usually described as one of the most effective ways to protect oneself from legal risk. The method and format for documenting calls is organizationally defined and should be consistently followed in daily practice (AAACN, 2009).

1. Basic encounter documentation should include:
   a. Date and time of the encounter.
   b. Patient's legal name with confirmed spelling.
   c. Date of birth.
   d. Name of person calling, if other than the patient, and relationship to patient.
   e. Person's reason for call.
      (1) In caller's own words, using quotations to indicate precise verbiage.
      (2) Stated expectations and/or perceived urgency.
   f. Phone number and location of patient/caller.
   g. The name and credentials of nurse processing the call.

2. Relevant history, including diagnosed health problems and health risks, current medications and use of any alternative treatments, allergies, recent injuries, procedures, and infection or exposure to infectious disease.

3. Assessment of symptom(s), including onset, location, duration, character, effect of symptom(s) on usual activities, history of similar symptoms, and associated or other symptoms. It is also helpful to know if any patient action has worsened or improved the symptoms.

4. Guideline selected for client's symptom(s).

5. Interventions, including suggested home care, disposition, and follow-up plans. It is important to consider any barriers that might limit the patient's/caregiver's ability to carry out suggested interventions, such as co-morbidity, emotional state, ability to understand, impact of symptoms on ability to carry out activities of daily living, and ability to access care. In the presence of such barriers, it is imperative that clinical decisions are made to best meet the patient's needs.

6. Verification of patient's understanding and intended action.

7. Prescriptions called in with time and name of pharmacy, if any (Buppert, 2009).

C. Staff education and performance management processes.
   1. Orientation.
   2. Formal training for preceptors.
   3. Competency verification.

4. Continuing education opportunities.
5. Ongoing competency and needs assessments.

D. Defined quality improvement process.
1. The IOM (1998) defined *quality* as "the degree to which health services for individual and populations increase the likelihood of desired health outcomes and are consistent with current professional knowledge" (p. 6).
2. Simply defined, outcomes measurement is the collection and reporting of information about the relationship of interventions to the results of care. The challenge is to define and measure outcome indicators for clinical effectiveness in telehealth nursing practice and to identify action plans for improvement of care.
3. Outstanding needs:
   a. Data and format standardization to support comparisons.
   b. Longitudinal as well as episodic data.
   c. Evaluation of variables that impact results.
4. Examples of effectiveness measures focusing on nurse-sensitive outcomes:
   a. Increased compliance with disposition recommendations.
   b. Improved rates of verifying appropriate pediatric dosing for over-the-counter medications per weights.
   c. Consistent disposition trending, including provider paging, over-riding and under-riding dispositions when applicable.
   d. Improved functional status.
   e. Earlier identification of condition-specific complications.
   f. Decreased readmission rates and frequency of emergency department visits for those with chronic illness.
   g. Improved transition of care from one care setting to another.
   h. Satisfaction with nursing care advice and customer service.
   i. Increased compliance with treatment plans.
   j. Increased participation in age appropriate screenings.

X. **Operational Elements of a Telehealth Nursing Service**
Each practice setting has unique services and patient populations. Key to an effective telehealth nursing service is determining its role as a value-added service in supporting the health care organization's strategic initiatives. It is important to identify both the essential components of a telehealth nursing program as well as the demand for telehealth nursing care to provide optimal services. Additional considerations include practice setting/workspace design and technological needs.
A. Foundational components of a telehealth nursing service/program.
1. Defined purpose and mission.
2. Defined scope of practice.
3. Formal orientation and continuing education.
4. Assessment of competencies for role performance.
5. Decision support tools.
6. Program-specific policies and procedures.
7. Continuous performance improvement processes.
8. Ability to perform call audits and monitoring with processes for assuring inter-rater reliability.
B. Identify the demands and needs for telehealth care.
1. Patient populations that will contact the service/provider.
2. Patient's expectation of a telehealth service (such as symptom assessment, clarification of instructions, reinforcement of education, and prescriptions).
C. Identify the specific populations being served.
1. Special patient needs (such as elderly patients, oncology patients, and behavioral health patients).
2. Cultural issues (such as language barriers, health values, and differences in self-care management practices).
3. Socio-economic issues (such as access to transportation, ability to purchase medication, and availability of support system).
D. Identify the telecommunication flow and prioritization of encounter handling.

1. Systematically sort encounters and develop internal triaging.
   a. Prioritize symptoms by acuity; handle symptom encounters before non-symptom/general encounters; use non-clinical personnel to "screen service requests" (URAC, 2008).
   b. Only registered nurses or physicians perform assessment and triage.
   c. All personnel recognize emergency encounters and notify appropriate personnel to handle immediately.
   d. Use of non-clinical and unlicensed assistive personnel appropriate to service.
2. Efficiently and effectively respond to telecommunication encounters.

E. Analyze telecommunication encounter data:
   1. Identify peak access days and times.
   2. Identify the "waiting time" for answering the initial encounter (also known as ASA or "average speed of answer").
   3. Identify the "holding time" after answering the encounter.
   4. Develop staffing models to meet encounter demands (e.g., remote on-call nurses).
   5. Identify reasons for abandoned encounters; measure abandon rates.
   6. Identify inappropriate messaging.
   7. Trend "blockage rates" to assure you have enough bandwidth to service patients and callers.

F. Create methods to decrease telecommunication demand.
   1. Develop educational materials for patients on care of illnesses.
   2. Provide ambulatory patients with written discharge instructions.
   3. Provide descriptors of when/how to contact the telehealth nursing service.

G. Determine the telehealth nursing service location/physical space.
   1. Identify the practice setting where patient confidentiality will be maintained (HIPAA and privacy considerations).
   2. Identify amount of work surface and storage needed to support type of work performed.
   3. Consider sound control/noise reduction (such as height of walls if cubicle design, acoustic wall paneling).
   4. Provide overhead lighting that is non-glare, as well as adjustable task lighting.
   5. Consider ergonomics when designing workspace (such as seating, monitor position, and keyboard).
   6. Determine type of headsets to be used if communication involves use of telephone.
   7. Assure all aspects noted above are considered for remote work-at-home sites where applicable.

H. Determine technological needs.
   1. Evaluate computer hardware/software needs to support documentation of encounter and use of decision support tools.
   2. Evaluate telecommunication device and system needs based on volume assumptions, hours of operation, and flow of encounter.

I. Apply essential components of a telehealth nursing program specific to organization's strategic goals to enhance the nursing care provided and ensure optimal services.

References

American Academy of Ambulatory Care Nursing (AAACN). (2009). *Telehealth nursing practice essentials* (3rd ed.). Pitman, NJ: Author.

American Academy of Ambulatory Care Nursing (AAACN). (2010a). *Ambulatory care nursing orientation and assessment competency guide* (2nd ed.). Pitman, NJ: Author.

American Academy of Ambulatory Care Nursing (AAACN). (2010b). *Scope and standards of practice for professional ambulatory care nursing* (8th ed.). Pitman, NJ: Author.

American Academy of Ambulatory Care Nursing (AAACN). (2011). *Scope and standards of practice for professional telehealth nursing* (5th ed.). Pitman, NJ: Author.

American Accreditation Healthcare Commission/URAC. (2008). *Health call center accreditation program*. Retrieved from https://www.urac.org/programs/prog_accred_HCC_po.aspx

American Nurses Association (ANA). (2010). *Nursing: Scope and standards of practice*. Washington, DC: Author.

Briggs, J.K. (1997). *Telehealth triage protocols for nurses*. Philadelphia: Lippincott, Williams & Wilkins.

Buppert, C. (2009). Guidelines for telephone triage. *Dermatology Nursing, 21*(1), 40-41.

Emergency Nurses Association (ENA). (2010). *Position statement telephone advice*. Retrieved from http://www.ena.org/about/position/

Institute of Medicine (IOM). (1998). *Crossing the quality chasm: The IOM health care quality initiative.* Washington, DC: The National Academies Press.

Institute of Medicine (IOM). (2008). *HHS in the 21st century: Charting a new course for a healthier America.* Washington, DC: The National Academies Press.

Institute of Medicine (IOM). (2011). *Clinical practice guidelines: What we can trust.* Washington, DC: The National Academies Press.

Joint Commission, The. (2011). *2011 comprehensive accreditation manual for standards for ambulatory care.* Retrieved from http://www.jointcommission.org/standards_information/standards.aspx

Jones, M.A. (Ed.). (2004). *Office nursing practice standards for quality care of patients* (2nd ed.). Montvale, NJ: American Association of Office Nurses (AAON).

National Association of School Nurses (NASN). (2010). *Position statement: The use of telehealth technology in the practice of school nursing.* Retrieved from http://www.nasn.org/Portals/0/positions/2002pstelehealth.pdf

Newberry, L. (Ed.). (2003). *Sheehy's emergency nursing principles and practice* (5th ed.). St. Louis, MO: Mosby.

Park, E. (2006). Telehealth technology in case/disease management. *Case Management 11*(3), 175-182.

URAC. (2008). *Health call center (HCC) standards.* Retrieved from https://www.urac.org/policyMakers/resources/HealthCallCenterv4.0.pdf

Vinson, M.H., McCallum, R., Thornlow, D.K., & Champagne, M.T. (2011). Design, implementation and evaluation of population-specific telehealth nursing services. *Nursing Economic$, 29*(5), 265-272, 277.

Waters, R.J. (2005). Legal advice for telehealth pioneers. *Caring, 24*(5), 32-38.

Additional Reading

Institute of Medicine (IOM). (2011). *The future of nursing: Leading change, advancing health.* Washington, DC: The National Academies Press.

The Professional Nursing Role In Ambulatory Care

Chapter 10

Leadership

Jane Westmoreland Swanson, PhD, RN, NEA-BC

OBJECTIVES – *Study of the information in this chapter will enable the learner to:*

1. Describe leadership characteristics and transformational leadership concepts.
2. Describe the importance of collaboration and conflict resolution in health care and relationships.
3. Describe the planning process for ambulatory care nursing interventions and programs.
4. Discuss various professional activities, associations, and national initiatives.

KEY POINTS – *The major points in this chapter include:*

1. Each ambulatory care nurse needs a variety of leadership skills to problem solve and develop relationships with patients and staff.
2. Conflict resolution and negotiation strategies are vital to building better relationships and quality of care.
3. Program evaluation and strategic planning are essential to accomplish goals and obtain desired outcomes.
4. Participation in professional associations enhances lifelong professional learning.

Magnet® hospital research indicates that a work environment that fosters professional nursing practice in which nurses are encouraged to use their expertise and judgment is an essential ingredient in increasing job satisfaction among nurses (Kramer, Maguire, & Brewer, 2011). It is the responsibility of every nursing leader to create a supportive infrastructure that encompasses trust and accountability, whereby nurses have the autonomy to make decisions and practice nursing in accordance with professional standards. Each ambulatory care nurse needs to be a leader. Nurses should use a variety of leadership skills to problem solve and develop relationships as they care for individual patients and families, supervise the work of others, and use evidence-based practice and the research process to plan and evaluate ambulatory care programs. This chapter is designed to provide the ambulatory care nurse with an outline of leadership concepts and with the knowledge and skills needed to understand and implement effective leadership and team building. Emphasis is placed on transformational leadership, team building, interdisciplinary collaboration, creating structures and processes to support evidence-based quality practice, and evaluating ambulatory care. Further reference and additional study references are included.

I. Transformational Leadership in Ambulatory Care

During rapid change, there is a tendency to revert to what one knows has worked in the past. Some leaders may default to a dictatorial command and control-type leadership. However, that style of non-participatory leadership in decision-making can result in further disengagement of workers, lack of teamwork, and less effective problem solving. To make the most effective progress, one needs to engage everyone involved. Utilizing transformation leadership with self-managed teams is far more productive, flexible, and resilient.

A. Major tasks of 21st century nursing leaders (Wheatley, 2005):
1. Remove barriers to health care and problem solving.
2. Alert staff regarding implications of practice.
3. Establish safety around developing new skills and practices.
4. Anticipate changes and trends early.
5. Translate changes so staff members understand the implications and their roles.
6. Articulate organizations as living systems where changes in one department impact reactions in other departments.
7. Develop clear core goals that are congruent with the overall mission and are understood by all.
8. Demonstrate personal engagement with the changes ("walk the talk").
9. Help others adapt to the demands of a changing health system.
10. Emphasize engagement: Individuals taking initiative and making changes.
11. Create a work environment that is safe and that provides worker satisfaction and constantly updated, relevant information.
12. Highlight small steps of progress and success while striving for overall change.
13. Celebrate accomplishments when goals are reached and help chart the next steps.
14. Recognize that "quick fixes" are oxymoron and usually do not address the root cause of a problem.

B. Transformational leadership is a long-term process.
1. It requires enormous amounts of self-awareness and support.
2. Change requires more time than one usually wants to acknowledge.
3. Real change is usually at least a three- to five-year process.

C. Leadership outcomes and maximized skills are evidenced by:
1. High-quality, evidence-based care is provided to patients and families.
2. Supervision of others' work is fostered in a collaborative, value-driven model.
3. Patient population programs involve multiple, interdependent systems with complexity-based models of design that are interdependent.
4. Services are provided efficiently to high volumes of patients in spite of unpredictable clinical and organizational issues.

D. Creating a culture of innovative and transformational leadership requires:
1. Focus on the power of creating a common vision that is held by all; everyone is focused on obtaining the same outcomes.
2. A clear vision that helps direct, align, and inspire actions for a large number of individuals.
3. Vision that motivates individuals to excel in their productivity and to achieve desired outcomes.
4. Creation of an environment in which individuals feel comfortable to take risks and communicate "out of the box" ideas (Melnyk & Davidson, 2009).
5. Work performed differently rather than the "perception of doing more with less."

E. Transformational leadership improves the outcomes of care.
1. The quality of nursing services has an impact on the overall outcomes of the health status of people served.
2. The emphasis on high-intensity, high-intervention, high-cost health services has little evidence of producing a higher quality of health (Porter-O'Grady, 2010).
3. However, these characteristics and involvement by staff and patients lead to mutual commitment and better outcomes:
   a. Multifocal rather than unilateral interests and goals.
   b. Strong alignment of all stakeholders versus allowing non-participation.
   c. Driven by mutual interest rather than self-interest.
   d. Focus on relatedness rather than function alone.
   e. Outcomes-driven rather than just competitive.
   f. Centered on improvement and thriving rather than survival focus.

II. Transformational Leadership Characteristics for Emotional Competence

Emotionally competent transformational leaders can connect with different groups of people in a variety of contexts and circumstances by increasing their emotional intelligence. Emotional intelligence is the ability to accurately perceive one's own and others' emotions, to understand the signals that emotions send about the relationship, and to manage one's own and others' emotions (Goleman, 2004; Swanson, 2000; Wheatley, 2005). A leader with emotional intelligence possesses the following traits:

A. Self-awareness.
   1. Recognition of feelings' impact on self, others, and job performance.
   2. Comfort discussing own strengths and areas for improvement.
   3. Appreciation and acceptance of differences.
B. Mindfulness or to "be present."
   1. Concentration on the present.
   2. Development of deep listening skills.
   3. Increased ability to detect trends or patterns.
C. Openness to new ideas.
   1. Appreciation of multiple perspectives.
   2. Development of the ability to listen without judgment.
   3. Development of trust.
D. Impulse control.
   1. Motivation to temper negative emotions or self-regulate.
   2. Ability to appropriately share emotions and maintain dignity.
   3. Preparedness to confront conflict and resolve with multiple strategies.
   4. Self-regulation and achievement motivation; equal ability to overcome frustration and setbacks.
E. Willingness to continually learn and unlearn.
   1. Display of humility and willingness to admit vulnerability of not knowing.
   2. Willingness to let go of old knowledge and accept new learning.
   3. Motivated to emulate best practices and incorporate into processes.
F. Willpower and courage.
   1. Readiness to explore new options and take risks.
   2. Aptitude to act on convictions and detect trends that are ahead of conventional practice.
   3. Display of integrity as defined by honest and moral actions.
   4. Ability to provide consistent feedback.
G. Compassionate and value-driven.
   1. Ability to express sincere empathy without needing to control the situation or solution.
   2. Skill to clarify and articulate values.
   3. Ability to empathize with others' needs, concerns, and goals.
H. Passionate optimism.
   1. Enthusiasm and energy regarding work.
   2. Positive mindset.
   3. Idealism sustains values.
   4. Pride in a job well done.
   5. Unflagging energy to improve performance.
I. Resilience and reflection.
   1. Motivated to accept and manage disappointment or setbacks.
   2. Supportive of others to cope with disappointments and grieve loss.
   3. Power to take time to nurture self and encourage others to live in balance.
   4. Capability to effectively use humor and relieve tension with mirth.

III. Strategies to Counter Negative Influences, Achieve Positive Outcomes, and Foster Collaboration

Working conditions in health care organizations are not always healthy, and it is important for the leader to stay open to cues of dysfunctional behaviors or toxicity. Dysfunctional behaviors make it more difficult to achieve positive outcomes and create working environments that are energizing and collaborative. The following suggestions help the leader to spot toxicity and initiate proactive steps that foster collaboration and focus upon outcomes central to the stated organizational mission and goals (Porter-O'Grady & Malloch, 2010).

A. Keep organizational mission, vision, and values the central focus.

1. What is the preferred outcome?
2. Are all plans and strategies focused on the goal?

B. Discuss disagreements.
   1. Encourage voicing diverse opinions that may provide better solutions and multiple options.
   2. Encourage time for discussion, especially from the doubters.

C. Cultivate truth tellers.
   1. Ensure individuals are present who will tell you what they really think.
   2. Create an environment where it is safe to voice unpopular or unpalatable opinions.

D. Treat others as you would like to be treated.
   1. Observe both actions and verbal responses.
   2. Set a good ethical climate.
   3. Have clear boundaries.

E. Honor your intuition.
   1. If your gut indicates you are being manipulated, you are probably right.
   2. Be honest with yourself.

F. Delegate, don't desert.
   1. Share control and empower staff.
   2. Remember who is ultimately responsible for outcome.
   3. Trust, but verify progress reports.

G. Performance coaching to develop leaders requires making constructive conversations with employees to enhance management relationships. In the role of coaching versus social conversation, the emphasis is focused on work and each person's performance (Tulgan, 2007).
   1. Coach performance steadily and persistently.
   2. Coach in enthusiastic, hands-on manner.
   3. Focus on improvement and accountability.
   4. Hold people accountable through clearly stated expectations.
   5. Tune into the uniqueness of the individuals you are coaching.
   6. Focus on specific instances of individual performance.
   7. Describe the employee's performance honestly and in detail.
   8. Develop concrete next steps.

9. "Close the loop," providing feedback regarding progress.

IV. Conflict Resolution, Negotiation Strategies, and Alternative Dispute Resolution

Conflict happens frequently in relationships and when different perceptions exist. When nurses do not feel supported in conflicts, either by their bosses, co-workers, or other health care providers, they may fear retribution and feel unsafe.

A. Conflict resolution.
   1. Conflict: A situation with multiple viewpoints and where perceptions are not shared, resulting in differing outcomes.
   2. Realities can be distorted or obstructed by imbalances in power.
   3. Negotiation is a process or activity to create a range of possibilities to resolve a conflict.

B. Guidelines for creating conditions for negotiation (Kritek, 2002).
   1. Develop an even playing field, although it may be very difficult to provide equal places for all parties.
   2. Acknowledge the dominant culture or worldview that is present in the situation.
   3. Creating alternative solutions and a range of possibilities.

C. Conflict management strategies and outcomes.
   1. Valentine (2001) reported a synthesis of research findings about nurses' conflict management strategies as identified by use of the Thomas-Kilmann Index (TKI).
   2. The TKI is a conflict mode index that identifies preferred conflict management strategies from a set of five options: Avoiding, compromising, collaborating, competing, and accommodating.
   3. Conflict strategies used predominantly by all levels of nurses, whether in direct patient care or administration, are avoiding, compromising, and accommodating, with avoiding used most frequently.
      a. Avoiding: One party does not pursue own concerns or those of the other party; uses withdrawal and suppression.

(1) Useful situations: As a cool-down mechanism when confronting issues so damaging as to outweigh benefits; need for information; for trivial issues or when one party is much more powerful.

(2) Outcomes: Lose-lose; unassertive; short-term resolution.

b. Compromising: One party gives up something to satisfy both parties; middle position.

    (1) Useful situations: Quick fix for temporary settlement of complex issues; for inconsequential issues; when goals are important but not worth major disruption; backup when collaboration and competition fail.

    (2) Outcomes: No-win, no-lose; moderately assertive, cooperative; short-term resolution.

c. Collaboration: One party works with the other party to find a solution that satisfies both parties; cooperative, confronting issues.

    (1) Useful situations: Merge insights from different perspectives for crucial issues; gains understanding; gains commitment for change; solves disruptive emotional issues; spreads responsibility and risk taking.

    (2) Outcomes: Win-win; fully assertive, cooperative; long-term resolution.

d. Accommodation: One party neglects own concerns to satisfy concerns of others; emphasizes similarities; minimizes differences; self-sacrificing.

    (1) Useful situations: For routine issues; when one is wrong; when the issue is more important to the other party; when outmatched; to build credits for later use; to preserve harmony; to teach others.

    (2) Outcomes: Lose-win; unassertive; cooperative; short-term resolutions.

e. Competing: One party wins, one party loses; power-oriented; high concern for self; low concern for others.

    (1) Useful situations: Quick decisions; unpopular causes – issues vital to the organization; defense against people who exploit noncompetitive behaviors; knowledgeable person able to make decision.

    (2) Outcomes: Win-lose; assertive; uncooperative; short-term resolution.

D. Suggestions to utilize to increase nurse conflict resolutions strategies (Kritek, 2002).

1. Be aware that nurses are conflict avoidant.

2. Avoid seeking "easy" answers or simple solutions for complex issues.

3. Recognize that conflicts are about relationships and values.

4. Refrain from snap judgments and conduct a conflict analysis.

5. Search for common ground, and avoid blaming and judging.

6. Seek to clarify the situation by asking questions and evoking more information.

7. Clarify the difference between accommodation and collaboration that smooth over a situation without resolving the conflict.

8. Recognize some of the structure inequities designed in health care systems that can place nurses in uneven positions in relationship to administration and physicians.

9. Seek the widest variety of options and choices that reinforce not rushing to a quick solution or settlement; investigate the consequence of each action.

10. Speak the truth. Keeping silent or compromising one's integrity diminishes one's authentic self and increases dissatisfaction with the profession.

11. Become more skilled at conflict resolution and obtain training in this area.

12. Ask peers and colleagues to critique one another's conflict skills and provide feedback on behaviors.

13. Form a coalition with other colleagues interested in improving their conflict man-

agement skills. Learn from one another and normalize dealing with conflict as a group expectation.

V. Planning Ambulatory Care Nursing Interventions and Programs

The objective of planning is to produce the best possible practical approach that will achieve organizational goals and specific program objectives, and that has the support of all stakeholders. The leader needs to build consensus among the stakeholders and align team members around shared goals.

A. These factors improve team relationships and collaboration:
  1. Trust among members.
  2. Sense of group identity.
  3. Sense of group efficacy or consistent goal direction.
  4. Development and coaching of leaders.
B. Strategic planning is the continuous process of systematically evaluating the nature of the organization, defining its long-term objectives, identifying quantifiable goals, developing strategies to reach these objectives and goals, and allocating resources to carry out these strategies. Strategic planning begins by addressing the following four questions (Porter-O'Grady & Malloch, 2010):
  1. Situational analysis: Where are we today?
  2. Program planning: Where do we want to go?
  3. Implementation of plan: How do we get there?
  4. Program evaluation: Have we achieved the desired outcomes?
C. Characteristics of effective goals:
  1. Recognized as important.
  2. Clear and easy to understand.
  3. Documented in specific terms.
  4. Measurable and framed in time.
  5. Aligned with organizational strategy.
  6. Achievable but challenging.
  7. Supported by appropriate rewards.
D. Prioritization of goals:
  1. Which goals are valued most by the organization?
  2. Which goals have the greatest impact on performance or profitability?
  3. Which goals are most challenging or difficult to obtain?
  4. Which goals best fit team members' talent or training?
  5. Highest priorities are goals of high value and primary concern.
  6. Next priorities are goals of medium value and secondary importance.
  7. Lowest priority goals have little value and minor importance.
  8. Next step is to prioritize highest-priority goals according to most important.
E. Four steps to accomplish goals by converting to realities.
  1. Break each goal into specific tasks with clear, measurable outcomes.
  2. Plan the execution of tasks with timetables to accomplish.
  3. Gather the required resources.
  4. Execute the plan.
F. General considerations involving various stakeholders with various agendas and priorities of outcomes.
  1. Are the proposed programs consistent with the organization's mission and strategic goals?
  2. Are the proposed programs consistent with the values of the stakeholders?
  3. Do the plans fit within the time frame and budget?
  4. Does the plan include consideration of all resources needed to support the program (such as money, time, staff, space, and goodwill of the community)?
  5. Is the proposed program evidence-based, and does it include the latest clinical practice guidelines as standard of care?
  6. Does the plan include evaluation criteria and standards to judge success/failure based on program goals and measured outcomes?
G. Needs assessment is the first step in planning ambulatory care nursing interventions and programs.

1. New programs may be triggered by perceived deficits in existing programs, changes in standard, or changing populations served.
2. Program decisions reflect organizational mission and values, and have fiscal benefit.

H. Needs assessment in ambulatory care is a process to reflect the needs of the community served (Anderson & McFarland, 2005). Sources of data include:
   1. What is the history of the community, and what can be gained by talking with members of the community?
   2. What are the demographics of the community that can be gathered from census data from local, state, and federal agencies regarding age, sex, racial, and ethnic distribution?
   3. What are the cultural and ethnicity indicators as gathered by interviews, local planning boards, and chamber of commerce?
   4. What values and beliefs are held by the community or population to be served?
   5. What is the physical environment impact (such as availability of housing, air quality, climate, water sources) on the population?
   6. What existing health and social services and resources outside of the immediate community are available?
   7. What is the economy of the population to be served with indications of employment, unemployment rates, and insurance availability?
   8. What are the transportation and safety issues of the community?
   9. Are there signs of political and government support?
   10. Is there common communication, or will language variations be a barrier?
   11. Are schools and educational resources available for distribution of information and gathering for health initiatives?
   12. What recreational areas are available for children to play, and what are the major forms of recreation?
   13. How do residents perceive their living conditions and community?

I. Action steps for a successful project.
   1. Secure approvals of stakeholders.
   2. Develop a budget and secure funding.
   3. Develop accounting, budgeting, and management information systems.
   4. Establish policy and procedures.
   5. Set standards and criteria for evaluation.
   6. Hire and train personnel.
   7. Plan marketing and celebration.

VI. Professional Nursing Association Membership and Magnet Recognition Program

A. Participation in professional associations is a very rewarding endeavor and helps a nurse mature in professional responsibilities and perspectives. Nursing professional associations do the following:
   1. Educate members through publications, research, conferences, and continuing education opportunities.
   2. Provide opportunities to present scholarly knowledge.
   3. Facilitate collegiality and networking.
   4. Seek to identify opportunities to be of service to the community and larger society.
   5. Advocate for change, providing evidence to shape policy.
   6. Develop and improve standards of practice.
   7. Provide learning about diverse methods and outcomes across communities.
   8. Co-create models of care delivery that remove the structural barriers to equitable health care for all.

B. Professional, community, scholarly, and specialty organizations are available on a local, state, and national level. The following are a few options and Web sites that provide more information.
   1. American Academy of Ambulatory Care Nursing (www.aaacn.org).
   2. American Nurses Association (www.ana.org).
   3. Sigma Theta Tau Honor Society of Nursing (www.nursingsociety.org).
   4. American Organization of Nurse Executives (www.aone.org).

5. The Alliance of Nursing Organizations (www.nursing-alliance.org) lists a number of specialty organizations.

C. Nurses in Magnet-recognized organizations have been shown to value professional autonomy, control over practice, and nurse-physician collaboration much more highly than nurses in non-Magnet facilities. Nurses in Magnet-recognized organizations tend to have higher membership in professional organizations and be certified in their nursing specialty (American Nurses Credentialing Center [ANCC], 2008).

1. In 1991, ANCC developed the Magnet Recognition Program® to recognize health care organizations that provide the very best in nursing care and uphold the tradition within professional nursing practice. In 2011, almost 400 of the nation's 5,000 hospitals and ambulatory facilities had achieved Magnet recognition (Frellick, 2011).

2. In 2010, the Magnet components were further refined to stress:

a. Transformation leadership.
   (1) Characteristics and involvement of senior nursing leader and strategic positioning (at the decision-making tables).
   (2) A structure for staff involvement in decision-making.
   (3) Evidence of strategic planning and involvement of nurses at all levels.
   (4) Support of leadership development for staff, mentoring, and performance reviews.

b. Structural empowerment.
   (1) Structure and process that encourages nurses at all levels to participate in decision-making, committees, councils, and task forces.
   (2) Commitment to professional development.
   (3) Support and processes to support nurses' roles as teachers to patients and colleagues.
   (4) Commitment to community involvement.
   (5) Recognition of nurses' contributions and value.

c. Exemplary professional practice.
   (1) Conceptual framework for nursing practice and interdisciplinary care.
   (2) A patient care delivery system that delineates nurses' authority and accountability for clinical decision-making and outcomes.
   (3) Nurses' involvement with staffing and budgeting to acquire necessary resources to assure consistent application of patient care.
   (4) Interdisciplinary collaboration across the continuum of care.
   (5) A work environment that provides a non-discriminatory climate for ethics, diversity, patients' rights, safety, and confidentiality.
   (6) Mechanism for quality care monitoring and improvements.

d. New knowledge, innovations, and improvement.
   (1) Conscientious integration of evidence-based practice and research into clinical and operational processes.
   (2) Infrastructures and resources in place to support the advancement of evidence-based practices and research in all clinical settings.
   (3) Innovation in patient care, nursing, and the practice environment: A hallmark of organizations receiving Magnet recognition.

e. Empirical outcomes.
   (1) The measurement used to evaluate the outcomes and impact on quality patient care.
   (2) Organizational measurements compared to national benchmarks.
   (3) Baseline measurements provided and tracked over time compared to baseline and national benchmarks.

(4) Measurement indicators include:
  (a) Total nursing care hours, skill mix, education, and experience level.
  (b) Nursing outcomes, such as job satisfaction and injuries from needlesticks or back injuries.
  (c) Patient outcomes, such as prevalence of pressure ulcers, restraint use, and falls.
  (d) Patient satisfaction as measured by perception of care and pain management (National Database of Nursing Quality Indicators [NDNQI], 2012).

VII. National Initiatives

In 2010, over 40 million Americans were uninsured, and millions more lacked adequate care (IOM, 2010). As noted in the National Association of Community Health Centers 2009 report, health care reform makes meaningful improvements in the accessibility and quality of primary health care, an explicit goal of health care reform. The Patient Protection and Affordable Care Act of 2010, passed by Congress and the President of the United States, is intended to provide access to care for 32 million additional Americans (Stolberg & Pear, 2010). The logistics of meeting this increased requirement are being debated in Congress at this time. The United States health care system is characterized by fragmentation across many sectors, which raises substantial barriers to providing accessible, quality care at an affordable price. National initiatives focus on strategies for improving health care delivery models, providing culturally competent care, and retaining the available supply of nurses, while striving to increase the capacity.

A. Strategies for health improvements and delivery models.
  1. Increasing attention to health care access for the working poor and uninsured.
  2. Improving access services in transportation, childcare, and social services.
  3. Advancing culturally competent health care.

B. Responses to changing workforce issues.
  1. Advocating for accessible, affordable health care with culturally competent providers.
  2. Promoting research that identifies modes of care to improve the health status of diverse populations.
  3. Increasing the number of ethnic minority nurse leaders in the areas of health policy, practice, education, and research.
  4. Increasing the number of ethnic minority nurses to reflect the nation's diverse population.

C. Nurses and nurse leaders can stay current through involvement with professional organizations, journals, and newsletters of professional organizations, computer access to group email lists, professional conference attendance, and participation in political action committees.

D. *The Future of Nursing* report sponsored by the Institute of Medicine (IOM) (2010).
  1. Nurses represent the largest sector of health professionals, with more than 3 million registered nurses in the United States. This study sought to answer the question regarding how nursing could help address the increasing demand for safe, high-quality, and effective health services.
  2. Four key recommendations of the report.
    a. Nurses should practice to the full extent of their education and training.
    b. Nurses should achieve higher levels of education and training through an improved education system that promotes seamless academic progression.
    c. Nurses should be full partners, with physicians and other health professionals, in designing health care across the United States.
    d. Effective workforce planning and policy-making require better data collection and an improved information infrastructure.
  3. Strategies recommended for achieving these recommendations.

a. Remove scope of practice barriers so advanced practice registered nurses can practice to the full extent of their education and training.

b. Expand opportunities for nurses to lead and diffuse collaborative improvement efforts with physicians and other members of the health care team to conduct research, and redesign and improve practice environment.

c. Implement nurse residency programs to support nurses' completion of a transition to practice program (nurse residency) after they have completed a pre-licensure or advanced practice degree program and when they are transitioning to a new clinical area.

d. Increase the proportion of nurses with a baccalaureate degree to 80% by 2020.

e. Double the number of nurses with a doctorate by 2020.

f. Ensure that nurses engage in lifelong learning.

g. Prepare and enable nurses to lead change to advance health across all levels of leadership positions.

h. Build an infrastructure for the collection and analysis of inter-professional health care workforce data.

References

American Nurses Credentialing Center (ANCC). (2008). *Application manual: Magnet Recognition Program*. Silver Springs, MD: American Nurses Association.

Anderson, E., & McFarland, J. (2005). Community as partner: Theory and practice in nursing (4th ed). Philadelphia: Lippincott, Williams & Wilkins.

Frellick, M. (2011, April). A path to nursing excellence. *Hospital and Health Networks*. Retrieved from http://www.hhnmag.com/hhnmag_app/jsp/articledisplay.jsp?dcrpath=HHNMAG/Article/data/04APR2011/0411HHN_FEA_workforce&domain=HHNMAG

Goleman, D. (2004). What makes a leader? *Harvard Business Review, 76*(7), 93-102.

Institute of Medicine (IOM). (2010). *The future of nursing: Leading change, advancing health*. Washington, DC: The National Academies Press.

Kramer, J.M., Maguire, P., & Brewer, B. (2011). Clinical nurses in Magnet hospitals confirm productive healthy work environments. *Journal of Nursing Management, 19*(1), 5-17.

Kritek, P. (2002). *Negotiating at an uneven table: Developing moral courage in resolving our conflicts* (2nd ed.). San Francisco: Jossey-Bass.

Melnyk, B., & Davidson, S. (2009). Creating a culture of innovation in nursing through shared vision, leadership interdisciplinary partnerships, and positive deviance. *Nursing Administration Quarterly, 33*(4), 288-295.

National Association of Community Health Centers. (2009). *Primary care access: An essential building block of health reform*. Retrieved from http://www.nachc.com/client/documents/pressreleases/PrimaryCareAccessRPT.pdf

National Database of Nursing Quality Indicators (NDNQI). (2012). *Home page*. Retrieved from http://www.nursingquality.org

Porter-O'Grady, T. (2010). Leadership for innovation: From knowledge creation to transforming healthcare. In T. Porter-O'Grady, & K. Malloch (Eds.), *Innovation leadership: Creating the landscape of healthcare*. Boston: Jones & Bartlett.

Porter-O'Grady, T., & Malloch, K. (2010). *Quantum leadership: Advancing innovation, transforming healthcare* (3rd ed.). Sudbury, MA: Jones & Bartlett.

Stolberg, S.G., & Pear, R. (2010). *Obama signs health care overhaul bill, with a flourish*. Retrieved from http://www.nytimes.com/2010/03/24/health/policy/24health.html

Swanson, J. (2000). Zen leadership: Balancing energy for mind, body and spirit harmony. *Nursing Administration Quarterly, 24*(2), 29-33.

Tulgan, B. (2007). *It's okay to be the boss: The step-by-step guide to becoming the manager your employees need*. New York: Harper-Collins Publishers.

Valentine, P. (2001). A gender perspective on conflict management strategies of nurses. *Journal of Nursing Scholarship, 33*(1), 69-74.

Wheatley, M. (2005). *Finding our way: Leadership for an uncertain time*. San Francisco: Berrett-Keohler.

Additional Reading

Moore, C. (2004). *The mediation process: Practical strategies for resolving conflict* (3rd ed.). San Francisco: Jossey-Bass.

Chapter 11

Evidence-Based Practice and Performance Improvement

Eileen M. Esposito, DNP, RN-BC, CPHQ

OBJECTIVES – *Study of the information in this chapter will enable the learner to:*

1. State the meaning of evidence-based practice and performance improvement, and their applicability to ambulatory care nursing and quality outcomes.
2. Describe the key steps of evidence-based nursing practice, discuss the quality and strength of the evidence, and identify strategies for facilitating the use of evidence-based clinical practice guidelines within an organization.
3. Develop an understanding of the importance of conducting nursing research using scientifically sound methodologies that contribute to the science of nursing and nursing theory, and provide the foundation for professional and ethical nursing practice.
4. Discuss the differences between quality assurance and performance improvement models.
5. Define the Institute of Medicine's (IOM) Six Aims and how they are used to enhance patient-centered care.
6. Identify different types of performance indicators and provide an example of when each would be used in measuring outcomes of processes and care.
7. Describe the P-D-C-A performance improvement model and how it is used to develop, monitor, and improve processes and outcomes of care.
8. Outline key performance indicators typically measured in an organization and displayed on a report card or dashboard.

KEY POINTS – *The major points in this chapter include:*

1. Evidence-based nursing practice and continually improving practice performance are two key components of professional nursing practice in all ambulatory settings.
2. Evidence-based practice and performance improvement are the cornerstones of safe, effective, efficient, timely, and appropriate patient-centered clinical practice.

Evidence-based nursing practice and continually improving practice performance are two critical components of professional nursing practice in all ambulatory care settings. Evidence-based initiatives are often central to the performance improvement process, and the improvement process is a cornerstone of total quality management programs. This chapter is designed to provide nurses with a basic understanding of evidence-based practice and performance improvement, and the naturally occurring link between the two processes. Used together, evidence-based practice and performance improvement can impact the quality of care delivered in ambulatory care settings.

Nursing research has its roots in the work of Florence Nightingale. Nightingale's *Notes on Nursing* (1860) described early nursing research, which demonstrated how a healthy environment can promote a patient's physical and mental well-being. Using data to document the improved outcomes, and statistical analysis to prove validity, Nightingale reported data in easy-to-read tables and pie charts. Nightingale's interventions resulted in decreased mortality from 43% to 2% during the Crimean War (Burns & Grove, 2009).

I. **Evidence-Based Practice**
   A. Definitions of evidence-based nursing.

---

1. "Evidence-based practice is the conscientious integration of best research evidence with clinical experience and the patient values and needs in the delivery of quality, cost-effective health care" (Burns & Grove, 2009, p. 16).
2. "Evidence-based practice guidelines are rigorous, explicit clinical guidelines that are based on the best research evidence available in that area" (Burns & Grove, 2009, p. 29).

B. Goals of evidence-based practice:
1. Integrating individual clinical expertise with the best available external evidence from systematic research.
2. Reducing wide variation in practice.
3. Eliminating worst practices.
4. Enhancing best practice.
5. Reducing cost and improving quality.

C. Key assumptions in evidence-based practice:
1. Clinicians directly involved in delivering patient care influence, either positively or negatively, patient outcomes.
   a. Clinicians assume full responsibility for their practice; in the case of nursing, some aspects of practice are dependent, interdependent, or independent.
   b. Clinicians draw on, as well as contribute to, a body of knowledge elucidating best evidence and optimum effectiveness (Kitson, 1997; National Association for Healthcare Quality [NAHQ], 2008).

II. Key Sources of Evidence-Based Nursing Practice Guidelines and Literature

There are many sources of nursing information, research, and evidence-based guidelines. These include:

A. Cumulative Index of Nursing and Allied Health Literature (CINAHL) – Provides comprehensive coverage of the English language journal literature for nursing and allied health disciplines.

B. Cochrane Database of Systematic Reviews and Cochrane Central Register of Controlled Trials – Includes the full text of the regularly updated systematic reviews of the effects of health care prepared by the Cochrane Collab-

oration (www.cochrane.org). This database includes the most rigorous studies available.

C. National Guideline Clearinghouse (NGC) – Publicly available electronic repository for clinical practice guidelines and related materials that provides online access to guidelines (www.guidelines.gov).

D. PubMed – The National Library of Medicine (www.nlm.nih.gov).
1. PubMed is a free database that allows easy access to the Medline database of references and abstracts on life sciences and biomedical topics maintained by the National Library of Medicine (NLM) at the National Institutes of Health (NIH).
2. Medical Subject Headings (MeSH) is the controlled vocabulary used for indexing articles in the MEDLINE subset of PubMed. MeSH provides a consistent way to retrieve information when several different terms may be used for the same concept (e.g., pressure ulcer, decubitus, bed sore).
3. PubMed has several sorting features that will help narrow down the returned literature.
4. Clinical Queries (a sorting feature of PubMed) will return only biomedical and life sciences articles that meet evidence-based practice criteria (will exclude editorials, opinions, newsletters).

E. Google Scholar (www.scholar.google.com) is a free online database that allows access to a wider variety of literature, including:
1. Peer-reviewed articles.
2. Dissertations and theses.
3. Guidelines.
4. Scientific books.
5. Proceedings, patents.
6. Publications from professional societies' Web sites.

F. Key differences in the ranking of material as displayed from the top of the list:
1. PubMed – The most currently added literature will display first.
2. Google Scholar – Displayed in the order of most cited:
   a. Article.
   b. Author.

c. Publication.

d. Organization.

(Hint: Click on related articles or most cited article by opening in a new tab. This will allow a drill down on a particular thread or topic without losing the original search list and will broaden the potential list of returns.)

G. Key differences in the strengths and limitations of PubMed and Google Scholar:

1. PubMed – Strengths:

   a. Well-organized database.

   b. Various search features allow for refinement of items returned.

   c. Many free, full-text articles.

   d. Subject searching with MeSH.

   e. Clinical queries sub-database returns only EBP articles.

   f. Most useful as the starting point of the search to answer a clinical question.

2. PubMed – Limitations:

   a. Not user-friendly.

   b. Covers articles and abstracts.

   c. Does not search the entire text.

   d. Does not provide reference lists.

3. Google Scholar – Strengths:

   a. Fast, easy, and convenient.

   b. Broad range of information sources.

   c. Searches the entire text.

   d. Is most useful at the end of a comprehensive search to fill any gaps.

4. Google Scholar – Limitations:

   a. Less organized than PubMed.

   b. Few limits or search features to limit search; can limit date field.

   c. Most full-text articles require paid access or password to retrieve.

   d. No subject searching.

   e. Not as current as PubMed.

H. Campbell Collaboration Database of Systematic Reviews: Includes the full-text of the regularly updated systematic reviews of the effects of interventions in the social, behavioral, crime and justice, and educational arenas prepared by the Campbell Collaboration (an international research network that relies on voluntary cooperation among researchers of a variety of backgrounds) (www.campbellcollaboration.org/index.html).

I. Federal government Web sites:

1. National Institutes of Health (NIH) (www.nih.gov).

2. Centers for Disease Control and Prevention (CDC) (www.cdc.gov).

3. Department of Health and Human Services (DHHS) (www.dhhs.gov).

4. *Morbidity and Mortality Weekly Report* (www.cdc.gov/mmwr).

5. Health Finder (consumer-oriented Web site) (www.healthfinder.gov).

6. U.S. Preventive Services Task Force (www. ahrq.gov/clinic/uspstfab.htm).

J. Professional associations:

1. American Academy of Ambulatory Care Nursing (AAACN) (www.aaacn.org).

2. American Nurses Association (ANA) (www.ana. org or www.nursingworld.org).

3. Sigma Theta Tau International (www.nursingsociety.org).

K. Voluntary health organizations:

1. American Lung Association (www.lungs.org).

2. American Heart Association (www.americanheart.org).

3. American Cancer Society (www.cancer.org).

III. Evaluating the Evidence

A. Critically appraise the evidence (Swan & Boruch, 2004).

1. What is the evidence?

2. Is the evidence valid?

3. If valid, is the evidence important?

4. If valid and important, can one apply this evidence when caring for the patient, family, or population?

B. Systematic review of research evidence is necessary to create evidence-based guidelines. When determining the appropriateness of the strength and appropriateness of the evidence, Craig and Smyth (2007) suggest the following steps for critically appraising the quality of systematic reviews:

1. Was the purpose or objective of the review clearly stated?

2. Did the reviewers report a systematic and comprehensive search strategy to identify relevant studies?

3. Were the inclusion and exclusion criteria clearly defined and were they appropriate to avoid selection bias?

4. Was the quality of the included studies assessed appropriately?

5. Were the results of the included studies combined systematically and appropriately?

6. Were the conclusions supported by data?

C. Levels of evidence are designed to help reviewers rate the quality and strength of the evidence and include the following characteristics:

1. Is there a scientific design?
2. Are the outcomes statistically significant?
3. Is the data valid and reliable?
4. Is there any bias? Amount of bias minimized?
5. Were time-controlled studies done?

D. Rating system for the hierarchy of evidence (Melynk & Fineout-Overholt, 2011, p. 12):

1. "Level I: Evidence from a systematic review or meta-analysis of all relevant randomized controlled trials (RCTs), or evidence-based clinical practice guidelines based on systematic reviews of RCTs."

2. "Level II: Evidence obtained from at least one well-designed RCT."

3. "Level III: Evidence obtained from well-designed controlled trials without randomization."

4. "Level IV: Evidence from well-designed case-control and cohort studies."

5. "Level V: Evidence from systematic reviews of descriptive and qualitative studies."

6. "Level VI: Evidence from a single descriptive or qualitative study."

7. "Level VII: Evidence from the opinion of authorities and/or reports of expert committees."

E. These levels are often translated into a triangle picture to increase understanding, with Level I at the top of the triangle and Level VII at the bottom (see Figure 11-1).

IV. Evidence-Based Clinical Practice Guidelines

A. "Clinical guidelines help define the standard of nursing care, are interdisciplinary, and are based on an extensive review of the literature focused on findings from previous studies" (Burns & Grove, 2009, p. 324).

B. Guidelines have been used to accomplish several major goals:

1. Improve clinical quality.
2. Reduce variability.
3. Improve outcomes.
4. Reduce cost of care.

C. Clinical practice guidelines indicate the optimal treatment plan or "gold standard" for patient care that promotes high-quality outcomes. Using the best research evidence that has been synthesized by subject matter experts, researchers, and clinicians allows for the development of strong evidence-based guidelines for practice (Burns & Grove, 2009).

D. Clinical practice guidelines can overcome the barriers to research utilization by reducing the need to access and critically appraise the literature and make general conclusions and recommendations. They do not eliminate clinical judgment regarding how well particular clients match the target population for the practice guideline (Melnyk & Fineout-Overholt, 2011).

E. The Agency for Healthcare Research and Quality (AHRQ) (www.ahrq.gov) initiated the National Guideline Clearinghouse (NGC) in 1998 to house evidence-based clinical guidelines. The guidelines are available online (www.guideline.gov).

V. Translating Evidence into Practice

A. "The focus of translation research has been the exploration of potentially useful strategies for enhancing the uptake or adoption of evidence and related guidelines into practice" (Stetler, 2003, p. 99).

1. "Not all improvements in practice or quality in general can be achieved by inducing or exhorting individual clinicians and managers to change their own practice."

Figure 11-1.
Hierarchy of Evidence

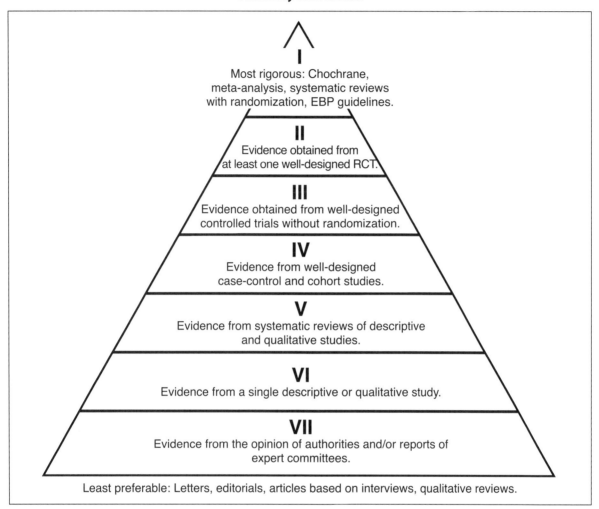

Source: Adapted from Melynk and Fineout-Overholt, 2011.

2. "Evidence-based change is not likely to be sustained over time without explicit system supports."

3. "Organizational context can have either a facilitative or hindering impact on the adoption of research findings."

4. "The process of implementing and using research findings must be institutionalized so that evidence-based practice and related implementation efforts become part of both the organization and the individual clinician's daily way of doing business" (Stetler, 2003, p. 98-99).

B. Several models have been developed to promote evidence-based practice in nursing:

1. Stetler Model of Research Utilization to Facilitate EBP (Stetler, 2001) – Model provides a comprehensive framework to enhance the use of research evidence by nurses to promote or facilitate evidence-based practice. The model contains five phases:

a. Preparation.
b. Validation.
c. Comparative evaluation/decision-making.
d. Translation/application.
e. Evaluation.

2. Iowa Model of Evidence-Based Practice to Promote Quality of Care (Titler et al., 2001).
   a. This model provides direction for development of evidence-based practice in a clinical agency and is responsive to the triggers that initiate a need for change.
   b. Examples of problem-focused triggers are risk management data, process improvement and benchmarking data, financial data, and clinical problems.
   c. Knowledge-focused triggers for change include new research findings, the national health agenda (*Healthy People 2020* [CDC, 2009]), professional society and agency findings, and guidelines and organizational standards.

3. Grove Model for Implementing Evidence-Based Guidelines in Practice (Burns & Grove, 2009). This model contains five steps for evaluating a guideline prior to implementation into practice. Practitioners should:
   a. Review the authors.
   b. Determine the significance of the health care problem.
   c. Examine the strength of the evidence.
   d. Determine the link to national standards.
   e. Review the cost-effectiveness (Burns & Grove, 2009).

VI. Definition of Nursing Research

A. *Research* is defined as the diligent, systematic inquiry or investigation undertaken to validate and refine existing knowledge and to generate new knowledge.

B. *Nursing research* is defined as "a scientific process that validates and refines existing knowledge and generates new knowledge that directly and indirectly influences the delivery of evidenced-based nursing practice" (Burns & Grove, 2009, p. 3).

1. Nursing research reflects science and theory, and includes philosophy, knowledge, abstract thought processes, reality testing, and the empirical world to bring learning from the abstract to the concrete.

2. Strategies for facilitating nursing research include:
   a. Create an environment of inquisitiveness in which nurses are free to question and evaluate current practice, seeking out research-based solutions to care problems, and testing them in pilot studies.
   b. Support nursing research committees, research presentations, and publication.
   c. Assure access to journals, online databases, and research librarians.
   d. Encourage and support nurses' research skills.
   e. Support from leadership, management, and administrators for nurses to conduct research, and to report and present their findings in multiple venues, including professional conferences.

VII. History of Nursing Research

A. Florence Nightingale initiated nursing research in 1850 and published *Notes on Nursing*, the first account of nursing research, in 1860. Nightingale used data to correlate environmental factors and mortality in hospitalized soldiers during the Crimean War. Her interventions demonstrated a decrease in mortality from 43% to 2% (Burns & Grove, 2009).

B. Nursing research was limited from 1900–1950.

C. 1950 – ANA initiated a 5-year study on nursing functions and activities.

D. 1957 – The first Department of Nursing Research was established at Walter Reed Army Institute of Research.

E. 1970s – Nursing research picked up momentum as the nursing process became a focus of many studies.

F. 1978 – *Research in Nursing & Health* was published.

G. 1983 – *The Annual Review of Nursing Research* was published.

H. 1988 – *Applied Nursing Research* was published.

I. 1992 – *Clinical Nursing Research* was published.

J. 1993 – The National Institutes of Health created the National Institute of Nursing Research (NINR). The NINR seeks to advance nursing science by supporting clinical, basic, and translational research that will enhance the scientific foundation for clinical nursing practice (www.nih.gov/ninr).

K. 2001 – Stetler published the Steps of Research Utilization to Facilitate Evidence-Based Practice Model.

L. 2007 – The National Institute for Nursing Research identified the mission and funding themes for the future of nursing research (Burns & Grove, 2009).

VIII. Nursing Research Methods

A. Four common types of research (Burns & Grove, 2009):
1. Quantitative:
   a. Descriptive.
   b. Correlational.
   c. Quasi-experimental.
   d. Experimental.
2. Qualitative:
   a. Phenomenological.
   b. Ethnographic.
   c. Grounded theory.
   d. Historical.
   e. Philosophical.
      (1) Ethical analysis.
      (2) Foundational inquiry.
      (3) Philosophical analysis.
   f. Critical social theory methodology.
3. Outcomes:
   a. Examines the outcomes or results of care.
   b. Measures the health status of patients.
4. Intervention – Examines the effectiveness of nursing interventions in achieving the desired outcome(s) in a natural setting.

IX. Ethics in Research
(Burns & Grove, 2009)

A. Ethical codes (for example, the Nuremberg Code) and regulations exist to provide guidelines for the selection of the study purpose, design and subjects, the collection and analysis of data, the interpretation of the results, and the presentation and publication of the results of the study.

B. The Nuremberg Code was created in 1949 in response to unethical treatment of human subjects during research studies, especially during the Third Reich/Nazi reign from 1933–1945. The Nuremberg Code contains guidelines for:
1. Subjects' voluntary consent to participation.
2. The right of subjects to withdraw from the study at any time and without penalty.
3. Protection of subjects from mental and physical suffering, injury, disability, and death during the study.
4. Risk and benefits disclosure.

C. Despite the Nuremberg Code, unethical treatment of human subjects continued to occur as evidenced by the Tuskegee Syphillis Study, the Willowbrook Study, and the Jewish Chronic Disease Hospital Study. These studies continued into the 1960s and early 1970s, and placed subjects at considerable health risk, and in some cases, death.

D. In 1973, the U.S. Department of Health Education and Welfare (DHEW) published regulations intended to protect human subjects, and in 1978, the National Commission for the Protection of Human Subjects of Biomedical and Behavioral Research was established as part of public law.

E. Belmont Report: Identified three ethical principles for human research, determined protected subjects, and established Institutional Review Boards as an oversight system to protect the rights of research participants.
1 Three ethical principles for human research:
   a. Respect for persons – The right to self-determination.
   b. Beneficence – Above all, do no harm.
   c. Justice – Treat subjects fairly.

2. Protected subjects:
   a. Legally and mentally incompetent subjects.
   b. Neonates.
   c. Pregnant women.
   d. Children.
   e. Prisoners.
   f. Terminally ill subjects.
3. Established Institutional Review Boards; all proposed studies must go though review prior to commencement.

X. Definition and Overview of Performance Improvement

A. Performance improvement is the systematic analysis of the structure, processes, and outcomes within systems for the purpose of improving the delivery of care (The Joint Commission, 2011).
   1. Performance improvement is one of the most critical endpoints in a quality model.
   2. The goal of performance improvement is to determine if the desired outcome is achieved through the implementation of appropriate processes, policies, procedures, guidelines, or any combination of the above.
B. The Institute of Medicine's (IOM) "Six Aims for Improving Healthcare" identifies key aspects of performance improvement used to guide the development and evaluation of quality initiatives as safe, effective, patient-centered, timely, efficient, and equitable (IOM, 2001).
C. The IOM's definition of health care quality in the 1990s set the framework for improvement as detailed in *To Err is Human* and *Crossing the Quality Chasm* (IOM, 1999, 2001). The definition of "quality" has morphed from "the degree to which health services for individuals and populations increase the likelihood of desired health outcomes and are consistent with current professional knowledge" (IOM, 1990, p. 21), to its more current version. Health care quality is currently defined as the extent to which health services provided to individuals and patient populations improve desired health outcomes and are based on the strongest clinical evidence and provided in a technically and culturally competent manner with good communication and shared decision-making (IOM, 1999, 2001).

D. History of quality assurance (QA), continuous quality improvement (CQI), quality performance improvement (QPI), and total quality management (TQM).
   1. Historically, performance improvement initiatives focused on QA.
      a. QA relies on principles of inspection and audit. It is frequently referred to as the "bad apple" approach, in which the bad apples are discarded, but there is no process to assure the production of only good apples.
      b. Using a QA approach, health care organizations focused on the performance of individuals or specific departments, and used audit methodologies to review areas of mortality review, transfusion utilization, and medical record review. This approach is problem-focused and tends to be defensive and reactive (Leebov & Ersoz, 1991).
   2. In 1986, The Joint Commission introduced a 10-step process that replaced the problem-focused QA approach with one that required systematic evaluation and monitoring of key aspects of patient care. Through the use of additional strategies, including the use of written specifications or guidelines and more rigorous statistical evaluations that focus on performance over time, the concept of CQI or continuous performance improvement emerged. CQI relies on the use of data, not anecdotal evidence, as the basis for comparison and performance over time, and data are tracked and trended through use of control charts and other statistical tools (NAHQ, 2008).
   3. To accomplish the transition from QA to CQI, organizations and businesses needed to adopt a new approach to both management principles and QA. One of the most influential quality "gurus" in this transition process was an American named W. Edwards Deming, PhD. Deming

(2000) believed that a culture of quality within an organization would influence the outcomes. Deming created a management philosophy based on 14 points for businesses to be competitive (NAHQ, 2008).

4. In the 1920s, Walter Shewhart introduced the concept of Plan-Do-See; Deming modified the Shewhart Cycle to Plan-Do-Study-Act (PDSA), and later to Plan-Do-Check-Act (PDCA). This cycle is the basis for many performance improvement programs. There are variations of the acronym, but all are intended to define a process of continuous assessment, evaluation, and action (NAHQ, 2008).

5. Deming, along with Philip B. Cosby and Joseph Juran, created a set of strategies in which the front line workers had as much input into process improvement as the managers, and as such, were held accountable for the outcomes of production (Juran Institute, 2003). The strategies also included soliciting and listening to the "voice of the customer" to understand requirements, needs, and desires, and aligning the performance improvement efforts with the mission, vision, and strategic plan of the organization. The "voice of the customer" is a key input in Six Sigma methodology.

6. Reduction of process variation is the hallmark of quality methodologies, such as Six Sigma. Performance improvement focuses on the processes of care, not the individual person's performance. This approach removes the placement of blame from an individual and seeks to improve processes of care to assure greater success among a wider cohort of employees (Pande & Holpp, 2002).

7. A classic model that acts as a mechanism to focus our quality efforts is the Donabedian Quality Trilogy Model: Structure, Process, and Outcomes (NAHQ, 2008). Successful improvement efforts require the integration of all three. Within the quality model, structure, process, and outcome can be defined as:

a. Structure – Factors within an organization that support the delivery of quality care (e.g., staff credentials, competencies, policies, procedures, and guidelines).

b. Process – The work that supports delivering quality care on behalf of the patient or health care consumer (e.g., medication reconciliation).

c. Outcome – The result of care processes that can be measured.

XI. Performance Improvement (PI) Indicators and Measurements

A. An indicator is a performance measure that provides an indication of an organization's performance in relation to a specified process or outcome. Basic types of indicators (Joint Commission on Accreditation of Healthcare Organizations [JCAHO], 2005):

1. Clinical indicators (such as Pap smear, mammography, and immunization rates) reflect the adherence to known standards of care or clinical guidelines.

2. Administrative indicators (such as revenue, expenses) reflect efficiency and productivity.

3. Operational indicators (such as visit volume data, no-shows, and cancellations) are measures of access to care.

4. Perception of care indicators (such as waiting time and attributes of caring by staff) are measures of patient satisfaction.

B. Measurement is the process of collecting and aggregating data. There are three fundamental purposes of measurement (JCAHO, 2005):

1. *Assessing current performance* – Measurement to assess current performance is often the first step in a structured performance improvement project. Such measurement produces data that illustrate the strengths and weaknesses of current processes and achieved outcomes, thereby providing a baseline. Practices can be "benchmarked" or compared to like practices to assess current performance in key areas.

2. *Verifying improved performance* – Measurement to demonstrate the effectiveness of improvement actions. For example, an organization that has added an advanced practice nurse to a group practice may use measurement to determine whether the addition has indeed met a high-volume community need, enhanced patient volume, and increased revenue.

3. *Control of performance* – Measurement can also be used to determine whether key processes are in control. It can provide an early warning system that identifies an undesirable change in performance and allow immediate corrective actions to be made.

C. Choosing an indicator or measure.

1. Performance improvement priorities are usually determined by the performance improvement coordinating group (PICG) or quality council, and may be based on needs identified through the PI process, sentinel events, The Joint Commission standards' compliance, Department of Health regulations, hospital agenda, or administrative direction (NAHQ, 2008).

2. Processes often chosen for review include:
   a. New techniques or equipment.
   b. High-risk.
   c. High-volume.
   d. High-cost.
   e. High-risk and low-volume.

XII. Priority Focus Areas

A. Priority focus areas are processes, systems, or structures in a health care organization that significantly impact the quality and safety of care.

B. The Joint Commission (2011), through the use of database analysis, expert literature, and expert opinion, has identified 14 priority focus areas that are most likely to ensure safe, high-quality care and are generally universal across health care organizations and settings. The 14 priority focus areas are:

1. Assessment and care/services.
2. Communication.
3. Credentialed practitioners.
4. Equipment use.
5. Infection control.
6. Information management.
7. Medication management
8. Organizational structure.
9. Orientation and training.
10. Patient safety.
11. Physical environment.
12. Quality improvement expertise/activities.
13. Rights and ethics.
14. Staffing.

C. When identifying performance improvement opportunities, it is crucial for organizations to consider the 14 priority focus areas in relation to their scope of services or scope of care; their high-risk, high-volume, problem-prone services; and newest technologies.

XIII. The Performance Improvement Process

Carey and Lloyd (1995) described the steps in a performance improvement process.

A. Identify the opportunity for improvement.
B. Organize a team.
C. Flowchart the process.
D. Determine if the process is standardized; if not, standardize the process.
E. If the process is standardized, identify the important aspects of the process.
F. Select the most important aspect in the process.
G. Define the most important aspect and develop a plan to collect data to study the most important aspect.
H. Analyze the data collected, and determine the degree of variation in the data and whether the variation is random (occurring by chance). If the variation is not occurring by chance, a special reason may be causing the variation.

1. Common-cause variation is variation that occurs due to chance. It represents the normal variation found in any process and is not indicative of a process that is out of statistical control (e.g., fluctuating oral/rectal temperatures around a set of normal limits) (NAHQ, 2008).

2. Special-cause variation occurs when a factor intermittently and unpredictably induces variation that is not a normal part of the process. It often appears as an extreme point beyond the control limits on a control

chart, or as a specific, identifiable pattern in the data (NAHQ, 2008).

  a. Example: A temperature spike caused by an infection. A spike significantly higher than most values would need to be questioned to determine if something unusual is occurring to cause the abnormally high temperature.

  b. Example: Patient satisfaction rates drop precipitously following a decrease in the number of clinicians who provide care, therefore causing the waiting room times to increase significantly.

3. Different performance improvement actions are taken depending on the type of variation.

  a. If data indicate a common-cause variation is present, the team must first decide if the degree of variation is acceptable. When using control charts to assess data, processes are considered in control when data remain within two standard deviations from the statistical mean and no data runs or trends are noted.

     (1) For example, if data indicate patient satisfaction varies between 80% and 85%, the team would ask, "Is that level acceptable?" (Should the team attempt to improve performance by raising the goal to 87% or 90%?)

     (2) The team would also consider what factors have the greatest influence on the process.

     (3) The most important factor influencing the process is then selected and an improvement strategy is implemented.

     (4) Data are collected to determine if the intended improvement was achieved.

     (5) If not, another factor is selected, actions are implemented to improve the process, and data are again collected.

     (6) When the action achieves the intended improvement, the action becomes a permanent part of the process.

  b. If data indicate a special cause is present, the team will work to eliminate it.

I. Specific mechanisms exist to improve quality; each mechanism serves a different purpose in the performance improvement process. This section discusses two of these mechanisms: benchmarking and root-cause analysis.

1. Benchmarking is a comparison measurement of a process, product, or service in comparison to those of the toughest competitor, to those considered industry leaders, or to those considered to have best practice (external benchmarking), or to similar activities in the organization (internal benchmarking). The information is used to change/improve practices, resulting in superior performance as determined by measured outcomes (NAHQ, 2008).

  a. Three types of benchmarking:

     (1) *Internal benchmarking*: Process of examining internal performance and gauging improvement over time.

     (2) *External or competitive benchmarking*: Measurement of performance of a given organization with reliable and valid indicators against that of another similar organization using identical indicators. Comparative reference databases (national, regional, or system level) as well as practice guidelines, critical paths, Care Maps®, and other recognized professional standards of practice and care used for benchmarking (NAHQ, 2008).

     (3) *Functional benchmarking*: Comparing a similar function or process, such as scheduling, in another industry.

  b. Potential outcomes of benchmarking (Ellis, 1995; Jeffries & Timms, 1998; Kobs, 1998; Spann, 1997):

(1) Quality improvement and practice development are accelerated.

(2) Quality measures are established.

(3) Motivation and enthusiasm among staff are improved as a result of recognition and reward for achievement and success.

(4) A structured forum for networking is provided.

(5) A systematic process for evaluating and improving care and service delivery to patients is developed.

c. Selecting what to benchmark (Kobs, 1998).

(1) Ask the question, "Have the best of the best been identified in any other organization?"

(2) Identify what services, products, and practices have been benchmarked internally and externally.

(3) Decide which services, products, and practices, if improved, would have the most impact within your organization.

(4) Agree on the most critical services, products, and practices for quality improvement.

2. Root-cause analysis is a method to determine the fundamental reason that causes variation in performance (Dlugacz, Restifo, & Greenwood, 2004).

a. Key characteristics of root-cause analysis include:

(1) A focus on systems rather than individuals.

(2) Analyzing special causes first, then common causes by repeatedly asking, "Can anything be causing this problem?" until no further logical answers can be found.

b. The steps of a root-cause analysis include:

(1) Define the event – What happened?

(2) Identify the proximate cause – Why did this happen? Proximate causes

may include human error, process deficiency, equipment breakdown, and environmental factors.

(3) Identify the underlying reason for the proximate cause by brainstorming to determine why the proximate cause happened.

(4) Collect and assess data on the proximate and underlying causes.

(5) Develop and implement interim changes (e.g., if one cause might be broken equipment, the team should not wait to fix the equipment).

(6) Identify the root-cause by asking key questions, including:

(a) What factors in the environment might have contributed to the errors? For example, was staffing adequate, was the activity level greater than normal, was the equipment working properly, and were breaks being taken?

(b) How is the flow of communication being managed? For example, does information flow freely, accurately, clearly? Is the information accessible?

(c) Is staff competent and is a system in place to objectively assess staff competency?

(d) How is competent performance maintained? Note: the *Ambulatory Care Nursing Orientation and Competency Assessment Guide* (AAACN, 2010) is a valuable resource for competency assessment.

(7) Once the factors have been identified, a performance improvement action plan is developed and implemented. The modified processes are assessed for positive change in the outcome, and additional modifications are made as necessary to prevent future occurrences.

XIV. Analyzing and Displaying Data

A. Balanced scorecards and dashboards.
1. A balanced scorecard or dashboard is a graphic or pictorial display of the organization's indicators chosen to support the strategic plan and vision of the organization.
2. The balanced scorecard allows for the examination of relationships among key performance measures (care, quality, financial, operational) to assure alignment with the strategic plan.
3. Key performance measures (Kedrowski & Weiner, 2003) in ambulatory care include:
   a. Access to care.
   b. Utilization and productivity.
   c. Financial operations.
   d. Quality and service (see Table 11-1).
B. Report cards. As health care costs increase, desire of consumers to know how an organization is performing is also increasing. Financial reimbursement and incentives may be tied to the organization's (and individual practitioner's) ability to meet the performance standards, benchmarks, and outcomes.
1. The demand for information about performance is driving a revolution that will profoundly affect health care providers and payers (IOM, 2002).
2. Variation in specific indicators will help consumers determine different values and will help organizations identify potential opportunities for improvement.
3. Example of an ambulatory report card:
   a. Healthcare Effectiveness Data and Information Set (HEDIS®).
      (1) HEDIS is a tool created by the National Committee on Quality Assurance (NCQA) to collect data about the quality of care and services provided by health plans.
      (2) Emphasis is quality of care, access to care, and patient satisfaction with health plans and providers.
      (3) The indicators are linked to nursing and provider performance (such as immunization, Pap smear, and satisfaction rates).
      (4) Data from this report card are used to determine health plan expenditures and performance accountabilities (NAHQ, 2008).

XV. Pay for Performance

The federal government and other providers of health care insurance are interested in standardization of care through the use of evidence-based guidelines that lead to improved patient outcomes. The Centers for Medicare and Medicaid Services (CMS) has established several initiatives and programs to measure adherence to the suggested guidelines (www.cms.gov). Compliance with the guidelines will be publicly reported in a report card format in the near future and will be subject to financial incentives and/or penalties.

A. Physician Quality Reporting System (PQRS).
1. Formerly known as Physician Quality Reporting Initiative (PQRI).
2. Voluntary program that provides financial incentives for physicians who adopt and demonstrate evidence-based practice.
3. Based on individual physician outcomes.
B. Group practice reporting option.
1. Introduced in 2010 as a way for physicians in group practice to work together to achieve compliance with PQRS measures.
2. Focuses on chronic condition measures (such as diabetes, hypertension, cardiac), as well as preventive measures (such as mammography and influenza vaccination).
C. Outpatient prospective payment system.
1. Selected indicators in selected settings.
   a. Ambulatory surgery.
      (1) Timing of antibiotics.
      (2) Appropriateness of antibiotic choice.
   b. Emergency department.
      (1) Cardiac core measures for "treat and release" patients (such as AMI, chest pain).
         (a) Fibrinolytic therapy received within 30 minutes of arrival.
         (b) Median time to transfer to another facility for acute coronary intervention.
         (c) Aspirin on arrival.

Table 11-1.
Key Performance Measures in Ambulatory Care

Access to Care	Utilization and Productivity	Financial Operations	Quality and Service
Appointment availability; for example, next vs. 2nd or 3rd available	Space/exam room utilization Visits per exam room	Charge timeliness and accuracy • Charge lag	Patient satisfaction
Bumped/rescheduled appointment rate	Number of specialty referrals	Co-payment and cash collection rate	Staff satisfaction
No show appointment rate	Number of ED visits	Rejection/denial rate	PI projects; site specific
Wait time • Exam room • Waiting room	Number of visits conforming to CPT codes	Accounts receivable days	Sedation outcomes
Cancellation rate	Staff mix per visit	Insurance/registration accuracy	Immunization rates
Referral request turnaround	Staff turnover rate	Total visit volume • New patient • Urgent/walk-in visits • Percent change to prior year visit variance to budget	Diabetes compliance • Hgb A1c • Annual eye exams • Foot care
Consult request turnaround	Support staff FTEs per MD	Total direct cost per visit	Point of care testing compliance
Availability of urgent or walk-in appointments	Expenses per visit	Revenue and expense per visit	Population-specific guidelines (e.g., CHF, COPD, CF)
Telephone access • Abandonment rate • Average time before answered • Total number of calls by agent • Response time for clinical triage	Relative Value Units (RVUs) • RVUs per visit • Total RVUs • RVU variance to budget	Billing timeliness and accuracy • Billing lag	Prevention of tobacco use

Source: Kedrowski & Weiner, 2003. Reprinted from *Nursing Economic$,* 2003, Volume 21, Number 4, pp. 188-193. Used with permission of the publisher, Jannetti Publications, Inc., East Holly Avenue, Box 56, Pitman, NJ 08071-0056; (856) 256-2300; FAX (856) 589-7463; Web site: www.nursingeconomics.net. For a sample copy of the journal, please contact the publisher.

(d) Median time to ECG.

(e) Troponin result turnaround time within 60 minutes of arrival.

(2) Throughput measures.

(a) Cycle time.

(b) Time to provider assessment.

(c) Discharge transition record given to patient.

(d) Left without being seen.

(3) Pain management for long bone fracture.

(4) Stroke assessment – Head CT or MRI performed and interpreted within 45 minutes of arrival.

c. Ambulatory radiology.

(1) Goal to reduce unnecessary CT scans with contrast for lower back pain.

(2) Assess screening mammography follow-up rates.

References

American Academy of Ambulatory Care Nursing (AAACN). (2010). *Ambulatory care nursing orientation and competency assessment guide* (2nd ed.). Pitman, NJ: Author.

Burns, N., & Grove, S. (2009). *The practice of nursing research: Appraisal, synthesis and generation of evidence* (6th ed.). St. Louis, MO: Saunders/Elsevier.

Carey, R.G., & Lloyd, R.C. (1995). *Measuring quality improvement in health care: A guide to statistical process control applications.* New York: Quality Resources.

Centers for Disease Control and Prevention (CDC). (2009). *Healthy people 2020.* Retrieved from http://www.cdc.gov/nchs/healthy_people/hp2020.htm

Craig, J.V., & Smyth, R.L. (2007). *The evidence-based practice manual for nurses* (2nd ed.). Edinburgh: Churchill Livingstone.

Deming, W.E. (2000). *Out of the crisis.* Cambridge, MA: The MIT Press.

Dlugacz, Y., Restifo, A., & Greenwood, A. (2004). *The quality handbook for health care organizations: A manager's guide to tools and programs.* San Francisco: Jossey-Bass.

Ellis, J. (1995). Using benchmarking to improve practice. *Clinical Quality Assurance, 9*(35), 25-28.

Institute of Medicine (IOM). (1990). *Medicare: A strategy for quality assurance* (Vol. I). Washington, DC: The National Academies Press.

Institute of Medicine (IOM). (1999). *To err is human: Building a safer health system.* Washington, DC: The National Academies Press.

Institute of Medicine (IOM). (2001). *Crossing the quality chasm: A new health system for the 21st century.* Washington, DC: The National Academies Press.

Institute of Medicine (IOM). (2002). In J.M. Corrigan, A. Greiner, & S.M. Erickson (Eds.), *Fostering rapid advances in health care: Learning from system demonstrations.* Washington, DC: The National Academies Press.

Jeffries, E., & Timms, L. (1998). Sharing good practice: Developing network forums. *Nursing Standard, 12*(50), 33-34.

Joint Commission on Accreditation of Healthcare Organizations (JCAHO). (2005). *Accreditation manual for ambulatory care.* Oakbrook, IL: Author.

Joint Commission, The. (2011). *Hospital accreditation standards.* Oakbrook, IL: Author

Juran Institute. (2003). *Juran Institute's Six Sigma breakthrough and beyond: Quality performance breakthrough methods.* Columbus, OH: McGraw-Hill Professional.

Kedrowski, S., & Weiner, C. (2003). Performance measures in ambulatory care. *Nursing Economics$, 21*(4), 188-193.

Kitson, A. (1997). Using evidence to demonstrate the value of nursing. *Nursing Standard, 11*(28), 34-39.

Kobs, A.E. (1998). Getting started on benchmarking. *Outcomes Management for Nursing Practice, 2*(1), 45-48.

Leebov, W., & Ersoz, C. (1991). *The health care manager's guide to continuous quality improvement.* Chicago: American Hospital Publishing, Inc.

Melynk, B.M., & Fineout-Overholt, E. (2011). *Evidence-based practice in nursing and healthcare: A guide to best practice* (2nd ed.). Philadelphia: Lippincott, Williams & Wilkins.

National Association for Healthcare Quality (NAHQ). (2008). *Q-Solutions – Essential resources for the healthcare quality professional* (2nd ed.). Glenview, IL: Author.

Nightingale, F. (1860). *Notes on nursing.* New York: D. Appleton and Company.

Pande, P., & Holpp, L. (2002). *What is Six Sigma?* New York: McGraw-Hill.

Spann, K. (1997). Benchmarking: Best practices. *MEDSURG Nursing, 6*(1), 5-6, 8.

Stetler, C.B. (2001). Updating the Stetler Model of Research Utilization to facilitate evidence-based practice. *Nursing Outlook, 49*(6), 272-279.

Stetler, C.B. (2003). Role of the organization in translating research into evidence-based practice. *Outcomes Management, 7*(3), 97-103.

Swan, B.A., & Boruch, R.F. (2004). Quality of evidence: Usefulness in measuring the quality of health care. *Medical Care, 42*(2), II-12-II-20.

Titler, M.G., Kleiber, C., Steelman, V.J., Rakel, B.A., Budreau, G., & Everett, L.Q. (2001). The Iowa Model of Evidence-Based Practice to promote quality care. *Critical Care Nursing Clinics of North America, 13*(4), 497-509.

Additional Reading

Institute of Medicine (IOM). (2010). *The future of nursing: Leading change, advancing health.* Washington, DC: The National Academies Press.

Chapter 12

Ethics

June Levine, MSN, RN

OBJECTIVES – *Study of the information in this chapter will enable the learner to:*

1. Recognize the importance of the 2001 American Nurses Association (ANA) *Code of Ethics for Nurses.*
2. Define an ethical dilemma.
3. Discuss the ethical principles that guide ethical decision-making.
4. List the essential steps in the process of ethical decision-making.
5. Identify ambulatory practice issues that may pose an ethical dilemma.
6. Define the concepts of moral uncertainty and moral distress.
7. Identify ways in which the registered nurse can advocate for patients in the ambulatory care setting.

KEY POINTS – *The major points in this chapter include:*

1. The nursing profession has always been concerned with the moral responsibility of its practitioners and the pivotal role registered nurses must play to improve patient care.
2. The ANA *Code of Ethics for Nurses* offers specific provisions and interpretive statements to clarify nursing's responsibilities to patients, other health team members, society, and the nursing profession.
3. There are several key ethical principles that guide decision-making.
4. Ethical decision-making occurs when a problem or concern is identified as an ethical dilemma and the nurse begins to sort out the right thing to do amidst personal, professional, and societal values.
5. Ethical decision-making can be a complex process that benefits from guidelines to help ensure a reasoned approach to ethical issues.

From its inception as a professional group, nursing has been concerned with the moral responsibility of its practitioners, has expressed a commitment to high ideals for providing service, and has professed a belief in the pivotal role nurses must play in improving patient welfare.

I. The Code of Ethics for Nurses

A. The American Nurses Association (ANA) House of Delegates first adopted a *Code of Ethics for Nurses* in 1950.

　　1. Since that time, the Code and/or its Interpretive Statements has been revised six times.

2. It has evolved as the social context in which registered nurse (RN) practice has changed and as the profession of nursing progressed.

3. The Code forms the ethical basis for professional practice and is a public statement of nursing's shared values, moral concerns, and responsibilities.

4. It provides an ethical framework to clarify nurses' responsibilities to patients, other health team members, society, and the nursing profession.

B. The most recent *Code of Ethics for Nurses* was adopted in 2001 and contains nine provisions with interpretive statements (ANA, 2001). The interpretive statements provide clarity to gain a deeper understanding of the meaning of each provision.

1. The first three provisions describe the most fundamental values and commitments of the nurse, such as practicing with compassion, respecting the individual, and demonstrating that the nurse's primary commitment is to the patient.
2. The second three provisions address the boundaries of duties and loyalty, such as accepting accountability for individual nursing practice, providing nursing care with integrity, and improving health care environments.
3. The last three provisions address aspects of duties that take professional nurses beyond individual patient encounters, such as participating in activities that advance the profession, promoting community efforts to meet health care needs, actively participating in professional associations, and promoting the implementation of the *Code of Ethics for Nurses.*

C. The 2001 Code's nine provisions apply to all RNs working in all settings.
D. For the Code to be a document that is utilized, nurses must understand what it says, use it in their daily practice, and ensure that the environments in which they work support the provisions of the *Code of Ethics for Nurses.*

II. **Ethical Dilemmas**
A. An ethical dilemma may occur when there is a conflict among duties, loyalties, rights, or values.
B. A nurse would experience an ethical dilemma when he or she does not know the right course of action, feels hampered by his or her own inability to adequately explain the concern, or feels that the organizational system or individual(s) prevent him or her from pursuing the action deemed correct.
1. When the dilemma is clinical and concerns a patient and/or family member, the issues usually have to do with determining the right thing to do in a specific patient care situation and/or determining who decides a certain treatment direction.

2. If everyone is in agreement about the choice of treatment or non-treatment and clear about who makes the treatment decisions, then there is usually no dilemma.
3. Disagreements may arise among health care professionals and between health care professionals and the patient/family about the plan of care or who actually should be making certain decisions.

C. Dilemmas may also arise in a non-clinical context when nurses encounter issues relating to scope of practice or competence of a team member, verbal abuse, sexual harassment, safety of equipment, and organizational systems that do not support the nurse's advocacy role.
D. Ethical questions that arise can be directly related to patients or health care staff or the environment where practice occurs, such as:
1. Can treatment be stopped once initiated?
2. Who should be giving consent?
3. Can patients be forced to go along with a treatment plan?
4. Who judges the quality of someone's life?
5. What should the nurse do when the information the patient or surrogate decision-maker received was not adequate for them to be fully informed?
6. How does the nurse stop the verbal abuse of a physician, manager, or another staff nurse?
7. What should the nurse do when a physician refuses to wash his or her hands?
8. How can a nurse require that individuals in a patient care environment adhere to scope of practice laws?

E. The existence of moral uncertainty and/or moral distress can complicate the issues.
1. Moral uncertainty can be described as a personal feeling that something is not right, perhaps decisions are being made too fast, without sufficient discussion or clarity, and/or with many unanswered questions.
2. Moral distress is a concept that is unique to the practice of nursing.
a. Conflicting loyalties to the patient, the physician, the organization, and the nursing profession often place nurses

in the middle, not knowing how to navigate the path of conflicting expectations.

   b. When the RN knows the right thing to do, but is organizationally prevented from doing so too many times, it may lead to burnout and perhaps worse, an uncaring, dispassionate attitude.

3. Andrew Jameton (1984) defined the concepts of moral uncertainty and moral distress in the following way:

   a. Moral uncertainty – When one is unsure of what principles or values apply or what the problem is.

   b. Moral distress – When one knows the right thing to do, but is prevented by institutional constraints (systems and/or individuals) from pursuing the right course of action.

III. Ethical Decision-Making

A. Ethical decision-making involves choosing a direction, a next step to process the issues, and understanding the best course of action.

1. Historically, the inpatient setting was the source of the majority of ethical issues, both clinical and non-clinical.

2. Although nurses in the ambulatory care setting are challenged by many of the same ethical concerns as inpatient nurses, the ambulatory environment has created new dilemmas. The increasing number of chronically ill patients and the performance of more complex procedures have raised old issues and brought new ones to deliberate:

   a. Scope of practice concerns related to the use of non-RNs.

   b. Insufficient RNs available to assure safety and quality.

   c. Limited time available to adequately teach patients to prevent harm.

   d. Insufficient numbers of RNs in patient care management positions.

   e. Access concerns presented by managed care protocols and organizational policies and procedures.

B. Historically, the physician made all treatment decisions for the patient. Patients and family members were often unaware of why some treatments were initiated and some were not.

1. As medical science grew in its ability to prolong the dying process, questions were raised about who actually should be making patient care decisions that involved choices about what treatments would be initiated, not initiated, and/or stopped.

2. A shift occurred from the paternalistic decision-making process to one in which the physician conceded authority to patients and families.

3. Ultimately, neither approach is adequate. A partnership between patients and families and their physician will be what leads to the best outcomes.

4. Leah Curtin (2010) stated it clearly when she emphasized that patients and families want to be guided in making decisions.

   a. Patients/families need the advice and council of their medical team.

   b. The RN can assist the process by helping team members use a process for decision-making that considers the important elements.

C. Ethical decision-making is a learned skill that needs to be practiced for the nurse to build confidence and competence. When viewing the steps involved in this decision-making model, it is not unusual to feel overwhelmed by the process itself.

1. The steps reflect the nursing process, which when used correctly, helps shed light on a reasoned approach to problem-solving.

2. The more ethical issues are addressed with a defined process for decision-making, the easier it is to critically think through the known concerns, put emotion aside, and identify the questions that still need clarification.

3. The model can be applied to issues that directly impact patients and families, as well as those that involve organizational concerns.

4. It is also important to note that although the model is presented as a step-by-step process, in reality, it is usually not so precise.
5. It is essential to consider all steps within the ethical decision-making process.

D. The steps of the ethical decision-making model are:
1. Define the dilemma – Defining the problem can be the hardest step.
   a. Nurses may struggle with finding the right words to describe their concern. Stating the problem in words that are comfortable helps in identifying the ethical issues.
   b. Some nurses, when defining the dilemma, utilize an ethical principle to help state the problem.
   c. Using their own words can be more helpful as they learn more about ethical decision-making.
      (1) For example, a nurse might say, "Mr. Jones told me he wanted to stop chemotherapy, but his daughter does not want this to happen. He now has no advance directive, and his daughter wants everything done."
      (2) Or the nurse can provide a broader understanding of her or his concern with this next statement: "Mr. Jones had once told me he wanted to stop his chemotherapy treatments, but his daughter persisted. At one visit, I suggested he let his daughter and the doctor know what he wants. I provided him with information on completing an advance directive and asked about it the next time I saw him. He had not done anything and continued to express frustration and sadness. I asked the social worker to see him next time he came to the infusion center. Mr. Jones is now not able to advocate for himself. The disease process and medications have made him confused and disoriented, and the daughter persists in having everything tried. No one has sat down with her to explain the goals of treatment. When I try to tell her what is going on, she does not listen. I cannot bear to continue with these infusions every week."
      (3) Some nurses might use the ethical principle of autonomy by saying this: "Mr. Jones told me he wanted to stop chemotherapy, but his daughter does not want this to happen. He now has no advance directive, and his daughter wants everything done. His ability to advocate for himself is limited by his current inability to make decisions. Thus, his autonomy is being compromised."
      (4) Each of these statements tells a story about a patient needing the medical team to come together and work with the daughter to have the patient's wishes realized and adhered to.
2. Identify the medical facts – Gather relevant information and confirm the identified facts.
   a. Managerial issues that pose ethical dilemmas usually do not require a review of medical facts. When working through clinical issues, the diagnosis and prognosis are critical components of this step.
   b. The nurse can support the patient by encouraging the medical team to focus on the broad goals of treatment and their impact on the patient's quality of life.
3. Identify the non-medical facts. There are two distinct groups:
   a. Facts that apply directly to the patient and family.
      (1) Religious beliefs.
      (2) Cultural issues.
      (3) Advance directives appointing a surrogate for decision-making and/ or the patient's written wishes about life-sustaining treatment.

(4) Patient's verbal statements about continuing treatment.

b. Facts external to the patient and family.
   (1) Organizational policies and procedures.
   (2) Applicable laws.
   (3) Regulatory requirements.
   (4) Ethical codes of professionals providing care.
   (5) Concern of the nurse or other provider about the benefits weighed against the suffering that may be caused or is being caused by the treatment.

4. Separate assumptions from facts – It is easy to make judgments without full consideration of all of the facts. However, these judgments may be incorrect and lead the nurse to the wrong conclusion.
   a. Verifying certain facts, such as diagnosis and prognosis, can be critical because different medical specialists can have different views.
   b. The issue for the nurse is to always focus on the patient and not a particular organ system.
   c. Discussing this issue with primary care providers can be helpful.
   d. It is important to confirm assumptions that others are making about what treatments people within a certain religious or ethnic group would want or not want. Within this context, it is important to understand differences that may be present between the patient and family members.

5. Identify items needing clarification – Information that is being questioned needs to be clarified so that better decisions can be reached.

6. Identify the decision-makers – Decision-making can be a complex issue when family members have differences, when patients with decision-making capacity do not want to upset their family by wanting something different than their family, when patients lacking decision-making capacity are not clear in writing or verbally what

their wishes would be at the end of life, or when a family member's guilt and/or sadness confuse the reality of the patient's diagnosis and prognosis.

a. Clarify if the patient has decision-making capacity and can tell the health care team what treatments he or she wants or does not want.
   (1) Patients having decision-making capacity can verbalize questions and comprehend what decisions need to be made for their own care.
   (2) Medical decisions are complex, and many patients may need to hear the information more than once before they are able to make any decisions.

b. The nurse and the physician or other health care professional (such as a social worker) should review an advance directive to assess its compliance with the state law where the document was executed and whether or not the information documented by the patient is still accurate. Critical areas to verify with the patient:
   (1) What type of treatments the patient wants or does not want, and under what conditions.
   (2) Whom the patient appointed as their surrogate.

c. Should there be a change, the nurse and primary care provider should understand the state laws to assist the patient. Unlike acute care, ambulatory practice provides more of an opportunity to encourage this type of planning and discussion with patients before they cannot speak for themselves.

d. RNs and other health care professionals should not assume that if there is no advance directive, then there is no legal decision-maker.
   (1) Most states have written into their health care decision laws the process of such recognition; they have identified a process where certain family members are given

the power of surrogacy in a certain order, such as spouse; if no spouse, adult children; if neither a spouse nor adult children, the parents.

e. Sometimes the decision-maker is the nurse. These questions may pose ethical dilemmas for some registered nurses:

    (1) Should I report the incompetent behavior of a colleague?

    (2) What do I do when a physician is attempting a procedure under the influence of drugs or alcohol?

    (3) Do I continue to cover for another RN who everyone likes, but should not be providing patient care?

    (4) What do I do when a physician shouts at me for clarifying his or her medical order?

    (5) What do I do when a patient and/or family has not been given full disclosure about treatment options?

7. Review underlying ethical principles:

a. The identification of the relevant ethical principles (often, more than one) helps to support a critical thinking approach by utilizing reasoning skills rather than bias, intuition, emotion, incorrect data, or the authority of another individual.

b. Ethical principles – Consideration of these ethical principles help to further guide the decision-making process.

    (1) Autonomy – Individual self-determination and freedom of choice.

        (a) Requires that health care professionals respect the rights of patients to make autonomous decisions.

        (b) Supports the patient who has decision-making capacity and implies that one is cognitively able to exercise this right.

        (c) Supports a patient's right to appoint a surrogate through verbal declaration or an advance directive (dependent on state law) to speak for the patient when he or she can no longer speak for him/herself (see Chapter 9, "Legal Issues").

        (d) To support the patient's autonomy, the surrogate ought to choose for the patient what the patient would want if he or she could speak for him or herself, not based on the surrogate's personal beliefs, guilt, or dynamics with the family or health care team.

           i. This can get complicated when surrogates make decisions based on their own personal beliefs, their attempt at trying to correct past relationship mistakes, and/or sometimes not being well supported or guided by the health care team.

           ii. These situations require a team that is capable of working through the issues with families and have a clear understanding of their own roles in providing treatment or not providing treatment.

           iii. Inpatient organizations have had these types of policies and procedures for many years. Because of the changes in ambulatory care, it is time to have these discussions and provide written direction for the health care team.

    (2) Beneficence – Relates to acts of doing good.

        (a) People differ in their definition of what is a good act.

(b) To do good requires the nurse to help patients receive the care they need to cope with the effects of disease and disability, and achieve their goals of health.

(c) To fully actualize the ethical principle of beneficence, the nurse must also be ready to prevent harms in order to do good.

(d) In *Nursing's Social Policy Statement*, ANA (2010) defines nursing as "the protection, promotion, and optimization of health and abilities, prevention of illness and injury, alleviation of suffering through the diagnosis and treatment of human response, and advocacy in the care of individuals, families, communities, and populations" (p. 10).

(3) Nonmaleficence – To not act in such a way that causes harm, either intentional harm or harm as an unintended outcome.

(a) Consideration must be given to the difficult situation when one may do harm in order to do good. For example, chemotherapy may have serious systemic consequences; the treatment may be as life-threatening as the illness. However, the benefits (goods) of such a treatment may outweigh the burdens (harms).

(b) The nurse needs to be aware of potentially harmful side effects, and assist the patient to weigh the benefits versus the burdens of potential or actual undesirable outcomes in making treatment choices. Sometimes, the difficult role for the nurse is to understand that each patient and/or family member may see benefits and burdens differently than the nurse or other members of the health care team.

(c) Nonmaleficence takes on other meaning when the nurse needs to decide whether he or she should intervene in a situation where the physician or another nurse is about to cause harm or is causing harm. For example, does the nurse tell a physician to stop what he or she is doing and wash his or her hands and risk possible anger and retribution? Does the nurse take over from another staff member who is doing a urinary catheterization incorrectly or wait until he or she is done to speak with the staff member? Ethically, both cases are clear: The nurse owes a duty first to the patient and to not speak up or act puts the patient in a situation of potential or actual harm.

(4) Veracity – Truth telling.

(a) Truth is the foundation of the development of trust between patient and nurse. All patients and their surrogate decision-maker are owed the duty of being fully informed about health conditions, treatment options, and prognosis, with as much completeness and accuracy as possible.

(b) Immediate attention without prejudgment must be given to situations in which a patient with decision-making capacity wants to turn over all decisions to a family member. The nurse must assure this is the patient's request and determine if he or she would like to be part of conversations with the surrogate decision-maker and the health care team. That determination may require the nurse to have a conversation with the patient.

(c) The patient should be made aware that if his or her wishes change, the health care provider or the nurse must be notified about the patient's desire to be more involved.

(5) Fidelity: Faithfulness.

(a) Fidelity involves the duty owed to patients, families, and colleagues to do what one says he or she will do.

(b) Professional fidelity requires the nurse to consistently act in accordance with the requirements of the state nurse practice act and the ethical standards of the profession.

(c) Honoring fidelity may be as simple as letting a patient know how much longer he or she needs to wait or to return a call to a patient when promised.

(6) Justice – The allocation of scarce resources.

(a) In health care, this principle is usually discussed when criteria need to be applied to the allocation of scarce resources, whether equipment, personnel, or access. Differing views about how to allocate scarce resources occur:

i. Discussion of the concept often evokes a sentiment of fairness. To be fair, one might think that all available resources need to be divided to give everyone an equal share. Yet that approach gives no consideration to differences in the amount of personnel and equipment that might be needed by different patients at different times.

ii. Although medical need is raised as the prevailing right direction, how that need is determined is debatable.

iii. Judgments have been based on an acceptance of such criteria as societal contribution, how much money a patient has, the age of the patient, or patient compliance with follow-up.

(b) Whether at the micro level or macro level of decision-making, the distribution of scarce health care resources requires critical examination in all organizations that are making such decisions daily, and nursing must be part of the decision-making process.

8. Define alternatives – The process of ethical decision-making may lead the nurse to one alternative or direction with which to proceed. However, there can be more than one next step to consider. In fact, more than one choice may be acceptable. Sometimes, there are two or more approaches to the problem, neither of which may be entirely satisfactory.

a. The benefits and burdens for each alternative should be discussed with the patient and/or family. In reality, in health care it is reasonable to present more than one alternative to a patient and help him or her in the decision-making process. When there is no clear direction, a patient care conference and/or a discussion with the health care team helps clarify direction and choice.

b. When issues are related to the organization and nurses must decide what to do, they may need to seek advice. The section on *Institutional Ethics Committees* (below) may help.

9. Follow-up – The most underused step in the process.

   a. In some situations, a family conference has occurred, and the family has been asked to let the health care team know about their choice, such as whether the patient wants chemotherapy or a particular surgery. The health professionals often do not reach out to ask how their decision-making is going and if they have additional questions.

      (1) Often in ambulatory care, patients are not in the immediate physical setting, and time may pass too quickly. Nurses must reach beyond the walls of the setting to assist patients and families with difficult choices.

      (2) RNs can provide care coordination, such as answering questions and arranging referrals.

   b. Additionally, when decisions are reached and the health care team is not satisfied with the process or the outcomes, it is helpful to sit down and discuss what occurred and how things can be improved the next time.

IV. Patient Advocacy

A. To advocate is to intercede on another's behalf. Thus, advocacy involves speaking up to state and/or clarify a patient's or family's decision.

B. Advocacy occurs when the nurse brings together the health care team to discuss the goals of treatment, helps families understand the prognosis and implications of further treatment, and contacts the physician to explain to the family again the rationale for a certain procedure.

C. The most effective advocacy happens when interventions focus on preventing future harms before issues arise.

D. Prevention, a key component of the principle of beneficence, is an effective strategy to advocate for the needs of patients. Providing information that helps patients and families understand the process before, during, and after surgery is an effective way of preventing the harms of miscommunications and misperceptions. Educating patients and families to take care of themselves at home minimizes complications and helps to assure a better outcome.

E. Regardless of the practice setting, every encounter a nurse has with a patient provides an opportunity for that nurse to serve as a patient advocate by assuring their autonomy, preventing harm, establishing trust, and treating them fairly.

F. Applications of nursing advocacy in ambulatory care are fully explored in Chapter 8, "Patient Advocacy and Use of Community Resources."

V. Institutional Ethics Committees

A. Organizations that have ethics committees are in a better position to assist patients, families, and health care professionals resolve ethical conflicts. The practice of ambulatory nursing has grown, and moral uncertainty and moral distress among nurses have become more evident as the patient care environment becomes more complex.

B. Ethics committees serve three major functions:

   1. Educate committee members on bioethical issues.

   2. Educate and provide guidance to health care professionals and other staff within the organization through the writing of policies and procedures and formal education.

   3. Perform case review, either concurrently or retrospectively.

C. Most organizational ethics committees encourage any staff member, patient, or family member to discuss a concern with the committee.

D. When an ethics committee does not exist within an organization, some sources for nursing information and support include:

   1. Position statements developed and published by specialty organizations, such as the American Academy of Ambulatory

Care Nursing (AAACN), state nurses' associations and state boards of nursing.

2. State board of nursing practice consultants who can offer advice.

3. Colleagues in academic nursing and/or ethics programs with expertise in health care ethics.

4. The *Code of Ethics for Nurses*, which provides the clarity needed to justify proceeding in a certain direction.

5. Educational conferences and journals on bioethics where issues related to the practice of nursing are discussed.

Summary

Nursing has an honorable and long tradition about caring for the health and welfare of its patients, whether as an individual, group, or community. Since the inception of nursing as a profession, it is no coincidence that nurses have written hundreds of books and articles about the ethical concepts touched on in this chapter. AAACN (2011) has made a commitment to continue this practice by clearly stating in its definition of ambulatory care nursing – "ambulatory care nurses apply the provision of the American Nurses Association *Code of Ethics for Nurses* to their professional obligations and for the patients entrusted to their care."

References

American Academy of Ambulatory Care Nursing (AAACN). (2011). *Definition of professional ambulatory care nursing.* Retrieved from http://www.aaacn.org

American Nurses Association (ANA). (2001). *Code of ethics for nurses with interpretive statements.* Washington, DC: Author.

American Nurses Association (ANA). (2010). *Nursing's social policy statement.* Silver Spring, MD: Author.

Curtin, L. (2010). Ethics for nurses in everyday practice. *American Nurse Today, 5*(2).

Jameton, A. (1984). *Nursing practice: The ethical issues.* Englewood Cliffs, NJ: Prentice-Hall.

Additional Readings

Burckhardt, M.A., & Nathaniel, A.K. (2008). *Ethics and issues in contemporary nursing.* Albany, NY: Delmar.

Catlett, S., & Lovan, S. (2011). Being a good nurse and doing the right thing. *Nursing Ethics, 18*(1), 54-63.

Levine-Ariff, J., & Groh, D. (1990). *Creating an ethical environment. Nurse managers bookshelf. 2:1.* Baltimore: Williams & Wilkins.

Murray, J.S. (2010). Moral courage in healthcare: Acting ethically even in the presence of risk. *The Online Journal of Issues in Nursing, 15*(3). Retrieved from http://www.nursingworld.org/MainMenuCategories/EthicsStandards/Courage-and-Distress/Moral-Courage-and-Risk.html

Chapter 13

Professional Development

Michelle Budzinski-Braunscheidel, BSN, RN
Sarah Jane Whalen-Espin, MSN, CCRN, RN-BC

OBJECTIVES – *Study of the information in this chapter will enable the learner to:*

1. Discuss key components of an orientation program for new staff in ambulatory care nursing settings.
2. Demonstrate knowledge of competence assessment requirements as mandated by accrediting agencies' standards and essential to performance of the nurse's professional role.
3. Discuss continuing education and professional growth and development needs.
4. Identify the value of nursing specialty certification.
5. Describe the value and characteristics of preceptor programs.

KEY POINTS – *The major points in this chapter include:*

1. The orientation plan should be flexible to meet the needs of both the new employee and the organization.
2. Competency assessment is an initial and ongoing process.
3. Preceptor programs are a vital aspect of a successful orientation program that aims to facilitate role transition. The ongoing evaluation of the orientee's performance, progression, and satisfaction with that program is a critical element in attaining those goals.
4. Continuing education should be available in a variety of formats, such as traditional classroom, Web-based interactive, CD-ROM, self-study modules, and distance learning.
5. Professional certification should be encouraged, facilitated, and rewarded.

Professional development is an essential element of the nursing profession. Individual commitment to the lifelong learning process is fundamental to the practice of nursing. This chapter outlines key components of the professional development of ambulatory care nurses that include orientation of new staff, competency assessment, precepting, continuing education, and professional nursing certification.

The primary purpose of orientation is to help staff acclimate to a new clinical setting and learn about the professional standards for practice in that organization (Hargreaves, Nichols, Shanks, & Halamak, 2010). Performance assessment of basic nursing skills and warranted supplemental training are essential components of orientation. This attention to the individual skillsets of a new employee allows for a more seamless transition into independent unit-specific practice. As the implementation and complexity of ambulatory care nursing has changed over recent years, so has the profile of its rank and file. Experienced nurses are moving from the acute care setting to positions in ambulatory care, along with new graduate nurses, fledglings in the nursing profession. Consequently, an effective orientation program must provide socialization, employee support, and clearly defined expectations of professional performance (Steffan & Goodin, 2010).

Competency assessment necessitates teamwork and collaboration. The stakeholders include the nurse educator, the unit manager, the preceptor, and the staff member, as well as the patient and family members who will be the recipients of the nurse's care. Competencies of staff must be assessed and documented according to standards set by regulating agencies and the employing institution. Ensuring the competence of staff is an ongoing process of initial assessment and development, maintenance of knowledge and skills, educational consultation, remediation, and revision (Whelan, 2006).

A culture of lifelong learning for nurses must be nurtured by health care organizations and regulatory agencies to ensure optimum care for diverse populations across the lifespan (Institute of Medicine [IOM], 2010). Professional nursing certification has become recognized as a symbol of enhanced commitment to excellence in nursing practice and has been linked to improved patient outcomes. The certification process validates qualifications for and knowledge of practice in a nursing specialty as well as a significant pledge to lifelong learning (Altman, 2011; Kaplow, 2011; Teal, 2011).

I. Orientation

Orientation is an organized plan created by the health care facility to prepare new staff to take on their assigned roles. Three distinct phases make up this process for nursing staff: Introduction to the organization, general and specific nursing department standards review, and unit orientation to precise job elements (Bowers, Bennett, Schneider, & Brunner, 2009). The objective is to guarantee that the new hire has the necessary skillset and knowledge to deliver quality patient care (American Academy of Ambulatory Care Nursing [AAACN], 2010a).

A. Organizational components (AAACN, 2010a; Bowers et al., 2009; Lott, 2006).
 1. The culture: Mission, vision, and goals of the organization.
 2. Human resources components.
 3. Professional expectations.
 4. Policies and procedures.
 5. Cultural diversity.
 6. Organizational chart/hierarchy.

 7. Environmental safety.
  a. Infection control.
  b. Patient rights.
  c. Emergency preparedness – Fire, safety, disaster, weather.
  d. Security and violence in the workplace.
B. Department-specific job duties and responsibilities.
 1. Position/job description.
  a. Role expectations.
  b. Performance measures.
  c. Safety/environment of care (related to equipment, physical risks).
  d. Department mission and goals.
  e. Department organizational chart.
  f. Specific skill training (e.g., computers, emergency equipment).
  g. Professional standards/performance criteria/clinical ladder.
 2. Competency.
  a. Age- and population-specific care, including medication administration safety.
  b. Knowledge of clinical practice guidelines, protocols, and evidence-based practice.
  c. Technical skill assessment and training.
  d. Critical thinking/priority setting.
  e. Process improvement.
  f. Communication/interpersonal skills.
C. Position-specific duties and responsibilities.
 1. Unique to professional ambulatory care nursing role.
  a. Interviewing and counseling patients, such as described in the Clinician Importance and Confidence Regarding Health Behavior Counseling (see Figure 13-1).
  b. Assisting patients to make health behavioral change, such as described in the Motivational Interviewing Skills Checklist (see Figure 13-2).
  c. Telehealth nursing.
 2. Requisite competencies – Exclusive to that particular unit and those needing additional instruction based on initial assessments.

Figure 13-1.
Clinician Importance and Confidence Regarding Health Behavior Counseling

I. For each of the following communication strategies, please provide your rating of its importance as a way for promoting patient health behavior change.

Please circle a number on the following scale:

	Not at All Important									Extremely Important
1. Making a personal connection with patients to establish rapport	0 1 2 3 4 5 6 7 8 9 10									
2. Eliciting patients' agendas and needs	0 1 2 3 4 5 6 7 8 9 10									
3. Eliciting patients' ideas, values, and feelings regarding health behavior change	0 1 2 3 4 5 6 7 8 9 10									
4. Reflecting patients' ideas, beliefs, and concerns	0 1 2 3 4 5 6 7 8 9 10									
5. Responding to and affirming patients' concerns and feelings	0 1 2 3 4 5 6 7 8 9 10									
6. Sharing information in small chunks	0 1 2 3 4 5 6 7 8 9 10									
7. Checking the patients' understanding	0 1 2 3 4 5 6 7 8 9 10									
8. Guiding patients toward healthy choices	0 1 2 3 4 5 6 7 8 9 10									
9. Setting goals collaboratively	0 1 2 3 4 5 6 7 8 9 10									
10. Assessing patients' confidence to follow through with a plan	0 1 2 3 4 5 6 7 8 9 10									
11. Exploring barriers	0 1 2 3 4 5 6 7 8 9 10									
12. Problem-solving to address barriers	0 1 2 3 4 5 6 7 8 9 10									

II. For each of the following communication strategies, please provide your rating of your confidence in using this skill to promote patient health behavior change.

Please circle a number on the following scale:

	Not at All Confident									Extremely Confident
1. Making a personal connection with patients to establish rapport	0 1 2 3 4 5 6 7 8 9 10									
2. Eliciting patients' agenda and needs	0 1 2 3 4 5 6 7 8 9 10									
3. Eliciting patients' ideas, values, and feelings regarding health behavior change	0 1 2 3 4 5 6 7 8 9 10									
4. Reflecting patients' ideas, beliefs, and concerns	0 1 2 3 4 5 6 7 8 9 10									
5. Responding to and affirming patients' concerns and feelings	0 1 2 3 4 5 6 7 8 9 10									
6. Sharing information in small chunks	0 1 2 3 4 5 6 7 8 9 10									
7. Checking the patients' understanding	0 1 2 3 4 5 6 7 8 9 10									
8. Guiding patients toward healthy choices	0 1 2 3 4 5 6 7 8 9 10									
9. Setting goals collaboratively	0 1 2 3 4 5 6 7 8 9 10									
10. Assessing patients' confidence to follow through with a plan	0 1 2 3 4 5 6 7 8 9 10									
11. Exploring barriers	0 1 2 3 4 5 6 7 8 9 10									
12. Problem-solving to address barriers	0 1 2 3 4 5 6 7 8 9 10									

Source: Veterans Health Administration (VHA) National Center for Health Promotion and Disease Prevention (NCP), 2011a. Used with permission.

Figure 13-2.
Motivational Interviewing Skills Checklist – Format for Observer

Which of the following skills/strategies were demonstrated? Comment or give examples of each and identify opportunities for use of these skills.

I. Engaging: OARS
• Open-ended questions and statements
• Affirmations
• Reflections
  ○ Simple (restatements)
  ○ Complex (reflect deeper meaning, feelings, values)
• Summaries
• Ratio of questions/reflections
 	
II. Focusing
• Ask about agenda
• Explore ambivalence
  ○ Reasons for change (DARN)
    – **D**esire
    – **A**bility
    – **R**easons
    – **N**eed
  ○ Reasons for status quo/sustain
• Share information
  ○ Ask permission to share information
  ○ Elicit understanding
  ○ Provide information
    – Small chunks
  ○ Elicit understanding
	III. Evoking Change Talk and Commitment Language
	• Importance ruler
	• Ask explicitly about DARN
	• Reinforce support change talk and commitment language though:
	  ○ Selective reflection
	  ○ Affirmation
	  ○ Selective summaries
	• Explore typical day
	• Querying about extremes ("What is the worst thing that could happen if you don't change?")
	• Hypothetical questions ("If you were to change, what would you do?")
	• Looking forward ("If you look ahead a few months, what might your life be like if you continue on the same path?")
	• Explore goals and values
	• Roll with resistance
	  ○ Open-ended inquiry
	  ○ Affirmation
	  ○ Reflection (especially double-sided; reflections of feelings)
	  ○ Summaries
	  ○ Shifting focus
	  ○ Emphasize autonomy/choice
	  ○ Coming alongside/empathy
		IV. Planning
		• Summarize with emphasis on change talk and taking steps toward change
		• Collaborative goal setting
		  ○ Offer options
		  ○ Seek commitment ("So, what are you willing to do?")
		  ○ Support choice
		• Explore confidence (open-ended questions)
		• Confidence ruler
		• Explore past successes Identify personal strengths/supports
		• SMART action planning
		  ○ **S**pecific
		    – What
		    – When
		    – How Often/How Long
		    – Where
		    – With Whom
		    – How
		  ○ **M**easurable
		  ○ **A**ction-oriented
		  ○ **R**ealistic
		  ○ **T**ime-specific
		• Explore barriers
		• Problem-solving strategies
		• Arrange follow-up

Source: Veterans Health Administration (VHA) National Center for Health Promotion and Disease Prevention (NCP), 2011b. Used with permission.

3. Essential job duties and scope of practice.
   a. Initial Orientation Competency Verification Checklist – Ambulatory RN/LPN (AAACN, 2010a).
4. Unit-based preceptors characteristics.
   a. Completed a preceptor workshop/training.
   b. Demonstrated exceptional communication.
   c. Dedicated to team excellence.

D. Education based on identified needs.
   1. Sub-standard or missing skills and/or competence remediation.
   2. New skills and/or competence development.
E. Regulatory requirements related to orientation.
   1. The Joint Commission requires that health care organizations provide an orientation process for each staff member that will:

a. Assess competence to perform specific job skills.
b. Clearly define key patient safety dimensions of job duties.
c. Certify safe and functional performance of specific duties.
d. Provide general summary of job specifics.

2. Accreditation Association for Ambulatory Health Care (AAAHC) (2009) requires the documentation of initial orientation and training according to position description. Standards direct that this training be:
   a. Completed within 30 days of commencement of employment.
   b. Provided annually thereafter and when there is an identified need.
   c. Provided by a qualified person(s) designated by the organization.

F. Measuring quality and value of orientation program.
1. Evaluate participant satisfaction.
2. Measure learning/practice outcomes.
3. Construct a continuous process improvement program from evaluations and survey results.
4. Benchmark best orientation practices.
   a. Benchmarking – A structured comparison of products, services, or operations of analogous organizations, divisions, or professionals to discern current best practices for the purpose of continuous quality improvement.
      (1) External – Outside organizations' process and procedure.
      (2) Internal – Within the organization (such as interdepartmental, site variance for process and procedure).

II. Competence Assessment

Competence assessment enables the organization to determine whether its staff has the ability to utilize specific skills and apply the necessary knowledge to perform their jobs (The Joint Commission & Joint Commission Resources, 2010). In accordance with The Joint Commission standards, competency of staff is initially assessed and documented during orientation, then subsequently followed up by ongoing education and training to maintain or enhance those competencies. Assurance of competence is the shared responsibility of the profession, individual nurses, professional organizations, credentialing and certification entities, regulatory agencies, employers, and other key stakeholders (American Nurses Association [ANA], 2008). Documentation of this process is mandated by accreditation agencies.

A. Customary aspects of competency activities (AAACN, 2010b; Bradley, 2010).
1. Focus on end result.
2. Adapt to diverse needs of employee and organizational standards.
3. Incorporate self-paced activities.
4. Utilize educator as a facilitator.
5. Schedule sufficient time.
6. Apply principles of adult learning.
7. Use a number of validation methods along with initial and ongoing assessment (such as return demonstration, teach-back, testing, observation in clinical situation).

B. Establish a starting point.
1. Self-assessment.
2. Validator assessment.

C. Evaluate all skill domains.
1. Psychomotor.
2. Interpersonal.
3. Critical thinking.

D. Offer learning/testing alternatives in the form of online modules and tests, skills laboratory testing, case scenario, quizzes, and individual validation of job-specific criteria.

E. Assure professionalism.
1. Applying nursing process.
2. Practicing in accordance with the ANA *Code of Ethics* (2001).
3. Supporting membership in professional organizations.
4. Maintaining credentials and proficiencies.

F. Concentrate clinical performance improvement (PI) initiatives on vital skills.

G. Promote ethical conduct.
1. Scope of practice.
2. Legal matters.
3. Organization's vision and goals.

H. Promote nursing leadership skills.
   1. Collaboration.
   2. Accountability.
I. Support the integration of research into practice.
   1. Evidence-based practice.
   2. Benchmarking.
J. Comply with regulatory directives.
   1. Governing body rules.
   2. Risk management.

III. Precepting

The art of precepting requires more than clinical expertise or seniority. Clinical expertise is important, but caring kindness is equally valuable. The literature indicates that organizations without good preceptor programs experience greater turnover and early nurse burnout, which may lead to nurses leaving the profession altogether (O'Shea, 2002; Yonge, Krahn, Trojan, Reid, & Haase, 2002).

A. The preceptor's role is to:
   1. Acclimate the new nurse to the ambulatory setting.
   2. Acclimate the new nurse to department specialty standards.
   3. Serve as a role model and resource for all nursing personnel.
   4. Develop a written plan:
      a. Policies and procedures.
      b. Essential skill sets.
      c. Competence to be validated initially and annually.
   5. Provide feedback, positive and negative, to improve preceptor program.
   6. Document completion of competency validations during probationary period and annually.
   7. Orient new graduate nurses.
      a. Increase understanding of the state's nurse practice act.
      b. Support development of leadership skills/career ladders, if applicable.
      c. Provide opportunities to lead.
      d. Encourage peer discussions.
      e. Foster critical thinking skills.
B. Training preparation for preceptor.
   1. Qualifications of preceptor. The smartest and "best" nurse may not make the best preceptor.
      a. Knowledgeable in various levels of nursing.
      b. Knowledgeable about the scope of practice for the orientee.
      c. Communicates and works well with others.
      d. Open to new staff and new ideas.
   2. Formal class preparation of preceptor.
      a. Validates competence levels of the preceptor.
      b. Addresses knowledge needed regarding adult learning theories and principles.
      c. Demonstrates adult learning theories in practice.
      d. Teaches on the roles and responsibilities of the preceptor and preceptee.
      e. Reinforces good communication skills.
      f. Teaches the handling of conflict resolution.
C. Accommodations for non-traditional precepting.
   1. Cross-training to other areas.
      a. Interdepartmental – Staff are competent to support and train for a department/unit where not usually assigned.
      b. Intradepartmental – Staff are competent to support and train team member positions.
   2. One-nurse practices.
      a. Write standards of expected practice.
      b. Identify support from other staff (such as physician, office manager).
      c. Encourage the nurse to participate in a professional organization to provide a network of peers and a larger context of specialty.
   3. Use of agency or per diem staff.
      a. Write a standard of expected practice.
      b. Provide formal orientation with a resource person.
      c. Maintain a working relationship with the agency or per diem pool.
         (1) Set key standards of preparation/competence expectations.
         (2) Attempt to utilize same agency/per diem staff.

4. Use of unlicensed assistive personnel (UAP) (American Association of Medical Assistants, 2009).
   a. Apply knowledge of the scope of practice of UAP for the specific state.
   b. Assess literacy level.
   c. Provide background information about reason skill/function is being performed.
   d. Define complex terminology.
   e. Simplify anatomical terms.
   f. Evaluate effectiveness of delegation processes.
   g. Determine complexity of the patient to be managed by UAP versus retained by a professional for care.
   h. Reinforce importance of rapport and communication between nurse and UAP.
D. Potential limitations of preceptor programs.
   1. Lack of administrative support.
      a. Clinical schedules.
      b. Lack of understanding and valuing of role by department personnel.
      c. Patient care loads/staffing constraints.
   2. Lack of educational support.
      a. Additional training required.
      b. Uninformed on methods of assessing learning needs.
      c. Inadequate tools available.
      d. Limited methods of evaluating the orientee's progress.

IV. Continuing Professional Education and Development

The goal of continuing education is to improve and expand the nurse's knowledge base and to allow him or her to maintain competence and further develop in a specific work setting. With the rapid pace of change in health care, nurses need ongoing education to understand and apply new knowledge and new technology. New graduates, as well as experienced professionals, benefit from continuing their education. Opportunities must meet the varied learning needs of professional nurses.
A. Agencies requiring continuing education activities for nurses:

1. Occupational Safety and Health Administration (OSHA).
   a. Bloodborne pathogens precautions.
   b. Preventing tuberculosis transmission.
   c. Handling hazardous chemicals.
2. The Joint Commission.
   a. Staff competency for job-specific responsibilities.
   b. Patient care standards.
   c. Population-specific competencies.
   d. Process improvement initiatives.
   e. Patient safety.
   f. Handling of medical emergencies.
   g. Fire safety.
   h. Disaster management internally and externally.
3. American Association for Ambulatory Health Care (AAAHC).
   a. Rights of patients.
   b. Quality of care provided – Includes staff competence.
   c. Quality management and improvement.
   d. Facilities and environment.
   e. Patient safety.
   f. Handling of medical emergencies.
   g. Fire safety.
   h. Disaster management.
   i. Health education and teaching.
4. State licensing board's rules and regulations:
   a. Some states require 20 or more continuing education hours be obtained for each registered nurse's re-licensure cycle.
   b. Continuing education credit may be accepted for teaching, participation in meetings, and attending academic programs, in addition to participation in continuing nursing education programs.
B. Facility-specific in-services.
   1. New equipment.
   2. Change in policy and procedure.
   3. Review of situations requiring low frequency, high-risk skills.

C. Continuing nursing education programs targeting development of skills used in the ambulatory care setting.
   1. Patient education issues.
   2. New trends in care and disease state management.
   3. Pharmacology updates.
   4. New technology.
   5. Clinical practice guidelines.
   6. Electronic medical records (EMRs).
   7. Evidence-based practice guidelines.
D. Factors that influence one's professional continuing development.
   1. Identifying and setting short- and long-term goals and objectives.
   2. Establishing measurable objectives.
   3. Building confidence and self-esteem.
   4. Finding time to devote to professional goals.
   5. Personal motivation.
      a. Self-knowledge and insight.
      b. Individual's desire for learning.
      c. Willingness to learn.
      d. Self-direction.
   6. Practice-related challenges.
   7. Ability to access presentations, lectures, readings, online classrooms.
   8. Personal learning preferences.
      a. Observation/written material – Visual learner.
      b. Doing – Psychomotor learner.
      c. Lecture/audio materials – Auditory learner.
   9. Personal attributes.
      a. Interest in subject matter.
      b. Availability of time.
      c. Resources/cost.
E. Learning and professionalism is enhanced by:
   1. Critical thinking.
   2. Confidence.
   3. Positive relationships.
   4. Appropriate timing.

V. Distance Learning

Nursing remains a high-touch profession, not just a high-tech one. Recent advances in technology allow creative educators to offer alternative methods for learning. In an age when information growth is expanding at an accelerated speed, it is difficult to keep pace. Readily available, easily accessed educational opportunities are a priority. Courses and faculty resources are now pooled together for wider distribution, which is a more effective use of resources. Distance learning/education has become the norm rather than the exception, as it once was.

A. Distance learning provides access to learning modalities, allowing nurses to remain in their hometown or work setting, and balance multiple responsibilities between work, family, and advancing their learning. Methods include:
   1. Correspondence-type courses.
      a. Individuals enroll in a correspondence course.
      b. Work on material at own pace.
      c. Submit results for grading/credit as applicable.
   2. Email and Internet, allowing for interchange with a quicker turn-around and increased teacher/learner feedback.
   3. Video capabilities, such as recorded programs online or to play in a computer or video system.
   4. Video-interactive capabilities.
   5. Internet access to references, persons, knowledge bases.
B. Era of information/knowledge explosion and instant communications.
   1. Increasingly, considering a college education as mastery of a body of knowledge or a complete preparation for a lifetime career is becoming outmoded. Instead, graduates need to have acquired skills, such as critical thinking, quantitative reasoning, and effective communication, along with abilities, such as the ability to find needed information and the ability to work well with others (Twigg, 1994).
   2. This shift has increased the need for learning environments and systems to integrate learning.
      a. Multimedia training systems.
      b. Web casts.
      c. Blogs.

d. Podcasts/PDAs.
e. Smartphones.
f. Increased theory classes' faculty-to-student ratios.

C. Availability of learning resources.
1. Once, the cost of technology was the limiting factor.
2. Charges needed to cover cost (such as program cost, materials, mailing costs, computer access/cost, video/audio capability).
3. Tools are now available – Do learners have the skills to use them?
4. Learning once occurred in a "place" – The environment is changing, and information can be sought wherever the tools are readily available by those with the critical thinking skills to put the tools to use (Peterson, 2004).
5. Virtual reality use of computers.
    a. Online chat.
    b. Audio over the Web.
    c. Practice lab simulators.
    d. Helmets with various stimuli and devices that modify as the user engages and changes the scenario.

D. Methods of implementation.
1. Self-initiated learning, not for credit.
2. Formalized distance learning for both continuing education credit and academic credit established by a traditional institution of learning.
3. Universities and colleges with distance programs offer credit and even degrees via distance learning.

E. Future considerations.
1. Language assimilation – Promote and demonstrate value of bilingual students/nurses.
2. Limits potentially placed on the Internet and access.
3. Capabilities of learners to use the tools effectively.
4. Cost of updates to software when older versions of the software are incompatible with the learning materials.
5. Establishing standards for new media.

6. Methods to validate learning, effectiveness, and outcomes.
7. Changing requirements for workers, leaders.
    a. Skill sets to include technology experience.
    b. Communication abilities not only verbal and non-verbal, but also electronic.
8. Partnership between academic institutions and health care informatics system vendors.
9. Nurse educator shortage.
    a. Students no longer being bound by location.
    b. Students may participate in online post-clinical conferences.
10. Updating the selected education delivery model to be congruent with the curriculum plan.

VI. Professional Certification

Certification is the formal recognition of the specialized knowledge, skills, and experience demonstrated by the achievement of standards identified by a nursing specialty to promote optimal health outcomes (American Board of Nursing Specialties [ABNS], 2005).

A. Several studies have demonstrated the positive benefits of nursing certification.
1. In a survey of nursing management, 86% of respondents indicated they would hire a certified nurse over a non-certified nurse if all else were equal. The most common reasons noted were that certified nurses have a proven knowledge base in a given specialty (85.8%) and demonstrate a greater professional commitment to lifelong learning (77.5%) (Stromborg et al., 2005).
2. A survey conducted by ABNS (2006) to validate nurses' perceptions of certification had over 11,000 respondents. Key findings on certification are:
    a. 84% agreed it indicates the level of clinical competence.
    b. 95% agreed it enhances professional credibility.
    c. 72% agreed it increases consumer confidence.

d. 78% agreed it enhances professional autonomy.

e. 84% agreed it provides evidence of accountability.

B. ABNS (2005) stated the following position about nursing specialty certification on March 5, 2005.

1. Registered nurses should seek certification in their specialty area of practice.

2. Certified nurses should promote their certification by publicly displaying their credentials and introducing themselves as certified nurses.

3. Health care consumers should be knowledgeable of the qualifications and credentials of the registered nurses caring for them.

4. Employers should seek certified nurses for their workforce, support individuals seeking and maintaining certification, inform patients and the public about the certification status of their workforce, encourage the display of the nurses' certified credentials on identification badges, and market the accomplishments of certified nurses.

5. Specialty nursing certification is an objective measure of knowledge that validates a nurse is qualified to provide specialized nursing care.

C. Certification in ambulatory care nursing.

1. Offered by the American Nurses Credentialing Center (ANCC) since 1999.

2. Addresses the broad scope of ambulatory care from clinics to HMOs, to group practices, to ambulatory surgery, to the diverse venues of telehealth nursing (AAACN, 2007).

3. Eligibility requirements (ANCC, 2012).

a. Hold a currently active registered nurse license (associate degree, diploma, baccalaureate, or higher degree in nursing) in the U.S. or its territories.

b. Have practiced the equivalent of two years full-time as a registered nurse.

c. Have a minimum of 2,000 hours of clinical practice in ambulatory care and/or telehealth nursing within the last three years.

d. Have completed 30 hours of continuing education in ambulatory care and/or telehealth nursing within the last three years.

4. Testing information (www.nurse credentialing.org).

It is the intent of the authors of this chapter for the readers to come away with the aforementioned key points of the content. The knowledge and expertise of the ambulatory care nursing experts cited in this material will serve as a model for professional development at all levels of clinical practice.

References

Accreditation Association for Ambulatory Health Care (AAAHC). (2009). *AAAHC standards.* Retrieved from http://www.aaahc.org/eweb/dynamicpage.aspx?site=aaahc_site&webcode=aaahc_standards

Altman, M. (2011). Let's get certified: Best practices for nurse leaders to create a culture of certification. *AACN Advanced Critical Care, 22*(1), 68-75.

American Academy of Ambulatory Care Nursing (AAACN). (2007). *AAACN holds telehealth visioning meeting.* Retrieved from https://www.aaacn.org/aboutaaacn/telehealthMtgSummary.pdf

American Academy of Ambulatory Care Nursing (AAACN). (2010a). *Ambulatory care nursing orientation and competency assessment guide* (2nd ed.). Pitman, NJ: Author.

American Academy of Ambulatory Care Nursing (AAACN). (2010b). *Scope and standards of practice for professional ambulatory care nursing* (8th ed.). Pitman, NJ: Author.

American Association of Medical Assistants. (2009). *Occupational analysis of the CMA (AAMA) 2007-2008.* Retrieved http://www.aama-ntl.org/resources/library/OA.pdf

American Board of Nursing Specialties (ABNS). (2005). *A position statement on the value of specialty nursing certification.* Retrieved from http://www.nursingcertification.org/pdf/value_certification.pdf

American Board of Nursing Specialties (ABNS). (2006). *Specialty nursing certification: Nurses' perceptions, values and behaviors.* Retrieved from http://www.nursingcertification.org/pdf/white_paper_final_12_12_06.pdf

American Nurses Association (ANA). (2001). *Code of ethics for nurses with interpretive statements.* Retrieved from http://www.nursingworld.org/MainMenuCategories/EthicsStandards/CodeofEthicsforNurses

American Nurses Association (ANA). (2008). *Professional role competence* [Position statement]. Washington, DC: Author.

American Nurses Credentialing Center (ANCC). (2012). *Ambulatory care nursing certification eligibility criteria.* Retrieved from http://www.nursecredentialing.org/Ambulatory-Eligibility.aspx

Bowers, B., Bennett, S.S., Schneider, S.K., & Brunner, B.W. (2009). A new approach to orientation: Professional entry into practice. *Journal for Nurses in Staff Development, 25*(3), E14-E18.

Bradley, D. (2010). Scope and standards. *Journal for Nurses in Staff Development, 26*(6), 290-293.

Hargreaves, L., Nichols, A., Shanks, S., & Halamak, L.P. (2010). A handoff report card for general nursing orientation. *The Journal of Nursing Administration, 40*(10), 424-431.

Institute of Medicine (IOM). (2010). *The future of nursing: Focus on education.* Retrieved from http://www.iom.edu/~/media/ Files/Report%20Files/2010/The-Future-of-Nursing/ Nursing%20Education%202010%20Brief.pdf

Joint Commission & Joint Commission Resources, The. (2010). *Accreditation process guide for hospitals: Includes the compliance assessment checklist.* Washington, DC: Author.

Kaplow, R. (2011). The value of certification. *AACN Advanced Critical Care, 22*(1), 25-32.

Lott, T. (2006). Moving forward: Creating a new nursing services orientation program. *Journal for Nurses in Staff Development, 22*(5), 214-221.

O'Shea, K.L. (2002). *Staff development nursing secrets.* Philadelphia: Hanley & Belfus, Inc.

Peterson, T. (2004). *Peterson's guide to distance learning programs.* Lawrenceville, NJ: The Thomson Corporation.

Steffan, K.P., & Goodin, H.J. (2010). Preceptor's perceptions of a new evaluation tool used during nursing orientation. *Journal for Nurses in Staff Development, 26*(3), 116-122.

Stromborg, M.F., Niebuhr, B., Prevost, S., Fabrey, L., Muenzen, P., Spence, C., … Valentine, W. (2005). Specialty certification: More than a title. *Nursing Management, 36*(5), 36-46.

Teal, J. (2011). Certifiably excellent. *AACN Advanced Critical Care, 22*(1), 83-88.

Twigg, C.A. (1994). *The need for a national learning infrastructure.* Retrieved from http://net.educause.edu/ir/libray/html/ nli0001.html

Veterans Health Administration (VHA) National Center for Health Promotion and Disease Prevention (NCP). (2011a). *Clinician importance and confidence regarding health behavior counseling.* Unpublished raw data.

Veterans Health Administration (VHA) National Center for Health Promotion and Disease Prevention (NCP). (2011b). *MI skills checklist – Format for observer* (VHA NCP 3.28.11). Unpublished raw data.

Whelan, L. (2006). Competency assessment of nursing staff. *Orthopaedic Nursing, 25*(3), 198-202.

Yonge, O., Krahn, H., Trojan, L., Reid, D., & Haase, M. (2002). Being a preceptor is stressful! *Journal of Nurses Staff Development, 18*(1), 22-27.

Additional Readings

Billings, D.M. (2007). Distance education in nursing: 25 years and going strong. *Computers, Informatics, Nursing, 25*(3), 121-123.

Bittner, N.P., & Gravlin, G. (2009). Critical thinking, delegation, and missed care in nursing practice. *Journal of Nursing Administration, 39*(3), 142-146.

Keating, S.B. (2006). *Curriculum development and evaluation in nursing.* Philadelphia: Lippincott, Williams & Wilkins.

Kendall-Gallagher, D., & Blegen, M.A. (2009). Competence and certification of registered nurses and safety of patients in intensive care units. *American Journal of Critical Care, 18*(2), 106-113.

Lee, T.Y., Tzeng, W.C., Lin, C.H., & Yeh, M.L. (2009). Effects of a preceptorship programme on turnover rate, cost, quality and professional development. *Journal of Clinical Nursing, 18*(8), 1217-1225.

Rebholz, M.O. (2006). A review of methods to assess competency. *Journal for Nurses in Staff Development, 22*(5), 241-245.

Simpson, R.L. (2003). Welcome to the virtual classroom. How technology is transforming nursing education in the 21st century. *Nursing Administrative Quarterly, 27*(1), 83-86.

Swan, B.A. (2007). Transitioning from acute care to ambulatory care. *Nursing Economic$, 25*(2), 130-134.

Valente, S. (2010). Improving professional practice through certification. *Journal for Nurses in Staff Development, 26*(5), 215-219.

Wayman, L.M. (2009). Staff development story: Tiered orientation: Easing the transition from being a novice to competent nurse. *Journal for Nurses in Staff Development, 25*(6), 304-314.

Wright, D. (2005). *The ultimate guide to competency assessment in health care* (3rd ed.). Minneapolis, MN: Creative Health Care Management, Inc.

Section Three

The Clinical Nursing Role
In Ambulatory Care

Chapter 14

Application of the Nursing Process In Ambulatory Care

Kathy Kesner, MS, RN, CNS
Wanda Mayo, BSN, RN, CPN

OBJECTIVES – *Study of the information in this chapter will enable the learner to:*

1. Outline the steps of the nursing process and how the steps promote critical thinking.
2. Identify the skills necessary for application of the nursing process in ambulatory care.
3. Apply the nursing process in ambulatory care.
4. Explain how to determine if outcomes are achieved.

KEY POINTS – *The major points in this chapter include:*

1. Collaborative and multidisciplinary approaches significantly impact the role of the nurse in the provision of nursing care.
2. Critical thinking is an essential nursing competency, and is applied to every step of the nursing process.
3. Planning and implementation are based on scientific principles that are congruent with the overall plan of care.
4. One goal of patient/family education is to empower the patient and family to be involved in the management of their care.
5. Outcomes are based on the established goals of care and are measured in the evaluation portion of the nursing process.

Health care in the 21st century involves the integration of knowledge, skills, and evidence to deliver care in a timely, efficient manner. It involves the interdisciplinary collaboration of health care professionals to provide patient- and family-centered care that is both cost effective and of high quality. Nursing care provided is captured in and communicated through the use of the nursing process.

The nursing process is a purposeful, problem-solving approach to meeting the needs of patients. It uses scientific reasoning and critical thinking to guide the plan of care. According to the American Nurses Association (ANA) (1980), the nurse uses the nursing process to diagnose and treat human responses to health and illness. Guided by professional standards and a code of ethics, the nursing process relies on cognitive, interpersonal, and psychomotor skills. All steps of the nursing process are interrelated, interdependent, and cyclical (see Figure 14-1).

I. The Nursing Process

A. Definition of the nursing process:
   1. Is guided by critical thinking.
   2. Leads to accurate and thorough data collection.
   3. Involves the integration of data and information at every step.
   4. Provides an organized framework for the delivery of nursing care.
   5. Is theory- and research-based.
   6. Is not static, fixed, or linear.
   7. Provides a feedback loop until the diagnosis is resolved.

Figure 14-1.
The Nursing Process

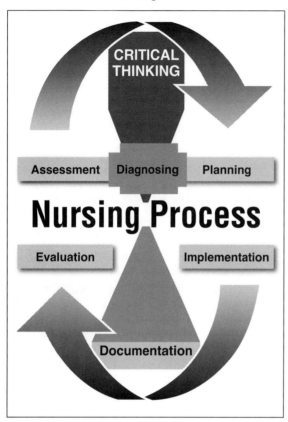

a. The disciplined, intellectual process of applying skillful reasoning as a guide to belief or action (Norris & Ennis, 1989).

b. The ability to think in a systematic and logical manner with openness to question and reflect on the reasoning process, used to ensure safe nursing practice and quality care (Heaslip, 2008).

c. Gathering, focusing, remembering, organizing, analyzing, generating, integrating, and evaluating (Staib, 2003).

2. Activities of the ambulatory care nurse require other types of thinking skills, such as clinical reflection (one asks questions of practices that need reform) and clinical reasoning (one reasons through a situation as it changes, taking into account context and concerns of the patient and family). Critical thinking is sometimes used to represent the myriad ways nurses interact with information and ideas (Benner, Sutphen, Leonard, & Day, 2010).

3. Critical thinking is applied to every step in the nursing process (Maiocco, 2010).

   a. Assessment: Is the data complete?

   b. Diagnosis: What else could be happening? Is there more than a single problem affecting the patient and family?

   c. Plan: What are the goals for this patient? Has the patient shared in the establishment of these goals? What are the best interventions to meet these goals?

   d. Implementation: Can the patient tolerate the intervention? Should the intervention be altered to meet the needs of the patient? If so, will it still be effective?

   e. Evaluation: Did the interventions achieve the desired outcomes? Do more data need to be collected?

8. Includes documentation, a crucial step in the process that has at times been identified as an additional step in the process (Healthcare Information and Management Systems [HIMSS], 2012).

B. The nursing process steps:

1. Assessment.
2. Diagnosis.
3. Plan.
4. Implementation.
5. Evaluation.

C. Critical thinking: Problem-solving and decision-making are crucial skills for a nurse. Critical thinking is an essential nursing competency.

1. There is no single, agreed upon definition of critical thinking. Some accepted definitions include:

D. Assessment: Systematic collection of data to determine the patient's health status and to identify any actual or potential health problems (Nettina, 2006). Through the assessment process, the deliberate collection of data is obtained by interviewing, observing, and examining the patient for evidence of health problems and risk factors. Incomplete or inaccurate data can lead to errors in decision-making. In the assessment phase of the nursing process, obtaining, classifying, and organizing data is the main function of critical thinking (Nettina, 2006).

1. Assessment occurs each time a patient enters the ambulatory care system, whether in person, on the telephone, through electronic communications, or via remote technological monitoring.
2. Situations in which assessment occurs:
   a. Comprehensive (such as pre-admission or pre-operative).
   b. Problem-focused (symptomatic visit or call).
   c. Emergency assessment (triage).
   d. Time-lapsed re-assessment: Chronic care management. Continuously monitoring responses to treatment.
3. Assessment includes:
   a. Collection of data: Continues with each nurse-patient interaction.
      (1) Objective: Data are observed or indirectly observed through measurement or physical examination using sight, touch, sound, and smell. Includes collection of data about the body, the mind, and the environment.
      (2) Subjective: Data that are stated, described, and verified by the patient and family through verbal and non-verbal communication. Can be collected during interviews, and portray the client's and family's point of view. Subjective data include the patient's feelings, perceptions, and concerns.
   b. Verification of data to validate the understanding of the problem and determine that all information is factual and complete.
      (1) Confirm observations through interview and examination.
      (2) Review data collected to identify if more in-depth or additional information is necessary using critical thinking skills.
      (3) Document data in a systematic manner.
   c. Organization and analysis of data to prioritize potential or actual problems by clustering data to identify patterns and assist with making inferences.
   d. Prediction, detection, prevention, and control of outcomes.
      (1) Consider cultural, spiritual, and environmental factors.
      (2) Assess patient and family wishes, strengths, and limitations.
   e. Documentation of data to form a database to communicate with other members of the health care team.

E. Diagnosis: Organize, synthesize, and summarize assessment data (Nettina, 2006). The analysis results in the identification of the patient's problems, which may be expressed as nursing diagnoses. A nursing diagnosis includes the etiology and forms the basis for the plan of care. According to the North American Nursing Diagnosis Association (NANDA) (2009), a nursing diagnosis is a clinical judgment about individual, family, or community responses to actual or potential health problems/life processes. Nursing diagnoses provide the basis for selection of nursing interventions to achieve outcomes for which the nurse is accountable.

1. Analyzes and synthesizes data collected for problem identification.
   a. Classifies data, grouping significant and related data.
   b. Creates a list of suspected problems.
   c. Identifies problems that must be managed by physicians or advanced practice nurses, or another member of the health care team (Alfaro-LeFevre, 2005).
   d. Rules out similar problems using critical thinking skills.
   e. Determines risk factors that must be managed.

f. Identifies resources, strengths, and areas for health promotion.

2. Defines the patient's problems, and problem characteristics and etiology.
   a. Development of nursing diagnosis using approved NANDA nursing diagnosis.
      (1) Excludes all non-nursing diagnoses.
      (2) Includes environmental stressors.
      (3) Includes data identified during assessment.

3. The nurse is accountable for actions that occur within the scope of the nursing diagnosis framework.

4. The nursing diagnosis provides criteria for quality improvement through review and evaluation.

5. Nursing diagnoses are intended to improve communication between health care professionals.

F. Nursing plan: Prioritizes identified nursing diagnoses, and identifies the action the nurse should take to achieve the desired goals and outcomes. It is aimed at solving or alleviating the problems identified in the assessment process by setting realistic goals that are clear, concise, and established with the patient. It includes a plan, short- and long-term client-centered goals, strategies for outcome achievement, and nursing measures for the delivery of care (Smith, Duell, & Martin, 2008).
   1. A plan of care (Alfaro-LeFevre, 2005):
      a. Promotes communication among caregivers.
      b. Provides continuity of care.
      c. Directs care and documentation.
      d. Includes advocacy by promoting the patient's right to autonomy.
      e. Incorporates evidence.
      f. Is patient- and family-centered.
   2. Clarification of goals and outcomes are guided by the use of:
      a. Protocols.
         (1) Provide basis for consistency.
         (2) Describe steps and actions in exact order.
         (3) Delineate responsibilities.
         (4) Do not supersede clinical judgment.
      b. Guidelines.
         (1) Based on standards of care that guide nursing actions.
         (2) Based on current best evidence.
         (3) Aimed at achieving outcomes.
         (4) Do not supersede clinical judgment.
      c. Patient outcomes are reflected in expected changes in the patient.
         (1) Should be specific, measurable, attainable, realistic, and time-sensitive.
         (2) Allow the nurse to evaluate outcome achievement and re-evaluate the plan of care as needed.

G. Implementation: Refers to priority nursing actions performed to accomplish a specified goal. Coordinates activities of the patient, family, nursing team, and other health care professionals (Nettina, 2006), and is the action component of the nursing process.
   1. Nursing interventions:
      a. May involve delegation.
      b. Assess patient response pre- and post-action.
      c. Weigh risks and consequences of each action.
      d. Resolve, prevent, or manage problems.
      e. Promote optimum sense of physical, psychological, and spiritual well-being.
      f. Should include safety, including fall prevention and identification of suicide risk.
   2. *Nursing Interventions Classification* (NIC) describes the interventions and treatments nurses perform (Bulechek, Butcher, & Dochterman, 2008).
      a. Include independent and collaborative interventions.
      b. Are used by nurses in all settings.
      c. Include illness treatment, illness prevention, and health promotion.
      d. The fifth edition (Bulechek et al., 2008) includes 542 research-based interventions.

e. Updated every four years.

f. Linked to NANDA nursing diagnoses.

3. Medically directed interventions include:

   a. Administering medications.

   b. Administering IV solutions.

   c. Providing wound care or other procedures.

   d. Following other orders as directed by a physician, physician's assistant, advanced practice nurse, or other person authorized to write orders.

4. Prior to performing a procedure, the nurse:

   a. Reviews the procedure, intervention, protocol, or guideline.

   b. Educates the patient and family.

   c. Allows time for questions.

   d. Ensures the safety of the patient.

H. Evaluation: The nurse analyzes the patient outcomes. The nurse assesses the patient's response to the plan of care by determining the effectiveness of the actions and the degree of goal attainment. If the patient is not satisfied, the plan is revised. Critical thinking questions at this time would be: "Have the patient's goals been met?" "Did the status of the problem change with the interventions?" "What else can be done to assist the patient?"

1. Collect assessment data.

   a. Compare the patient's actual outcome with expected outcomes to determine to what extent the goals have been met.

   b. Include the patient, family, and other health care team members in the evaluation.

   c. Identify alterations that need to be made in the goals and in the nursing plan of care.

2. Nursing Outcomes Classifications (NOC): Standardized classification for patient outcomes to evaluate the effects of nursing interventions (Donahue & Brighton, 1998).

   a. Developed for use in all settings and with all patient populations.

   b. Provide a list of indicators to evaluate patient status in relation to outcomes.

   c. Yield more information than just whether or not a goal was met.

d. Linked to NANDA.

e. Continually updated based on new research and published in a four-year cycle.

3. Evaluation is an ongoing process. The professional nurse will continue all steps of the nursing process until all patient goals and outcomes are met to the nurse's and patient's satisfaction.

I. Triage: Based on the concept of prioritizing the needs of the patient. After immediate needs are identified, the level of treatment is further defined based upon referrals to the appropriate level of care and resources available. Telephone triage is defined as "an interactive process between nurse and client that occurs over the telephone and involves identifying the nature and urgency of client health care needs and determining appropriate disposition" (Greenberg, Espensen, Becker, & Cartwright, 2003, p. 8). The goal of triage is safe patient care and appropriate disposition of the patient. Triage includes:

1. Assessment based in interviews, use of protocols, guidelines, algorithms, critical thinking, clinical judgment, and resource assessment.

2. Verification of information.

3. Prioritization of the patient's needs.

4. Development of a collaborative plan of care, taking into account the context, evidence, and the preference of the patient.

5. Nursing interventions, to include care advice over the telephone.

6. Determination of disposition.

7. Accurate and complete documentation.

8. Evaluation of outcomes and quality measurement.

II. Invasive Procedures: Applying the Nursing Process to Interventions

An invasive procedure is one in which the normal protective barrier of the skin or mucus membrane is broken or compromised. When broken, there is an increased risk for pathogenic microorganisms to enter the body, causing a reaction to tissues and the toxins generated by them. When performing an invasive procedure, physical and chemical control of microorganisms is required. Medical or surgical asepsis makes the environment and objects free of microorganisms (deWit, 2008). For invasive procedures, the use of surgical asepsis is practiced for preparing and handling materials. This involves using sterile supplies and techniques for procedures that enter the body.

A. Venipuncture for diagnostic testing is used for the screening of early signs of alterations to the patient's health or the course of disease, or to monitor response to treatment.

   1. Assessment:
      a. Review purpose.
      b. Review orders.
      c. Determine if special conditions are needed: Previous vaso-vagal response, privacy for disrobing, communications issues, or restraint by adult for child.
      d. Assess patient for risks; fragile veins, or signs of infection.
      e. Assess patient understanding of procedure.
      f. Assess contraindications that exclude certain sites: Site has signs of infection, infiltration, thrombosis, or patient is post-mastectomy.

   2. Plan:
      a. Venipuncture procedure completed per policy of institution.
      b. Patient is free of discomfort.
      c. No complications.
      d. Document date, time, specimen collected, site, and patient response.
      e. Report abnormal findings.

   3. Implementation (Smith et al., 2008):
      a. Assemble equipment.
      b. Review and plan the sequence for drawing the tubes.
      c. Identify correct patient and explain procedure.
      d. Position patient and select site.
      e. Place protection pad under site.
      f. Perform hand hygiene.
      g. Apply tourniquet on arm at least 4–6 inches above site. The tourniquet should remain on no longer than 1 minute and should not be so tight as to occlude arterial blood flow.
      h. Reassess site for suitability.
      i. Don gloves.
      j. Cleanse site according to agency policy.
      k. Stabilize the skin approximately 2 inches below insertion site.
      l. Perform venipuncture according to agency policy, inserting needle at a 15- to 30-degree angle.
      m. Release tourniquet and withdraw needle.
      n. Apply pressure to site until bleeding stops. Keep arm in extended position. Bending the arm permits blood to escape into surrounding tissues, causing a bruise or hematoma.
      o. Assess site and patient response, and apply dressing.
      p. Write date, time, and patient identifiers (such as name and date of birth or registration number) on tubes according to agency policy.
      q. Remove gloves and perform hand hygiene.
      r. Record procedure as stated by agency policy.

   4. Evaluation:
      a. Re-inspect site for evidence of bleeding or hematoma.
      b. Patient response for pain or discomfort.
      c. Specimen collected and obtained properly according to agency guidelines.

   5. Teaching:
      a. Regarding procedure – Purpose and how blood will be obtained.
      b. Allow questions and reassurance to decrease anxiety; use age-appropriate guidelines.
      c. Post-procedure – Continue pressure at site until bleeding stops; report any discomfort, pain, or bruising at site. If known, when results will be available and how they will be communicated.

B. Venipuncture for intravenous therapy – For medication or fluid administration to correct or prevent fluid and electrolyte disturbances.
  1. Assessment:
     a. Review purpose.
     b. Review orders.
     c. Determine if special conditions are needed; privacy for disrobing, communications issues, or restraint by adult for child.
     d. Assess patient for risks; fragile veins or signs of infection.
     e. Assess patient understanding of procedure.
     f. Assess contraindications.
     g. Check intravenous (IV) bag for outdating, tears, and leaks by applying gentle pressure to bag.
     h. Check the IV medication against order and appropriateness for peripheral intravenous infusion.
     i. Hold bag up to dark and light background to examine for discoloration, cloudiness, or particulate matters.
     j. Determine if the patient is allergic to IV solution or medication.
     k. Check for drug incompatibilities if more than one solution is to be hung.
  2. Plan:
     a. Venipuncture procedure.
     b. Patient free of discomfort.
     c. No complications.
     d. Documentation of date, time, IV solution, site, and patient response.
     e. Report abnormal findings.
  3. Implementation (Smith et al., 2008):
     a. Identify correct patient and explain procedure.
     b. Assemble equipment.
     c. Hang IV bag on IV pole.
     d. Prepare IV bag/tubing according to agency policy.
     e. Position patient and select site.
     f. Place protection pad under site.
     g. Perform hand hygiene.
     h. Apply tourniquet on upper arm at least 4–6 inches above site.
     i. Reassess site for suitability.
     j. Don gloves.
     k. Cleanse site according to agency policy.
     l. Stabilize the skin approximately 2 inches below insertion site.
     m. Use appropriate methodology for pain management per order (such as EMLA, ELA-max, lidocaine).
     n. May use dry heat to dilate veins for difficult IV starts; do not use microwave ovens to heat wraps because serious burns can occur.
     o. Perform venipuncture, verify blood return prior to beginning fluid or administering medications, and begin IV according to agency policy. If an intradermal bleb is used, sodium chloride 0.9% with benzyl alcohol preservative has been determined to be the safest.
     p. Reduce flow rate of IV to keep open until taped needle and tubing are in place.
     q. Apply occlusive transparent dressing over infusion site. Do not place anything under occlusive dressing (no tape, no gauze).
     r. Assess site and patient response while applying dressing.
     s. Write date, time, and needle gauge on label, along with nurse's initials according to agency policy.
     t. Remove gloves and perform hand hygiene.
     u. Set drip rate according to order by pump or calculated gravity flow drips per minute.
     v. Immobilize infusion site in functional position. Capped IV should be flushed before and after medication administration. Vigorously clean hub of cap prior to accessing cap.
     w. Clean up supplies and make the patient comfortable.
     x. Record procedure as stated by agency policy.
     y. Change cannula/tubing as stated by agency policy.

z. Peripheral line discontinuation.
   (1) Gather equipment, perform hand hygiene, don gloves, and discontinue all infusates.
   (2) Remove dressing and inspect catheter skin junction.
   (3) Disinfect junction and remove IV catheter.
   (4) Verify catheter is intact.
   (5) Hold pressure until bleeding stops. Secure site with gauze and cover with occlusive dressing.
   (6) Document removal of IV catheter, intactness of catheter, date and time, and condition of site.
   (7) If swelling is present, measure and document.
   (8) Remove gloves and perform hand hygiene.

4. Evaluation:
   a. Re-inspect site for evidence of bleeding, infiltration, hematoma, phlebitis, and extravasation. Inspect dressing and change if damp, loose, or soiled.
   b. Assess patient response for pain or discomfort. Record pain assessment prior to, during, and post-procedure.
   c. Verify the solution is running at the correct rate into vein without pain and IV cannula is secure.

5. Teaching:
   a. Regarding procedure – Purpose of and how IV access will be obtained.
   b. Allow questions and reassurance to decrease anxiety; use age-appropriate guidelines.
   c. Post-procedure – Report and document any discomfort, pain, or bruising at site; signs and symptoms of infiltration; and complications.

C. Tuberculin skin testing (TST) (Centers for Disease Control and Prevention [CDC], 2003) – Tuberculosis is an infection typically of the lungs caused by *Mycobacterium tuberculosis*, an acid-fast bacterium. Tubercle bacillus may be communicated to others by means of inhalation of droplets, ingestion, or inoculation. Testing determines the antibody response to tubercle bacillus. In the United States, the Mantoux tuberculin skin test has been the standard method for detecting latent tuberculosis (TB).

1. Predisposing factors to tuberculosis infection include:
   a. Alcoholism.
   b. Cardiovascular disease.
   c. HIV infection.
   d. Diabetes mellitus.
   e. Cirrhosis.
   f. End-stage renal disease.
   g. Cancers of the upper gastrointestinal tract or oropharynx.
   h. Poor nutrition.
   i. Crowded living conditions.
   j. Adverse social-economic conditions.
   k. Persons known to inject illicit drugs.
   l. Foreign-born individuals from countries with a high prevalence of TB.
   m. Low-income populations that are medically underserved.
   n. Patients who are non-compliant with appropriate drug therapy.
   o. Close contact with persons who are known or suspected to have TB.
   p. Residents and employees of high-risk congregate settings.
   q. Health care workers who serve high-risk patients.

2. Assessment for disease:
   a. Subjective: Malaise, pleuritic pain, easily fatigued.
   b. Objective: Fever, night sweats, cough that progressively becomes worse, hemoptysis, and weight loss.

3. Assessment prior to testing.
   a. Review purpose for obtaining test.
   b. Review orders.
   c. Determine if special conditions needed; disrobing, adult assistance with child.
   d. Know expected reactions.
   e. Check date of expiration of tuberculin purified protein derivative (PPD). Store the PPD at a temperature between 35 and 46 °F. Avoid prolonged exposure to light.

f. Assess the patient's knowledge of procedure and its purpose. Ensure patient's ability to return within 48–72 hours for reading.
g. Assess patient allergies.
h. Do not administer to patients who have a documented history of a positive Mantoux test; such testing has no diagnostic utility.
i. Review with the patient, as indicated, that potential cross reactions with antigens shared between Mycobacteria and prior vaccination with *Bacillus Calmette-Guerin* (BCG) may occur, but the test is still administered.

4. Plan:
    a. Administer test.
    b. Observe reaction.
    c. Teach patient about test and when/how to read test.
    d. Administer safely and correctly; no impaired skin integrity, no injury.
    e. Use aseptic technique.
    f. Follow CDC recommendations to prevent accidental exposure to blood and body fluids.
    g. Document amount and type of testing substance, date, time, site, appearance of skin, any undesirable effects from administration, and the patient's response.
    h. If live vaccines (such as measles-mumps-rubella [MMR], varicella, and herpes zoster) are indicated, also give live vaccines with TST concurrently or delay TST for 4–6 weeks because live vaccines given in a shorter time frame prior to a TST may interfere with the TST response.

5. Implementation:
    a. Verify order and properly identify patient.
    b. Assemble supplies and select site. The inside forearm is the standard location.
    c. Assess the patient's understanding of the test and when/how to read.
    d. Position patient, perform hand hygiene, and don gloves.

e. Follow agency policy for administration of intradermal injection.
f. Mantoux test is the standard method of testing in the United States.
    (1) Administer 0.1 mL of PPD containing 5 Tuberculin units (TU) on the ventral surface of the forearm, 2–4 inches below the elbow, using a 27-gauge needle with a short bevel. Area selected should be free of barriers to placing and reading, such as heavy hair, scars, muscle margins, and sores.
    (2) Administer injection intradermally, with the bevel of the needle facing upward. Injection should produce a pale, discrete 6 mm to 10 mm wheal on the skin. Do not massage area or cover the test site with an adhesive bandage because the adhesive could cause irritation and interfere with test results.
g. Remove gloves and perform hand hygiene.
h. Document date and time of test, name and manufacturer of the injected solution, lot number, dose administered, expiration date of solution, forearm used, name of person administering the test, and the reason for administering the test.
i. Interpret results as described in the *Evaluation* section (see below).

6. Teaching:
    a. Purpose of test.
    b. How the test is administered, low concentration of medication.
    c. Positive test may indicate exposure, but not active disease.
    d. Return for reading between 48 and 72 hours (see *Reading the Results* in the *Evaluation* section, below – C 7 i)

7. Evaluation:
    a. Verify bleb remains.
    b. Patient experiences no discomfort.
    c. Safe and correct administration.
    d. Timely documentation.

e. A positive skin test necessitates additional workup.

f. Reactions may wane with age, but can be restored by repeated testing. The "booster" phenomenon may occur at any age, but frequency increases with age, highest among persons older than 55 years of age and/or among persons who have had prior BCG vaccination. This "booster" effect of patients who undergo repeat testing may be falsely considered a new conversion of the skin test from non-reactive to reactive if the second test is administered at some later interval, such as in health care workers getting a second test a year after employment. The CDC (1995) recommends a two-step procedure for the initial screening of residents and employees of long-term care facilities.

    (1) The two-step procedure – If the first Mantoux test result is non-reactive, perform a second test one to two weeks later.

    (2) Reaction to the "booster" test usually indicates old, not new, TB infection.

g. Absence of a tuberculin reaction does not exclude a diagnosis of TB infection, when symptoms suggest the presence of active disease.

h. A small percentage of tuberculin reactions may be caused by errors in administering the test or reading the results.

i. Reading the results (CDC, 2005):

    (1) Skin test should be read between 48 and 72 hours.

    (2) The patient who does not return within 72 hours will need to be retested.

    (3) Basis for reading the test is the presence or absence of induration.

    (4) Erythema should not be measured.

    (5) Reactions at injection site can range from no induration to a large, well-defined induration.

    (6) Induration is not always visible; palpate with fingertips for induration.

    (7) With a light, gentle motion, sweep the surface of the forearm in a 2-inch diameter in all four directions to locate margins of induration.

    (8) Mark and measure, using the millimeter ruler, the longest diameter across the forearm.

    (9) Document the measurement and record any blistering. Do not record as positive or negative. Actual measurement is needed. If no induration, then record as "0 mm."

    (10) Positive reading: Greater than 5 mm with risk factors; greater than 10 mm without risk factors, but in high-incidence group; greater than 15 mm without risk factors and in low-incidence group.

    (11) Check agency policy regarding patient reading of TST.

    (12) The CDC (2003) offers educational materials for TST and provides directions for administering and reading the test.

III. Noninvasive Procedures

Noninvasive procedures are diagnostic or therapeutic techniques that do not require the skin to be broken or the body to be entered. Noninvasive procedures reduce discomfort to the patient and the spread of microorganisms. Medical asepsis, or the clean technique, is used for these procedures. Proper hand hygiene and disinfecting anything that may have been contaminated while performing a noninvasive procedure reduces the risk for transmission of organisms from person to person or to items in the environment (deWit, 2008).

A. Vital signs – The measurements of 5 vital signs provide important indications regarding the state of health of an individual. The term "vital" is used because of the clear correlation of vital signs to overall health status. Vital signs provide baseline data that reflect the status of several body systems, thus deviations or changes can be more easily recognized. Many therapeutic decisions are made based on vital signs, thus accuracy is important. Vital signs are not assessed in isolation, but in addition to assessing signs, symptoms, patient's medications, laboratory tests, history, and records.

1. Factors that may influence vital signs:
   a. Age.
   b. Gender.
   c. Race and heredity.
   d. Medications.
   e. Pain.
   f. Time of day.
   g. Caffeine, nicotine.
   h. Exercise.
   i. Emotions.
   j. Pregnancy.
   k. Presence of disease.
   l. Blood loss.
   m. Degree of hydration.
   n. Environmental temperature.

2. Blood pressure – Measuring arterial blood pressure provides important information about the overall health of the patient. The systolic pressure provides information about the condition of the heart and great arteries. The diastolic pressure indicates arteriolar or peripheral vascular resistance. The difference between the systolic and diastolic pressure provides information about cardiac function and blood volume. A series of blood pressure readings should be taken to establish a baseline to provide adequate data. Seven factors affect blood pressure: Cardiac output, peripheral vascular resistance, elasticity of arteries, blood volume, blood viscosity, chemo receptors, and hormones (Smith et al., 2008). It is important that the nurse evaluates blood pressure in the context of the total view of the patient.
   a. Assessment:
      (1) Blood pressure reading initially and whenever patient status changes. The frequency of blood pressure checks should be individualized to the patient.
      (2) Size of cuff needed for accurate reading.
         (a) Bladder width should cover 40% of arm circumference at midpoint; bladder length should cover 80–100% of upper arm or thigh circumference. Bladder ends should not overlap.
         (b) Improper cuff size:
            i. Too small or narrow will result in falsely elevated measurements.
            ii. Too large or wide will result in falsely depressed measurements.
      (3) Presence of factors that can alter readings (such as smoking or ingesting caffeine within prior 30 minutes).
      (4) Any changes from prior readings.
   b. Planning – Measure the blood pressure in both arms, at least initially. A difference of 5–10 mmHg between arms is normal (Nettina, 2006).
      (1) Determine if reading is within normal range for the patient.
      (2) Establish a baseline for further evaluation.
      (3) Identify alternations in reading results from changes in the patient's condition.
      (4) Correlate readings with pulse and respirations.
      (5) Frequency of measurement is individualized.
      (6) Manage and minimize vascular complications.
      (7) Assess for contraindications to taking blood pressure on either arm (such as mastectomy, serious injury, lymph node dissection, or arteriovenous fistula).
      (8) Blood pressure is dependent on the position of body and arm.
      (9) A validated electronic device meeting the requirements of the American National Standard for

Electronic Advancement of Medical Instruments may be used. A list of approved devices is available from the U.S. Food and Drug Administration (FDA) (2012).

c. Implementation.
   (1) Identify the patient.
   (2) Provide privacy.
   (3) Provide a quiet environment. Have the patient sit and rest for 5 minutes.
   (4) For pediatric patients, use play therapy appropriate for age or distraction technique to decrease stress and encourage cooperation.
   (5) Obtain blood pressure reading after assessing heart rate and respirations.
   (6) Perform hand hygiene.
   (7) Expose upper part of patient's arm and position palm up, arm slightly flexed, and arm supported at heart level. Blood pressure should always be taken over bare skin. Wrinkled clothing prevents correct placement of cuff. Patient should be sitting upright, with feet flat on the floor, and legs and ankles uncrossed.
   (8) Wrap deflated cuff snugly and smoothly around arm (lower border of cuff 1 inch above antecubital space, center of cuff over brachial artery). Make sure pressure dial is at zero. Apply the cuff firmly. If it is too loose, it will give a false high reading.
   (9) Apply stethoscope lightly to the antecubital fossa. Close valve on sphygmomanometer pump.
   (10) Inflate cuff rapidly to a level 30 mmHg above point where the radial pulse is no longer palpable.
   (11) Deflate cuff gradually at a constant rate by opening valve on pump no more than 2–3 mmHg per second until first Korotkoff's sound is heard (systolic pressure).
   Note reading. Continue to deflate cuff. Note the disappearance of Korotkoff's sound (diastolic pressure).
   (12) Deflate cuff completely, remove from arm. Check that patient is comfortable. Perform hand hygiene.
   (13) Document systolic/diastolic reading, position, limb used, and cuff size for consistency.

d. Teaching.
   (1) Educate using age-appropriate guidelines regarding procedure and what is expected.
   (2) Discuss risks of hypertension and importance of blood pressure monitoring.
   (3) Develop education plan for self-measurement, if indicated.
   (4) Describe signs and symptoms that must be reported to health care professionals.
   (5) Educate patient self-management strategies, as appropriate, including optimal nutrition and activity (see Chapter 21, "Care of the Chronically Ill Patient," for more information about hypertension).

e. Evaluation.
   (1) Blood pressure for adults 18 years of age or older within normal range less than 120 systolic and less than 80 diastolic. High blood pressure is usually defined as a systolic pressure of 140 or higher or a diastolic pressure of 90 or higher (U.S. Preventive Services Task Force, 2007).
   (2) The normal range of blood pressure in children and adolescents is based on sex, age, and height, and is classified according to body size (National Heart, Lung, and Blood Institute [NHLBI], 2005). *Hypertension* is defined as blood pressure that is on repeated measurement at the 95th per-

centile or greater when adjusted for age, height, and gender (NHLBI, 2005).

   (3) *Blood Pressure Tables for Children and Adolescents* (NHLBI, 2004).

   (4) Alterations are identified early, and appropriate treatment is initiated.

   (5) Severely altered readings are rechecked on another limb, different equipment used, or validated by another health care professional.

   (6) Initial visit – Use the average of at least 2 readings. Permit the blood to be released from veins by waiting 1–2 minutes before repeated readings.

   (7) Altered readings are reported to physician or provider.

3. Pulse – The palpable bounding of blood flow noted at various points on the body. Each time the heart contracts to force blood into an already full aorta, the arterial walls in the vascular system must expand to accept the increased pressure. The pulse rate is determined by counting each pulsation of the arterial wall (deWit, 2008). The radial and apical pulses are the most common sites for assessment of vital signs.

  a. Assessment:

   (1) Appropriate site, rate, rhythm, volume, and quality.

   (2) Obtaining baseline.

   (3) Any changes from prior readings.

   (4) Consider factors that normally influence pulse character: Age, exercise, postural changes, medications, emotional status.

  b. Plan:

   (1) Determine if pulse rate is within the normal range.

   (2) Monitor for health changes.

   (3) Take apical rate before administration of cardiac medication.

   (4) Apical pulse is used to assess in infant or child, or if there is question about radial pulse in adolescent or adult.

  c. Implementation (radial pulse):

   (1) Assess radial pulse at rest to allow for comparison of values.

   (2) Identify the patient.

   (3) Perform hand hygiene.

   (4) Patient sitting – Bend elbow 90 degrees and support lower arm on chair, slightly extending wrist with palm down.

   (5) Place tips of first two fingers of your hand over groove along radial (thumb side) of patient's inner wrist.

   (6) Lightly compress against radius so that pulse is easily palpable.

   (7) Begin to count with zero. If pulse is regular, count rate for 30 seconds and multiply by 2. If pulse is irregular, count for one full minute.

   (8) Determine rate, strength, and rhythm of pulse.

   (9) Palpate with two fingers along course of artery toward wrist to determine elasticity of arterial wall.

   (10) If irregular or skipped beats, two people need to assess radial and apical pulse at the same time.

   (11) Document pulse rate, rhythm, and intensity. Perform hand hygiene.

  d. Teaching:

   (1) Teach the patient to assess his or her own pulse if taking certain medications or if there is a need to assess response to exercise.

   (2) Describe signs and symptoms to report to health care professional.

   (3) Normal adult pulse range is 60–80 beats per minute (Nettina, 2006).

  e. Evaluation:

   (1) Palpated pulse without difficulty.

(2) Pulse within normal range and easily detected (Nettina, 2006).

(3) Response to activities of daily living or exercise.

(4) Cardiac status is stable; radial artery is patent.

4. Respirations – Involve the processes of ventilation, diffusion, and perfusion. Accurate assessment of respirations depends on recognizing normal thoracic and abdominal movements. Monitoring respirations assists in the detection of abnormal conditions or diseases in the pulmonary or metabolic system.

    a. Assessment:
        (1) Risk factors of disease or illness on respiratory functions.
        (2) Health factors causing alterations in respirations, including fever, pain, anxiety, smoking, medications, postural changes, chest or abdominal dressings, or gastric distention.
        (3) Signs and symptoms of respiratory alterations: Dyspnea at rest or on exertion, cyanosis, labored breathing with use of accessory muscles, pain, wheezing, stridor, audible adventiuous sounds, paradoxical chest wall movement, or coughing.
        (4) Utilization of supplemental oxygen: Flow rate, pattern of use.

    b. Plan:
        (1) Determine previous baseline rate, if available.
        (2) Analyze in relationship to other vital signs.
        (3) Note changes from previous readings.

    c. Implementation:
        (1) Assess after pulse measurement while patient is not aware.
        (2) Observe complete respiratory cycle of one inspiration and one expiration.
        (3) Count one with first full respiratory cycle.
        (4) Count respiratory rate for a full minute.
        (5) Assess the three objective qualities: Rate, depth, and rhythm.
        (6) Assess the ratio of inspiration to expiration.
        (7) Document time, respiratory rate, and any abnormalities.

    d. Teaching:
        (1) Effective breathing techniques.
        (2) Signs or symptoms to report to health care professional.
        (3) Lifestyle modifications, if indicated (see *Asthma, Heart Failure,* and *Chronic Obstructive Pulmonary Disease* sections in Chapter 21, "Care of the Chronically Ill Patient").

    e. Evaluation.
        (1) Compare with patient's baseline.
        (2) Regular rate and effortless breathing.
        (3) Respirations are effective, relaxed, and of normal depth.
        (4) Normal respiratory rate for an adult is 16 respirations per minute (Nettina, 2006), with a normal range of 12–20 (Perry & Potter, 2010).

5. Temperature – The balance of body temperature is regulated by physiological and behavioral mechanisms. Temperature control mechanisms keep the body's core temperature in a relatively constant range. The core body temperature is the temperature of the deep tissues of the body, not of the skin temperature. For the body to function on a cellular level, a core temperature between 36.5 °C and 37.7 °C (96.0 °F and 99.9 °F) must be maintained (Weber & Kelley, 2011). Variations of heat loss and gain in individuals are influenced by body surface, peripheral vasomotor tone, and quantity of subcutaneous tissue.

    a. Assessment (deWit, 2008):
        (1) Methods of obtaining.

(a) Oral – Glass thermometer (non-mercury) or electronic.

(b) Electronic digital – For oral, rectal, axillary.

   i. Readings appear in seconds.

(c) Tympanic – Portable, electronic auditory canal probe.

   i. Readings appear in seconds.

   ii. Accurate, good indicator of core body temperature.

   iii. Measures heat radiated from infrared energy; same blood vessels that serve hypothalamus.

(d) Temporal: Non-invasive, more accurate than tympanic.

(2) Orders or unit guidelines for when temperature should be assessed.

(3) Temperature in relationship to time of day and age of patient.

(4) No single normal temperature for all patients.

b. Plan:

(1) Factors that influence site chosen.

(a) Safety.

(b) Accuracy.

(c) Convenience.

(d) Age.

(e) Patient cooperation.

(2) Reliability of temperature depends on:

(a) Accurate temperature-taking technique.

(b) Minimization of variables that influence.

(c) Site chosen.

(3) Determine if patient has consumed hot or cold liquids or smoked within 15–30 minutes prior to taking orally.

c. Implementation:

(1) Measurements at any site include:

(a) Most appropriate site chosen.

(b) All equipment assembled prior to procedure. Electronic devices checked for charge.

(c) Patient identified.

(d) Patient positioned properly and privacy ensured.

(e) Explanation of purpose and method.

(f) Perform hand hygiene and don gloves.

(g) After removing device, wipe from stem to bulb tip.

(h) Assist the patient to a comfortable position.

(i) Document temperature, time, and method used.

(2) Oral – Electronic.

(a) Used for alert, cooperative clients.

(b) Place probe with proper cover/sleeve under tongue, to the right or left of the frenulum.

(c) Ask the patient to keep lips tightly closed around thermometer. Open-mouth breathing will result in lower readings.

(d) Remove probe when light or audible signal occurs.

(e) Read temperature.

(f) Push ejection button of probe, dispose of disposal cover/sleeve.

(3) Axillary – Electronic.

(a) Reliable for skin temperature.

(b) Used if oral/rectal/tympanic contraindicated. Temporal preferred over axillary, if possible.

(c) Hold under axilla firmly.

(d) Remove when light or audible signal occurs.

(e) Read temperature.

(f) Push ejection button of probe, dispose of disposal cover/sleeve.

(4) Rectal – Electronic.

(a) Do not use if contraindicated (e.g., coagulation disorders).

(b) Switch to rectal probe attachment.

(c) Used if other routes not practical.
  i. If patient cannot cooperate.
  ii. If patient cannot close mouth.
(d) Use disposable sleeve or lubricate according to agency protocol.
(e) Insert probe 1 inch into rectum; never force probe into rectum.
(f) Remove when light or audible signal occurs.
(g) Read temperature.
(h) Push ejection button of probe; dispose of disposal cover/sleeve.
(i) Assist patient by cleansing area, repositioning.

(5) Tympanic – Electronic auditory canal probe.
(a) Measures body heat radiating from tympanic membrane.
(b) Do not use in infected or draining ear.
(c) Place probe gently at opening of auditory canal.
(d) Remove when light or audible signal occurs.
(e) Read temperature.
(f) Push ejection button of probe; dispose of disposal cover/sleeve.

(6) Temporal.
(a) Disinfect probe.
(b) Place probe flush on center of forehead.
(c) Depress and hold button to read temperature.
(d) Slide probe across forehead to hairline.
(e) Lift probe from forehead (or slide behind ear) and touch the neck just behind the earlobe; keep button depressed throughout procedure.

(f) Release button and read temperature.

d. Teaching:
  (1) Need to monitor.
  (2) Appropriate site.
  (3) How to obtain and positioning.
  (4) Glass thermometers should be disinfected in 70–90% isopropyl alcohol, then rinsed with clear water, dried, and stored in dry container.
  (5) Signs and symptoms of fever.
  (6) Caution against use of mercury thermometers at home.

e. Evaluation:
  (1) Comparison to normal range.
  (2) Normal ranges (deWit, 2008):
    (a) Oral – 36.4 $^\circ$C to 37.5 $^\circ$C (97.5 $^\circ$F to 99.5 $^\circ$F).
    (b) Axillary – 0.5 $^\circ$C (1 $^\circ$F) lower than oral temperature.
    (c) Rectal – Between 0.4 $^\circ$C and 0.5 $^\circ$C (0.7 $^\circ$F to 1 $^\circ$F) higher than oral.
    (d) Tympanic – 0.8 $^\circ$C (1.4 $^\circ$F) higher than oral.

6. Pain – It is estimated that more than 75 million people suffer from pain. Pain is the feeling of distress, suffering, and/or discomfort that has long been regarded as a symptom of a condition to be diagnosed and treated (deWit, 2008). One classic definition of pain was offered by McCaffery in 1968 (p. 95): "Pain is whatever the patient experiencing pain says it is." Today, pain is often regarded as the "fifth" vital sign. It is subjective and individualized, and involves psychosocial and cultural factors. The Joint Commission has established standards that recognize the right of patients to appropriate assessment and management of pain, require that one screens patients for pain during their initial assessment, and when clinically required, during ongoing, periodic re-assessments, and further require that one educate patients suffering from pain and their families about pain management (The Joint Commission, 2011).

a. Assessment:
  (1) Type of pain: Acute or chronic.
  (2) Characteristics of pain:
    (a) Location – Diffuse or localized.
    (b) Quality – Description, use patient's words.
    (c) Intensity – Rating with an instrument appropriate to developmental stage of patient and according to agency guidelines.
    (d) Precipitating factors – Fears, anxiety, trauma, disease state.
    (e) Aggravating factors – Position change, environment, fatigue, inadequate pain relief measures.
    (f) Relieving factors, including use of pharmaceutical and non-pharmaceutical interventions.
    (g) Frequency and duration.
  (3) Nonverbal indication of pain.
  (4) Patient's ability or reluctance to report pain.
  (5) Patient's beliefs and fears, including cultural.
  (6) Cognitive status.
  (7) Assess pain prior to and after procedures that may cause pain.
b. Plan:
  (1) Review patient history.
    (a) Assessment.
    (b) Management strategies.
    (c) Relevant medical, surgical, and family history.
    (d) Psychosocial history.
    (e) Impact of pain on patient's daily life.
    (f) Patient expectations and goals.
  (2) Establish a positive relationship. Advocate for the patient.
  (3) Identify appropriate pain scale.
    (a) Numeric – 0 to 10 rating; 0 = no pain to 10 = worst pain.
    (b) Verbal – Word; no pain to worst pain.
    (c) Visual (visual analog scale, a horizontal line anchored by words or numbers); categorical scale (such as the Faces Pain Scale).
    (d) Multidimensional pain assessment tools; Brief Pain Inventory; Initial Pain Assessment Inventory; McGill Pain Questionnaire.
    (e) Non-verbal assessment tools for infants or the nonverbal client (Pain Attitudes and Beliefs Scale [PABS], Neonatal Infant Pain Scale [NIPS]).
  (4) Set realistic goals with the patient for pain management.
  (5) Use time frames.
  (6) Identify pharmacologic and non-pharmacologic therapies.
c. Implementation.
  (1) Use appropriate pain scale for baseline and reassess, as appropriate.
  (2) Implement providers' orders, which may include pharmacologic treatment.
  (3) Implement non-pharmacologic treatments for pain.
    (a) Patient education.
    (b) Psychological approaches.
    (c) Physical rehabilitative approaches.
    (d) Surgical approaches, if indicated.
  (4) Document the patient's preferred pain assessment tool and goals.
  (5) Document using common language across the continuum of care.
d. Teaching:
  (1) Educate about pain assessment, use of pain scales.
  (2) Explore misconceptions of pain.
  (3) Identify signs and symptoms to report to the health care provider.
  (4) Review physical and psychological consequences of unrelieved pain.

(5) State importance of following medication schedules and plan of care. Reinforce length of action of various medications and which can be taken together or alternately.

(6) Identify cautions to be taken in narcotic medications are prescribed, such as increased fall risk.

(7) Instruct to observe for behavioral changes, if applicable for medication prescribed.

(8) Provide written information and contact persons.

(9) Give patient permission to report pain.

e. Evaluation:
(1) Patient's satisfaction with pain control.
(2) Patient report of decreased anxiety.
(3) Patient reaction, tolerance, and dependence.
(4) Activities of daily living achieved to the patient's expectations.
(5) Patient report of unrelieved or new appearance of pain.

B. Physical assessment – Provides a picture of the physiologic functioning of the patient. It is conducted in a systematic way, beginning with measuring the height, weight, and vital signs. A patient's health status assessment is formed by combining health history with the above measures plus the physical examination techniques of inspection, palpation, percussion, and auscultation (deWit, 2008).

1. Inspection and observation.
a. Scrutinize and observe the patient's body and behavior in an organized manner (Nettina, 2006).
b. Perform first in the physical examination.
c. Involves senses of sight, smell, and hearing to detect normal and abnormal characteristics and findings.
d. Includes general appearance, color, patterns, size, location, consistency, symmetry, movement, behavior, odors, and sounds.

2. Palpation.
a. Use sense of touch to feel various parts of the body.
b. Includes texture, temperature, moisture, mobility, consistency, strength of pulses, size, shape, and degree of tenderness.
c. Perform in an organized sequence.
d. Determine areas of tenderness using light palpation.
e. Examine condition of organs using deep palpation.

3. Percussion.
a. Lightly tap on the body structures to produce sound waves. Percussing hollow structures produces tympany and percussing solid structures produces dullness.
b. Use to elicit pain, detect abnormal masses, and elicit reflexes.
c. Used to determine location, size, and density of underlying structures.
d. Type of tapping:
(1) Direct – Using one or two fingertips to check tenderness.
(2) Indirect – One hand flat; with fist of other hand to strike back of hand or place the middle finger of non-dominant hand and strike with finger of dominant hand.
(3) Sounds produced – Tympany, resonance, hyperresonance, dullness, and flatness.

4. Auscultation.
a. Listen to sounds produced in the body by use of a stethoscope.
b. Use to listen to lungs, assess heart sounds, detect presence of bruits, and detect presence and character of bowel sounds.

5. Abdominal examination.
a. Differs slightly from other assessments because ausculating bowel sounds should be performed prior to percussion or palpation of bowel, which may stimulate sounds.

b. Order of assessment of abdomen is inspection, auscultation, percussion, and palpation.

C. Electrocardiogram (EKG/ECG) – A graphic representation of electrical impulses generated by the heart.

1. Assessment:
   a. Determine preexisting cardiac disease.
   b. Identify rationale for obtaining EKG/ECG.
   c. Identify pharmacologic agents currently prescribed.
   d. Determine subjective complaints.
   e. Identify electrolyte abnormalities.
   f. Assess patient's knowledge of procedure.
   g. Obtain baseline vitals.
   h. Determine ability to lie supine.

2. Plan:
   a. Obtain an accurate 12-lead EKG/ECG.
   b. Determine EKG/ECG abnormalities and/or changes.
   c. Identify electrolyte abnormalities.
   d. Determine cardiac irregularities.
   e. Identify and report potentially dangerous rhythms.
   f. Determine if relationship exists between subjective complaints and EKG/ECG changes.

3. Implementation:
   a. Obtain tracing (Smith et al., 2008).
      (1) Follow the EKG/ECG machine's own set of operating instructions and agency protocol.
      (2) Check the color coding on the manufacturer's directions before placing electrodes to ensure they are placed on correct wires.
      (3) Review order and identify patient.
      (4) Provide privacy and determine if skin site care is necessary.
      (5) Attach electrodes to wires before pressing on patient's chest.
      (6) Perform hand hygiene.
      (7) Place electrodes on fleshy areas, avoiding bone and muscle.
      (8) Place four limb leads according to color coding.
      (9) Place the chest leads as follows:
         (a) V1 – Fourth intercostal space, right sternal border.
         (b) V2 – Fourth intercostal space, left sternal border.
         (c) V3 – Midway between V2 and V4.
         (d) V4 – Fifth intercostal space, left midclavicular line.
         (e) V5 – Fifth intercostal space, anterior axillary line.
         (f) V6 – Fifth intercostal space, left midaxillary line.
      (10) Assist patient to supine position. Head of bed may be slightly elevated.
   b. Run and monitor EKG/ECG.
   c. Remove electrodes; assist the patient with cleansing; ensure privacy.
   d. Assist the patient to a comfortable position.
   e. Perform hand hygiene.
   f. Provide for interpretation of EKG/ECG strip.
   g. Document and record a 12-lead EKG/ECG, vital signs, date, time, and patient's response.
   h. Monitor any patient complaint or discomfort.
   i. Report any unexpected outcomes immediately.
   j. Perform right-sided EKG as ordered to confirm inferior heart attacks or for use on patients with dextrocardia.
   k. Children 14 and under, V3 is moved to the right side.

4. Teaching:
   a. Explain purpose and steps of procedure.
   b. Reassure that electric current is from patient to machine; therefore, no danger of electric shock.
   c. Contact physician or health care provider regarding test results.

5. Evaluation:
   a. EKG/ECG performed accurately.
   b. Abnormal findings interpreted accurately.
   c. Patient's tolerance of procedure noted.
   d. Vital signs remain stable.
   e. Clear EKG/ECG strip obtained.
D. Body mass index (BMI) – Describes weight relative to height. It is used to assess overweight and obesity, and to monitor changes in body weight. The calculation and classification of BMI provides the most current evidence-based guidelines on the identification, evaluation, and treatment of adults and children who are overweight and obese (U.S. Preventive Services Task Force, 2010). BMI is a reliable indicator of body fatness for most children and teens. BMI is age- and gender-specific in children. The CDC BMI-for-age growth charts for girls and boys take into account these differences and allow translation of a BMI number into a percentile for a child's/teen's gender and age (U.S. Preventive Services Task Force, 2010).
   1. Assessment:
      a. Frequency of measurement in adults is based on clinical discretion.
      b. Formula for calculation: Weight (kg)/ Height (m)^2.
      c. BMI values for adults (National Institutes of Health [NIH], 2011):
         (1) Underweight = below 18.5.
         (2) Normal = 18.5 to 24.9.
         (3) Overweight = 25.0 to 29.9.
         (4) Obese = 30.0 and above.
         (5) Children and adolescents ages 6 to 18 years, overweight is defined as an age- and gender-specific BMI between the 85th and 95th percentiles; obesity is age- and gender-specific BMI at 95th or greater percentile (U.S. Preventive Services Task Force, 2010).
      d. Determine need for BMI measurements.
      e. Review disease conditions, cardiovascular risk factors, physical inactivity, and patient motivation.

   f. Other measures of adiposity: Waist circumference, bioelectrical impedence, dual-energy X-ray absorptiometry, and total body water are less practical for routine use.
   2. Plan:
      a. Establish baseline data.
      b. Identify excess or deficit fluid balance.
      c. Determine patient's expectations.
   3. Implementation:
      a. Obtain height, weight, and calculation of BMI.
      b. Document height, weight, BMI, vital signs, and general appearance.
   4. Teaching:
      a. Normal range of BMI.
      b. Weigh at same time each day.
      c. Diet.
      d. Exercise.
      e. Medication.
   5. Evaluation:
      a. Indication of losses/gains.
      b. Assessment of nutritional status by presence/absence of body fat.
      c. Possible indication of growth disorder.
      d. Possible indication for referral to treatment program.
E. Visual acuity – The purpose of the eye and vision examination is to identify any changes in vision or signs of eye disorders (U.S. Department of Health and Human Services, 2004).
   1. Assessment:
      a. Age.
      b. History of difficulty with vision.
      c. History of ocular pain, disease, trauma, diabetes, hypertension, or eye surgery.
      d. Risk factors for cataracts: Smoking, alcohol use, exposure to ultraviolet light, corticosteroid use, Black race.
      e. Risk factors for age-related macular degeneration: Smoking, family history, and White race (U.S. Preventive Services Task Force, 2009).
      f. Subjective complaints.
      g. Use of glasses or contacts.
      h. Medications used.
      i. Computer usage.
      j. Date of last eye examination.

2. Plan:
   a. Determine visual acuity with or without correction.
   b. Patient denies discomfort during exam; identification of visual problems.
3. Implementation:
   a. If glasses/contacts are worn at all times, they are to be used for test.
   b. Vision of each eye is tested individually and in both eyes.
   c. Identify patient, and explain purpose and procedure.
   d. Test visual acuity using appropriate chart (U.S. Public Health Service, 1997).
      (1) Snellen (letters or numbers) – The patient reads as many of the symbols as possible, reading each line and proceeding down from the top.
      (2) Tumbling E – Used if the patient is not familiar with western alphabet.
      (3) HOTV Eye Chart (National Institute of Standards and Technology [NIST], 2011).
      (4) Allen figures.
      (5) Leah Hyvarinen (LH) test.
   e. Test for visual acuity at 10, 15, or 20 feet using the appropriate chart.
   f. Document results and chart used.
4. Teaching:
   a. Importance of regular eye examination.
   b. Signs and symptoms of eye disease.
   c. Safety precautions for visual deficits.
   d. Signs and symptoms to report to health care professional.
5. Evaluation:
   a. Compare results to other findings (if available) and report abnormal results to health care provider.
   b. Patient safety and self-care measures reviewed with patient.
   c. Home environment assessment completed, if indicated.
   d. If visual acuity is at 20/40 or less with corrective lenses, refer to eye care specialist.

F. Peak flow rate monitoring – Peak flow meter is designed for monitoring of airflow in patients. The peak expiratory flow rate represents the maximum flow rate generated during a forceful exhalation. Peak flow rates can be accurately performed by most patients who are at least 5 years of age. The most frequent usage of peak flow measurement is in the home environment to monitor asthma. If peak flow measurement is used, then the suggested written plan of action is to utilize the patient's personal best peak flow (Neuspiel, 2011). The 2007 Expert Panel of the National Asthma Education and Prevention Program suggests that measuring flow rate in acute asthma episodes helps to determine the severity of exacerbations and assist in guiding therapeutic decisions in the home, school, practitioner's office, and emergency department (Neuspiel, 2011).

1. Assessment:
   a. Obtain medical, social, and family history.
   b. Review lifestyle and patient cooperation.
   c. Assess signs of airway obstruction.
   d. Perform respiratory history and physical assessment.
   e. Review of aggravating factors and how they are managed.
   f. Assess functional status and quality of life.
   g. Describe current pharmacotherapy.
2. Plan:
   a. Allow for individualized plan of action to address changes.
   b. Monitor for signs and symptoms of distress.
   c. Maintain near normal pulmonary function.
   d. Maintain normal activities.
   e. Prevent chronic and troublesome symptoms.
   f. Meet patient/family expectations.
3. Implementation.
   a. Review orders.
   b. Educate about the use of a peak flow meter and proper procedure.

c. Observe the patient properly using peak flow meter (NHLBI, 2001).
   (1) Move the indicator to the bottom of the number scale.
   (2) Stand up.
   (3) Take a deep breath, filling lungs completely.
   (4) Place mouthpiece in mouth, close lips around it.
   (5) Blow out as hard and fast as possible.
   (6) Write down the number.
   (7) Repeat two more times.
   (8) Write down the best (highest) number of three blows. Peak flow meter interpretation is based on personal best reading:
       (a) Green 80–100% – Indicates good control of asthma.
       (b) Yellow 50–80% – Signals caution, take quick relief medicine.
       (c) Red less than 50% – Signals danger, take quick relief medicine, and seek medical care if not returned to yellow or green immediately.
   (9) Assist patient with setting realistic goals with a written action plan.
   (10) Document patient understanding, use, tolerance, time, and results (see *Asthma* section of Chapter 21, "Care of the Chronically Ill Patient").

4. Teaching.
   a. Discuss disease process.
   b. State signs and symptoms to report to health care professionals.
   c. Educate patient and/or family members on the asthma action plan.
   d. Keep scheduled follow-up appointments.
   e. Maintain adequate hydration.
   f. Review proper use of hand-held nebulizer, oxygen therapy, and inhalers, if prescribed.
   g. Provide clear directions on how to use the peak flow meter.

5. Evaluation:
   a. Vital signs stable and within normal range.
   b. Patient able to breathe with normal inspiratory capacities.
   c. Realistic short- and long-term goals set.
   d. Understanding of follow-up care and medication plan as ordered.

IV. Onsite Testing

Onsite testing is also referred to as "point of care testing" (POCT). POCT is medical testing at or near the patient site of care. The test is conveniently brought to the patient. POCT allows for the test results to be seen immediately, thereby allowing for immediate clinical decisions to be made by the provider. POCT includes (but is not limited to) blood glucose testing, blood gas and electrolyte analysis, rapid coagulation testing, rapid cardiac markers diagnostic, drugs of abuse screening, urine strip testing, pregnancy testing, fecal occult blood analysis, food pathogen screenings, hemoglobin diagnostics, infectious disease testing, and cholesterol screening. Listed below are a few of the most common tests performed in the ambulatory care setting.

A. Blood glucose testing – Essential in the diagnosis and control of diabetes (deWit, 2008).
   1. Assessment:
      a. Understanding and purpose of test.
      b. Determine if specific conditions need to be met (e.g., oral glucose tolerance test).
      c. Area of skin to be used.
      d. Fasting or non-fasting state.
      e. Check to see if test is routine or urgent.
   2. Plan:
      a. Obtain an uncontaminated blood specimen.
      b. To obtain accurate blood glucose level at specific time ordered.
      c. Review laboratory parameters.
      d. Obtain blood sample without complications.
   3. Implementation.
      a. Review physician's order.
      b. Gather equipment.

c. Identify patient and explain purpose of test and procedure.

d. Choose puncture site.

e. Have patient hold selected finger in dependent position. If hand is cold, have patient warm hand under warm water.

f. Perform hand hygiene and don gloves.

g. Cleanse chosen fingertip with an alcohol swab.

h. Turn the machine on, place lancet in holder, and remove lancet cover.

i. If using an automatic blade retraction device, cock the lancet device.

j. Check the control number on the screen with the control number on test strips.

k. Remove a test strip and insert the metal strip end into machine. Follow manufacturer's directions on machine.

l. Place the finger-stick device firmly on skin and push the release button, allowing lancet to penetrate the skin.

m. Lightly squeeze the finger, gently milking down toward the tip.

n. Lightly apply the drop of blood to the test strip pad and apply a cotton ball to the puncture wound.

o. Follow manufacturer's directions regarding timing for test. When complete, record the reading and turn machine off.

p. Assess the patient's finger.

q. Dispose of test strip, lancet, and supplies in appropriate waste receptacles.

r. Remove gloves and perform hand hygiene.

s. Document procedure and results.

t. Report abnormal levels.

u. Determine level of instruction needed.

4. Teaching:

a. Review of disease process.

b. Review and update goals.

c. Review of risk factors.

d. Management of hyperglycemia and hypoglycemia.

5. Evaluation:

a. Specimen obtained without complications.

b. Patient understanding of home monitoring, disease, nutrition, and physical activity (see *Diabetes* in Chapter 21, "Care of the Chronically Ill Patient").

B. Fecal occult blood – A guaiac test is a common laboratory test that can be done in the office following a rectal examination or at home. This test measures microscopic amounts of blood in the feces.

1. Assessment:

a. Patient's ability to cooperate.

b. Medical history for bleeding or gastrointestinal disorders.

c. Medications; note drugs that can cause gastrointestinal bleeding.

d. Diet.

e. Use of laxatives.

f. Exercise.

2. Plan:

a. Monitor for signs and symptoms of gastrointestinal bleeding, anemia, pain.

b. Patient instructed (if performed at home) to:

(1) Not collect if obvious hematuria, rectal bleeding, or menstruation.

(2) Avoid aspirin and non-steroidal anti-inflammatory drugs (NSAIDs) 7 days prior to test.

(3) Not consume vitamin C in diet or supplemental, red meats, and raw fruits or vegetables for at least 3 days.

(4) In home setting, collect two separate samples from each of three separate bowel movements.

3. Implementation (in ambulatory care setting).

a. Identify patient and explain procedure.

b. Prepare necessary equipment.

c. Check if dietary or medication restrictions were followed.

d. Perform hand hygiene and don gloves.

e. Obtain uncontaminated stool specimen.

f. Use tip of applicator to obtain a small portion of feces.

g. Perform Hemoccult® slide test:

(1) Open flap of slide and apply thin smear of stool in first box.

(2) Obtain second feces specimen from different portion of stool and apply to second box.

(3) Close slide cover and turn over, opening flap.

(4) Apply 2 drops of Hemoccult® developing solution on each box of guaiac paper.

(5) Read results of test after 30–60 seconds, note color changes.

(6) Dispose of supplies, remove gloves, and perform hand hygiene.

(7) Document results.

4. Teaching:

a. Regarding effect of diet and medications on test result.

b. Importance of following instructions of test, if sending specimens from home.

c. Risk factors for colon cancer, warning signs, and screening tests.

5. Evaluation.

a. Test completed and returned as instructed.

b. Results recorded.

Summary

In summary, the nursing process is an integral component of nursing because it guides the nurse to use a systematic, holistic, problem-solving approach to partner with the patient and family. The nursing process is also a method or language used to communicate with other health care providers. It can be applied in any and all situations, and support an evolving, cyclical approach to care. The nursing process consists of five components by which a person's health status and needs are identified (assessment and diagnosis), plans are developed (planning), care is delivered (implementation), and outcomes are evaluated (evaluation). Regardless of the field of nursing in which one may practice, the common thread that unites nurses is the nursing process – The essential core of practice for the registered nurse to deliver holistic, patient-focused care (ANA, 2011).

References

Alfaro-LeFevre, R. (2005). *Applying nursing process a tool for critical thinking* (6th ed.). Philadelphia: Lippincott, Williams & Wilkins.

American Nurses Association (ANA). (1980). *Nursing: A social policy statement*. Washington, DC: Author.

American Nurses Association (ANA). (2011). *The nursing process: A common thread amongst all nurses*. Retrieved from http://ana.nursingworld.org/EspeciallyForYou/Student Nurses/Thenursingprocess.aspx

Benner, P., Sutphen, M., Leonard, V., & Day, L. (2010). *Educating nurses: A call for radical transformation*. Stanford, CA: Jossey-Bass.

Bulechek, G.M., Butcher, H.K., & Dochterman, J.M. (Eds.). (2008). *Nursing interventions classification* (5th ed.). St. Louis, MO: Mosby.

Centers for Disease Control and Prevention (CDC). (1995). Screening for tuberculosis and tuberculosis infection in high-risk populations: Recommendations of the Advisory Committee for the elimination of tuberculosis. *Morbidity and Mortality Weekly Report, 44*(No. RR-11), 19-34.

Centers for Disease Control and Prevention (CDC). (2003). *Tuberculosis education and training resource guide*. Retrieved from http://www.cdcnpin.org/Guides/tbguide.pdf

Centers for Disease Control and Prevention (CDC). (2005). *Mantoux tuberculosis skin test facilitator guide*. Retrieved from http://www.cdc.gov/nchstp/tb/pubs/Mantoux/part2.htm

deWit, S. (2008). *Fundamental concepts and skills for nursing*. Philadelphia: W.B. Saunders.

Donahue, M.P., & Brighton, V. (1998). Nursing outcome classification: Development and implementation. *Journal of Nursing Care Quality, 12*(5).

Greenberg, M., Espensen, M., Becker, C., & Cartwright, J. (2003). Telehealth nursing practice SIG adopts teleterms. *ViewPoint, 25*(1), 8-10.

Healthcare Information and Management Systems (HIMSS). (2012). *Nursing informatics*. Retrieved from http://www.himss.org/ASP/topics_nursingInformatics.asp

Heaslip, P. (2008). *Critical thinking: To think like a nurse*. Retrieved from http://www.criticalthinking.org/pages/critical-thinking-and-nursing/834

Joint Commission, The. (2011). *Facts about pain management*. Retrieved from http://www.jointcommission.org/pain_management/

Maiocco, G. (2010). *Nursing process*. Retrived from http://www.wright.edu/nursing/shareableobjects/bedside_assessment/Bedside_Nursing_Process_notes.pdf

McCaffery, M. (1968). *Nursing practice theories related to cognition, bodily pain, and man-environment interactions*. Los Angeles: University of California LA Student Store.

National Heart, Lung, and Blood Institute (NHLBI). (2001). *Controlling your asthma* (NIH Publication No. 01-2339). Bethesda, MD: U.S. Government Printing Office.

National Heart, Lung, and Blood Institute (NHLBI). (2004). *Blood pressure tables for children and adolescents*. Retrieved from http://www.nhlbi.nih.gov/guidelines/hypertension/child_tbl.htm

National Heart, Lung, and Blood Institute (NHLBI). (2005). *The fourth report on the diagnosis, evaluation, and treatment of high blood pressure in children and adolescents* (NIH Publication No. 05-5267). Bethesda: U.S. Government Printing Office.

National Institute of Standards and Technology (NIST). (2011). *Standards for visual acuity*. Retrieved from http://www.nist.gov/el/isd/ks/upload/Visual_Acuity_Standards_1.pdf

National Institutes of Health (NIH). (2011). *Clinical guidelines on the identification, evaluation, and treatment of overweight and obesity in adults: The evidence report*. Retrieved from http://www.nhlbi.nih.gov/guidelines/obesity/ob_gdlns.pdf

Nettina, S.M. (Ed.) (2006). *Lippincott manual of nursing practice* (8th ed.). New York: Lippincott, Williams & Wilkins.

Neuspiel, D.R. (2011). *Peak flow rate measurement*. Retrieved from http://emedicine.medscape.com/article/1413347-overview

Norris, S.P., & Ennis, R.H. (1989). *Evaluating critical thinking*. Pacific Grove, CA: Midwest Publications, Critical Thinking Press.

North American Nursing Diagnosis Association (NANDA). (2009). *Nursing diagnoses: Definitions and classification 2009-2011*. Philadelphia: Author.

Perry, A.G., & Potter, P.A. (2010). *Clinical nursing skills and techniques* (7th ed.). St. Louis, MO: Mosby.

Smith, S., Duell, D., & Martin, B. (2008). *Clinical nursing skills: Basic to advanced skills* (6th ed.). Upper Saddle River, NJ: Prentice Hall Health.

Staib, S. (2003). Teaching and measuring critical thinking. *Journal of Nursing Education, 42*(11), 498-507.

U.S. Department of Health and Human Services (DHHS). (2004). *Vision screening for children*. Retrieved from http://www.uspreventiveservicestaskforce.org/uspstf11/vischildren/vischildrs.htm

U.S. Food and Drug Administration (FDA). (2012). *Medical devices*. Retrieved from http://www.fda.gov/MedicalDevices/default.htm

U.S. Preventive Services Task Force. (2007). Screening for high blood pressure: U.S. Preventive Services Task Force reaffirmation recommendation statement. *Annals of Internal Medicine, 147*(11), 783-786.

U.S. Preventive Services Task Force. (2009). *Screening for visual impairment in older adults: Systematic review to update the 1996 U.S. Preventive Services Task Force recommendations*. Retrieved from http://www.uspreventiveservicestaskforce.org/uspstf09/visualscr/viseldes.pdf

U.S. Preventive Services Task Force. (2010). *Screening for obesity in children and adolescents*. Retrieved from http://www.uspreventiveservicestaskforce.org/uspstf/uspschobes.htm

U.S. Public Health Service. (1997). *Put prevention into practice: Clinicians's handbook of preventive services* (2nd ed.). Germantown, PA: International Medical Publishers.

Weber, J., & Kelley, J. (2011). *Health assessment in nursing*. Philadelphia: Lippincott, Williams & Wilkins.

Additional Readings

Aiken, T.D. (2004). *Legal, ethical, and political issues in nursing*. Philadelphia: F.A. Davis Company.

American Nurses Association (ANA). (2004). *Nursing scope and standards of performance and standards of clinical practice*. Washington, DC: American Nurses Publishing.

Centers for Disease Control and Prevention (CDC). (2011). *About BMI for children and teens*. Retrieved from http://www.cdc.gov/healthyweight/assessing/bmi/childrens_bmi/about_childrens_bmi.html

Dochterman, J., & Bulechek, G. (Eds.). (2004). *Nursing interventions classification* (4th ed.). St. Louis, MO: Mosby.

Hewitt-Taylor, J. (2003). Developing and using clinical guidelines. *Nursing Standard, 18*(5), 41-44.

Infusion Nurses Society. (2006). *Policies and procedures for infusion nursing* (3rd ed). Norwood, MA: Author.

LaGuardia Center for Teaching and Learning. (2011). *Implementing technology in the nursing curriculum*. Retrieved from http://faculty.lagcc.cuny.edu/ctl/journal/pdf/InTransit_v1n1_TechnologyInNursingCurriculum.pdf

National Heart, Lung, and Blood Institute (NHLBI). (1998). *Obesity* (NIH Publication No. 98-4083). Bethesda, MD: U.S. Government Printing Office.

National Heart, Lung, and Blood Institute (NHLBI). (2003). *The seventh report of the Joint National Committee on Prevention, Detection, Evaluation, and Treatment of High Blood Pressure*. Retrieved from http://www.nhlbi.nih.gov/guidelines/hypertension/

National Heart, Lung, and Blood Institute (NHLBI). (2007). *Guidelines for the diagnosis and treatment of asthma*. Retrieved from http://www.nhlbi.nih.gov/guidelines/asthma/

Pasero, C., & McCaffery, M. (2011). *Pain assessment and pharmacologic management*. New York: Mosby.

Wagner, G. (2008). *Marriott's practical electrocardiography* (11th ed.). Philadelphia: Lippincott, Williams & Wilkins.

Waltz, C., & Jenkins, L. (2001). *Measurement of nursing outcomes*. New York: Springer.

Chapter 15

Transcultural Nursing Care

Patricia D. Chambers, BHScN, RN
Candia Baker Laughlin, MS, RN-BC

OBJECTIVES – *Study of the information in this chapter will enable the learner to:*

1. Describe the concept of culturally competent care.
2. Discuss cultural factors that are involved in the nurse/patient encounters.
3. Explain the concepts of cultural safety, cultural competency, cultural knowledge, and skill.
4. Identify health care disparities that occur within the context of culture.
5. Identify guidelines and resources to use for further exploration of this topic.

KEY POINTS – *The major points in this chapter include:*

1. The U.S. population is increasingly more culturally diverse.
2. Racial and ethnic minorities in the U.S. receive a lower quality of health care.
3. Culturally competent nursing care means that one takes into consideration the patient's cultural background, beliefs, values, and traditions.
4. Culturally competent care involves sensitivity to many attributes of patients and groups.
5. Disease incidence and management vary among different cultures.

Human beings come together in groups and sub-groups as they modify and organize their social and physical environments in ways that improve their quality of life. The resulting cultural patterns of behavior, beliefs, values, knowledge, morals, law, customs, and habits guide their worldview and decision-making. These patterns may be explicit or implicit, are primarily learned and transmitted within the family, are shared by most members of the culture, and change over time in response to various global phenomena. *Culture* refers to the processes that happen between individuals and groups within organizations and society, and that confer meaning and significance. Culture affects a person's way of perceiving the world, and serves as a guide for beliefs and practices related to health and illness (Giger & Davidhizar, 2008; Varcoe & Rodney, 2009).

Providing culturally competent health care is a professional and social mandate in modern health care. It is a component of quality practice environments that leads to improved health outcomes for clients, health care professionals, and systems. Underlying values for cultural competence include respect, inclusivity, equity, commitment, and valuing differences (Canadian Nurses Association [CNA], 2010). In today's increasingly multicultural environment, it is essential that health care providers consider the potential impact of the culture of patients and their families, the health care system, and health care providers themselves. Culture influences beliefs about how to prevent and treat illness and what constitutes good care (Leininger & MacFarland, 2002). In the health care setting, it is vitally important that providers develop cultural expertise that will enhance relationships, processes, and outcomes for consumers and providers. Cultural competence is the application of knowledge, skills, attitudes, or personal attributes required by health care professionals to maximize respectful relationships with diverse populations of clients and co-workers.

This chapter describes the importance of cultural competency in providing ambulatory care nursing services. With the increasingly diverse population in the United States, the nurse must have a working understanding of cultural factors that can be involved in the nurse/patient encounter. Current disparities in health for minority groups, potential causes for those differences, and suggestions for improvement are addressed. In addition, this chapter describes guidelines and resources for further exploration of pertinent information.

I.   **Increasing Diversity of the Population**
A.   Cultural diversity is growing because minority populations have been increasing in the U.S. in recent years.
1.   As of August 2008, individuals who were minorities made up roughly one third of the U.S. population and are expected to be the majority by 2042 (U.S. Census Bureau, 2010a) (see Table 15-1).
a.   Members of the most prevalent racial group of the U.S. population are Caucasian (having origins in the original people of Europe, the Middle East, or North Africa).
b.   Members of the second most prevalent racial group in the U.S. are those who are Black or African American.
c.   People who identify their origin as Hispanic, Latino, or Spanish may be any race. The 2010 U.S. Census found almost 36 million persons to be those who currently identify themselves ethnically as Hispanic, but racially identified themselves as either White or Black. The Hispanic/Latino population is projected to steadily increase as a percentage of the U.S. population through 2050, rising from 12.6% in 2000 (about one in seven persons) to 30.2% in 2050 (one in every three persons) (U.S. Census Bureau, 2011).

Table 15-1.
2010 U.S. Census by Race

	Estimated Census	Percentage
Total	309,349,689	
White alone	229,397,472	74.15%
Black or African American alone	38,874,625	12.57%
American Indian and Alaska Native alone	2,553,566	0.83%
Asian alone	14,728,302	4.76%
Native Hawaiian and Other Pacific Islander alone	507,916	0.16%
Some other race alone	14,889,440	4.81%
Two or more races	8,398,368	2.71%

Source: U.S. Census Bureau, 2010b. Used with permission.

2.   The overall patient population is projected to increase by 41.5% between 2010 and 2050, with Asians and "All Other Races" (American Indian and Alaska Native alone, Native Hawaiian and other Pacific Islander alone, and persons of two or more races) both more than doubling in that interval (see Table 15-2).
B.   Other faces of diversity that need to be considered for culturally competent care include (Campinha-Bacote, 2011):
1.   Gender.
2.   Religious affiliation.
3.   Sexual orientation.
4.   Language.
5.   Physical size.
6.   Age.
7.   Mental and physical disability.
C.   While the population has become increasingly diverse, the nursing population has remained fairly homogenous.

Table 15-2.
Projected U.S. Population by Race: 2000–2050

Population	2000	2010	Percent Change	2050	Percent Change
Total	282,125 (100%)	310,233 (100%)	9.7%	439,010 (100%)	41.5%
White alone	228,584 (81.0%)	246,630 (79.5%)	7.9%	324,800 (74.0%)	31.7%
Black alone	35,818 (12.7%)	39,909 (12.9%)	11.4%	56, 944 (13%)	42.7%
Asian alone	10,684 (3.8%)	14, 415 (4.6%)	34.9%	34, 399 (7.8%)	138.6%
All other races*	7,075 (2.5%)	9,279 (3.0%)	31.2%	22,867 (5.2%)	146.4%

Notes: In thousands, except as indicated. As of July 1, 2008. Resident population. Numbers may not add due to rounding.
* Includes American Indian and Alaska Native alone, Native Hawaiian and other Pacific Islander alone, and persons of two or more races.
Source: Adapted from U.S. Census Bureau, 2004, 2008.

1. In the 2004 National Sample Survey of Registered Nurses, 10.6% of all registered nurses (RNs) were minorities, while the total U.S. population of ethnic minorities rose to 32% (Health Resources & Services Administration, 2006).
2. The diversity gap between the RN population and the U.S. population has been responsive to efforts to change it (Noone, 2008).
3. Even if the nursing population is racially/ethnically similar to the patient population in a locality, there may be differences in language, place of birth, and ancestry that still represent cultural differences (McGinnis, Brush, & Moore, 2010).
4. Transcultural nursing requires that nurses are sensitive, knowledgeable, and competent to provide care across cultures, which may be independent of the RN's own racial or ethnic background.

II. **Cultural Disparities in Health and Health Care**

A. Perception of illness and disease and their causes vary by culture, influencing how people seek health care and how they behave toward care providers, among other things.

B. According to the Institute of Medicine (IOM) in *Unequal Treatment: Confronting Racial and Ethnic Disparities in Health Care*, racial and ethnic minorities experience a lower quality of health services and are less likely to receive even routine medical procedures than Caucasian Americans, even when studies control for insurance status, income, age, co-morbid conditions, and symptom expression (Smedley, Stith, & Nelson, 2003). In 1966, Dr. Martin Luther King, Jr. stated, "Of all the forms of inequality, injustice in health care is the most shocking and inhumane."

1. Sources of disparities include (Smedley et al., 2003):
   a. Historic inequities.
   b. Health systems' processes.

c.   Time pressures.

d.   Cost containment.

e.   Language and literacy barriers.

f.   Geography and distribution of resources.

2.   When compared with Caucasians, African Americans are less likely to receive:

a.   Appropriate cardiac medications.

b.   Cardiac bypass surgery.

c.   Peritoneal dialysis.

d.   Kidney transplantation.

e.   Quality basic clinical services including intensive care (Smedley et al., 2003).

C.   Racial differences have been found with:

1.   Cancer diagnostic tests, treatments and analgesics, and disparities in cancer care are associated with higher death rates among minorities.

2.   HIV treatment and survival rates.

3.   Diabetes care.

4.   End-stage renal disease and kidney transplants.

5.   Pediatric care.

6.   Maternal and child health.

7.   Mental health.

8.   Rehabilitation and nursing home services.

9.   Surgical procedures (Smedley et al., 2003).

D.   Minorities are more likely to undergo procedures that are less desirable, such as bilateral orchiectomy and amputation.

E.   IOM's review of research studies found the reasons that minority patients have different care may include (Smedley et al., 2003):

a.   Patient characteristics.

(1) Minority patients more likely to refuse recommended services, delay seeking care, and not follow prescribed treatment regimens because of differences between the cultural backgrounds of the patient and provider, mistrust, misunderstanding of instructions, problems with previous interactions with the health care system, or lack of knowledge of how to access the health care system.

(2) Patients presenting their symptoms/disease in different ways.

b.   Health care system characteristics.

(1) Lack of appropriate interpreter services, creating language barriers that may prevent patients from using a facility or negatively affect care.

(2) Time pressures of the provider, hindering complete assessment that takes into account appropriate language and cultural aspects of the patient's situation.

(3) Services may be geographically remote or not be available to minorities.

(4) Financial barriers.

c.   Health care provider characteristics.

(1) Bias or prejudice against minorities.

(2) Clinical uncertainty when interacting with minority patients.

(3) Beliefs or stereotypes about the behavior or health of minorities.

(4) Misinterpretation of behaviors or responses of patients to the provider.

F.   Recommendations from the IOM report (IOM, 2002).

1.   Broader awareness of the scope, causes, and effective strategies to reduce health disparities.

2.   Systems that ensure financial incentives do not restrict minority patients' access to care.

3.   Provision of interpretive services.

4.   Financial incentives that reward appropriate screening, preventive services, and evidence-based care.

5.   Increased numbers of minority health care professionals.

6.   Culturally appropriate education of patients to improve access to care and participation in decision-making.

7. Continuing education for health care providers that addresses current research on disparities in health, the role of unintentional bias and stereotyping, and clinical research related to differences in health responses related to ethnic and cultural factors.
8. Resources — The IOM report. The 780-page published report is available either as hard copy or in electronic format (Smedley et al., 2003).

G. Insurers, regulatory and purchasing groups.
1. Since the IOM report, many insurance groups have made efforts to improve culturally disparate care (Betancourt, Green, Carrillo, & Park, 2005).
   a. Kaiser Permanente has provided educational monographs in cultural competence and "Centers of Excellence in Cultural Competence," targeting specific populations.
   b. Aetna has collected race and ethnicity data on its members, developed culturally competent disease management programs, and mandated cultural competence training for its internal medical directors, nurses, and case managers.
   c. Blue Cross Blue Shield in some states has initiated programs that include internal diversity training and cultural competence education for providers.
2. Health care purchasing coalitions have been informing their members about cultural competence and racial/ethnic disparities in health care.

H. Agency for Healthcare Research and Quality (AHRQ, 2011).
1. Since 2003, AHRQ has studied and reported annually on the disparities in health care access and quality, and the progress toward improvement.
   a. Priority populations include:
      (1) Racial and ethnic minority groups.
      (2) Low-income groups.
      (3) Women.
      (4) Children (under age 18).
      (5) Older adults (age 65 and over).
      (6) Residents of rural areas.
      (7) Individuals with special health care needs, including individuals with disabilities and individuals who need chronic care or end-of-life care.
   b. Eight priority areas are monitored (AHRQ, 2011):
      (1) Patient and family engagement.
      (2) Population health.
      (3) Safety.
      (4) Care coordination.
      (5) Palliative care.
      (6) Overuse of services.
      (7) Access to care.
      (8) Health system infrastructure.
   c. Of the core measures, fewer than 20% faced by African Americans, American Indians/Alaska Natives, Hispanics, and poor individuals have improved, and about 30% of the gaps have narrowed for Asian Whites (AHRQ, 2011).
2. Details of the findings, including information about risk factors, screening, treatment, management, and mortality for high-priority diseases (such as breast cancer, diabetes mellitus, end-stage renal disease, heart disease, maternal and child health) of the priority population groups are included in the second report of the AHRQ (2011).

III. Cultural Competency

A. Cultural competence is "an ongoing process in which the health care professional continually strives to work effectively within the cultural context of the patient (individual, family, and community)" (Campinha-Bacote, 2011, p. 3).
B. Culturally competent nursing care requires the nurse to take the patient's cultural background, beliefs, values, and traditions into consideration when planning and delivering nursing care.

C. Cultural competence should not only be employed when caring for immigrants, ethnic minority groups, and marginalized populations (homeless, the working poor), but also in encounters with all patients.

D. Developing cultural competence requires the integration of cultural desire, cultural awareness, cultural knowledge, cultural skill, and cultural encounters (Campinha-Bacote, 2011).
   1. Cultural desire: Internal motivation of the nurse to "want to" become culturally competent.
   2. Cultural awareness: Conscious learning process through which the individual becomes appreciative of and sensitive to the cultures of other people.
   3. Cultural knowledge: Process of understanding the key aspects of a group's culture, especially related to interpretations of health and illness, and health care practices.
   4. Cultural skill: Ability to collect relevant data regarding health histories and performing culturally specific assessments.
   5. Cultural encounter: Process that encourages individuals to engage directly in cross-cultural interactions with people from culturally diverse backgrounds.

E. Purnell and Paulanka (2003) described cultural competence as encompassing the following:
   1. Developing and appreciating an awareness of one's own existence, sensations, thoughts, and surroundings without letting it have an untoward influence on others.
   2. Demonstrating knowledge and understanding of the cultural preferences of others (e.g., patients, family, and colleagues).
   3. Accepting and respecting the cultural differences of others.
   4. Avoiding ethnocentric responses.
   5. Being open to cultural encounters.
   6. Adapting professional practice so it is congruent with the culture of others.

F. To meet the needs of culturally diverse groups, health care providers must engage in the process of becoming culturally competent.

1. Using guides to cultural assessment, such as *Transcultural Communication in Nursing* (Munoz & Luckman, 2005), can facilitate this nursing process.
2. Exploring one's own cultural background, values, and beliefs, as well as examining one's own cultural biases toward people who differ from oneself, are important to becoming culturally competent.

G. Cultural competence is also necessary for communication, collaboration, and effective working relationships among members of the health care team who have cultural differences.

IV. Cultural Safety

A. Cultural safety is predicated on understanding power differentials inherent in health service delivery and addressing these imbalances through education.

B. Over the last decade, this concept has gained increasing international influence across professional and political organizations and associations concerned with addressing health inequities and achieving social justice.

C. The idea of cultural safety holds value for nursing practice, research, and education when used to underscore critical self-reflection, assessment of structures, discourses, power relations, and assumptions (Browne et al., 2009; CNA, 2010).

D. Key concepts of cultural safety:
   1. Unsafe cultural practices are actions undertaken by a person from the more powerful cultural group to diminish, demean, or disempower a person of the less powerful cultural group.
   2. People who receive the care decide what is safe or unsafe.
   3. Providing culturally safe care requires nurses to be respectful of nationality, culture, age, sex, and political and religious beliefs.
   4. By establishing trust with the patient, the nurse empowers him or her, reinforcing that each person's knowledge and reality is valid and valuable.

5. Each nurse is the bearer of his or her own culture and attitudes, and nurses consciously or unconsciously exercise power over patients.
6. Health care professionals need to examine their own realities and attitudes that are brought to each new person they encounter in practice, and to be open-minded and flexible in their attitudes toward people who are different from themselves.
7. Typically practiced by RNs who are well-educated, self-aware health care professionals are deemed culturally safe as defined by the people they serve.
E. The concept of cultural safety provides a critical lens for examining health policy. It is incumbent on those involved in health care to critically consider if his or her attitudes and actions may place others at risk for cultural harm (Smye, Rameka, & Willis, 2006).

V. Strategies to Improve Cultural Knowledge, Skill, and Encounters
A. Improving cultural knowledge (Campinha-Bacote, 2003, 2011).
1. Learning basic general information about the predominant cultural groups in the geographic area of the ambulatory care setting.
2. Becoming aware that many belief systems exist.
3. Exploring Web sites and cultural pocket guides as resources for general information.
4. Finding research studies available describing cultural differences in respected nursing, medical, and health care journals.
5. Reading or viewing documentaries about cultural groups.
6. Reviewing the ambulatory care facility's cultural competence framework and training available to staff.
B. Improving cultural skill.
1. Exploring and understanding one's own worldviews and those of the patient.

2. Adapting to different cultural beliefs and practices with flexibility and a respect for others' viewpoints.
3. Learning and understanding culturally influenced health behaviors.
4. Being alert for unexpected responses of patients, especially as they relate to cultural issues.
5. Being aware that individuals have their own belief system about causes of illness, what the illness does to them, and how it may be cured. For example:
   a. A Hispanic mother may believe that her child has *Mal d'ojo* or has been cursed with the "evil eye."
   b. An Asian patient may believe she is having a difficult birth because of an imbalance between hot and cold in her body, and believing that pregnancy is a "cold" condition, she may request drinks of hot water for balance (Pediatric Pulmonary Centers, 2005).
6. Developing cultural assessment skills, such as by asking patients what they call their problem, what they think caused it, if they believe it is serious, how long they think it will last, what they fear about their illness, what treatment they think they need, what they expect to receive, and whether they have received what they think, will help them feel better (Campinha-Bacote, 2011).
C. Strategies to improve cultural encounters.
1. Creating opportunities to interact with predominant cultural groups.
2. Visiting cultural events, such as religious ceremonies, significant life passage rituals, social events, and cultural practice demonstrations.
3. Visiting markets and restaurants in ethnic neighborhoods.
4. Exploring ethnic neighborhoods.
5. Listening to different types of ethnic music.
6. Visiting or volunteering at health fairs in local ethnic neighborhoods.

7. Learning more about prominent cultural beliefs and practices and incorporating this knowledge into planning nursing care.

VI. Attributes to Consider When Planning for Culturally Competent Care

A. Communication skills/culturally and linguistically appropriate care.
1. National Standards on Culturally and Linguistically Appropriate Services (CLAS).
   a. Developed in 2000 by the U.S. Department of Health and Human Services (DHHS) Office of Minority Health (OMH).
   b. Intended to address and correct inequities that exist in the provision of health care to culturally and ethnically diverse groups, and should be considered when planning culturally competent care.
   c. Available at the OMH Web site (www.omhrc.gov/CLAS).
2. Communication styles and patterns differ vastly among people from different cultures.
3. Approximately 52 million people in the U.S. (19% of the population) speak languages other than English, including:
   a. Spanish (62%).
   b. Chinese (4%).
   c. French (3%).
   d. Tagalog (3%).
   e. Vietnamese (2%).
   f. German (2%).
   g. Korean (2%) (Andrews & Boyle, 2008).
4. Appropriate linguistic health care is sensitive to different standards for loudness, speed of delivery, spatial distance, silence, eye contact, gestures, attentiveness, and response rate during communication. Some examples:
   a. Arab people may avert their eyes when listening or talking to a superior.
   b. Someone from South America may consider it impolite if you speak with your hands in your pockets.

c. A Chinese or Japanese patient may present with a facial expression that could be recognized as conveying happiness; in reality it may actually express anger or mask sadness; expressions which would be culturally unacceptable to overtly display (Andrews & Boyle, 2008).
5. Even if an interpreter is used, some words used in one language may have nuances that do not easily translate into another. Some languages have no equivalent for the English word "pain."
   a. A patient might describe pain as "like electric shocks," a family member/interpreter could translate this as "twinges," the nurse could interpret this to indicate mild pain when, in fact, on a numeric scale, the pain would rate as high.
   b. A Native American patient presented with a linear numerical scale may choose a "favorite" or "sacred" number to represent their pain instead of a number that correctly indicates their level of pain (Narayan, 2010).
6. To improve interactions with patients from different cultures, one should assess each patient's level of understanding rather than assume that a patient understands what is being said (Munoz & Luckman, 2005).
   a. Use a certified medical interpreter, whenever possible.
   b. Use common words versus medical jargon or slang.
   c. Repeat basic ideas without shouting.
   d. Use active listening skills, such as paraphrasing important ideas to check for mutual understanding.
7. To develop and apply culturally competent communication, encourage health professionals and agencies to:
   a. Modify communication patterns to adapt to the style of the individual or group addressed.
   b. Identify and avoid using gestures that individuals or groups might find threatening or insulting.

c. Use clarifying and validating techniques.

d. Utilize team members from different cultures as resources in learning about and using culturally sensitive behaviors.

e. Employ trained interpreters, as appropriate. Avoid use of family, friends, or hospital workers who are not trained as professional interpreters.

f. Provide translated patient instructions and handouts in different languages.

B. Cultural dimensions of space, social organization, and time.

1. Space, in terms of cultural behavior, is defined as the physical distance in personal interactions and the intimacy techniques utilized when relating to others, both verbally and nonverbally.

a. Assessing the relevance of space includes acknowledging that space has distinct zones for different interactions: Intimate, personal, and public.

b. Culturally appropriate communication acknowledges that distance has different meanings in different cultures.

c. Health care providers need to honor these space differences and preferences.

2. Social organization refers to the values that individuals place on important support groups in their life, such as family, friends, or religious leaders.

a. Health care providers need to value, respect, and integrate individual differences for preferred social organization in professional interactions with individuals and groups.

b. One needs to understand where men and women and family rank fit in the clients' society.

(1) In some cultures, the primary decision-maker of the rest of the family is the oldest male.

(2) Among many traditional Chinese, it is the eldest son.

(3) In some Muslim cultures, it may be the husband or the father.

c. Health care professionals should ask who the decision-maker is and make sure he or she is included in the patient's care.

3. In the time dimension, cultures may be oriented to past, present, or future.

a. Past-oriented cultures have a tendency to value tradition and stability. An example would be an Asian culture where remedies of the ancestors are honored and valued. This may cause conflict with modern western medical care.

b. Present-orientated people tend to focus on activities that meet current demands, and they may not see the importance of immunizations or treatments of asymptomatic diseases, such as hypertension.

c. Future-orientated people tend to conduct activities in light of their contributions to achieving goals, such as taking steps to promote health or use preventive care services.

C. Environmental cultural variations.

1. Environmental control refers to an individual's perceived ability to control external occurrences; the degree to which they control events has an internal or external locus of control.

a. Someone with an internal locus of control believes his or her actions can evoke events.

b. A person with an external locus of control believes that events occur by chance, karma, luck, or fate, and that he or she has little control over what happens.

c. Assessing the patient's perceptions about his or her ability to control external events allows the health care provider to understand beliefs about the cause of a health condition and the patient's perceived ability to influence outcomes by his or her own actions.

d. If the patient believes that a condition is caused by fate or as a result of his or her own bad behavior, the prescribed treatment interventions may not be carried out.

e. Framing interventions and programs in a way that facilitates comfort levels of patients is more likely to lead to successful outcomes.

D. Biological variation as a dimension in cultural competence (bio-cultural ecology) refers to the genetic differences among individuals.

1. Genetic biological variations among specific ethnic, gender, or cultural groups is increasingly being associated with risk factors for specific diseases or responses to therapeutic pharmaceuticals or regimens.

2. Ethnopharmacology is an emerging field of research that describes the following:

    a. How physiological and genetic differences between racial and ethnic groups impact the effectiveness of pharmacological products.

    b. How a person's cultural beliefs about his or her health have an impact on the medications used and how to use them.

    c. How racial bias and cultural attitudes affect the development and prescribing of certain drugs (Wessling, 2007).

3. Clinical trials on medications, until recently, have been conducted on primarily the white population, mostly men, and the results are generalized to women and minorities.

4. Fillers of medications vary, such that brand name drugs and generics may be metabolized differently based on genetic makeup of the patient.

5. Genetic variations in certain enzymes may lead to different responses to medications in some cultural subgroups (Munoz & Hilgenberg, 2005).

    a. Many Chinese patients cannot convert codeine into morphine-like metabolites that give the drug its analgesic properties, making them less likely to receive adequate pain relief with opioid medication and more likely to experience gastrointestinal side effects (Narayan, 2010).

    b. Some antihypertensive drugs, such as captopril and losartan, may be less effective in African Americans than in Caucasians, while others, such as thiazide diuretics, are more effective in African Americans than in Caucasians (Munoz & Hilgenberg, 2005).

E. Ambulatory care nurses should take into account the potential variations in effects of treatments, the potential effect of patients discontinuing their therapies based on side effects, and the effects of beliefs and previous experience in planning and delivering care for all patients, including those from diverse cultural backgrounds.

VI. Cultural Differences in Disease Incidence and Management

A. For health care providers to positively impact health care outcomes and guide treatment decisions, health education, screening, and treatment programs, they need to have accurate epidemiological data, knowledge of bio-cultural ecology, and ethnic pharmacology (Campinha-Bacote, 2003).

B. Culture influences how people seek health care, how they behave toward health care providers, and how they respond to care.

C. Obesity.

1. Obesity is prevalent among Native Hawaiians.

2. The relationship between Hawaiian-style food and perceptions of health and well-being can create a challenging struggle.

3. Native Hawaiians can be encouraged to expend consumed calories in physical activity as their ancestors did (Lassetter, 2011).

4. Nurses may find it effective to discuss nutrition from a family framework.

D. The Arab Muslim population in the United States is at increased risk for several diseases and faces many barriers to accessing American health care.

1. Arab Muslims' barriers to effective health care include modesty, gender preference in health care providers, illness causation misconceptions, and lack of culturally competent service (Yosef, 2008).
2. Health care providers are encouraged to integrate Islamic teachings into their interventions to provide appropriate care and to motivate healthy behaviors.

E. Hepatitis.
1. Effectiveness of interferon treatment for chronic hepatitis C varies in racial and ethnic groups, with African Americans having the lowest effectiveness rates (Gaglio et al., 2004):
    a. White, non-Hispanic – 24%.
    b. Hispanic – 12%.
    c. African American – 4%.
2. Individuals with chronic hepatitis B are at high risk of developing liver cancer.
    a. Immigrants from some countries, such as China, where hepatitis B is endemic, have higher rates of hepatitis B.
    b. Screening programs should be in place to screen for liver cancer in these groups because studies indicate that early detection and treatment of cancer improves the survival rate.
    c. Screening programs in rural areas, such as the Alaska Native populations, have proven to be cost effective.

F. Asthma and other lung diseases.
1. African Americans have the highest asthma prevalence of any racial/ethnic group in the U.S. The asthma prevalence rate in African American children was found to be almost 59% higher than that in Caucasian children, while the rates in adults are much more similar (Centers for Disease Control and Prevention [CDC], 2006).
2. Data from some studies indicate that American Indians/Native Americans may have equal if not greater rates of asthma than other racial groups.

G. Pain management.
1. Culture influences how one experiences pain because pain has psychological, social, spiritual, and physical dimensions.
2. Green and colleagues (2003) of the American Pain Society performed a metaanalysis that revealed disparities in pain management for varieties of conditions, types of pain, and treatment settings.
    a. Minority patients are more likely to be underinsured or otherwise have limited financial resources for accessing medications.
    b. Some clinicians associate minority populations with drug-seeking and may inadequately treat pain out of fear of illicit use of the drugs.
3. Managing pain in culturally diverse populations can be a challenge because there are differences in beliefs about how to prevent and treat illness and what constitutes quality care, as well as how the individual experiences and responds to pain (Narayan, 2010).
    a. Stoicism versus expressivity.
        (1) Over their lifetimes, people learn cultural norms about masking their pain, relieving pain by moaning or screaming, or getting attention and support when they are in pain.
        (2) Some patients believe they will be perceived as "good" by not complaining to their caregivers about their pain, so they underreport it.
    b. Frameworks for describing pain.
        (1) While numeric rating scores for pain are widely used (rate pain from 0–10), some cultural groups would more readily describe the full nature of their pain as a constellation of feelings, symptoms, and consequences of the pain. Some cultures also respond to pain in stoic or very expressive ways, and these, too, do not fit readily on the standard scales.

Figure 15-1.
Resources for Cultural Competence and Knowledge about
Disease Management in Various Cultural Groups

Alzheimer's Disease: The Alzheimer's Association Web site includes information on cultural variations.

www.alz.org/diversity/overview.asp

Respiratory: The American Lung Association provides information on incidence, causes, and treatment of respiratory problems in cultural populations.

http://www.lung.org/

Cancer: The Office of Minority Health, Health Resources and Services Administration published an 84-page handbook to guide heath care providers who want to decrease cancer health disparities, available through the Intercultural Cancer Council Web site.

http://iccnetwork.org

Developing Cultural Competence: The "Cross Cultural Health Care-Case Studies" program is an online interactive self-study program consisting of a series of 5 tutorials in cultural competence. The tutorials are available at no charge.

http://ppc.mchtraining.net

Working with Minority Patients and Health Care Providers: The Minority Nurse Web Site and journal are valuable resources for minority nurses and provide insight into working with nurses from various cultural backgrounds. The journal, *Minority Nurse,* provides information that will help any nurse improve care for patients from different cultural backgrounds.

http://minoritynurse.com

Transcultural Nursing: The mission of the Transcultural Nursing Society is "to enhance the quality of culturally congruent, competent, and equitable care that results in improved health and well-being for people worldwide."

http://www.tcns.org

The journal of this society (*Journal of Transcultural Nursing: A Forum for Cultural Competence in Health Care*) publishes research that explores the influence of culture on nursing practice and the delivery of health care.

http://intl-tcn.sagepub.com

National Center for Cultural Competence: *Online Journal of Cultural Competence in Nursing and Healthcare.*

http://www.cultural-competence-project.org/ojccnh/1(1).shtml

The Provider's Guide to Quality and Culture: This Web site is designed to assist health care organizations throughout the U.S. in providing high quality, culturally competent services to multi-ethnic populations.

http://erc.msh.org/quality&culture

Center for Healthy Families and Cultural Diversity (CHFCD), Department of Family Medicine/UMDNJ, Robert Wood Johnson Medical School: CHFCD "is dedicated to leadership, advocacy, and excellence in promoting culturally-responsive, quality health care for diverse populations. CHFCD recognizes that persisting racial and ethnic health care disparities in health care are major clinical, public health, and societal problems."

www2.umdnj.edu/fmedweb/chfcd/INDEX.HTM

Cross Cultural Health Care: A training and consulting organization whose mission is to "serve as a bridge between communities and health care institutions to ensure full access to quality health care that is culturally and linguistically appropriate."

www.xculture.org

DiversityRx: This Web site provides information about significant cross cultural health care issues and topics. Links to CLAS resources, a database of organizations and resources related to cross cultural health care, and an insightful blog are some of the key features of this Web site.

www.diversityrx.org

Initiative to Eliminate Racial & Ethnic Disparities in Health: U.S. Department of Health & Human Services, Office of Minority Health.

http://raceandhealth.hhs.gov

continued on next page

Figure 15-1. (continued)
Resources for Cultural Competence and Knowledge about
Disease Management in Various Cultural Groups

National Standards on Culturally and Linguistically Appropriate Services (CLAS): www.omhrc.gov/clas *Transcultural and Multicultural Health Links:* http://web.nmsu.edu/~ebosman/trannurs/index.shtml	*Transcultural Care Associates:* www.transculturalcare.net *Cultural Competence Resources for Health Care Providers:* http://www.hrsa.gov/culturalcompetence/index.html

(2) Language barriers and differences in non-verbal communication also make it difficult to assess pain.

c. Beliefs about managing pain:

(1) Some may believe that suffering from pain is part of life, punishment for misdeeds, or beyond their ability to influence (fatalistic view), while others see it as an important sign of serious illness needing immediate and serious attention.

(2) Beliefs about pain treatments also vary, so some immediately turn to medication while others prefer herbs, yoga, meditations, touch, acupuncture, or other complementary and alternative therapies.

(3) Many are reluctant to use opioids because of cultural beliefs.

H. Other disease incidence and health practices.

1. Many diseases affect different cultural groups disproportionately.

a. The prevalence of arthritis is lower in African Americans and Hispanics than among Caucasians, but the impact is worse (Bolen et al., 2010).

b. Among men who have sex with men, African Americans and Hispanics had a higher incidence of HIV/AIDS diagnoses than Caucasians, and African Americans had a lower three-year survival rate than both Cau-

casians and Hispanics (Hall et al., 2008).

2. Health practices are also highly diverse among different cultural groups.

a. In a study of infants from 2002–2004, it was found that non-Hispanic Blacks had a lower prevalence of breast-feeding initiation than non-Hispanic Whites; Hispanics generally had lower prevalence than non-Hispanic Whites in western states and higher in eastern states (Ruowei, Darling, Maurice, Barker, & Grummer, 2005).

b. Asian American women have the lowest cancer screening rates of all ethnic populations (Kagawa-Singer, 2006).

3. Specific disease incidences and health practices continue to be the source of significant volumes of research and targeted education and other public health interventions.

4. Health care services that are respectful of and responsive to the health beliefs, practices, and cultural and linguistic needs of diverse patients can help bring about positive health outcomes for all patients.

VII. Resources for Cultural Competence and Knowledge about Disease Management In Various Cultural Groups

See Figure 15-1 for a listing of resources for cultural competence and knowledge about disease management in various cultural groups.

References

Agency for Healthcare Research and Quality (AHRQ). (2011). *Disparities in healthcare quality among racial and ethnic minority groups: Selected findings form the 2010 National Healthcare Quality and Disparity Reports.* Retrieved from http://www.ahrq.gov/qual/nhqrdr10/nhqrdrminority10.htm#moreinfo

Andrews, M.M., & Boyle, J.S. (2008). *Transcultural concepts in nursing care* (5th ed.). St. Louis: Mosby Year Book.

Betancourt, J.R., Green, A.R., Carrillo, I.E, & Park, E.R. (2005). *Cultural competence and health disparities: Key perspectives and trends.* Retrieved from http://content.health affairs.org/content/24/2/499.full

Bolen, J., Schieb, L., Hootman, J.M., Helmick, C.G., Theis, K., Murphy, L.B., & Langmaid, G. (2010). Differences in the prevalence and impact of arthritis among racial/ethnic groups in the United Sates, National Health Interview Survey, 2002, 2003, and 2006. *Preventing Chronic Disease 7*(3), A64. Retrieved from http://www.cdc.gov/pcd/issues/2010/may/10_0035.htm

Browne, A.J., Varcoe, C., Smye, V., Reimer-Kirkham, S., Lynam, M.J., & Wong, S. (2009). Cultural safety and the challenges of translating critically oriented knowledge in practice. *Nursing Philosophy, 10*(3), 167-179.

Campinha-Bacote, J. (2003). *Many faces: Addressing diversity in health care.* Retrieved from http://www.nursingworld.org/MainMenuCategories/ANAMarketplace/ANAPeriodicals/OJIN/TableofContents/Volume82003/No1Jan2003/AddressingDiversityinHealthCare.html

Campinha-Bacote, J. (2011). *Delivering patient-centered care in the midst of a cultural conflict: The role of cultural competence.* Retrieved from http://www.nursingworld.org/MainMenuCategories/ANAMarketplace/ANAPeriodicals/OJIN/TableofContents/Vol-16-2011/No2-May-2011/Delivering-Patient-Centered-Care-in-the-Midst-of-a-Cultural-Conflict.html.

Canadian Nurses Association (CNA). (2010). *Promoting cultural competence in nursing.* Retrieved from http://www2.cna-aiic.ca/CNA/documents/pdf/publications/PS114_Cultural_Competence_2010_e.pdf

Centers for Disease Control and Prevention (CDC). (2006). *The state of childhood asthma, United States, 1980–2005. Table B.* Retrieved from http://www.cdc.go v/nchs/data/ad/ad381.pdf

Gaglio, P.J., Rodriguez-Torres, M., Herring, R., Anand, G., Box, T., Rabinovitz, M., & Brown, R.S. (2004). Racial differences in response rates to consensus interferon in HCV infected patients naïve to previous therapy. *Journal of Clinical Gastroenterology, 38*(7), 599-604.

Giger, J.N., & Davidhizar, R.E. (2008). *Transcultural nursing: Assessment and intervention* (5th ed.). St Louis, MO: Mosby.

Green, C.R., Anderson, K.O., Baker, T.A., Campbell, L.C., Decker, S., Fillingam, R.B., … Vallerand, A.H. (2003). The unequal burden of pain: Confronting racial and ethnic disparities in pain. *Pain Medicine, 4*(3), 277-294.

Hall, I., Rulguang, S., Rhodes, P., Prejean, J., Qian, A., Lee, L., … Janssen, R. (2008). Estimation of HIV incidence in the United States. *JAMA, 300*(5), 520-529.

Health Resources and Services Administration. (2006). *Preliminary findings: The registered nurse population: National sample survey of registered nurses March 2004.* Washington, DC: Author.

Institute of Medicine (IOM). (2002). *Guidance for the national healthcare disparities report.* Washington, DC: The National Academies Press.

Kagawa-Singer, M. (2006). *A socio-cultural perspective on cancer control issues for Asian Americans.* Retrieved from http://www.ncbi.nlm.nih.gov/pmc/articles/PMC1618773/

King, M.L., Jr. (1966, March 25). Presentation at the Second National Convention of the Medical Committee for Human Rights. Chicago, IL.

Lassetter, J. (2011). The integral role of food in native Hawaiian migrants' perception and well-being. *Journal of Transcultural Nursing, 22*(1), 63-70.

Leininger, M., & MacFarland, M.R. (2002). *Transcultural nursing: Concepts, theories, research and practice* (3rd ed.). New York: McGraw-Hill.

McGinnis, S., Brush, B., & Moore, J. (2010). Cultural similarity, cultural competence, and nurse workforce diversity. *Western Journal of Nursing Research, 32*(7), 894-909.

Munoz, C., & Hilgenberg, C. (2005). Ethnopharmacology. *American Journal of Nursing, 105*(8), 40-49.

Munoz, C., & Luckman, J. (2005). *Transcultural communication in nursing* (2nd ed.). Clifton Park, NY: Delmar Learning.

Narayan, M. (2010). Culture's effects on pain assessment and management. *American Journal of Nursing, 10*(4), 38-47.

Noone, J. (2008). The diversity imperative: Strategies to address a diverse nursing workforce. *Nursing Forum, 43*, 133-143.

Pediatric Pulmonary Centers (PPC). (2005). *Cross cultural health care.* Retrieved from http://ppc.mchtraining.net

Purnell, L.D., & Paulanka, B.J. (2003). *Transcultural health care.* Philadelphia: FA Davis.

Ruowei, L., Darling, N., Maurice, E., Barker, L., & Grummer, L. (2005). Breastfeeding rates in the United States by characteristics of the child, mother, or family: The 2002 national immunization survey. *Pediatrics, 115*(1), e 31-37.

Smedley, B.D., Stith, A.Y., & Nelson, A.R. (Eds.). (2003). *Unequal treatment: Confronting racial and ethnic disparities in health care.* Washington DC: The National Academies Press.

Smye, V., Rameka, M., & Willis, E. (2006). Indigenous health care: Advances in nursing practice. *Contemporary Nurse: A Journal for the Australian Nursing Profession*, 22(2), 142-154.

U.S. Census Bureau. (2004). *Population projections: U.S. interim projections by age, sex, race, and Hispanic origin: 2000-2050.* Retrieved from http://www.census.gov/population/ www/projections/usinterimproj/

U.S. Census Bureau. (2008). *Population projections: Projections of the population by sex, race, and Hispanic origin for the United States: 2010-2050.* Retrieved from http://www.census.gov/population/www/projections/summarytables.html

U.S. Census Bureau. (2010a). *2008 population estimates.* Retrieved from http://www.census.gov/popest

U.S. Census Bureau. (2010b). *2010 census data.* Retrieved from http://2010.census.gov/2010census/data/

U.S. Census Bureau. (2011). *Overview of race and Hispanic origin.* Retrieved from http://www.census.gov/prod/cen2010/briefs/c2010br-02.pdf

Varcoe, C., & Rodney, P. (2009). Constrained agency: The social structure of nurses' work. In B.S. Bolaria, & H. Dickinson (Eds.), *Health, illness and health care in Canada* (4th ed., pp. 122-151). Scarborough, Ontario, Canada: Nelson Thomas Learning.

Wessling, S. (2007). *Ethnopharmacology: What nurses need to know.* Retrieved from http://www.minoritynurse.com/minority-health-research/ethnopharmacology-what-nurses-need-know

Yosef, A. (2008). Health beliefs, practice, and priorities for health care of Arab Muslims in the United States: Implications for nursing care. *Journal of Transcultural Nursing, 19(3),* 284-291.

Additional Readings

International Council of Nurses. (2004). *Minutes of the International Council of Nurses Workforce Forum, September 20-22, 2004, Wellington, New Zealand.* Geneva: Author.

Nursing Council of New Zealand. (2005). *Guidelines for cultural safety, the treaty of Waitangi and Maori health in nursing education and practice.* Retrieved from http://www.nursing council.org.nz

Ramsden, I. (2000). Cultural safety/Kawa Whakaruruhau ten years on: A personal overview. *Nursing Praxis in New Zealand, 15(1),* 4-12.

Spector, R.E. (2004). *Cultural diversity in health and illness* (6th ed.). Upper Saddle River, NJ: Pearson Education.

Chapter 16

Patient Education and Counseling

Christina Watwood, MPH/MHA, BSN, RN

1. Describe factors that influence the educational process in ambulatory care.
2. Identify teaching strategies used for patient education and counseling in ambulatory care.
3. Compare traditional patient education to self-management education.
4. List challenges faced in providing patient education within the ambulatory care setting.
5. Evaluate the nursing process as a method for tailoring patient education.
6. Discuss major health topics for education and counseling that promote healthy behaviors.

1. Ambulatory care nurses are uniquely qualified to influence care delivery in the outpatient setting, specifically regarding patient education and coordination of services.
2. Ambulatory care nurses serve as advocates and facilitators of teaching processes that promote awareness, influence attitudes, and identify needs and opportunities, as well as increase aptitude for healthy living.
3. Teaching patients is not only a legal mandate for the practice of nursing, but also an essential part of health care management.
4. Standards for patient education are found in The Joint Commission and The National Committee for Quality Assurance (NCQA) guidelines.

I. Patient Education in Ambulatory Care: Historical Foundations and Mandates

A. Historical foundations.
　1. The nurse as educator (Bastable, 2008).
　　a. Mid 1800s: Florence Nightingale educates those who deliver health care.
　　b. Early 1900s: Public health nurses in the United States teach prevention of disease and maintenance of health.
　　c. 1918: The National League of Nursing Education (now the National League for Nursing [NLN]) recognizes health education as a component of the scope of nursing practice.
　　d. 1950: The NLN's course content aims to prepare nurses upon completion of its basic program to assume the teaching role.
　　e. 1970s: The American Hospital Association (AHA) develops the *Patients' Bill of Rights*, which establishes guidelines for how patients receive medical information.
　　f. 1993: The Joint Commission, then the Joint Commission on Accreditation of Healthcare Organizations (JCAHO), establishes standards for patient education.
　　g. 2006: NLN creates the first certified nurse educator examination (CNE).
　　h. Both the American Nurses Association (ANA) and the International Council of Nurses have long identified the importance of the teaching component in nursing practice.

B. Mandates.
1. Legal mandates.
   a. All state nurse practice acts include teaching within the scope of nursing practice.
   b. The *Patient Self Determination Act of 1990* defines informed consent (see Chapter 8, "Legal Aspects of Ambulatory Care Nursing," for more details).
2. Accreditation mandates.
   a. The Joint Commission (2011) standards require evidence that patients have been taught as well as understand what they have been taught.
   b. The Joint Commission (2011) standards also define what is required for patient education in ambulatory care. The patient's needs are assessed, and as appropriate to the patient's condition and the specific setting, the patient is educated about:
      (1) The plan of care, including treatments and services.
      (2) Basic health practices.
      (3) Basic safety.
      (4) Safe and effective use of medications.
      (5) Nutrition, modified diets, oral health.
      (6) Safe and effective use of medical equipment or supplies.
      (7) Habitation or rehabilitation techniques to reach maximum independent functioning.
      (8) Fall reduction strategies.
      (9) Pain, including:
         (a) What it is.
         (b) The risk for pain.
         (c) Importance of pain management.
         (d) How to evaluate for pain and measure it.
         (e) Methods for pain management.
3. Professional mandates.
   a. The National Committee for Quality Assurance (NCQA) (2011) *Health Plan Accreditation Requirements* pro-

vides several performance measures regarding patient self-management tools, wellness, and prevention, as well as health information.
   b. *The Patient Care Partnership: Understanding Expectations, Rights and Responsibilities*, which replaces the previous AHA (2011) version (*Patients' Bill of Rights*), informs patients about what they should expect during their hospital stay.
   c. *Healthy People 2020* outlines health education topics and objectives specific to programs outside of traditional health care settings, including community-based worksites and health care facilities (U.S. Department of Health and Human Services [DHHS], 2011b).
   d. The American Academy of Ambulatory Care Nursing (AAACN) (2010a) *Conceptual Framework for Ambulatory Care Nursing* lists patient education as the first element in the clinical nursing role.
   e. AAACN (2010b) includes integration of patient and family education into the delivery of care in its *Scope and Standards of Practice for Professional Ambulatory Care Nursing*.

II. **Patient Education in Ambulatory Care: Process, Theories, and Teaching Strategies**
A. Education process.
   1. Definitions (Bastable, 2008).
      a. *Education process* – A systematic, planned course of action consisting of two major interdependent operations: Teaching and learning.
         (1) *Teaching* – A deliberate intervention to meet intended learner outcomes.
         (2) *Learning* – An action by which knowledge, skills, and attitudes are consciously or unconsciously acquired so that behavior is altered in some way that can be observed or measured.

b. *Patient education* – A process of assisting people to learn health-related behaviors (knowledge, skills, attitudes, and values) so they can incorporate them into their everyday lives.

2. Factors that influence the educational process.

a. Learner developmental stage (see *Developmental Stages*).

b. Learner level of literacy:

(1) Health literacy: Capacity to obtain, process, and understand basic information and services needed to make appropriate decisions regarding health (Institute of Medicine [IOM], 2004).

(2) Skills include word recognition, comprehension, numeracy, and knowledge of common health-related vocabulary and medical abbreviations, as well as social and cultural factors that influence individual expectations and preferences (The Joint Commission, 2007).

(3) Test of Functional Health Literacy in Adults (TOFHLA) (Nurss, Parker, Williams, & Baker, 2001) uses health care-related materials, such as appointment instructions, prescriptions labels, and informed consent documents to measure patient literacy skills. Test administration takes about 20 minutes. The form is also available in Spanish (TOFHLA-S) and takes less than 10 minutes to administer.

(4) Rapid Estimate of Adult Literacy in Medicine (REALM) uses word recognition and pronunciation, but does not assess comprehension, nor is it available in other languages (Agency for Healthcare Research and Quality [AHRQ], 2009). REALM takes 2–5 minutes to administer and works best for screening purposes when time is limited.

(5) Patients do not always see the same provider each time they seek care, which creates a more challenging situation for assessing health literacy.

(6) Three factors affect an individual's performance on health literacy tasks.

(a) The characteristics/literacy demands of the task.

(b) The reader's literacy skills.

(c) The appropriateness of the written material to the reader's level of literacy (White, 2008).

(7) *Healthy People 2020* (DHHS, 2011b) health literacy objectives include increasing the proportion of people who report that their health care providers:

(a) Always give easy-to-understand instructions about what to do to care for their illness/ health condition.

(b) Always ask them to describe how they will follow instructions.

(c) Always offer help in filling out a form.

c. Learner readiness to learn.

(1) Physical readiness: Physical ability, health status, gender, sensory or communication needs (patients with pre-existing hearing, visual, or speech impairments), environment.

(2) Emotional readiness: Acceptance of need to learn, level of anxiety, support systems, motivation.

(3) Experiential readiness: Cultural background, past coping mechanisms, short- and long-term goals.

(4) Knowledge readiness: What is already known, cognitive ability, learning style, presence or lack of learning disability.

d. Environment in which education takes place.
e. Learner cultural and language preferences.
f. Time allotted for education.
  (1) The episodic nature of outpatient visits makes providing comprehensive care challenging.
  (2) Pressure is increasing for health care providers to see more patients each day, which makes it difficult to determine and adequately address knowledge gaps during shortened medical interviews and examinations (Egbert & Nanna, 2009).
B. Learning theories: Learning theory is a framework that describes, explains, or predicts how people learn. There are several theories of learning, and each provides its own perspective. The testing of these theories has made significant contributions to understanding how people acquire knowledge and change their ways of thinking, behaving, and feeling. The major learning theories form the foundation, not only for education, but also for psychological counseling, from which many principles of behavioral change have been developed (Bastable, 2008). This has implications for nurses teaching patients, because the principles of behavioral change are utilized in counseling patients regarding healthy lifestyle choices. Learning theories are useful as a guiding approach to education, and no single theory dominates health promotion research or professional practice. This section will briefly review the most frequently used models for understanding behavior and behavior change.
  1. Health Belief Model (HBM).
    a. Origin: In the 1950s, U.S. Public Health Service social psychologists developed the HBM to help explain lack of participation in disease prevention programs (Glanz, Rimer, & Lewis, 2008).
    b. Core assumption: An individual will take a health-related action if he or she perceives susceptibility to/severity of an illness can be avoided or re-

duced by a personal ability to successfully take a recommended action.
    c. Definitions and actions for the educator to apply for model concepts (Glanz et al., 2008).
      (1) *Perceived susceptibility* – An individual's belief of risk in developing a condition. The educator must define and determine the level of risk, personalize the risk based on the individual's behavior, and match the perceived susceptibility and actual risk.
      (2) *Perceived severity* – An individual's belief concerning the seriousness of contracting an illness and/or the consequences of leaving it untreated. Specify the consequences and conditions of the risk.
      (3) *Perceived benefits* – An individual's beliefs regarding the effectiveness of actions to reduce the risk or impact of illness. Define the characteristics of the action to take (how, when, where) and clarify the positive effects expected.
      (4) *Perceived barriers* – An individual's belief about the tangible and psychological costs of recommended actions. Identify and reduce perceived barriers by providing assistance, incentives, and reassurance. It is also important to correct misinformation.
      (5) *Cues to action* – Strategies for activating readiness to take action (perceived susceptibility and perceived benefits). Provide how-to information, promote awareness, and set up reminders.
      (6) *Self-efficacy* – An individual's confidence in his or her ability to take action. Provide training, verbal reinforcement, and guidance for progressive goal setting and performance, as well as demonstrate desired behaviors.

d. Opportunities for use: Mammography screening behaviors, AIDS-related behaviors.

2. Motivational interviewing (MI) (Miller, 1983):
   a. Originated from psychological counseling for substance use.
   b. Intended to guide an individual's exploration of his or her ambivalence about changing behavior.
   c. Miller (2008) updated the definition of MI to depict a more collaborative and patient-centered guiding technique to strengthen motivation for change (Baer, 2010).
   d. Individuals play the experts in evaluating their own behavior and generating solutions; they do most of the talking.
   e. The interviewer looks for discrepancies between current behavior and goals, as well as the individual's value placed on the behavior change (Redman, 2007).
   f. Expressing empathy, avoiding argumentation, and supporting self-efficacy are helpful methods during interviews.
   g. The interviewer must also practice guiding rather than directing, develop strategies to encourage the individual to talk about his or her motivation to change, and use active listening skills to encourage change talk (see Table 16-1) (Rollnick, Butler, Kinnersley, Gregory, & Mash, 2010).

3. Social Cognitive Theory (SCT).
   a. Origin: During the late 1970s, Albert Bandura developed a framework for understanding, predicting, and changing behavior – An interaction of individual factors, behavior, and environment.
   b. Core assumption: Critical factors include an individual's ability to demonstrate certain behaviors, anticipate outcomes, learn by observing others, perform behaviors with confidence, self-regulate behavior, and reflect on the change experience (Glanz et al., 2008).

Table 16-1.
Ten Useful Motivational Interviewing Questions

1.	What changes would you most like to discuss?
2.	What have you noticed about…?
3.	How important is it for you to change…?
4.	How confident do you feel about changing…?
5.	How do you see the benefits of…?
6.	How do you see the drawback of…?
7.	What will make the most sense to you…?
8.	How might things be different if you…?
9.	In what way…?
10.	Where does this leave you now?

Source: Adapted from Rollnick et al., 2010. Used with permission.

c. Definitions and applications of (major) model concepts (Glanz et al., 2008).
   (1) *Behavioral capability* – An individual's knowledge and skill to complete an action. Skills training with demonstration promotes mastery of learning.
   (2) *Expectations* – The anticipated outcomes from a performed behavior. Model positive outcomes of healthy behavior.
   (3) *Expectancies* – An individual's value placed on a given outcome (incentives). Present outcomes from the proposed change that have meaning to the individual.
   (4) *Self-control* – An individual's personal regulation of goal-directed performance. Present opportunities for decision-making, goal-setting, and problem-solving with self-monitoring and reward.
   (5) *Emotional coping responses* – An individual's strategies for dealing with emotional stimuli. Provide stress management techniques and training that include senarios for practicing skills in emotionally arousing situations.

(6) *Self-efficacy* (as defined within this chapter) – Plan an approach with small steps to ensure success and provide specificity regarding recommended action.

d. Opportunities for use: Community-wide programs for preventing and reducing alcohol use among adolescents, health education programs to increase vegetable and fruit consumption by elementary school-age children.

4. The Transtheoretical Model and Stages of Change (TTM).

a. Origin: James Prochaska and Carlo DiClemente (late 1970s to early 1980s) integrated leading theories from psychotherapy and behavior change to study smoking habits.

b. Core assumption: Most at-risk populations are not ready for action-oriented prevention programs. Behavior change is a process that occurs over time through a sequence of stages that are both open and stable.

c. Definitions and applications of model concepts (Glanz et al., 2008).

(1) Stages of change.

(a) *Precontemplation* – An individual has not yet acknowledged a problem behavior needing change. There is no intention to take action within the next six months.

(b) *Contemplation* – An individual acknowledges a problem behavior, but remains unsure about making a change. The intention is to take action within the next six months.

(c) *Preparation* – An individual is getting ready to make a change. The intention is to take action within the next 30 days and some behavioral steps have been taken.

(d) *Action* – An individual has changed overt behavior for less than six months.

(e) *Maintenance* – An individual has changed overt behavior for more than six months.

(f) *Termination* – An individual demonstrates total self-efficacy with little/no temptation to relapse, but may relapse.

(2) Processes of change.

(a) *Consciousness raising* – Increased awareness of causes and consequences. Provide feedback, confrontations, and media/literature (information).

(b) *Dramatic relief* – Experiencing the negative emotional experiences tied to unhealthy behavior. Use role-playing, grieving, and personal testimonies to evoke emotion.

(c) *Self-re-evaluation* – Assessing self-image by comparing life with and without behavior. Use imagery techniques, healthy role models, and value clarification.

(d) *Environmental re-evaluation* – Assessing how the presence or absence of behaviors affects an individual's social environment (e.g., the effect of smoking on others). Incorporate empathy training (seeing oneself as a positive or negative role model), interviews and/or interventions (significant other, family).

(e) *Self-liberation* – Believing one can change and making a commitment or recommitment to change. The individual takes a strong stand and becomes an advocate/spokesperson. Encourage resolutions, public testimonies, volunteering/advocacy opportunities.

(f) *Helping relationships* – Combining acceptance, trust, and caring to build an individual's own social support network. Create or find sources of social support, such as follow-up calls and buddy/cohort system(s).

(g) *Counter-conditioning* – Adopting healthier behaviors as substitution for problem behaviors. Teach strategies, such as positive self-statements, relaxation techniques, nicotine replacement, healthy food choices (how to read a nutrient label).

(h) *Reinforcement management* – Increasing rewards for positive behavior change and decreasing rewards for unhealthy behavior (self-changers rely on rewards much more than punishment). Acknowledge success through group recognition, reinforcements, contingency contracts, and individualized rewards.

(i) *Stimulus control* – Exchanging reminders or cues from unhealthy behaviors for those that encourage healthy behavior (e.g., holding a nicotine-free/electric inhaler instead of a cigarette). Reduce relapse risk through self-help groups, environmental reengineering, and avoidance, replacing cues.

(j) *Social liberation* – Recognizing changes in society that support healthy behavior change (e.g., smoke-free zones). Use advocacy, empowerment, and policies.

(3) Decisional balance.
  (a) An individual weighs the pros (benefits) and cons (costs) of changing behavior.

(4) Self-efficacy.
  (a) Situation-specific confidence that an individual has to cope with high-risk situations.
  (b) Temptation to engage in unhealthy behaviors in difficult/challenging situations. The three most common factors found in tempting situations include stress, positive social situations, and cravings.

d. Opportunities for use: Developing smoking cessation interventions, exercise, mammography, alcohol abuse, and condom use.

5. Theory of Reasoned Action (TRA) and Theory of Planned Behavior (TPB).
  a. Although these theories are not discussed in detail within this chapter, they are important to consider in an effort to understand the relationship between beliefs, attitudes, intentions, and behavior. Fishbein and Ajzen (1975) are credited with the origin of these theories. Both TRA and TPB focus on individual motivational factors as determinants of the likeliness that an individual will perform a specific behavior (Glanz et al., 2008).

C. Teaching strategies and instructional methods: Teaching strategies encompass a wide range and are chosen based on patient factors, setting, skill of the educator, and available resources.
  1. Parameters to consider in developing teaching strategies (Centers for Disease Control and Prevention [CDC], 2009b):
    a. Target audience, including secondary audience (influencers), if appropriate.
      (1) Utilize all appropriate information sources: Medical records, patient/support.
    b. Goals and objectives.
      (1) Goals are broad statements about the expected outcome(s).
      (2) Objectives are specific and detailed (SMART).

(a) **S**pecific – Concrete and well-defined terms.

(b) **M**easureable – Quantifiable with a specified source of measurement.

(c) **A**ttainable/achievable – Possible for the given time frame and resources.

(d) **R**elevant/realistic – Related to the overarching goal.

(e) **T**imebound – Set deadlines.

c. Learner needs.

(1) Three learning domains from Bloom's Taxonomy (1956).

(a) *Cognitive* – Knowledge; storing and recalling information.

(b) *Affective* – Attitude; changes in values, feelings, and outlook.

(c) *Psychomotor* – Skills; behaviors achieved through physical practice.

d. Readiness to learn (see *Learning Theories,* above). Self-management teaching strategies must consider:

(1) Learning domains.

(2) Sexual and psychosocial changes related to age.

e. Teaching approaches related to learner developmental stage; developmental stages and application (Bastable, 2008; Redman, 2007).

(1) Infant and toddler (0–2 years of age). Stages combined trust vs. mistrust; autonomy vs. shame (Erikson, 1963).

(a) Focus instruction toward parents.

(b) Allow older toddlers, if appropriate, to participate to some extent in the process (e.g., perform procedures on a teddy bear or doll first to help the child comprehend, keep teaching lessons brief, avoid analogies, and explain in simple terms).

(2) Early childhood (3–5 years of age). Initiative vs. guilt (Erikson, 1963).

(a) Instruct about health promotion and disease prevention, emphasizing importance of this to parents. Parents are strong role models for a variety of health habits.

(b) Allow the child to handle equipment and play with dolls to learn about body parts. There are special kidney, ostomy, and stoma dolls, as well as those which can have splints and traction attached.

(c) Use praise, approval, and tangible rewards, such as stickers and badges, as reinforcement for a successful learning experience.

(3) Middle to late childhood (6–11 years of age). Industry vs. inferiority (Erikson, 1963).

(a) Encourage independence and active participation.

(b) Use analogies to make invisible processes real, as well as drawings and models. Also consider group activities and play therapy.

(4) Adolescent (12–19 years of age). Identity vs. role (Erikson, 1963).

(a) Recognize that language skills of adolescents and their ability to conceptualize mean a wide variety of teaching methods and instructional tools may be used.

(b) Assure confidentiality by using one-on-one instruction about sensitive information.

(c) Provide for control by sharing decision-making whenever possible, and suggest options to help provide choices. Including the adolescent in determining the best way to master information helps to support his or her sense of autonomy.

(d) Anticipate negative responses when adolescent self-image/self-integrity is threatened. Approach with respect, flexibility, and openness to encourage responsiveness to teaching-learning situations.

(5) Young adulthood (20–40 years of age). Intimacy vs. isolation (Erikson, 1963). Adult learning principles suggest that the adult learner is the center of the activity, not the end point at which teaching is directed. Teaching strategies should be based on principles that guide adult learning (Bastable, 2008).

(a) What is to be learned must be related to an immediate need.

(b) Learning is voluntary, self-initiated, person-centered, and problem-centered.

(c) Learning is self-directed.

　i. Motivation theories explain causes for learning engagement in two categories: Extrinsic (earning rewards and avoiding punishment) and intrinsic (curiosity and mastery).

　ii. As a goal-directed behavior, motivation is heightened through feedback, modeling, support, and successful experiences (Glanz et al., 2008).

(d) The role of the teacher is that of facilitator.

(e) Learning new material draws on past experience and is related to something the learner already knows.

(f) Information and assignments must be relevant.

(g) Learning is reinforced by prompt feedback and application.

　i. A potential obstacle is health literacy. According to the National Assessment of Adult Literacy (NAAL), only about 12% of adults have proficient health literacy, with an average overall reading proficiency at the 5th grade level (National Center for Education Statistics [NCES], 2007). This indicates a high likelihood of low or limited health literacy skills for most patients seeking medical services.

　ii. Correlation may exist between increased risk for hospital readmission and very low health literacy, especially if patients leave the clinical setting without understanding their medical treatment (e.g., how to take prescriptions, when to call for medical attention, how to make lifestyle changes).

　iii. Careful attention must be paid by the educator to recognize reading or vocabulary difficulties because these may be hidden due to feelings of shame or embarrassment (DHHS, 2011a). The American Medical Association (AMA) outlines some behaviors and responses that may indicate limited literacy: Incomplete or inaccurately completed forms; frequently missed appointments; patients indicate they are taking medication or treatments as recommended, but tests do not reflect expected readings; patients verbalize a preference to read written information at home or ask a clinician to read it to them instead (Weiss, 2007).

(6) Middle-aged adulthood (41–64 years of age). Generativity vs. self-absorption and stagnation (Erikson, 1963).

    (a) Concerned with physical changes, while re-examining goals and values.

    (b) Demonstrates confidence in abilities and desire to modify unsatisfactory life aspects. Provide information that relates to concerns and assess for any potential sources of stress. Focus on reestablishing normal patterns.

(7) Older adulthood (65 years and over). Integrity vs. despair (Erikson, 1963).

    (a) Cognitive changes with decreased ability to think abstractly.

    (b) Sensory-motor deficits, difficulty hearing high-pitched tones, decreased visual adaptation (night-vision, peripheral perception).

    (c) Build on past life experiences with relevant and meaningful applications. Keep explanations brief with analogies and repetition. Speak slowly.

    (d) Use white backgrounds with black ink and large letters, while avoiding blue, green, purple, and yellow color-coding.

2. For a summary of instructional methods, see Table 16-2. Barbara Klug Redman's (2007) work regarding the practice of patient education remains a respected reference for learning theories and teaching strategies.

III. Patient Education in Ambulatory Care: Health Promotion and Disease Prevention and Counseling

A. Health promotion and disease prevention.

1. With the Patient Protection and Affordable Care Act signed into law on March 23, 2010, a unique opportunity has arisen for prevention practice (DHHS, 2010a). This encourages health care providers to focus on efforts such as implementing evidence-based education programs, as well as supporting initiatives that encourage patient self-efficacy and self-management.

    a. *Self-efficacy:* A person's perception of their ability to attain certain goals (most commonly recognized theory from the work of Albert Bandura). With regard to education, this means learners will be more likely to attempt, to persevere, and to be successful at tasks at which they have a sense of efficacy.

    b. *Self-management:* The concept of self-management is not new, and depending upon the work and focus, there may be many different definitions. Because of continuing efforts to decrease the burden of illness and improve the public's health status (IOM, 2011b), evolving perspectives of self-management have gained a threshold in many health care organizations. Current self-management recognizes the central role played by the patient in preventing and managing illness. This is a shift from traditional patient education (see Table 16-3).

2. Health promotion: By increasing the scope of health plans to cover preventive services and wellness care, government programs aim to help make services more affordable

Table 16-2.
Instructional Methods

Method	Advantages	Disadvantages	Approach and Key Points
Group Discussion	• Increases interaction • Keeps individual focus • Learning exchange/ sharing experiences • Encourages Q & A	• Not all voices may be heard • Must enforce ground rules • Limited information retention	• Instructor steers discussion • Use questions • Prep-work required • Participants share at least one similar factor (age, disease, language, etc.) • Keep energy high
Simulation/ Exercises	• Works well for small to mid-sized groups • Supports all levels of ability	• Props and equipment are usually required	• Look for existing plans/curriculum for simulation scenarios • Use explanations, demonstrations, and return-learner practices
Printed Materials	• Increases retention (especially with pictures and cartoons) • Takes information home/ may revisit	• May decrease amount of interaction • Risk of missing health literacy issues	• Use SMOG readability formula (< 100 words) • FOG (> 100 words) • Include pictures, cartoons, simple models • Read aloud • Circle/highlight key points
Online/Web Site	• Allows interactive participation • Supports taking action • Can be used with mid to low literacy rate	• Online access (may be difficult for remote areas)	• Computer does not replace person-person communication • Present information simply with a straightforward delivery
Video/DVD/ Slideshow	• Professional presentation of information • Stimulates discussion • (Printed) doubles as notes/handout • Enhances confidence by demonstration	• May distract from a concise message • Most effective with discussion • Difficult to generate full audience participation	• Plan for equipment set-up • Prep-work required for discussion • Audio-visual sensory method
Virtual/ Role-Playing	• Dramatizes problem situation • Assigns roles • Increases empathy • Highlights alternative points-of-view • Explores creative solutions • Acts out and practices skills	• Puts individuals on the spot, may feel threatened • Not intended for large groups • May require additional equipment	• Requires clear instructions with pre-defined roles
Case Study/ Application	• Focuses on problem-solving • Explores creative solutions	• Requires analytical thinking/ability to apply relevance • Coordinate information to fit everyday routine	• Use reliable and tested case studies • Clearly defined purpose with prep

continued on next page

Table 16-2. (continued)
Instructional Methods

Method	Advantages	Disadvantages	Approach and Key Points
Teach-Back	• Applies new knowledge/ skills • Increases engagement • Repeats demonstration • Improves information retention/understanding • Uses open-ended questions by replacing • *Do you understand?*	• Increases time demand for teaching • Accountability is placed on the educator • Requires patience	• Practice re-teaching strategies with clarifying statements • Educator assumes communication responsibility • Use repetition • Allow restating of information in their own words

Ask Me 3 (National Patient Safety Foundation, 2011)	• Provides patient-provider dialogue
	• Time-efficient
	• Reduces embarrassment
	• Promotes three simple questions:
	  • *Why is it important for me to do this?*
	  • *What do I need to do?*
	  • *What is my main problem?*
		• Relies on provider adoption
		• Small/no effect on populations with higher-level health literacy
			• Materials may be downloaded/ordered
			• Simple statements with visuals help support clear communication

Sources: Adapted from AHRQ, 2011; Bastable, 2008; Lowenstein, 2008; Redman, 2007.

Table 16-3.
Shift to Self-Management Education

Traditional Patient Education	Self-Management Education
Provides information and technical skills	Fosters/incorporates problem-solving
Specific disease-driven	Patient (self)-driven
Educator: Health care professional	Educator: Patients/peers, community groups, health care professionals
Knowledge determines behavior change	Self-efficacy determines behavior change
Goal is compliance	Goal is increasing confidence

Sources: Adapted from Bastable, 2008; Redman, 2007.

and accessible; therefore, people receive preventive health care they need to stay healthy, avoid or delay the onset of disease, lead productive lives, and reduce health care costs (DHHS, 2010a).

    a. For ambulatory nurses, this means serving as an advocate and facilitator of teaching processes that promote awareness, influence attitudes, and identify needs and opportunities, as well as increase aptitude for healthy living. Several nursing theories support and outline this practice.

    (1) Nola Pender's Theory of Health Promotion – Nurses and other health care providers (in addition to family and peers) are important sources of interpersonal influence

that can impact commitment and engagement in health-promoting behavior (Reed & Shearer, 2009).

(2) Dorothea Orem's Theory of Self-Care – Nursing action compensates for patients' self-care limitations (Reed & Shearer, 2009).

(3) Virginia Henderson's Theory – The role of the nurse is to support the patient in meeting health needs until he or she is able to do for him/herself (Reed & Shearer, 2009).

(4) All relate to the concepts of health promotion and health maintenance, and reinforce the individual's and family's responsibility for health care and encourage participation of family and significant others whenever possible.

b. *The Nurse's Toolbook for Promoting Wellness* provides wellness assessment tools with specific instructions and potential interventions (Miller, 2008). Some teaching methods may or should include:

(1) Shared decision-making with patient and/or family/caregiver involvement.

(2) Teach-back method or closing-the-loop technique (Dancel, 2009).

(3) Focus on everyday life context, rather than just disease-specific management.

(4) Patient advocacy that extends into the wider community.

3. Disease prevention: Best explained as a proactive commitment to wellness and conscientious desire to prevent illness or disease. As a leading authority, the U.S. Preventive Services Task Force (2010) provides a clinical pocket guide with recommendations on screening, counseling, and preventive topics. Other resources to consider include *Recommendations for Preventive Pediatric Health Care* (American Academy of Pediatrics [AAP], 2008) and

Quick Reference Information: Medicare Preventive Services (Centers for Medicare and Medicaid Services [CMS], 2011). The term *prevention* may have different definitions depending upon the area of health. For the purpose of this work, the classic definitions as set out by the field of public health are used, which distinguish between primary, secondary, and tertiary prevention (Commission on Chronic Illness, 1957).

a. *Primary prevention* – The prevention of a disease before it occurs. Examples of primary prevention measures include health education and counseling, immunizations (both passive and active), hand washing, water purification, and wearing seatbelts and bicycle helmets.

b. *Secondary prevention* – The prevention of exacerbations or recurrences of disease already present but without symptoms and dysfunction (not clinically apparent). *Stedman's Medical Dictionary* describes secondary prevention as the interruption of the disease process before the emergence of signs or diagnostic findings (Stedman, 2008). Further, the World Health Organization's (2009) well-recognized definition of *health,* which underscores the importance of seeing health not just as the absence of disease or illness. Secondary prevention measures include early detection with screening examinations, such as blood pressure, mammography, and sigmoidoscopy.

c. *Tertiary prevention* – Tertiary prevention occurs when a long-term disease or disability is already diagnosed. Prevention methods aim to achieve the highest level of function, minimize complications, and reduce disability. Examples of tertiary prevention measures include occupational and physical therapy after a stroke, wearing proper shoes with diabetic neuropathy, and assigning appropriate diet post-surgery to promote healing.

Figure 16-1.
Nursing Process as a Method for Tailoring Patient Education

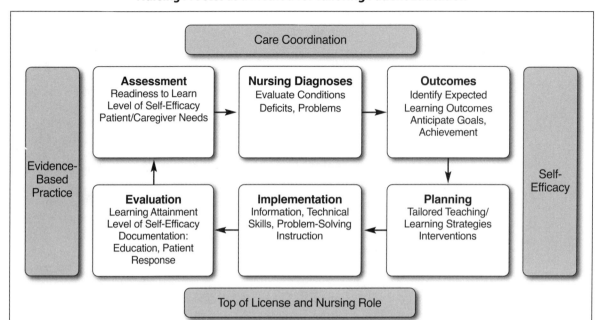

4. Impact on the nurse role: Ambulatory care nurses are uniquely qualified to influence care delivery in the outpatient setting, specifically regarding patient education and coordination of services (AAACN, 2010a). Understanding the patient health care experience and looking for opportunities to provide timely and planned education are critical.
   a. The ambulatory care nurse role requires several elements of care coordination:
      (1) Continuum planning (preparing patients/family/caregivers for transitions between health care settings) and education (instructing patients/family/caregivers about available services).
      (2) Collaborating with health care team resources as needed (interdisciplinary team approach).
      (3) Anticipating barriers to learning and self-management (level of health literacy and self-efficacy).
      (4) Providing patient-tailored teaching strategies with appropriate instructional methods.
   b. Further, educational interventions must combine current evidence-based research, clinical expertise, and patient preferences with instruction on navigating the health care system. The nursing process remains a fundamental method for addressing patient education needs (see Figure 16-1).
5. Challenges for educating patients in ambulatory care:
   a. Episodic nature of visits.
      (1) Aligning comprehensive care and team coordination: Continuity.
      (2) Opportunity for feedback and "closing the loop."
   b. Time constraints.
      (1) *New Health Partnerships Initiative* toolkit (Schaefer, Miller, Goldstein, & Simmons, 2009).
         (a) "Ask-Tell-Ask" technique.

      i. Ask permission: "There are a few things I'd like to tell you about your new medication. Ready?"

     ii. Tell the information: Use simple explanations (omit medical jargon), use pictures and models when possible, and encourage family/caregiver involvement.

    iii. Ask for understanding: "What questions do you have about your medication? When you go home, how will you explain the medication changes to your family/caregiver? What will you do if you have these symptoms…?"

  (2) Capturing "readiness to learn" during patient visit, small window of time.

  (3) Quick and experienced assessment skills are key.

c. Range of patient socio-demographic and community characteristics.

  (1) Wide geographic catchment area.

  (2) Cultural considerations.

  (3) Age-grouped patients/aging population.

  (4) Gender and sex.

  (5) Race and ethnicity.

  (6) Economic and educational characteristics.

  (7) Social, community, and familial support.

  (8) Disease complexity and chronicity.

  (9) Health status.

  (10) Access to health care and health insurance.

  (11) Endemic health and geographic environmental issues.

6. Looking ahead: The IOM's (2011a) collaborative report, *The Future of Nursing: Leading Change, Advancing Health*, depicts an upcoming health care system that purposefully promotes wellness and disease prevention, improved health outcomes, and carefully planned care across the health continuum. This picture places outpatient care and disease prevention as core drivers of the health care system, where interprofessional collaboration and coordination is routinely practiced (IOM, 2011a). Nurses practicing at the top of their license and supporting the environment of preventive care will influence how patient education is delivered in ambulatory care settings. A handful of developments in this area include:

a. Creating outpatient learning centers as repositories of information.

b. Direct-care nurses evolving into coordinators of care and information, transition managers (following and educating patients from one level of care to another), and navigators of the health care system.

c. Nurses and care providers using social networking to educate and remain in contact with patients on a day-to-day basis (CDC, 2009b).

d. Increasing the number of nurse-managed practice sites.

e. Growth of nurse telehealth call centers and expansion of virtual assessment opportunities.

  (1) Expanding technology capabilities: Mobile applications and devices that assess and send health status updates to health care providers for real-time feedback and education opportunities (A1c/glucose, blood pressure).

B. Patient counseling for health promotion and disease prevention: Defining health for an individual Involves assessing the complex interaction between mind, body, spirit, and environment. This holistic approach considers each of these elements to help make lifestyle changes and reach an optimal state (Edelman & Mandle, 2006). Using the nursing process within a holistic framework assumes an individual is related to his or her environment and takes an increasing amount of accountability for maintaining his or her health. As care providers aim to promote health and prevent disease, this view becomes critical in seeing the whole patient picture and understanding the value an individual places on his or her wellness.

In the ambulatory care setting, the nurse plays a central role in providing health promotion and disease prevention education and counseling. According to ANA's (2010) *Standards of Professional Nursing Practice*, the registered nurse must demonstrate competence in providing "health teaching that addresses such topics as healthy lifestyles, risk-reducing behaviors, developmental needs, activities of daily living, and preventive self-care" (p. 41). The following section identifies content for providing counsel to patients. Topics and strategies presented parallel those described in *The Guide to Clinical Preventive Services 2010–2011* (recommendations of the U.S. Preventive Services Task Force), *HealthyPeople 2020*, the National Center for Chronic Disease Prevention and Health Promotion, and updates from the Agency for Healthcare Research and Quality (AHRQ). A number of health behaviors and environmental factors that contribute to premature death in the U.S. have been identified, including smoking tobacco, poor diet, physical activity patterns, alcohol consumption, toxic agents, firearms, sexual behavior, motor vehicles, and illicit use of drugs (U.S. Preventive Services Task Force, 2010). *Healthy People 2020* objectives and interventions also consider social determinants of health and health-related quality of life/well-being.

1. Counseling for child and adolescent health.
    a. Alcohol and prescription drug abuse.
        (1) The National Institute on Alcohol Abuse and Alcoholism (NIAAA) (2011) reported 40% of children have tried alcohol before reaching 8th grade (75% by 12th grade). Children and adolescents tend to drink heavily in an episodic man-

ner. Each year, about 5,000 deaths involve underage drinking (under the age of 21); most occur from unintentional injuries, such as motor vehicle crashes, homicides, and suicides (NIAAA, 2011).
        (2) According to *Healthy People 2020*, prescription drug abuse continues to rise, with higher usage rates of hydrocodone bitartrate and acetaminophen (Vicodin®) and oxycodone (OxyContin®) (DHHS, 2011b). About 8% of adolescents ages 12–17 abuse prescription drugs; the overwhelming majority are painkillers (National Institute on Drug Abuse [NIDA], 2009). More than alcohol or tobacco, painkillers are more commonly abused by teens. Availability of these drugs and belief that prescription medication is safer than street drugs may be two factors related to these findings.
        (3) Topics to include in counseling.
            (a) Physical effects of drug and/or alcohol use.
            (b) Psychosocial effects of drug and/or alcohol use.
            (c) Dangers of drinking alcohol and driving.
            (d) Parental role in educating about the dangers of drug and alcohol use.
            (e) Dangers of using prescription drugs.
            (f) Encourage adoption of stress-relieving techniques and coping measures.
                i. Long-term stress indicators: Headaches, change in eating and sleep patterns, persistent feelings of anger (CDC, 2011a).
                ii. Techniques from the CDC's *Body and Mind* Web site: Physical activity,

increasing healthy food choices and eating breakfast, talking to someone trustworthy, having fun and laughing, consistent sleep patterns, keeping a journal, volunteering.

    (g) Review signs and symptoms of depression.

        i. The National Institute of Mental Health (NIMH, 2011) outlines common questions about depression, including impact on daily activities, duration of symptoms, and physical manifestations such as aches, pains, or digestive problems that persist.

    (h) Encourage parents to speak with their children frequently about drinking.

    (i) Children are more likely to avoid drinking when a trusting relationship exists with their parental figure(s) (NIAAA, 2011).

  (4) Resources.

    (a) NIAAA (2011) interactive teen Web site, *The Cool Spot: Facts about Alcohol.*

    (b) NIDA (2011) teen fact Web site with blog, *NIDA for Teens.*

    (c) National Clearinghouse for Alcohol and Drug Information (NCADI, 2012) resource Web site for clinicians and general public.

b. Dental and oral health.

  (1) According to the CDC (2006), dental caries or tooth decay affect children more than any other chronic infectious disease (25% of children 6–11 years of age; 59% of adolescents 12–19 years of age). From 2005 to 2008, about 16% of children 6–19 years of age presented with untreated dental caries, and less than 1 of 3 children enrolled in Medicaid received at least one preventive dental service in a recent year. More than 50% of children and adolescents experienced dental caries in at least one primary or permanent tooth in a study from 1999–2004 (DHHS, 2011b).

  (2) Topics to include in counseling (CDC, 2006).

    (a) Strategies preventing tooth decay and improving oral hygiene.

    (b) Proper technique for brushing teeth, including toothbrush replacement every three to four months and after experiencing a cold or bacterial infection.

    (c) Importance of consulting a dental health professional regarding use of dental floss, fluoridated drinking water, and dental sealants on permanent molars.

    (d) The impact of dietary habits on oral health: Avoiding foods high in simple sugars or starches, encouraging the consumption of raw fruits and vegetables, avoiding tobacco products.

c. Nutrition.

  (1) In 2008, the prevalence of obesity among children ages 6–11 was approximately 20% (CDC, 2009c). Today, many children have an excessive intake of saturated fat paired with a physically inactive lifestyle. According to the Dietary Guidelines Advisory Committee (DGAC) (2010) *Dietary Guidelines Report*, current research findings show diets high in energy but low in nutrients. This commonly found pattern among young Americans results in an over-

weight but undernourished health status and, in the longer-term, increases risk for developing heart disease, Type 2 diabetes, joint problems, and sleep apnea, as well as social and psychological problems (DGAC, 2010). In recent years, the School Health Policies and Programs Study has supported implementation of school-based programs that provide healthier food and beverage choices, health screenings, and health education on topics related to preventing obesity and other chronic diseases (CDC, 2009c).

(2) Topics to include in counseling.

    (a) Inadequate nutrition during infancy and childhood prevents proper growth and development: Discuss benefits of breastfeeding infants for the first 6–12 months of life, introduce one food at a time at 3- to 5-day intervals, use iron-rich foods, such as iron-fortified cereal and infant formula.

    (b) Coordinate with Dietary/Nutrition Counseling as needed to educate parents and children about choosing a balanced diet.

       i. Review the Dietary Guidelines for Americans (over 2 years of age). Eat a variety of foods; balance food consumption with physical activity; do not skip breakfast (especially adolescents); increase intake of grains, vegetables, and fruits; decrease saturated fat and cholesterol; limit sugary foods; and moderate sodium (DGAC, 2010). Further recommenda-

tions from the 2010 *Dietary Guidelines Advisory Committee Report* include greatly reducing intake of sugar-sweetened beverages, infrequently consuming meals from quick service (fast food), spending fewer hours in front of a screen (television, computer), and adding more hours of active play.

    (c) Advise parents about community-based food supplementation programs (food pantries; food stamps; Women, Infants, and Children [WIC]).

    (d) Assess for stress-related causes, low or impaired body image and self-esteem. Offer appropriate stress-reducing techniques and consult with counselor/social worker as needed.

    (e) Measure body mass index (BMI) and review results with parent(s). Discuss the importance of maintaining a healthy weight with physical activity.

d. Physical activity.

    (1) Despite all the well-demonstrated benefits of physical activity, most American children and adolescents are not physically active. The CDC's (2009c) *Youth Risk Behavior Surveillance* found only 18% of high school students had participated in at least 60 minutes of daily physical activity. Pairing the increasing amount of calories consumed with decreasing physical activity results in weight gain. The *Physical Activity Guidelines for Americans* (DHHS, 2008) outlines the first-ever physical activity plan from the federal government (see *Topics*, below, for detail).

(2) Topics to include in counseling.
    (a) Children and adolescents (ages 6–17):
        i. 60 minutes or more of physical activity daily.
        ii. Majority of the activity should be moderate- or vigorous-intensity aerobic exercise.
        iii. Exercise should include vigorous-intensity at least three days per week with muscle-strengthening and bone-strengthening focus.
        iv. Limit exposure to screen activities, such as watching television.
    (b) Importance of engaging in a variety of activities to help with the development of a range of abilities.
    (c) Importance of safety equipment, such as helmets, guards, and pads, and protection against sunburn for outdoor activities with use of sunscreens, lip balm, and protective clothing.

e. Safety.
    (1) Unintentional injuries are the leading cause of death for children and adolescents 5–19 years of age.
        (a) Approximately 48% from motor vehicle injuries (occupants and pedestrians combined).
        (b) 21% from all other unintentional injuries (falls, poisoning, choking, drowning, firearms, and sports).
        (c) 16% from homicides.
        (d) 14% from suicides (CDC, 2010a). Violent injuries (homicide and suicide) among adolescents 15–19 years of age account for the second-leading cause of death.

(2) Of the estimated 300,000 females forcibly raped each year in the U.S., more than half are less than 18 years of age, and approximately 20% are less than 12 years of age when first raped (CDC, 2010a).

(3) Two important issues will emerge within the next decade for adolescents:
    (a) Growing ethnic diversity (requires cultural responsiveness to health care needs and attention to disparate health and academic outcomes).
    (b) An increasing focus on utilizing positive youth development interventions to prevent risk behaviors (DHHS, 2011b).

(4) Topics to include in counseling.
    (a) Teaching children to use the community emergency response system (9-1-1 and other emergency numbers).
    (b) Importance of parents, family, and peers learning life-saving skills, such as cardiopulmonary resuscitation (CPR) and the Heimlich maneuver.
    (c) Parents and dependents using appropriate child safety seats and seatbelts in automobiles.
    (d) Discussing parents' role in modeling safety (wearing seatbelts and bike helmets, not driving after drinking alcohol, refraining from texting or cell phone use while driving).
    (e) How to avoid and protect children from choking and suffocation, drowning, electrocution, falls, firearms, motor vehicle accidents, poison ingestion, and sudden infant death syndrome (SIDS).

(f) Importance of having a dating safety plan (Alabama Coalition Against Domestic Violence [ACADV], 2011; Rape, Abuse and Incest National Network [RAINN], 2011).

f. Sexually transmitted diseases and HIV infection.

(1) In 2009, the CDC's (2009c) *Youth Risk Behavior Surveillance* found many high school age students engaging in sexual risk behaviors that may result in negative health outcomes.

    (a) 46% reported having sexual intercourse (14% had four or more partners).

    (b) 39% did not use a condom.

    (c) 77% did not use birth control pills the last time they had sex.

(2) The consequences of sexually transmitted diseases can be very serious for teenagers.

    (a) Because of the histology of their cervix, female adolescents are more susceptible to certain sexually transmitted diseases (STDs) than older women.

    (b) Pelvic inflammatory disease and sterility can result from gonorrhea and chlamydia infections.

    (c) Human papillomavirus (HPV), which may be the most prevalent STD in adolescents, can lead to cervical cancer.

    (d) The presence of other STDs may increase susceptibility to the HIV virus.

    (e) Untreated STDs during pregnancy can lead to serious consequences for the fetus or newborn child (U.S. Preventive Services Task Force, 2010).

(3) An estimated 8,300 youths (13–24 years of age) were included in state reports to the CDC as having an HIV infection, and nearly 50% of the 19 million new STD cases each year comprise individuals ages 15–24 (CDC, 2009a).

(4) Topics to include in counseling.

    (a) Risk of STDs and HIV infections.

    (b) Routes of transmission of STDs and HIV infections.

    (c) Importance of communication between parents and their adolescents regarding responsible, safe sexual behavior.

    (d) Abstinence as the most effective way to prevent STDs and HIV infection.

    (e) Importance of using condoms to prevent STDs and HIV infection.

    (f) The proper way to use condoms.

    (g) How to access resources about specific topics related to sexual activity and STDs/HIV infection.

    (h) Availability of HPV vaccine (see Chapter 17, "Care of the Well Client: Screening and Preventive Care").

g. Tobacco use.

(1) Passive exposure to tobacco smoke is a potential health hazard for infants and children, exacerbating the symptoms of asthma and allergies, and decreasing pulmonary function. Additionally, parental smoking poses a higher risk factor for adolescents adopting a smoking habit. Health consequences of smoking (including smokeless or chewing tobacco): Risk for multiple types of cancer, heart disease, and respiratory disease. According to the CDC (2009c), current tobacco and cig-

arette use declined in both middle and high school-age students from 2000–2009. The number of onscreen tobacco incidents in youth-rated movies decreased by 72% from 2005–2010 (CDC, 2009c).

(2) Topics to include in counseling.

    (a) Importance of a smoke-free home environment.

    (b) Parental role modeling and its effect on children and adolescents.

    (c) Negative health consequences of parental smoking on the child.

    (d) Importance of beginning to discuss tobacco use and its negative effects when children are of early elementary school age.

    (e) Negative cosmetic and athletic effects of smoking (in discussions with children and adolescents).

h. Unintended pregnancy.

(1) Data for 2008 and 2009 indicate a decline in U.S. teen pregnancy; however, the overall rates are still substantially higher than those in other western-industrialized nations (CDC, 2009a). More than 50% of 18- and 19-year-olds, as compared with half of all adults, describe their pregnancies as being unintended.

    (a) Adolescent pregnancy has a higher incidence of low birth weight, prematurity, and neonatal death than for adult pregnant women.

    (b) Psychosocial complications of adolescent pregnancy include school interruption and/or lack of completion of education. Slightly more than 50% of teen mothers earned a high school diploma by 22 years of age, versus nearly 90% who had not given birth during high school years (Perper, Peterson, & Manlove, 2010). This may indicate longer-term effects in terms of the socioeconomic future for both parent and child.

(2) Topics to include in counseling.

    (a) Options for contraception for a sexually active adolescent.

    (b) How to support an adolescent's decision of abstinence (for parents).

    (c) Importance of using condoms for preventing STDs and HIV infection, even if another form of contraception is used.

    (d) Importance of sexually active adolescents talking freely with their partners about STDs, HIV, and hepatitis B infection, as well as the use of contraceptives.

    (e) Importance of adolescents assertively discussing contraception use and protective measures against STDs with their partners.

    (f) Importance of follow-up with a health care provider after initiating use of contraceptives. Provides opportunity to clarify any misconceptions and address any concerns, thus promoting continued use.

i. Violent behavior and firearms.

(1) Violence is a major health problem for children and adolescents in the U.S. Homicide is the second leading cause of death among individuals ages 15–24, and for African American males and females and Hispanic males in this age group, it is the leading cause of death. Violence to females, in the form of dating violence, sexual assault, and rape, is also a con-

cern (U.S. Preventive Services Task Force, 2010).
(2) Topics to include in counseling.
  (a) Risk factors for violent injury (history of violent injury to the child or other family members, history of alcohol or other drug abuse by the child or other family members, guns or other weapons kept in the house, prevalence of violence-related injury in the community).
  (b) Dangers of keeping a gun in the home.
  (c) For those who do have a gun in the home, review the specifics of gun safety.
  (d) Availability of guns in places where children spend time, such as school, friends' homes, and recreational facilities.
  (e) Discuss methods of addressing and diffusing anger.
  (f) Importance of developing and communicating a dating safety plan.
  (g) Provide resources for information about violence prevention.
  (h) Provide and review resources for reporting potentially violent behavior in peers.
2. Counseling for adult and older adult health.
  a. Alcohol and other drug abuse.
    (1) Alcohol and drug abuse are physically damaging and are associated with other major causes of death, including suicide, traffic accidents, homicide, and HIV infection (U.S. Preventive Services Task Force, 2010). Consumption of alcohol during pregnancy can lead to the development of fetal alcohol syndrome, which can produce a wide variety and severity of physical and mental problems in infants.

    (2) Definition of alcohol misuse: "Risky" or "hazardous" drinking has been defined as:
      (a) For men, more than 14 drinks per week or more than 4 drinks per occasion.
      (b) For women, more than 7 drinks per week or more than 3 drinks per occasion (U.S. Preventive Services Task Force, 2010).
    (3) Illicit drug use.
      (a) Highest between the ages of 18 and 20 years.
      (b) Marijuana is most common, and cocaine is second most common.
      (c) Abuse of prescription painkillers, tranquilizers, stimulants, and sedatives is a growing health problem in the U.S. (U.S. Preventive Services Task Force, 2010).
    (4) Topics to include in counseling.
      (a) Importance of discontinuing alcohol/substance abuse.
      (b) Information about the negative impact on health of alcohol/substance abuse.
      (c) Risks of HIV infection, hepatitis B or hepatitis C infection, and other disorders associated with shared needle use.
      (d) Resources to assist with discontinuing alcohol/substance abuse.
  b. Dental and oral health.
    (1) The most common adult oral health problems consist of tooth decay and periodontal diseases. Personal oral hygiene measures can help control plaque, decay, and gingivitis in most individuals; however, certain segments of the adult population (lower socioeconomic, racial or ethnic minority groups, and elderly) suffer severe and often untreated dental decay.

According to CDC reports, over 40% of adults in lower socio-economic groups, compared to 16% of adults in middle to high socio-economic groups, present with at least one untreated tooth decay (CDC, 2006). With a goal to eliminate disparities in oral health, the federal government has sought strategic partnerships with national organizations, while also arranging cooperative agreements with the Association of State and Territorial Dental Directors (ASTDD) and the Children's Dental Health Project (CDHP) to strengthen state and community oral health programs (CDC, 2011c). About 75% of oral and pharyngeal cancers are attributed to tobacco (both smokeless and smoked). The overall survival rate from these cancers has not improved during the last 16 years.

(2) Topics to include in counseling.
    (a) Regular preventive health care with an oral health professional.
    (b) Importance of brushing and flossing daily.
    (c) Dietary considerations: Limiting intake of refined sugars, especially for patients with a history of dental carries.
    (d) Risks associated with tobacco and alcohol use.
    (e) Recognition of oral cavity irregularities that last for more than two weeks: Color changes, sores that fail to heal and bleed easily, persistent ulcers, gum bleeding, swelling or thickening in lips, cheeks, tongue, gums, or roof of the mouth, difficulty chewing or swallowing food.

    (f) Discuss early detection through periodic medical and dental examinations, especially for patients with heavy alcohol and tobacco use.
    (g) Provide information on endocarditis prophylaxis with regard to dental or operative procedures, as applicable.
    (h) Review oral effects and complications of medication and other treatments.
    (i) Provide resources for those with limited or no dental insurance.

c. Injury and domestic violence.
    (1) The fifth leading cause of death in the U.S. is unintentional injuries, with motor vehicle crashes and alcohol being a factor in both fatal and non-fatal injuries.
        (a) Nationwide seatbelt use estimates at 85%; however, 1 in 7 adults do not wear a seatbelt on every trip (CDC, 2010b).
        (b) Falls, especially in older adults, are a leading cause of injury death, with hip fractures being the most common fall-related injury leading to hospitalization. Roughly half of all persons sustaining hip fractures never regain full function.
        (c) Domestic violence is a health risk, especially for women and older adults (U.S. Preventive Services Task Force, 2010).
        (d) The amount of death and disability caused by preventable injuries and violence warrant a discussion of these topics with every patient.
    (2) Topics to include in counseling.
        (a) Questions about safety, including seatbelt and helmet use.

(b) Reinforcement that seatbelt use reduces serious injury and death by about 50% (CDC, 2010b).

(c) Importance of not consuming alcohol prior to driving or operating equipment.

(d) Importance of installing and maintaining smoke and carbon monoxide detectors in homes.

(e) Dangers of hazards and importance of safety rules at worksites.

(f) Importance of safety in the home. Encourage use of home safety checklists. This list reviews such things as adequate lighting, conditions that may result in falls, and presence of handrails and traction strips on stairs and in bathtubs.

(g) Unacceptability of violence when abuse is disclosed (must be reported).

(h) Information on community, social, and legal resources available to abuse victims.

d. Nutrition.

(1) Obesity among adults has increased significantly over the last 20 years. Over 30% of U.S. adults are obese. This increasing rate is concerning because being overweight or obese increases the risk of many diseases and health concerns: Heart disease, stroke, high blood pressure, Type 2 diabetes, cancers (especially breast and colon), high cholesterol/triglycerides, liver and gallbladder disease, sleep apnea and respiratory issues, joint degeneration/osteoarthritis, reproductive problems (including infertility), and mental health conditions.

(2) Recent reports from the CDC (2011b) show substantial differences among the groupings of race/ethnicity, gender, and sex in regards to obesity prevalence:

(a) 50% of non-Hispanic Black women age 20 or older were obese.

(b) 43% of Mexican-American women.

(c) 33% of White women.

(3) Obesity has become a major health problem in the U.S. and is attributed to over-consumption of calories and low levels of physical activity. Good nutrition is essential to good health throughout the lifespan, and it is also a component in the prevention and treatment of many diseases. Patients also rely on their primary care providers to give them adequate and appropriate dietary information.

(4) Topics to include in counseling.

(a) Dietary habits.

(b) Basic information about maintaining a healthy diet (see *Dietary Guidelines for Americans* in the previous *Nutrition* section related to children).

(c) Importance of women consuming adequate amounts of calcium and folic acid, including options for assuring adequate intake.

(d) Dietary strategies for weight reduction (fewer total calories, increase fruits and vegetables, decrease fat intake), for overweight patients.

(e) Low cholesterol diet for patients with borderline or high cholesterol.

(f) Resources to assist with weight reduction for patients who wish to lose weight.

e. Physical activity.
   (1) Regular exercise has been shown to reduce the risk of cardiovascular disease, the leading cause of death in the U.S. In addition, it helps prevent diabetes, control weight, improve musculoskeletal functioning, and decrease stress; it may also help prevent bone loss associated with aging. Despite the many benefits of exercise, according to the 2008 National Health Interview Survey, more than 60% of adults are not regularly exercising, and 36% report no physical activity at all (DHHS, 2011b).
   (2) When considering the benefits of regular exercise, counseling patients on this particular lifestyle change may have the greatest positive affect on the health of American adults. A goal outlined by *Healthy People 2020* is to increase the proportion of clinic visits that include counseling and patient education related to physical activity.
   (3) Patients unable or unwilling to engage in regular exercise should at least increase physical activity in their usual routine by parking farther away from a destination, walking to the supermarket, and taking the stairs rather than the elevator.
   (4) Topics to include in counseling.
       (a) Importance of moderate- (at least 2 hours and 30 minutes a week) to vigorous-intensity (1 hour and 15 minutes a week) exercises.
           i. Moderate-intensity examples. Walking briskly (3 miles/hour), water aerobics, tennis (doubles), ballroom dancing, general gardening.
           ii. Vigorous-intensity examples: Jogging, race-walking, swimming laps, tennis (singles), aerobic dancing, heavy gardening (continuous digging with increased heart rate), hiking uphill.
       (b) Exercise programs should include: Medically safe, enjoyable, convenient, structured, and realistic characteristics.
       (c) Review the importance of developing a daily routine that gradually increases intensity and/or builds in modifications to meet physical limitations.
       (d) Encourage follow-up with ongoing support and reinforcement for patients beginning a new regimen.
f. Sexually transmitted diseases (STDs) and HIV infection.
   (1) While substantial progress has been made in preventing, diagnosing, and treating certain STDs in recent years, STDs remain a major public health challenge in the U.S. The CDC (2008) estimates that 19 million new infections occur each year, almost half of them among young people ages 15–24. In addition to the physical and psychological effects of these diseases, a tremendous economic toll exists; it is estimated that direct medical costs associated with STDs in the U.S. are approximately $16 billion per year (CDC, 2008).
   (2) Topics to include in counseling.
       (a) Information about STD and/or HIV transmission.
       (b) Information about how to prevent STD and/or HIV infection.

(c) Risks of sex with partners who use injected drugs, multiple or anonymous sex partners, or STD-positive within the last 10 years, even if symptom-free.

(d) Health consequences of injection drug use, if indicated.

g. Smoking cessation.

(1) The 2010 Surgeon General's report on health consequences of smoking concluded that smoking harms nearly every organ in the body, causing diseases and reducing the health of smokers in general; smoking cigarettes with lower machine-measured yields of tar and nicotine provide no clear health benefit; even occasional smoking or secondhand smoke causes immediate damage to the body (DHHS, 2010b). Smoking causes more than 85% of lung cancers and can cause cancer almost anywhere in the body. The list of diseases caused by smoking has been expanded to include abdominal aortic aneurysm; acute myeloid leukemia; cataract; cervical, kidney, pancreatic, and stomach cancers; pneumonia; and periodontitis. Quitting smoking has immediate as well as long-term benefits, reducing risks of diseases caused by smoking and improving health in general. This last finding gives added importance to counseling on smoking cessation (DHHS, 2010b).

(2) Counseling strategies.

(a) Fiore and colleagues (2008) provided updates to the previous clinical practice pocket guide for smoking cessation. The following counseling strategies are based on the "5 As" approach to cessation intervention.

i. *Ask* about tobacco use at every visit.

ii. *Advise* tobacco users to quit. Use tailored materials, both print and Web-based, as well as self-help materials.

iii. *Assess* readiness to quit. If ready to quit, provide resources and assistance. If unwilling to quit, provide resources, help identify barriers, and use motivational intervention techniques.

iv. *Assist* tobacco users with a quit plan. Combine counseling and medication as a more effective approach. The plan should also include specific goals of setting a quit date; obtaining support from family, friends, and co-workers; and using past experiences to identify what worked and what did not. Provide advice on successful quitting, encourage the use of pharmacotherapy if not contraindicated, and provide resources.

v. *Arrange* for follow-up visits and provide information about appointments. If possible, make the appointment with the individual's input before leaving the clinic. If relapse occurs, encourage a repeat quit attempt; explain that relapse is part of the quitting process.

h. Unintended pregnancy.

(1) The CDC (2008) defines *unintended pregnancy* as a pregnancy either mistimed or unwanted at the

time of conception. Half of all pregnancies in the U.S. are unintended, and the U.S. has set a national goal of decreasing unintended pregnancies by 30% in the next few years (CDC, 2008).

    (a) The two groups of women with the highest percentages of unintended pregnancies were those younger than 18 years, and those 40 years of age or older (CDC, 2009a).

    (b) The main goal of counseling is to make sure family planning is a part of primary care for all sexually active patients.

(2) Topics to include in counseling.

    (a) Culturally and ethnically specific family planning.

    (b) Include topics specific to men's needs.

    (c) Explain forms of contraception and important characteristics of each.

    (d) Discuss contraceptive methods that provide protection against STDs and HIV infection. Stress use of two birth control forms, and condoms must be used if he or she is not in a mutually monogamous relationship with a person known to be infection-free.

    (e) Provide specific, in-depth information about the contraception method: How it works, theoretical vs. actual effectiveness, advantages, disadvantages, how to use the method, side effects, warning signs, and back-up methods.

    (f) Importance of early follow-up to evaluate the use of the method and to deal with any difficulties, misinformation and/or impediments to proper use.

i. Osteoporosis.

    (1) Osteoporosis is a slowly developing condition that causes loss of bone mass and fractures; 80% of the 10 million Americans with osteoporosis are women (National Osteoporosis Foundation [NOF], 2011). Of the individuals with hip fractures, 20% die within a year, while half of the survivors never walk again (Eldelman & Mandle, 2006).

    (a) Although osteoporosis is well-recognized and more common in women, 1 in 5 men over the age of 50 will experience an osteoporotic fracture. However, at one year post-fracture, the injury will result in almost twice the mortality as that which occurs in women (Bord-Hoffman & Donius, 2005).

    (b) Osteoporosis is largely preventable. The NOF (2011) recognizes several risk factors for osteoporosis: Increased age, female, Asian and Caucasian women, history of fracture, low body weight, smoking, use of oral corticosteroids for more than three months, estrogen deficiency before age 45, dementia, and poor health/frailty.

    (2) Topics to include in counseling.

        (a) Review daily-recommended calcium and Vitamin D, including nutrient-rich foods.

        (b) Discuss impact of smoking and excessive amounts of alcohol on bone health.

        (c) Point out importance of regular weight-bearing exercise.

        (d) Outline benefits and risks of hormone replacement therapy in menopausal women.

(e) Assess home safety for the prevention of falls. May need a social work consult or arrange a home visit.

(f) Review medications prescribed for the prevention/treatment of osteoporosis, as indicated.

References

Agency for Healthcare Research and Quality (AHRQ). (2009). *Health literacy measurement tools: REALM.* Retrieved from http://www.ahrq.gov/populations/sahlsatool.htm

Agency for Healthcare Research and Quality (AHRQ). (2011, September 20). *AHRQ initiative encourages two-way communication between clinicians and patients* [Press release]. Retrieved from http://www.ahrq.gov/news/press/pr2011/questionspr.htm

Alabama Coalition Against Domestic Violence (ACADV). (2011). *Dating violence.* Retrieved from http://www.acadv.org/dating.html#safety

American Academy of Ambulatory Care Nursing (AAACN). (2010a). *Conceptual framework for ambulatory care nursing: The role of the registered nurse in ambulatory care position statement.* Pitman, NJ: Author.

American Academy of Ambulatory Care Nursing (AAACN). (2010b). *Scope and standards of practice for professional ambulatory care nursing* (8th ed.). Pitman, NJ: Author.

American Academy of Pediatrics (AAP). (2008). *Recommendations for preventive pediatric health care: Committee on practice and ambulatory medicine and bright futures steering committee.* Retrieved from http://pediatrics.aappublications.org/content/120/6/1376.full.html

American Hospital Association (AHA). (2011). *The patient care partnership: Understanding expectations, rights and responsibilities.* Retrieved from http://www.aha.org/advocacy-issues/communicatingpts/pt-care-partnership.shtml

American Nurses Association (ANA). (2010). *Nursing scope and standards of practice* (2nd ed.). Silver Spring, MD: Author.

Baer, J.S. (2010). *Motivational interviewing in chronic care: A brief overview.* Retrieved from http://conferences.thehillgroup.com/obssr/di2008/02_Speaker%20Presentations/Concurrent%20Session%20II/CCII_Room%20C1C2_Baer_Think%20Tank.pdf

Bastable, S.B. (2008). *Nurse as educator: Principles of teaching and learning for nursing practice* (3rd ed.). Boston: Jones & Bartlett Publishers.

Bloom, B.S. (1956). *Taxonomy of educational objectives, handbook I: The cognitive domain.* New York: David McKay Company, Inc.

Bord-Hoffman, M.A., & Donius, M. (2005). Loss in height: When is it a problem? *ViewPoint, 27*(5), 1, 14-15.

Centers for Disease Control and Prevention (CDC). (2006). *Oral health for adults.* Retrieved from http://www.cdc.gov/oralhealth/publications/factsheets/adult.htm

Centers for Disease Control and Prevention (CDC). (2008). *Sexually transmitted disease surveillance.* Retrieved from http://www.cdc.gov/std/general/DSTDP-Strategic-Plan-2008.pdf

Centers for Disease Control and Prevention (CDC). (2009a). *Healthy youth: Sexual behaviors.* Retrieved from http://www.cdc.gov/healthyyouth/sexualbehaviors/

Centers for Disease Control and Prevention (CDC). (2009b). *School connectedness: Strategies for increasing protective factors among youth.* Atlanta: U.S. Department of Health and Human Services.

Centers for Disease Control and Prevention (CDC). (2009c). Youth risk behavior surveillance. *Morbidity and Mortality Weekly Report, 59*(SS-5), 1-142.

Centers for Disease Control and Prevention (CDC). (2010a). *Healthy youth: Injury and violence.* Retrieved from http://www.cdc.gov/healthyyouth/injury/facts.htm

Centers for Disease Control and Prevention (CDC). (2010b). *National Center for Injury Prevention and Control. Web-Based Injury Statistics Query and Reporting System (WISQARS).* Retrieved from http://www.cdc.gov/ncipc/wisqars.

Centers for Disease Control and Prevention (CDC). (2011a). *Body and mind (BAM!): Your life. Got butterflies?* Retrieved from http://www.bam.gov/sub_yourlife/index.html

Centers for Disease Control and Prevention (CDC). (2011b). *Obesity: Halting the epidemic by making health easier.* Retrieved from http://www.cdc.gov/chronicdisease/resources/publications/aag/obesity.html

Centers for Disease Control and Prevention (CDC). (2011c). *Oral health program: Strategic plan 2011-2014.* Retrieved from http://www.cdc.gov/OralHealth/pdfs/oral_health_strategic_plan.pdf

Centers for Medicare and Medicaid Services (CMS). (2011). *Quick reference information: Medicare preventive services.* Retrieved from http://www.cms.hhs.gov/MLNProducts/downloads/MPS_QuickReferenceChart_1.pdf

Commission on Chronic Illness. (1957). *Chronic illness in the United States: Chronic illness in a large city* (Vol. 4.). Cambridge, MA: Harvard University Press.

Dancel, R. (2009). *The teach-back method: One solution to improving health literacy.* Retrieved from http://www.prevention.va.gov/HealthPOWER_Prevention_News_Summer_2009_Prevention_Practice_and_Policy.asp

Dietary Guidelines Advisory Committee (DGAC). (2010). *Report of the Dietary Guidelines Advisory Committee on the dietary guidelines for Americans.* Retrieved from http://www.cnpp.usda.gov/dgas2010-dgacreport.htm

Edelman, C.L., & Mandle, C.L. (2006). *Health promotion through the lifespan* (6th ed.). St. Louis, MO: Mosby.

Egbert, N., & Nanna, K. (2009). Health literacy: Challenges and strategies. *The Online Journal of Issues in Nursing, 14*(3), 1.

Erikson, E.H. (1963). *Childhood and society* (2nd ed.). New York: Norton.

Fiore, M.C., Jaén, C.R., Baker, T.B., Bailey, W.C., Benowitz, N.L., Curry, S.J. …, Wewers, M.E. (2008, May). *Treating tobacco use and dependence: 2008 update. Clinical practice guideline.* Rockville, MD: U.S. Department of Health and Human Services.

Fishbein, M., & Ajzen, I. (1975). *Belief, attitude, intention, and behavior: An introduction to theory and research.* Reading, MA: Addison-Wesley Publishing Company.

Glanz, K., Rimer, B.K., & Lewis, F.M. (Eds.). (2008). *Health behavior and health education: Theory, research, and practice* (4th ed.). San Francisco: Jossey-Bass.

Institute of Medicine (IOM). (2004). *Health literacy: A prescription to end confusion*. Washington, DC: The National Academies Press.

Institute of Medicine (IOM). (2011a). *The future of nursing: Leading change, advancing health*. Washington, DC: The National Academies Press.

Institute of Medicine (IOM). (2011b). *Leading health indicators for Healthy People 2020: Letter report*. Washington, DC: The National Academies Press.

Joint Commission, The. (2007). *What did the doctor say?: Improving health literacy to protect patient safety*. Oakbrook Terrace, IL. Retrieved from http://www.jointcommission.org/assets/1/18/improving_health_literacy.pdf

Joint Commission, The. (2011). *Comprehensive accreditation manual for ambulatory care*. Oakbrook Terrace, IL.

Lowenstein, N. (2008). Teaching with groups. In A. Lowenstein (Ed.), *Teaching strategies for health education and health promotion: Working with patients, families, and communities* (pp. 129-139). Boston: Jones & Bartlett Publishers.

Miller, C. (2008). *The nurse's toolbook for promoting wellness* (1st ed.). Columbus, OH: McGraw-Hill.

Miller, C. (2012). *Nursing for wellness in older adults* (6th ed.). Philadelphia: Wolters Kluwer/Lippincott, Williams & Wilkins.

Miller, W.R. (1983). Motivational interviewing with problem drinkers. *Behavioural Psychotherapy, 11,* 147-172.

National Center for Education Statistics (NCES). (2007). *The health literacy of America's adults: Results from the 2003 National Assessment of Adult Literacy*. Washington, DC: U.S. Department of Education.

National Clearinghouse for Alcohol and Drug Information (NCADI). (2012). *Professional and research topics*. Retrieved from http://www.store.samhsa.gov/facet/Professional-Research-Topics

National Committee for Quality Assurance (NCQA). (2011). *Health plan accreditation requirements*. Washington, DC: Author. Retrieved from http://www.ncqa.org/tabid/1405/Default.aspx

National Institute of Mental Health (NIMH). (2011). *Depression and high school students*. Retrieved from http://www.nimh.nih.gov/health/publications/depression-and-high-school-students/depression-and-high-school-students.shtml

National Institute on Alcohol Abuse and Alcoholism (NIAAA). (2011). *The cool spot: Facts about alcohol*. Retrieved from http://www.thecoolspot.gov/facts.asp

National Institute on Drug Abuse (NIDA). (2009). *InfoFacts: Prescription and over-the-counter medications*. Bethesda, MD: NIDA, National Institutes of Health (NIH), & U.S. Department of Health and Human Services (DHHS). Retrieved from http://www.teens.drugabuse.gov/peerx/the-facts/prescription#faq

National Osteoporosis Foundation (NOF). (2011). *Fast facts*. Retrieved from http://www.nof.org/node/40

National Patient Safety Foundation (NPSF). (2011). *Ask me 3 presentation*. Retrieved from http://nchealthliteracy.uncg.edu/docs/askme3presentation.ppt

Nurss, J.R., Parker, R., Williams, M., & Baker, D. (2001). *TOFHLA: Test of functional health literacy in adults*. Snow Camp, NC: Peppercorn Books & Press.

Perper, K.B., Peterson, K., & Manlove, J. (2010). *Fact sheet: Diploma attainment among teen mothers*. Washington, DC: Child Trends. Retrieved from http://www.childtrends.org/files/child_trends-2010_01_22_FS_diploma attainment.pdf

Rape, Abuse and Incest National Network (RAINN). (2011). *Safety planning*. Retrieved from http://www.rainn.org/get-information/sexual-assault-prevention/safety-plan

Reed, P.G., & Shearer, N.C. (2009). *Perspectives on nursing theory* (5th ed.). Philadelphia: Lippincott, Williams & Wilkins.

Redman, B.K. (2007). *The practice of patient education: A case study approach* (10th ed.). St. Louis, MO: Mosby, Inc.

Rollnick, S., Butler, C.C., Kinnersley, P., Gregory, J., & Mash, B. (2010). Competent novice: Motivational interviewing. *British Medical Journal, 340,* c1900. Retrieved from http://www.stephenrollnick.com/index.php/all-commentary/69-motivational-interviewing-article-in-the-british-medical-journal

Schaefer, J., Miller, D., Goldstein, M., & Simmons, L. (2009). *Partnering in self-management support: A toolkit for clinicians*. Cambridge, MA: Institute for Healthcare Improvement.

Stedman, T.L. (2008). *Stedman's medical dictionary for the health professions and nursing*. Philadelphia: Wolters Kluwer Health/Lippincott, Williams & Wilkins.

U.S. Department of Health and Human Services (DHHS). (2008). *Physical activity guidelines for Americans*. Retrieved from http://www.health.gov/paguidelines/guidelines/default.aspx

U.S. Department of Health and Human Services (DHHS). (2010a). *The Affordable Care Act's new rules on preventive care and you*. Retrieved from http://www.healthcare.gov/news/factsheets/2010/07/preventive-care-and-you.html

U.S. Department of Health and Human Services (DHHS). (2010b). *Exposure to tobacco smoke causes immediate damage: Surgeon General (fact sheet)*. Retrieved from http://www.surgeongeneral.gov/library/tobaccosmoke/factsheet.html

U.S. Department of Health and Human Services (DHHS). (2011a). *Health literacy and health outcomes*. Retrieved from http://www.health.gov/communication/literacy/quickguide/factsliteracy.htm

U.S. Department of Health and Human Services (DHHS). (2011b). *Healthy people 2020*. Retrieved from http://odphp.osophs.dhhs.gov/

U.S. Preventive Services Task Force. (2010). *Guide to clinical preventive services, 2010–2011*. Retrieved from http://www.ahrq.gov/ clinic/pocketgd1011/

Weiss, B.D. (2007). *Health literacy and patient safety: Help patients understand. Manual for clinicians* (2nd ed.). Chicago: American Medical Association Foundation.

White, S. (2008). *Assessing the nation's health literacy: Key concepts and findings from the National Assessment of Adult Literacy (NAAL)*. Retrieved from http://www.ama-assn.org/ama1/pub/upload/mm/367/hl_report_2008.pdf

World Health Organization (WHO). (2009). *Milestones in health promotion: Statements from global conferences*. Retrieved from http://www.who.int/healthpromotion/en

Additional Readings

Cornett, S. (2009). Assessing and addressing health literacy. *OJIN: The Online Journal of Issues in Nursing, 14*(3). Retrieved from http://www.nursingworld.org/MainMenuCategories/ANAMarketplace/ANAPeriodicals/OJIN/TableofContents/Vol142009/No3Sept09/Assessing-Health-Literacy-.html

Learning Theories. (2011). *Erikson's stages of development.* Retrieved from http://www.learning-theories.com/eriksons-stages-of-development.html

Straus, S.E., Richardson, W.S., Glasziou, P., & Haynes, R.B. (2005). *Evidence-based medicine*: *How to practice and teach EBM* (3rd ed.). Edinburgh: Churchill Livingstone.

Chapter 17

Care of the Well Client: Screening and Preventive Care

Carol Jo Wilson, PhD, FNP-BC
Gail DeLuca, MS, FNP-BC

OBJECTIVES – *Study of the information in this chapter will enable the learner to:*

1. Explain the clinical guidelines for regular health screening.
2. Describe primary, secondary, and tertiary prevention.
3. Identify resources for a healthy diet and exercise guidelines.
4. Explain nutritional status assessment tools.
5. Identify resources for immunization education.
6. Describe methods of contraception, STD prevention and treatment, and abnormal Pap guidelines.

KEY POINTS – *The major points in this chapter include:*

1. Nurses in the 21st century will partner with individuals and families to focus on illness and injury prevention and health promotion.
2. Dietary changes that should be promoted include increasing intake of soluble fiber, plant sterols/stanols, whole grains, and fish, as well as decreasing intake of saturated fats, trans fats, cholesterol, sodium, and refined grains/sugars.
3. Lifestyle behaviors consisting of weight management, diet (as above), regular exercise, moderate caffeine intake, moderate to no alcohol intake, and smoking cessation should be stressed to help prevent certain cancers, diabetes, hypertension, and other chronic conditions.
4. Health care providers should regularly consult U.S. Preventive Services Task Force Screening guidelines to provide evidence-based nursing care.
5. Nurses should consult the CDC (www.cdc.gov/vaccines/schedules) for the latest recommendations for children, adolescents, and adults regarding protection from communicable diseases.

Health care in the United States is undergoing revolutionary changes at an increasingly accelerated pace. In the 19th century, health care focused on illnesses caused by unsanitary conditions and epidemics. As our agrarian culture became industrialized in the 20th century, the population looked first to employers and then to the government to provide basic necessities, such as health care. The 1960s saw the federal government addressing inequities in health care with the implementation of Medicare and Medicaid. In 2010, Congress passed the Patient Protection and Affordable Care Act (PPACA) to provide health care to an estimated 31 million uninsured Americans. Health care in the 21st century has become focused on illness and injury prevention and health promotion. The comprehensive plan for U.S. health care, *Healthy People 2020*, is aimed at increasing lifespan and access to preventive services while decreasing disparities in health in the United States (U.S. Department of Health and Human Services [DHHS], 2011). This chapter will present care of the well client and address current issues regarding primary, secondary, and tertiary prevention; child, adolescent, and adult screening; immunizations; prevention of pregnancy and sexually transmitted diseases (STDs); and protocols for the abnormal Pap test.

I. **Wellness, Health Promotion, and Disease Prevention**

A. Consumers are increasingly knowledgeable and interested in health promotion. The relationship between stress and illness, the importance of wellness care (rather than disease-focused care), and the need to treat the whole person are increasingly recognized as essential elements of health care in society today.

B. The family unit teaches health/illness beliefs, values, and behaviors. It is known that family functioning affects an individual's health, while an individual's lifestyle, practices, and health affect the family. Family systems are foundational for learning culture, values, and health, and these behaviors impact the health of each family member. Promotion of family health is important to society. By incorporating health promotion strategies within families, current problems may be averted and future problems alleviated. Nurses in ambulatory settings can positively influence the family's quality of life with health promotion.

C. Life-lengthening habits include:
1. Abstaining from tobacco use.
2. Consuming limited or no alcohol.
3. Sleeping 7–8 hours nightly.
4. Eating regular, frequent, nutritionally dense, small meals.
5. Eating breakfast daily.
6. Maintaining a normal weight.
7. Exercising moderately, 30 minutes most days of the week (DHHS, 2011).

II. **Primary, Secondary, and Tertiary Prevention**

A. Primary prevention includes health promotion and specific measures to keep people free from disease and injury.

B. Secondary prevention consists of early detection, diagnosis, and treatment.

C. Tertiary prevention includes recovery and rehabilitation, and specific measures to minimize disability and increase functioning.

D. The following example of smoking and lung cancer illustrates the three forms of prevention:

1. Primary prevention would be patient education about refraining from use of tobacco products.
2. Secondary prevention would be patient education about signs and symptoms of lung cancer or emphysema, smoking cessation information, and using cessation products/methods resulting in early diagnosis of disease.
3. Tertiary prevention would be smoking cessation and pulmonary rehabilitation.

III. **U.S. Preventive Services Task Force Recommendations**

The U.S. Preventive Services Task Force is a non-governmental expert panel of primary care, evidence-based medicine experts to review current preventive services and make practice recommendations. The Agency for Healthcare Research and Quality (AHRQ, 2010) supports the U.S. Preventive Services Task Force by providing administrative, technical, and research assistance. It publishes and circulates the U.S. Preventive Services Task Force recommendations for screenings and clinical preventive services, also providing the strength of these recommendations as guided by research (Trinite, Loveland-Cherry, & Marion, 2009). The categories of recommendation strength are classified as A, B, C, D, or I, incorporating research strength, as well as evaluation of risk vs. benefit.

A. Category A indicates the service; practice or screening is strongly recommended because beneficial health outcomes from screening are evident.

B. Category B indicates the service; practice or screening has fair evidence of improved health outcomes. In both categories A and B, benefit of the screening outweighs the risk incurred.

C. Category C practices also indicate fair evidence of benefit, but the risk involved in the screening vs. the benefit is increased. Therefore, recommendation for general screening is not justified. Some targeted patients, however, may benefit from the screening.

D. Category D practices indicate that the service or screening is either ineffective or that the harm exceeds any benefits; therefore, it recommends against the routine screening of asymptomatic patients.

E. Category I indicates the practice is inconclusive; either the strength of the recommendation is poor or conflicting data exist, and making a decision of benefit to harm is undeterminable (AHRQ, 2010).

IV. Adult Screening: Blood Pressure and Lipids

Poor control of blood pressure and dyslipidemia both have interrelated adverse effects on the cardiovascular system; thus, screening and treatment of these conditions will be discussed together. Guidelines for blood pressure and lipid management are under current review, and new guidelines are anticipated for publication in 2012. Blood pressure guidelines may be quickly accessed by performing an Internet search for Joint National Committee on Prevention, Detection, Evaluation, and Treatment of High Blood Pressure (JNC 8). New guidelines for high blood cholesterol are also expected for publication in 2012. These may be accessed by an Internet search for Adult Treatment Panel IV (ATP 4).

A. Blood pressure screening – Normal blood pressure in adults is defined as systolic measurements of less than 140 mmHg with diastolic measurements of less than 80 mmHg (National Heart, Lung, and Blood Institute (NHLBI, 2003).
   1. Currently in the U.S., of the 25% of adults with hypertension, only 25% are at or below this goal.
   2. As blood pressure increases, risk for cardiovascular, renal, and cerebral disease increases (NHLBI, 2003).
   3. Benefits of lowering blood pressure include reductions of stroke incidence by up to 40% and heart failure by greater than 50% (U.S. Preventive Services Task Force, 2007).
   4. Lifestyle and genetic predisposition are risk factors for hypertension.
B. Lipid screening – Hyperlipidemia or dyslipidemia refers to an elevation of any lipid in blood plasma. The association between hyperlipidema, hypertension, and cardiovascular disease is well documented (Ruixing et al., 2009).

1. Blood lipids can be fractionated into:
   a. Triglycerides.
   b. Total cholesterol (TC).
   c. High density lipoproteins (HDL).
   d. Low density lipoproteins (LDL).
   e. Very low density lipoproteins (VLDL).
2. HDLs are cardio-protective, and low levels are an independent cardiac risk factor.
3. Patients having both elevated cholesterol and hypertension have a 7–8 times greater risk of coronary heart disease and stroke.
4. Control of TC, as well as a reduction in LDL, has led to significant reductions in cardiovascular disease.

C. Risk factors in hypertension and dyslipidemia.
   1. Family history.
   2. Smoking.
   3. Sedentary lifestyle.
   4. Drinking alcohol excessively (more than 2 drinks per day for men, more than 1 drink per day for women).
   5. Being overweight.
   6. Having diabetes.
D. Excess sodium intake is associated with hypertension. Diets rich in saturated fats play a role in the development of both hypertension and dyslipidemia.
E. Normalizing risk indicators, such as hypertension and abnormal lipid profiles, contributes to the overall reduction of cardiovascular disease, because the greater the number of cardiovascular risk factors, the greater the probability of future disease (Lloyd-Jones, 2010).
F. Anatomy and physiology.
   1. Development of hypertension is a complex interplay of modulating factors and still remains poorly understood. Essential or idiopathic hypertension represents about 95% of all hypertension cases. Hypertension is categorized as essential when a secondary cause cannot be identified. Secondary hypertension has an identifiable cause and represents less than 5% of all hypertension cases. Stroke volume, heart rate, cardiac output, and peripheral vascular resistance all affect blood pressure (Riaz, 2011).

2. The body's baroreceptors, chemoreceptors, fluid status, renin-angiotensin system, and vascular autoregulation are control mechanisms of arterial blood pressure.
3. Different mechanisms for the development of hypertension have been described.
   a. While the actual cause remains unidentified, it is believed to be a result of environmental as well as genetic factors, including:
      (1) Increased angiotensin II.
      (2) Mineralocorticoid excess.
      (3) Salt sensitivity by the kidney.
      (4) Genetic predisposition (Riaz, 2011).
4. The left ventricle hypertrophies as a compensatory mechanism. As the left ventricle strains under greater pressures, the actual muscle cells of the left ventricle increase in size and/or number. The left ventricular wall thickens, and the cavity of the left ventricle may enlarge, causing poor left ventricular performance.
5. The vascular effects occur in all areas of the body, compromising blood flow and damaging the tissues over time. This effect can be seen especially in:
   a. Heart (hypertensive cardiomyopathy, congestive heart failure).
   b. Brain (stroke, vascular dementia).
   c. Kidneys (chronic renal insufficiency to end-stage renal disease).
6. While much of dyslipidemia is lifestyle-induced, other factors can contribute to its origin. Known potential causes of dyslipidemia include:
   a. Diabetes.
   b. Alcohol abuse.
   c. Hypothyroidism.
   d. Chronic renal insufficiency.
   e. Genetic factors.
   f. Some medications.
7. In dyslipidemia, increased levels of LDL incorporate themselves into fatty plaque developments on the intima, the inner layer of the blood vessel causing inflammation, plaque formation with fibrous cap overlay, subsequent blood vessel remodeling, and blood flow reductions to vital organs similar to the vessel and organ damage of hypertension (Fowler, Kelly, Ruh, & Johnson-Wells, 2007).

G. Metabolic syndrome is a constellation of cardiovascular risk factors that places patients at increased risk for all cardiovascular diseases. Patients are classified as having metabolic syndrome when they possess three or more of the following:
1. Waist circumference greater than or equal to 35 inches in women, or 40 inches in men.
2. Triglycerides greater than 150 mg/dl.
3. HDL cholesterol less than 50 in women, 40 in men.
4. Blood pressure greater than 130/85 mmHg.
5. Fasting glucose greater than 100 (American Heart Association, 2011).

H. Nursing assessment/screening recommendations.
1. Blood pressure (U.S. Preventive Services Task Force, 2007).
   a. Recommendation strength – A.
   b. Normotensive individuals – Every two years.
   c. Individuals with systolic blood pressure greater than 120 – At more frequent intervals.
2. Lipid screening (U.S. Preventive Services Task Force, 2008b).
   a. Recommendation strength – A.
   b. Optimal screening interval – Every five years, beginning at 20 years of age.
   c. Individuals whose lipid levels are elevated may be screened at closer intervals, depending on the cholesterol levels and presence or absence of other coronary artery disease risk factors.
3. Nursing history.
   a. Duration of hypertension and/or dyslipidemia.
   b. Co-morbid conditions.
      (1) Diabetes.
      (2) Gout.
      (3) Peripheral vascular disease.

(4) Renal disease.

(5) Sexual dysfunction.

c. Nutritional history. Dietary interventions are part of lifestyle management in the treatment of hypertension. The DASH Diet eating plan, sponsored by the National Institutes of Health (NIH) lowers blood pressure and endorses moderation of caffeine, alcohol, and sodium reduction. It also recommends greater intake of fruits and vegetables (NHLBI, 2006). Sodium intake is associated with hypertension. Some individuals are more sodium-sensitive and obtain greater degrees of blood pressure control with reductions in sodium intake (Kaplan, Bakris, & Forman, 2011b). When screening for hypertension, the following components are included in a comprehensive nutritional intake.

(1) Caffeine.

(2) Sodium.

(3) Alcohol.

(4) Fats.

(5) Fruits and vegetables.

d. Family history.

(1) Hypertension.

(2) Cardiovascular disease.

(3) Dyslipidemia.

(4) Stroke.

(5) Diabetes.

(6) Kidney disease.

e. Lifestyle questions.

(1) Smoking, including amount and number of years.

(2) Alcohol consumption as number of drinks per week/month.

(3) Patterns of exercise.

(4) Weight gain.

f. Medication.

(1) Prescription.

(2) Over-the-counter.

(3) Herbal preparations.

g. Psychosocial.

(1) Stress from work or family.

(2) Coping mechanisms.

4. Physical assessment.

a. Height, weight, body mass index, waist circumference.

(1) Abdominal fat is correlated with increased risk of cardiovascular disease.

(2) Body mass index (BMI) higher than 27 kg/m^2 is associated with elevations in blood pressure.

b. Blood pressure measurement.

(1) Description of blood pressure measurement is addressed in Chapter 14, "Nursing Process." Blood pressure must be confirmed on three separate visits to establish the diagnosis of hypertension.

(2) Ambulatory blood pressure monitoring.

(a) Necessary for evaluation of "white-coat" hypertension.

(b) Provides 24-hour information about blood pressure and variances.

(3) Self-measurement of blood pressure.

c. Heart.

(1) Rhythm, rate, and regularity.

(2) Abnormal sounds.

(a) Murmurs.

(b) Extra heart sounds (S3, S4).

d. Lungs: Auscultate for rales or wheezing.

e. Peripheral vascular.

(1) Carotid, abdominal, or femoral bruits.

(2) Edema of the lower extremities.

(3) Temperature or color changes of the lower extremities.

(4) Presence and quality of pulses.

5. Diagnostic studies.

a. Laboratory evaluation.

(1) Urinalysis.

(2) Blood glucose.

(3) Electrolytes.

(4) Lipid profile.

(5) Liver function tests if on lipid-lowering medication.

b. Optional laboratory tests.
   (1) Urine protein.
   (2) Urine albumin/creatinine ratio.
   (3) Urine microalbumin.
c. Optional diagnostic studies: Electrocardiogram for men over 40 years of age and women over 50 years of age.

I. Physiologic alterations.
   1. Clinical manifestations.
      a. Most patients are asymptomatic.
      b. May have morning occipital headache with hypertension.
      c. May have evidence of target organ damage (TOD).
         (1) Brain: TOD may be manifested with conditions such as dementia and stroke.
         (2) Kidneys: TOD in the kidneys may present as nephropathy and all stages of chronic kidney disease.
         (3) Heart: TOD of the heart includes left ventricular hypertrophy, myocardial remodeling, and heart failure.
         (4) Blood vessels: TOD to the blood vessles is diffuse, causing myocardial infarction, hypertensive retinopathy as well as other illnesses (Kaplan et al., 2011a).
   2. Lifestyle recommendations.
      a. Weight management. Caloric intake should approximate physical activity.
      b. Regular aerobic physical activity 30–45 minutes most days of the week.
      c. Alcohol intake less than two drinks per day.
      d. Tobacco cessation.
      e. Diet components.
         (1) Reduced intake of saturated fats, trans fats, and cholesterol and refined grains.
         (2) Increased intake of fish, whole grains, soluble fiber, and plant stanols/sterols (Centers for Disease Control and Prevention [CDC], 2011).

V. **Adult Screening: Cancer**
A. Overview.
   1. Certain cancers have a hereditary predisposition and increasing incidence with age. Consideration must be given to the age at which certain cancers become more prevalent, and screening should be tailored appropriately.
      a. In the age group 25–64 years, malignant neoplasms rank first in the leading causes of death followed by heart disease.
      b. In the age group older than 65 years, heart disease is the leading cause of death followed by malignant neoplasms (CDC, 2010b).
B. Anatomy and physiology.
   1. Cancers are a dysregulation of tissue growth in which cell growth and differentiation of cell tissue becomes abnormal. While most causes of cancer remain unknown, there are certain risk factors for cancer, including genetic predisposition, environmental toxins, obesity, excess sunlight, radiation, excess alcohol, and tobacco. The three most common cancers occurring in men are prostate, lung, and colon cancer, while in women, breast, colon, and lung cancer are most common (National Center for Biotechnology Information [NCBI], 2011).
C. Nursing assessment/monitoring.
   1. Nursing history.
      a. Any past medical history of cancer.
      b. Any family history of cancer.
      c. Lifestyle risk assessment.
         (1) Blood pressure.
         (2) Lipids.
         (3) Exercise.
         (4) Diet.
      d. Current chronic conditions.
      e. Any unintended weight loss.
      f. Fever, fatigue.
      g. Pain.
      h. Skin changes.
      i. Changes in bowel or bladder function.
      j. Lesions that change or do not heal.
      k. Thickening or a lump in the breast.

l. Indigestion, change in swallowing.

m. Nagging cough or hoarseness.

n. Change in bowel or bladder habits.

o. White patches in the mouth or on the tongue (American Cancer Society, 2010).

2. Physical examination – A thorough physical examination would be necessary to screen for all types of cancer.

D. Screening recommendations.

1. While not all U.S. Preventive Services Task Force recommendations merit a strong level-A recommendation, targeted screening may reduce morbidity and improve quality of life for some individuals. Release date of recommendations vary as the evidence receives comprehensive review cyclically or when a major change is suggested by new research findings.

a. Cancer (U.S. Preventive Services Task Force, 2011a).

(1) Bladder cancer (U.S. Preventive Services Task Force, 2011b).

(a) Increased incidence among smokers.

(b) The U.S. Preventive Services Task Force recommends against routine screening.

(c) Strength of recommendation: D.

(2) Breast cancer (U.S. Preventive Services Task Force, 2010a).

(a) The U.S. Preventive Services Task Force recommends mammography every 2 years for women ages 50–74 years old.

(b) Strength of recommendation: B.

(c) Insufficient evidence in screening women older than 75 years.

(d) Strength of recommendation: I

(3) Cervical cancer (U.S. Preventive Services Task Force, 2012).

(a) The U.S. Preventive Services Task Force recommends cervical cancer screening in women with a cervix every 3 years from the age of 21 through 65.

(b) Screening intervals may be lengthened to every 5 years for women from age 30 through 65 by using both cytology and human papillomavirus (HPV) testing.

(c) Strength of recommendation: A.

(d) Recommendation against routine Pap screening in women older than 65 years if previous Pap screens were normal and in women who have had a hysterectomy for benign disease.

(4) Colorectal cancer (U.S. Preventive Services Task Force, 2009c).

(a) The U.S. Preventive Services Task Force strongly recommends screening of both men and women ages 50–75.

(b) Strength of recommendation: A.

(c) Screening options:

i. Fecal occult blood testing (FOBT) annually.

ii. Flexible sigmoidoscopy every 5 years with high sensitivity FOBT every 3 years.

iii. Colonoscopy every 10 years.

(d) Screening earlier than 50 years may be reasonable in persons with greater risk, such as those with a family history of colorectal cancer in a first-degree relative.

(e) Screening intervals should be individualized in persons ages 76–85.

(f) Strength of recommendation: C.

(g) Evidence is insufficient to recommend use of CT colonography or fecal DNA testing.

(5) Lung cancer (U.S. Preventive Services Task Force, 2011a).
    (a) The U.S. Preventive Services Task Force has insufficient evidence to recommend screening for lung cancer in asymptomatic persons.
    (b) Strength of recommendation: I.

(6) Ovarian cancer (U.S. Preventive Services Task Force, 2011a).
    (a) The U.S. Preventive Services Task Force recommends against routine screening.
    (b) Strength of recommendation: D.
    (c) No evidence exists that earlier diagnosis reduces mortality.

(7) Pancreatic cancer (U.S. Preventive Services Task Force, 2011a).
    (a) The U.S. Preventive Services Task Force recommends against routine screening in asymptomatic adults.
    (b) Strength of recommendation: D.

(8) Prostate cancer (U.S. Preventive Services Task Force, 2011a).
    (a) The U.S. Preventive Services Task Force finds evidence insufficient to recommend for or against routine prostate specific antigen (PSA) or digital rectal examination.
    (b) Strength of recommendation: I.
    (c) Benefit-to-harm ratio is uncertain.
    (d) If screening is desired, screening should target men 50–70 years of age with average risk, or men over age 45 with increased risk.

(e) Older men or those with a life expectancy of less than 10 years of age may not benefit from screening.
(f) Increased death from prostate cancer occurs in older men, African American men, and men with family histories of prostate cancer.
(g) Men should be advised about evidence gaps and be encouraged to make shared decisions with their health care provider.

(9) Skin cancer (U.S. Preventive Services Task Force, 2011a).
    (a) The U.S. Preventive Services Task Force finds evidence insufficient to recommend for or against routine counseling to prevent skin cancer.
    (b) The U.S. Preventive Services Task Force finds evidence insufficient to recommend for or against routine skin cancer screening utilizing a total body skin examination.
    (c) Strength of recommendation: I.

(10) Testicular cancer (U.S. Preventive Services Task Force, 2011a).
    (a) The U.S. Preventive Services Task Force does not recommend routine screening in asymptomatic adolescent or adult males.
    (b) Strength of recommendation: D.
    (c) No evidence exists to confirm that teaching testicular self-exam improves health outcomes.

VI. Adult Screening: Vision and Hearing

A. Overview.
   1. In the aging adult, both central acuity and peripheral vision may be diminished.
      a. Presbyopia, or difficulty with near vision, occurs as early as 40-years-old.

As individuals age, more light is necessary to see due to poorer adaptation to darkness.

b. Refractive errors, such as myopia, hyperopia, presbyopia, anisometropia, and astigmatism, can be corrected with glasses or contact lenses.

c. The incidence of cataracts, glaucoma, and macular degeneration increases with age.

d. Open-angle glaucoma affects more than two million individuals in the U.S. Without treatment, it can gradually reduce peripheral visual fields and cause blindness (National Eye Institute, 2004).

e. Macular degeneration is a loss of central vision and is the most common cause of blindness.

2. Hearing loss commonly occurs in the aging population because of reduced sound wave transmission due to increasing stiffening of cilia motion in the ear canal or by gradual nerve degeneration in the inner ear. Individuals may begin to notice these changes in their fifth decade. Previous lifestyle or environmental factors, such as chronic exposure to noise pollution or previous ear infections, can also contribute to hearing loss in older adults (Jarvis, 2007).

B. Anatomy and physiology.
   1. Glaucoma: Most common is open-angle where there is an obstruction to the outflow of aqueous humor from the anterior to posterior chamber. This results in increased intraocular pressure, damaging the optic nerve and causing loss of peripheral vision, eye pain, and redness. Other less common forms are low-tension (normal-tension), angle-closure (medical emergency), congenital, and secondary.
   2. Cataract: Opacification of the lens resulting in diminished vision, poor night vision, and sensitivity to glare.
   3. Age-related macular degeneration (AMD): Can be wet (abnormal blood vessels behind the retina grow and leak) or dry (light-sensitive cells in the macula slowly break down).

C. Nursing assessment/monitoring.
   1. Vision history (Jarvis, 2007).
      a. Eye pain.
      b. Double vision.
      c. Redness, swelling, or watering.
      d. Vision difficulty.
         (1) Visual acuity, blurred vision.
         (2) Halos or blind spots.
         (3) Night blindness.
         (4) Unilateral or bilateral.
         (5) Gradual or sudden.
      e. Past history of:
         (1) Ocular problems.
         (2) Cataracts.
         (3) Glaucoma.
         (4) Macular degeneration.
         (5) Hypertension.
         (6) Diabetes.
         (7) Trauma to the eye.
      f. Use of corrective lenses or contacts.
      g. Last eye examination.
   2. Hearing history (Jarvis, 2007).
      a. Ear pain.
      b. Ringing.
      c. Past ear infections.
      d. Discharge.
      e. Hearing loss.
         (1) Onset.
         (2) Ask if it is worse with background noise.
      f. Environmental noise exposure.
      g. Vertigo.
      h Last hearing examination.
   3. Physical assessment of vision (Jarvis, 2007).
      a. Snellen chart or Snellen E chart.
         (1) Provides assessment of visual acuity.
         (2) Vision may be examined with corrective lenses or contacts.
         (3) Each eye is tested individually at a distance of 20 feet.
      b. Jaeger card.
         (1) Tests for near vision.
         (2) Each eye is tested individually at a distance of 14 inches.
         (3) Vision may be examined with corrective lenses or contacts.

c. Amsler grid.
  (1) Tests for macular degeneration.
  (2) Vision may be examined with corrective lenses or contacts.
  (3) Each eye is tested individually.
  (4) While looking at the center dot, surrounding lines should appear straight.
  (5) Amsler Web site (www.amd.org) (Macular Degeneration Partnership, 2012).
4. Physical examination of hearing.
  a. Note if the individual is lip reading, asks to repeat, misunderstands questions, and/or turns a favored ear to hear.
  b. Whispered hearing test.
    (1) Have the person occlude one ear.
    (2) Whisper a two-syllable word, standing 3 feet behind the person on the unoccluded side.
  c. Otoscopic examination for cerumen occlusion.
D. Screening recommendations (U.S. Preventive Services Task Force, 2009d).
  1. Hearing.
    a. Routine screening for asymptomatic adults is not recommended.
    b. Screening of older adults for hearing impairment is recommended by:
      (1) Asking them about their hearing.
      (2) Educating about hearing aid devices.
      (3) Referrals, as needed.
  2. Vision.
    a. The U.S. Preventive Services Task Force (2009d) finds evidence insufficient for or against screening for glaucoma in adults.
    b. Strength of recommendation: I.
    c. The U.S. Preventive Services Task Force (2009d) finds evidence insufficient for or against screening for visual acuity in older adults.
    d. Strength of recommendation: I.

VII. Adult Body Measurement

A. Overview.
  1. Body measurements yield some objective measures of nutritional status. Nutritional screening can be done quickly and easily by evaluating an individual's:
    a. Height.
    b. Weight.
    c. Weight history.
    d. Diet history.
    e. Food preferences.
    f. Nutritional risk factors for patterns for under-nutrition or over-nutrition.
  2. If nutritional risk is identified through screening, obtain a full nutritional assessment including:
    a. History.
    b. Physical examination, including body measurements, oral cavity, and teeth.
    c. Examination for any clinical signs of adequate or altered nutrition.
    d. Laboratory evaluation may be warranted (Jarvis, 2007).
  3. Nutritional status reflects the balance between the intake of essential nutrients and the body's metabolic requirements for basic needs, plus activity and growth or healing.
  4. Under-nutrition occurs when the nutrient intake does not meet these needs; thus, nutritional stores are exhausted over time.
  5. Over-nutrition, a condition far more prevalent in the U.S., is an imbalance in nutrients where nutrient requirements are exceeded by an excess of food intake. Frequently, this excess consists of calories dense in fats, sugars, and sodium, but not dense in nutrients.
  6. Obesity affects approximately one-third of the American population and is a growing epidemic.
  7. Obesity is classified by body mass index (BMI) according to the World Health Organization (WHO).
    a. Desirable body weight: BMI of 18.5–24.9.
    b. Class I Obesity (overweight): BMI of 25–29.9.

c. Class II Obesity (obese): BMI of 30–39.9.

d. Class III Obesity (severe or morbid obesity): BMI over 40.

8. Obesity affects:
   a. Both genders.
   b. All age groups, though incidence increases with age.
   c. All socioeconomic statuses, though it has a disproportionate prevalence among certain ethnic groups and lower socioeconomic levels.

9. Obesity is a chronic disorder with multifactorial etiologies and is a risk factor for other disorders, including:
   a. Degenerative joint disease.
   b. Hypercholesterolemia.
   c. Type 2 diabetes mellitus.
   d. Hypertension.
   e. Heart disease.

10. Measurements defining obesity include:
    a. Body weight 120% of ideal.
    b. BMI equal to or greater than 30 (CDC, 2010a).
    c. Adipose deposition patterns.
    d. Percent body fat for men greater than 25% or over 33% for women.
    e. Anthropometric measurements.
       (1) Skin thickness measured in the triceps, biceps, suprailiac, or subscapular areas.
       (2) Waist or hip circumference.

11. Adequate nutrition is crucial to the maintenance of health and prevention of major chronic diseases. This is achieved by caloric intake to match nutritional needs from the five basic food groups, as well as regular exercise. The five food groups include:
    a. Bread, cereal, rice, and pasta group (5–11 servings per day).
    b. Vegetable group (3–5 servings per day.
    c. Fruit group (2–4 servings per day).
    d. Milk, yogurt, and cheese group (2–3 servings per day).
    e. Meat, poultry, fish, dry beans, eggs, and nuts group (2–3 servings per day).

f. Fats, oils, and sweets are to be used sparingly (U.S. Department of Agriculture [USDA], 2010).

12. Optimal health benefits occur from regular exercise most days per week completed in either 30 minutes of continuous activity or an accumulation of 30 minutes daily in divided activity. Both aerobic weight-bearing exercises as well as strengthening resistance exercises contribute to cardiovascular health, maintenance of ideal body weight, and prevention of bone demineralization with resultant osteoporosis. Endurance for aerobic types of activities can be initiated at any age and increased gradually over time; it provides excellent benefits to all age groups (National Institutes of Health [NIH], 2010).

13. The USDA (2010) food plate graphic, MyPlate.gov, provides a visual key to the proper dietary balance of the five food groups. Proper adaptation of the food plate into eating habits necessitates understanding of portion or serving size. In order for patients to familiarize themselves with proper portion size, food measurement may be utilized until visual estimation of portion sizes can be established.

14. The USDA (2010) recommends a minimum daily consumption of the following:
    a. Three- to four-ounce equivalents of grain foods per day, with 50% from whole-grain products.
    b. One-half to two cups of fruit and two to three cups of vegetables daily.
    c. Three cups per day of fat-free or low-fat milk or milk products, especially for adolescents, and pregnant or postmenopausal women.

15. The following is generally recommended:
    a. Maintenance of ideal body weight (IBW).
    b. Accurate interpretation of food label content.
    c. Balanced dietary intake following www.choosemyplate.gov.
    d. Regular exercise to increase caloric demand, lessen bone demineralization, and prevent lean tissue loss.

16. General dietary guidelines:
    a. Nutrient-dense, low-calorie, high-fiber foods.
    b. Water according to the individual's needs, gauged by thirst. Water is an essential nutrient, but most get sufficient water from all fluids and water-dense foods (USDA, 2011).
    c. Increasing sources of complex carbohydrates (without added sugar or fat).
    d. Slowly increasing fiber between 25 and 30 grams per day.
    e. Limiting sources of concentrated sugars.
    f. Limiting fat intake to less than 30% of the total calories.
17. Refer to www.choosemyplate.gov for individualized diet and exercise plans.

B. Nursing assessment/monitoring.
    1. Nursing history.
        a. Weight milestones, including weight in late childhood, high school and college graduation, marriage, and pre- and post-pregnancies.
        b. Diet history including 24-hour food recall.
        c. Past-dieting history and results.
        d. Family history of obesity, diabetes, cardiovascular disease, and sudden death.
        e. Amount and type of physical activity weekly.
        f. Psychosocial history including stressors and coping mechanisms.
            (1) Identification of maladaptive behaviors contributing to over- or under-nutrition.
                (a) Food as a coping mechanism.
                (b) Food as a reward.
                (c) Food as entertainment.
            (2) Identification of environmental cues to eat.
        g. Sleep apnea and snoring.
        h. Medications, tobacco, and alcohol use.
    2. Physical assessment.
        a. Height and weight. Review the record for weight history over the past 6 months and past year, noting any patterns/trends.
        b. Ideal body weight is based on the 1983 Metropolitan Life Insurance Tables (Health Check Systems, 2012).
        c. Percent ideal body weight = Current weight ÷ Ideal weight X 100.
            (1) 80–90% of ideal body weight indicates mild malnutrition.
            (2) Greater than 120% ideal body weight is obesity.
        d. Percent usual body weight = Current weight ÷ Usual weight X 100. Significant weight loss is unintentional weight loss of more than 5% over 1 month, 7.5% over 3 months, or more than 10% over 6 months (Jarvis, 2007).
        e. BMI = Weight (kilograms) ÷ Height (meters)^2, or Weight (pounds) ÷ Height (inches)^2 X 703.
            (1) BMI less than 18.5 is underweight, 18.5–24.9 is normal weight, 25.0–29.9 is overweight, 30.0–39.9 is obesity, greater than 40 is extreme obesity (CDC, 2010a).
            (2) BMI may overestimate body fat in people with muscular builds.
            (3) BMI may underestimate body fat in people who have diminished muscle mass or older persons.
        f. Waist-hip ratio (WHR) = Abdominal girth ÷ Hip circumference.
            (1) Values greater than 1.0 for men or 0.8 for women indicate upper body obesity.
            (2) Upper body obesity predicts future risk of diabetes, hypertension, heart disease, and stroke.
        g. Waist circumference.
        h. Desirable body weights (University of Washington, 2011).
            (1) Men: 106 pounds plus 6 pounds for each inch of height over 5 feet.

(2) Women: 100 pounds plus 5 pounds for each inch of height over 5 feet.
   i. Bioelectric impedance analysis measures both fat and lean body mass.
3. Diagnostic studies.
   a. Fasting lipid profile.
   b. Fasting glucose.
   c. Comprehensive metabolic profile.
   d. Thyroid studies.
C. Physiologic alterations.
   1. Clinical manifestations.
      a. Fatigue.
      b. Decreased energy.
      c. Weakness.
      d. Joint pain.
      e. Depression.
      f. Weight gain.
   2. Common therapeutic modalities.
      a. Nursing interventions.
         (1) Identification of at-risk individuals.
         (2) Obesity prevention counseling for non-obese family members.
         (3) Nutritional and weight trend screening.
         (4) Encouragement of lifestyle changes including physical activity.
         (5) Follow general dietary guidelines.
         (6) Create a partnership with the individual.
            (a) Mutually set achievable goals.
            (b) Help the individual modify problem behaviors.
         (7) Referral to appropriate support groups.
   3. Continued care and rehabilitation.
      a. Emphasize that proper body composition results from daily strategies.
      b. Emphasize the pitfalls of perfectionism.
D. Pharmacologic interventions. In addition to the following interventions, behavioral change is paramount for permanent results. Many antidepressants affect appetite. Up to 25% of patients will experience varying amounts of weight gain on selective serotonin reuptake inhibitors (SSRIs). Behavioral modification may help patients stay weight neutral.

1. Weight loss.
   a. Antidepressants (partial list).
      (1) SSRIs (most common).
         (a) Sertraline (Zoloft®).
         (b) Paroxetine (Paxil®).
         (c) Fluoxetine (Prozac®).
         (d) Citalopram (Celexa®).
         (e) Escitalopram (Lexapro®).
      (2) Serotonin norepinephrine reuptake inhibitors (SNRIs).
         (a) Venlafaxine (Effexor®).
         (b) Duloxetine (Cymbalta®).
      (3) Side effects (partial list) include nausea, nervousness, fatigue, and orgasmic dysfunction.
      (4) Contraindicated within 14 days of MAO inhibitor.
      (5) Bupropion (Wellbutrin®).
         (a) Atypical antidepressant.
         (b) May be used with SSRIs or SNRIs.
         (c) Side effects (partial list) include insomnia, dry mouth, headache, and seizures.
   b. Anti-obesity drugs.
      (1) Phentermine.
         (a) Sympathomimetic recommended for short-term use only.
         (b) Adverse effects include tachycardia, insomnia, change in libido, dizziness, dry mouth, and headache. May increase blood pressure or cause psychosis.
      (2) Orlistat.
         (a) Blocks fat absorption in the intestine.
         (b) Available by prescription as Xenical® or over the counter as Alli®.
         (c) Side effects include oily stains on the underwear, rectal urgency or incontinence, abdominal pain.
         (d) Patients lose an average of 2–3 kg more per year than with diet and exercise modifications alone.

c. Bariatric surgical interventions (American Society for Metabolic and Bariatric Surgery [ASMBS], 2004).
   (1) Must meet medical criteria.
   (2) Restrictive procedures limit the size of the gastric pouch.
      (a) Laparoscopic adjustable gastric banding.
      (b) Vertical banded gastroplasty.
   (3) Malabsorptive procedures diminish nutrient absorption.
      (a) Biliopancreatic diversion.
      (b) Duodenal switch.
   (4) Combination restrictive and malabsorptive.
      (a) Roux gastric bypass in combination with vertical banded gastroplasty.
2. Weight gain.
   a. Antidepressants.
      (1) SSRIs.
      (2) SNRIs.
   b. Other medications, such as mirtazapine (Remeron®), are sometimes used because weight gain is a common side effect of these drugs.

VIII. Adult Immunization

A. Overview.
   1. In contrast to childhood immunizations, which are required by law (unless exempt for religious or medical reasons), immunization of adults is voluntary. Health professionals should routinely review each adult's immunization status annually to reduce risks of communicable diseases. Middle-aged and older adults may have had actual diseases, such as varicella, measles, and mumps. Detailed histories must be obtained for immigrants because vaccine type, schedules, and/or disease exposure vary from country to country. With this understanding, the health care provider should inquire about both immunization status and past occurrence of actual diseases.
B. Nursing assessment/monitoring.

1. Nursing history: Immunization. Refer to the CDC (2012c) for most recent guidelines and updates.
   a. Influenza: Date of last immunization.
      (1) Annually for all adults, including pregnant women.
      (2) Live vaccine (FluMist®) may be given to healthy, non-pregnant adults free of chronic illness up through age 49; otherwise, inactivated vaccine is recommended.
      (3) High-dose influenza (Fluzone High-Dose®) is optional for those 65 years and older.
   b. Pneumococcal Polysaccharide vaccine (PPSV): Date of last immunization.
      (1) Recommended for those 19–64 years of age in one of the following risk groups:
         (a) Persons with medical or occupational indications, residents of nursing homes or long-term care facilities, or smokers.
         (b) Household contacts of persons with indications.
         (c) Those who have serious long-term health problems, such as chronic cardiovascular, renal, liver, and lung disease (including asthma); sickle cell disease; alcoholism; leaks of cerebrospinal fluid; diabetes; or liver cirrhosis.
         (d) Those whose resistance to infection is lowered due to Hodgkin's disease, multiple myeloma, cancer treatment with X-rays or drugs, treatment with long-term steroids, bone marrow or organ transplant, kidney failure, HIV/AIDS, nephrotic syndrome, damaged spleen or no spleen, and lymphoma, leukemia, or other cancers.
      (2) Those age 65 and older.

(3) One dose with a second dose in 5 years for those at risk.

c. Tetanus/diphtheria/acellular pertussis (Td/Tdap): Date of last immunization. Substitute a single dose of Tetanus Toxoid, Reduced Diphtheria Toxoid, and Acellular Pertussis Vaccine (Tdap) for adults to replace a single dose of Td booster, then boost with Td every ten years.

d. Hepatitis B (HBV): Give or complete a 3-dose series of hepatitis B vaccine to those persons not fully vaccinated (series of 3 doses at 0, 1, and 6 months): Dates of initial immunization or results of titer.

    (1) Recommended for:

        (a) Sexually active persons not in a long-term, mutually monogamous relationship; persons seeking evaluation or treatment of STDs; current or recent injection-drug users; men who have sex with men.

        (b) Health care personnel and other public safety workers who are exposed to blood or other potentially infectious body fluids.

        (c) Persons with end-stage renal disease (including those on hemodialysis), persons with HIV infection or chronic liver disease.

        (d) Household contacts and sex partners of persons with chronic HBV infection, clients and staff members of institutions for persons with developmental disabilities and international travelers to countries with high or intermediate prevalence of chronic HBV infection (check http://www.nc.cdc.gov/travel/).

        (e) Persons present in any testing/treatment facility for conditions stated above.

        (f) All previously unvaccinated adults ages 19 through 59 years with diabetes mellitus (Type 1 and Type 2) as soon as possible after a diagnosis of diabetes is made (recommendation category A) (CDC, 2011).

e. Hepatitis A: Series of 2 doses; one at initial injection and the second dose after 6–12 months.

    (1) Date of last immunization.

    (2) Completion of the series.

    (3) 19 years of age and older: Only indicated for persons with medical, behavioral, occupational, travel to countries where hepatitis A is endemic, or other indications.

f. Measles, mumps, rubella (MMR). This is a live vaccine.

    (1) Determine if the patient has had past history of these diseases. Adults born before 1957 are considered immune. Those born in 1957 or later need documentation of one or more doses of MMR, unless there is a medical contraindication, titer demonstrating immunity, or documentation of provider-diagnosed measles or mumps. Documentation of rubella by a provider is not sufficient.

    (2) Date of last immunization, if applicable.

    (3) Any past blood titers drawn.

    (4) Age 19–49 years: 1–2 doses, if the individual:

        (a) Lacks documentation of vaccination.

        (b) Has no prior history of disease.

        (c) Second dose is administered a minimum of 28 days after the first dose.

    (5) Age 50 or older: 1 dose if other risk factors are present.

(6) Contraindicated in pregnant women or women planning to become pregnant in the next 4 weeks.

(7) Contraindicated in long-term immunosuppressive therapy or people who are severely immunosuppressed.

g. Varicella. This is a live vaccine. All adults without evidence of immunity to varicella should receive two doses of single-antigen varicella vaccine if not previously vaccinated or the second dose (if they only need one), unless they have a medical contraindication. Ask about:

(1) Any past history of chicken pox.

(2) Date of last immunization, if applicable.

(3) Any past blood titers drawn.

(4) 19 years of age and older: 2 doses – Initial and at 4–8 weeks, if the individual:

    (a) Lacks documentation of vaccination.

    (b) Has no prior history of disease.

(5) 50 years of age and older; 19 years of age and older: 2 doses – Initial and at 4–8 weeks, if some other risk factor is present.

(6) Contraindicated in pregnant women or women planning to become pregnant in the next 4 weeks, and in persons with severely depressed immune systems.

h. Meningococcal conjugate vaccine (MCV4).

(1) One dose for persons with medical or other indications.

    (a) Persons without a spleen.

    (b) Adults with HIV should receive a 2-dose series even if prior vaccination.

    (c) Certain occupational exposures.

    (d) As indicated for travel.

(2) All unvaccinated college freshmen living in dorms (MCV4 or MPSV4, meningococcal polysaccharide vaccine).

i. Human papillomavirus vaccine: Given in three doses (second dose 1–2 months after first, third dose 6 months after first dose). Vaccines are HPV4 (Types 6, 11, 16, and 18) or HPV2 (Types 16 and 18).

(1) Recommended for females at ages 11–12 years and catch-up vaccinations for females at 13–26 years of age.

(2) Males ages 9–26 may receive HPV4.

j. Herpes zoster vaccine: One dose. Recommended at age 60 or older regardless of prior episodes of herpes zoster.

2. Nursing interventions.

a. Monitor for any adverse reactions.

b. Report vaccine reactions to Vaccine Adverse Event Reporting System (VAERS) at www.vaers.hhs.gov or 800-822-7967.

IX. Adult Aspirin Prophylaxis

A. Overview.

1. Aspirin therapy has been used for some time in persons with known coronary heart disease, but only recently has been approved for primary prevention of cardiovascular events. Cardiovascular disease, including stroke, coronary artery disease, and peripheral vascular disease, is a leading cause of morbidity and mortality in the U.S., claiming 194 lives per 100,000 people with an estimated cost in excess of $145 billion annually (Hayden, Pignone, Phillips, & Mulrow, 2002). Based on the evidence review of Hayden and colleagues (2002), the U.S. Preventive Services Task Force concluded that aspirin chemoprophylaxis decreases incidence rates of coronary heart disease in adults at risk and should be offered as the primary prevention of cardiovascular events. Because aspirin is known to increase risk of

gastrointestinal bleed and hemorrhagic stroke, the benefit-to-risk ratio is too low to recommend to all adults.

B. Screening.
1. The U.S. Preventive Services Task Force strongly recommends that clinicians discuss both potential benefits and harms of aspirin chemoprophylaxis with adults who are at increased risk for coronary heart disease.
2. Strength of recommendation: A.
3. Persons to consider aspirin therapy (U.S. Preventive Services Task Force, 2012).
   a. Men ages 45–79.
   b. Post-menopausal women, ages 55–79.
   c. Younger adults with risk factors for coronary heart disease.
      (1) Diabetes.
      (2) Hypertension.
      (3) Smoking.

C. Nursing history.
1. Ask about past medical history of:
   a. Heart disease.
   b. Stroke.
   c. Peripheral vascular disease.
   d. Dyslipidemia.
   e. Hypertension.
   f. Diabetes.
   g. Rectal bleeding.
   h. Gastric bleeding.
   i. Smoking.
2. Family history of heart disease, stroke, peripheral vascular disease, dyslipidemia, hypertension, and diabetes.
3. Nutritional history.
   a. Intake of caffeine.
   b. Sodium.
   c. Alcohol.
   d. Fats.
   e. Fiber.
4. Lifestyle questions.
   a. Smoking, including amount and number of years.
   b. Alcohol consumption as number of drinks per week/month.
   c. Patterns of exercise.
   d. Weight gain.
5. Medication.
   a. Prescription.
   b. Over-the-counter.
   c. Herbal preparations.
6. Psychosocial.
   a. Stress from work or family.
   b. Coping mechanisms.

D. Physical assessment.
1. Height, weight, BMI, waist circumference.
   a. Abdominal fat is correlated with increased risk of cardiovascular disease.
   b. BMI higher than 27 is associated with elevations in blood pressure.
2. Blood pressure measurement: See *Blood Pressure and Lipid Screening* in the *Adult Screening* section of this chapter.
3. Heart.
   a. Rhythm, rate, and regularity.
   b. Abnormal sounds.
      (1) Murmurs.
      (2) Extra heart sounds (S3, S4).
4. Lungs: Auscultate for rales or wheezing.
5. Neurological examination.
6. Abdomen.
   a. Masses, abnormal pulsations.
   b. Stool hemoccult for occult bleeding.
7. Peripheral vascular: Carotid, abdominal, or femoral bruits.

E. Diagnostic studies.
1. Stool hemoccult for gastrointestinal bleeding.
2. Complete blood count may be indicated.

F. Physiologic alterations.
1. Clinical manifestations.
   a. Most are asymptomatic.
   b. Some may complain of gastric upset.
2. Common therapeutic modalities.
   a. The U.S. Preventive Services Task Force (2009a) recommends use of aspirin for stroke prevention in women ages 55–79 and for myocardial infarction protection in men ages 45–79 when potential benefits outweigh potential harm due to an increase in gastrointestinal hemorrhage.
   b. Incidence of gastrointestinal bleeding is higher in older adults.

c. Some clinicians may add a proton pump inhibitor to the medication regime for gastric protection.

G. Pharmacotherapeutics: Aspirin.
1. Classification: Nonsteroidal anti-inflammatory drug (NSAID).
2. Route of administration: Usually by mouth. Rectal suppositories are available.
3. Adverse effects: Gastrointestinal bleed, ulcer, or perforation; angioedema; anaphylaxis; prolonged bleeding time; gastric upset; nausea; dyspepsia; abdominal pain (partial list).
4. Contraindicated with MMR vaccine, varicella vaccine; and use with other NSAIDS. Causes gastrointestinal bleed (partial list).

X. **Adult and Adolescent Screening: Pap Smears, Sexually Transmitted Diseases, Pregnancy Prevention**
A. Overview.
1. The scope of ambulatory women's health care offers opportunities to provide individualized, comprehensive nursing care to women of all ages from the onset of menses through the completion of menopause. Many women see only their obstetrics and gynecology provider for health care during their childbearing years. However, women also need information about cancer warning signs, adult immunizations, Papanicolaou (Pap) smears, blood pressure, sexually transmitted disease (STD) prevention, and additional health promotion information. Professional nurses in women's health care provide many facets of nursing care, including patient assessment, education, counseling, prevention of diseases and complications, diagnosis, treatment, and evaluation of care.
B. Pap smears.
1. The goal of screening with the Pap smear is to detect cancerous or precancerous lesions, and to detect the earliest changes in the cervix in which treatment modalities are less invasive.

2. 50–55 million Pap smears are completed annually in the U.S. and have reduced death rates from cervical cancer significantly. In 2007 in the U.S., women who were diagnosed with cervical cancer numbered 12,280, and 4,021 women died from cervical cancer (CDC, 2012a).
3. The Bethesda system is used for the categorization of Pap smears for standardized reporting on individual specimens, provides descriptive reports to use for clinical decisions (http://www.ahrq.gov/clinic/pocketgd1011/gcp10s2.htm).
4. Human papillomavirus infection (HPV) is associated with cervical cancer. While many strains of HPV exist, subtypes HPV 16 or 18 are frequently present in diagnoses of cancer of the cervix.
5. Other risk factors for abnormal Pap include sexual activity prior to age 18, multiple sexual partners, a sex partner who has had multiple sex partners, other STD(s), smoking, and increasing age.
C. Sexually transmitted diseases (STDs).
1. STDs are very common, affecting 1 in 5 adults of all socioeconomic levels in the U.S. (SmarterSex Organization, 2011).
2. Women of all age groups have more risk than men, and young women have a greater risk than older women.
3. Untreated, STDs in women may lead to pelvic inflammatory disease (PID), resulting in potential infertility and increased risk for ectopic pregnancy.
4. Encouraging communication about sexual history between sexual partners; counseling for STDs, including HIV; and providing assurance of the confidentiality of the patient's treatment and testing are critical in meeting the patient's health care needs.
D. Pregnancy prevention.
1. About 37% of births in women ages 15–44 between 2006 and 2010 were unintended at the time of conception (Mosher, Jones, & Abma, 2012).
2. For women to make informed choices about their reproductive care, they must be informed and understand each type of

contraceptive (the safety, efficacy, and risk profile of each).

3. Individual birth control choices are made based on many factors, including a person's health, religious beliefs, desire for children (currently or in the future), number of sexual partners, frequency of sexual activity, and the cost, safety, and efficacy of the contraceptive option.

4. The U.S. Food and Drug Administration (FDA, 2011) states that abstinence is the most effective means to avoid unintended pregnancy and STDs.

E. Screening recommendations.
1. Recommends Pap smears every 1–3 years. This can be delayed until 3 years after onset of sexual activity or age 21, whichever comes first.
2. May discontinue at age 65 if previous smears have been normal.

F. Nursing assessment/monitoring.
1. Nursing history.
   a. Sexual and gynecological history.
      (1) Number of lifetime sexual partners.
      (2) Past history of STDs, abnormal Pap, domestic violence.
      (3) Any partner history of STDs, intravenous drug use.
      (4) Number of total pregnancies.
      (5) Number of abortions (spontaneous or elective).
      (6) Age at first intercourse.
      (7) Condom use and consistency of use.
      (8) Contraceptive methods.
      (9) Last Pap date and results.
      (10) Any history of abnormal Pap.
         (a) Number.
         (b) Treatment.
         (c) Follow-up.
      (11) Abnormal vaginal discharge.
         (a) Amount.
         (b) Character.
         (c) Color, odor.
      (12) Pelvic pain.
      (13) Back pain.
      (14) Genital lesions.
      (15) Vaginal burning, itching.
   b. Menstrual history.
      (1) First day of last normal menstrual period.
      (2) Cycle length.
      (3) Number of days of flow.
      (4) Character of flow.
      (5) Cramping/pelvic pain.
   c. Lifestyle history.
      (1) Tobacco use.
      (2) Caffeine, alcohol, illicit drug use.
   d. Pregnancy history: The entire sexual, gynecological, menstrual history, plus:
      (1) Fatigue.
      (2) Breast tenderness.
      (3) Change in menses.
         (a) Ask about implantational bleeding: Light bleeding with mild cramping that may appear 12–15 days after fertilization.
         (b) Ask about amenorrhea.
      (4) Results of any home pregnancy testing.
      (5) Urinary frequency (occurs at 6–8 weeks).
      (6) Nausea or morning sickness.
      (7) Headache.
2. Physical assessment.
   a. Vital signs.
   b. Height, weight, general appearance.
   c. Nutritional status, BMI.
   d. Thyroid enlargement.
   e. Heart.
      (1) Rhythm, rate.
      (2) Murmurs, extra sounds.
   f. Breast exam.
      (1) Abnormal skin changes.
      (2) Nipple discharge.
      (3) Lymph node enlargement.
   g. Abdomen.
      (1) Enlargement.
      (2) Tenderness.
   h. Gynecological examination.
      (1) Private setting.
      (2) Proper draping of the patient.
      (3) Patient education.
      (4) Tray set up for provider.

3. Diagnostic studies.
   a. Urine chorionic gonadotropin (based on assessment).
   b. Serum human chorionic gonadotropin (based on assessment, to exclude ruptured ectopic pregnancy).
   c. Gonorrhea/chlamydia cultures for all sexually active and pregnant women at increased risk of infection.
   d. Potassium hydroxide (KOH) and normal saline (NS) wet preps of vaginal secretions for evidence of clue cells and trichomoniasis, respectively.
   e. Pap smear.
   f. Human papillomavirus (HPV) testing.
   g. HIV testing (based on risk assessment).
   h. Other testing (based on indications).
      (1) Culture of genital lesions.
      (2) Herpes simplex virus IGG, IGM.
      (3) Rapid plasma reagin (RPR) for syphilis testing.

G. Physiologic alterations.
   1. Clinical manifestations: The patient may be asymptomatic or present with any of the following:
      a. STD and/or abnormal Pap.
         (1) Abnormal vaginal discharge.
         (2) Post coital bleeding or irregular vaginal bleeding.
         (3) Pelvic pain, back pain (may indicate extensive disease).
         (4) Weight loss (may indicate extensive disease).
      b. Pregnancy.
         (1) Fatigue.
         (2) Breast tenderness.
         (3) Change in menses.
            (a) Implantational bleeding.
            (b) Amenorrhea.
         (4) Results of any home pregnancy testing.
         (5) Urinary frequency (occurs at 6–8 weeks).
         (6) Nausea or morning sickness.
         (7) Headache.
   2. Common therapeutic modalities.
      a. Medical testing and interventions.
         (1) Gonorrhea, chlamydia, syphilis.
            (a) Culture or blood testing.
            (b) Antibiotic treatment.
            (c) Education to complete full treatment spectrum.
            (d) Education regarding partner treatment.
         (2) Genital herpes.
            (a) Genital culture or HSV IGG, IGM blood tests.
            (b) Antiviral therapy.
            (c) Possibly give at each outbreak or continuous suppressive therapy.
         (3) HIV.
            (a) Laboratory studies.
            (b) Antiviral therapy.
            (c) Teach importance of adherence to therapy.
         (4) Abnormal Pap.
            (a) May be referred for colposcopy.
            (b) Teach importance of follow-up.
      b. Nursing interventions: Education. High-intensity behavioral counseling is recommended for all sexually active adolescents and for adults at increased risk for STDs (Grade B Recommendation) (U.S. Preventive Services Task Force, 2008a).
         (1) Encourage regular health checks.
         (2) Patient education.
            (a) Communication with present and past sexual partner if indicated.
            (b) Pregnancy prevention.
               i. Abstinence.
               ii. Choice of contraceptive method.
            (c) Condoms for STD reduction.
            (d) Signs and symptoms of infection.
            (e) Signs and symptoms of pregnancy.
            (f) Behavioral counseling to prevent STDs.
            (g) Domestic violence.

(3) Education about the need for evaluation, testing, and treatment of sexual partners.

c. Nursing interventions: Screening.
(1) Encourage sexually active asymptomatic persons for screening.
(2) Encourage partner screening.
(3) Reporting requirements.
(a) Report according to individual state law.
(b) Assure confidentiality.

d. Nursing interventions: Advocacy.
(1) Resources and referrals as needed.
(2) Social and community resources.
(3) Nurse as the informational resource.

XI. Newborn and Infant Screening and Measurement

A. Screening tests.
1. Requirements vary by state.
2. All states require screening for:
   a. Phenylketonuria (PKU).
   b. Hypothyroidism.
   c. Sickle cell anemia.
3. Many also recommend screening for galactosemia, hyperbilirubinemia, and hemoglobinopathies.
4. Vision testing consists of coordinated eye movements, tracking, and presence of red light reflex.
5. Hearing screening before discharge is mandatory in about half the states, and is recommended by the U.S. Preventive Services Task Force (2008c) (Grade B Recommendation).

B. Measurements: Measure and plot on age- and sex-appropriate standardized growth charts. Growth indicates nutritional status and overall health.
1. Length.
   a. Measure on flat surface with infant on back.
   b. Length generally increases by 50% by 1 year of age.
2. Weight.

a. Measure on infant scale. Adjust for any additional materials like a blanket.
b. Initial weight loss of 10% from birth weight. Weight generally doubles by age 6 months, triples by 1 year of age.
3. Head circumference.
   a. Measure broadest part across forehead and occiput.
   b. Average growth is 1 cm/month for first year.

XII. Child and Adolescent Screening

A. Overview – See *Anatomy and Physiology, Nursing History, Physical Examination, Diagnostic Studies*, and *Physiologic Alterations* under the *Adult Screening* section of this chapter.
1. Hypertension is defined for children and adolescents as an average systolic and/or diastolic blood pressure that is over or equal to the 95th percentile for gender, age, and height on three or more separate occasions (NHLBI, 2004).
2. Approximately half a million children in the U.S. have elevated lead levels in their blood (CDC, 2012b). Lead can cause anemia, hearing loss, kidney problems, physical and developmental delays, seizures, and death.
3. Approximately 1–5% of preschool children have vision problems (Chou & Bougatsos, 2011).
   a. Strabismus (misalignment of the visual axis) is the most common cause of amblyopia. Ideally, both eyes move together in unison, focusing the retinal image on the macula.
   b. If the retinal image is distorted due to strabismus or other condition, such as cataracts or refractive differences between the eyes, over time, the brain learns to suppress the poorer image, leading to permanent visual impairment (amblyopia). Early treatment in children ages 3–5 leads to improved vision outcomes. The earlier this condition is treated, the more likely a full recovery will occur.

4. Hearing loss can result in speech delays and school performance issues. Infants should be checked before one month of age and every three years thereafter (U.S. Preventive Services Task Force, 2008c). Indicators for hearing loss include:
   a. Caregiver concern regarding hearing, speech, language, and/or developmental delay.
   b. Family history of childhood hearing loss.
   c. Syndromes associated with hearing loss.
   d. Postnatal infections and hyperbilirubinemia.
   e. In-utero infections.
   f. Neurodegenerative disorders.
   g. Head trauma.
   h. Recurrent otitis media.
5. Dental caries affect 19% of children ages 2–5 years and 52% of children from 5–9 years. There is a higher prevalence and severity of caries in minority and economically disadvantaged children.
6. Childhood obesity affects approximately 12–18% of 2- to 19-year-old children and adolescents. Obesity is defined as having a BMI greater than or equal to the 95th percentile on age- and gender-specific CDC growth charts; Overweight is defined as being between the 85th and 94th percentile (U.S. Preventive Services Task Force, 2010b). Obesity increases the risk for Type 2 diabetes mellitus, asthma, non-alcoholic fatty liver disease, cardiovascular risk, and anesthesia risk, and can lead to mental health issues such as depression and low self-esteem.
7. Major depression disorder (MDD) is disabling, with long-term morbidities and risk of suicide. The majority of depressed youth are undiagnosed or untreated.

B. Nursing assessment/screening recommendations.
1. Blood pressure screening: Blood pressure screening is recommended for children ages 3 years and older at every health care encounter (NHLBI, 2004).

2. Vision screening.
   a. Ocular history, vision assessment, external inspection, ocular motility assessment, pupil examination, red reflex examination, visual acuity measurement, and ophthalmoscopy recommended for ages 3–5 years (U.S. Preventive Services Task Force, 2011c).
   b. Insufficient evidence to recommend screening 3-year-olds or younger for vision; however, commonly check acuity, strabismus, and stereoacuity.
3. Hearing screening.
   a. All ages should be screened for hearing loss as needed, requested, mandated, or when conditions place them at risk for hearing disability.
   b. All infants should have hearing screening before one month of age.
   c. Preschoolers need to be screened for hearing impairment, especially for common middle ear disease at this age.
   d. School-age children should be screened on first entry into school. Every year from kindergarten through the 3rd grade, in 7th grade, in 11th grade, upon entrance into special education, and upon grade repetition (American Speech-Language-Hearing Association [ASHA], 2011).
4. Dental screening: First dental visit is recommended at age 1. Prescribing oral fluoride supplementation to preschoolers over 6 months of age is recommended when the water source is deficient in flouride (U.S. Preventive Services Task Force, 2004).
5. Obesity screening: Obesity screening by BMI is recommended for 6 years of age and older. Offer or refer for comprehensive intensive behavioral interventions to improve weight status (U.S. Preventive Services Task Force, 2010b).

6. Major depressive disorders (MDDs): Screening is recommended for adolescents ages 12–18 for MDD when systems are in place to ensure accurate diagnosis, psychotherapy (cognitive-behavioral or interpersonal), and follow-up (U.S. Preventive Services Task Force, 2009b).

7. Lead screening. Specific lead screening guidelines are set by county health departments; however, the U.S. Preventive Services Task Force (2006) recommends against routine screening for elevated blood lead levels in asymptomatic children between the ages of 1 and 5 (Grade D Recommendation).

XIII. Childhood Immunizations

Review current CDC information for most up-to-date immunization schedules. This science is continually evolving, and recommendations change often.

A. Hepatitis B (HepB): Vaccinate all children ages 0 through 18 years. First dose is given to all infants soon after birth. Second dose is given at age 1 or 2 months; third dose at age 6–18 months. The last dose should not be administered before age 24 weeks. Check special recommendations if mother is HBsAg-positive.

B. Rotovirus (live virus vaccine): Administer orally first dose at 6 through 14 weeks of age. Do not initiate vaccine for infants ages 15 months 0 days. Maximum age for final dose is 8 months 0 days. If Rotarix® (rather than Rotateq®) is administered at ages 2 and 4 months, a dose at 6 months is not indicated.

C. Diphtheria, tetanus, and acellular pertussis (DTaP): Doses at 2, 4, 6, and 15–18 months, and at 4–6 years of age. Do not give DTaP/DT to children age 7 or older. Give Tdap to all children and teens 11–18 years of age who have not received previous Tdap; then boost every 10 years with Td.

D. Haemophilus influenzae type b (Hib) conjugate vaccine: Given at 2, 4, 6, and after 12 months of age.

E. Measles, mumps, rubella (MMR) (live virus vaccine): Give first dose at age 12–15 months. Give second dose at age 4–6 years. MMR in combination with varicella may be used in children ages 12 months through 12 years.

F. Varicella (live virus vaccine): Give first dose at age 12–15 months. Give second dose at age 4–6 years. Give a second dose to all older children and adolescents with history of only one dose.

G. Pneumococcal conjugate (PCV): Given at 2, 4, 6, and after 12 months of age. If underlying medical conditions in children over 2 years, including cochlear implant, administer pneumococcal polysaccharide vaccine (PPSV) at least 2 months after the last PVC dose.

H. Meningococcal: Administer MCV4 at age 11 through 12 years with a booster dose at age 16 years. Administer 1 dose at age 13 through 18 years if not previously vaccinated. Administer 1 dose to previously unvaccinated college freshmen. Check recommendations for immunocompromised individuals and those traveling to countries with highly endemic or epidemic infections.

I. Influenza.
   1. Vaccinate all children and teens ages 6 months through 18 years. Give two doses to first-time vaccinees age 6 months through 8 years, spaced 4 weeks or more apart.
   2. Live, attenuated influenza vaccine (LAIV) is an intranasal alternative to the intramuscular trivalent inactivated influenza (TIV) vaccine for healthy people ages 2–49 years.
   3. If live virus vaccines (such as LAIV, MMR, Varicella, Rotovirus and/or yellow fever vaccine) are not given on the same day, space them at least 28 days apart.

J. Hepatitis A: Administer to all children age 1 year, 2 doses separated by at least 6 months. Recommended for previously unvaccinated children older than 23 months who live in areas where vaccination programs target older children, who are at increased risk of infection, or for whom immunity against hepatitis A is desired.

K. Poliovirus, inactivated: 4 doses at 2, 4, 6 to 18 months, and a fourth dose at 4–6 years.

References

Agency for Healthcare Research and Quality (AHRQ). (2010). *Guide to clinical preventive services, 2010-2011: Recommendations of the U.S. Preventive Services Task Force.* AHRQ Publication No. 10-05145. Retrieved from http://www.ahrq.gov/clinic/pocketgd1011/

American Cancer Society (ACS). (2010). *Learn about cancer.* Retrieved from http://www.cancer.org/cancer/cancer basics/signs-and-symptoms-of-cancer

American Heart Association. (2011). *Metabolic syndrome.* Retrieved from http://www.americanheart.org/presenter.jhtml?identifier=4756

American Society for Metabolic and Bariatric Surgery (ASMBS). (2004). *Consensus statement.* Retrieved from http://www.asmbs.org/2012/06/consensus-statement/

American Speech-Language-Hearing Association (ASHA). (2011). *Hearing screening.* Retrieved from http://www.asha.org/public/hearing/

Centers for Disease Control and Prevention (CDC). (2010a). *Overweight and obesity.* Retrieved from http://www.cdc.gov/obesity/defining.html

Centers for Disease Control and Prevention (CDC). (2010b). *Ten leading causes of death and injury.* Retrieved from http://www.cdc.gov/injury/wisqars/LeadingCauses.html

Centers for Disease Control and Prevention (CDC). (2011). *Vaccines & immunizations.* Retrieved from http://www.cdc.gov/ vaccines

Centers for Disease Control and Prevention (CDC). (2012a). *Cervical cancer statistics.* Retrieved from cdc.gov/cancer/cervical/statistics

Centers for Disease Control and Prevention (CDC). (2012b). *Lead.* Retrieved from http://www.cdc.gov/nceh/lead

Centers for Disease Control and Prevention (CDC). (2012c). *Recommended adult immunization schedule – United States 2012.* Retrieved from http://www.cdc.gov/vaccines/schedules/downloads/adult/mmwr-adult-schedule.pdf

Chou, R., & Bougatsos, C. (2011). Screening for vision impairments in children ages 1–5. *Pediatrics, 127,* e442-e479.

Fowler, S., Kelly, M., Ruh, D., & Johnson-Wells, D. (2007). Management of lipid disorders for stroke prevention. *The Journal of Neuroscience Nursing, 38*(4), 282-287.

Hayden, M., Pignone, M., Phillips, C., & Mulrow, C. (2002). Aspirin for the primary prevention of cardiovascular events: A summary of the evidence for the U.S. Preventive Services Task Force. *Annals of Internal Medicine, 136*(2), 161-172.

Health Check Systems. (2012). *Height and weight charts.* Retrieved from http://www.healthchecksystems.com/height weightchart.htm

Jarvis, C. (2007). *Physical examination and health assessment* (5th ed.). Philadelphia: W.B. Saunders.

Kaplan, N.M., Bakris, G., & Forman, J.P. (2011a). *Overview of hypertension.* Waltham, MA: UpToDate.

Kaplan, N.M., Bakris, G., & Forman, J.P. (2011b). *Salt intake, salt restriction, and essential hypertension.* Waltham, MA: UpToDate.

Lloyd-Jones, D.M. (2010). Cardiovascular risk prediction: Basic concepts, current status, and future direction. *Circulation, 121*(15), 1768-1777.

Macular Degeneration Partnership. (2012). *The Amsler grid.* Retrieved from http://www.amd.org/living-with-amd/resources-and-tools/31-amsler-grid.html

Mosher, W.D., Jones, J., & Abma, J.C. (2012). Intended and unintended births in the United States: 1982-2010. *National Health Statistics Reports, 55.* Retrieved from http://cdc.gov/nchs/data/nhsr/nhsr055.pdf

National Center for Biotechnology Information (NCBI). (2011). *Cancer.* Retrieved from http://www.ncbi.nlm.nih.gov/pubmedhealth/PMH0002267

National Eye Institute (NEI). (2004). *Statistics and data: Prevalence of open-angle glaucoma among adults in the United States.* Retrieved from http://www.nei.nih.gov/eyedata/pbd5.asp

National Heart, Lung, and Blood Institute (NHLBI). (2003). *JNC 7 express. The seventh report of the Joint National Committee on Prevention, Detection, Evaluation and Treatment of High Blood Pressure.* Retrieved from http://www.nhlbi.nih.gov/guidelines/hypertension/express.pdf

National Heart, Lung, and Blood Institute (NHLBI). (2004). *The fourth report on the diagnosis, evaluation, and treatment of high blood pressure in children and adolescents.* Pressure. Retrieved from http://www.nhlbi.nih.gov/guidelines/hypertension/

National Heart, Lung, and Blood Institute (NHLBI). (2006). *The DASH eating plan.* Retrieved from http://www.nhlbi.nih.gov/health/public/heart/hbp/dash/new_dash.pdf

National Institutes of Health (NIH) – Senior Health. (2010). *Exercise and physical activity for older adults.* Retrieved from http://nihseniorhealth.gov/exerciseforolderadults/toc.html

Riaz, K. (2011). *Hypertension.* Retrieved from http://emedicine.medscape.com/article/241381-overview

Ruixing, Y., Jinzhen, W., Weixiong, L., Yuming, C., Dezhai, Y., & Shangling, P. (2009). The environmental and genetic evidence for the association of hyperlipidemia and hypertension. *Journal of Hypertension, 27*(2), 251-258.

SmarterSex Organization. (2011). *STI stats.* Retrieved from http://www.smartersex.org/stis/sti_stats.aso

Trinite, T., Loveland-Cherry, C., & Marion, L. (2009). U.S. Preventive Services Task Force: An evidence-based prevention resource for nurse practitioners. *Journal of the American Academy of Nurse Practitioners, 21*(6), 301-306.

U.S. Department of Agriculture (USDA). (2010). *Dietary guidelines.* Retrieved from http://www.choosemyplate.gov/dietary-guidelines.html

U.S. Department of Agriculture (USDA). (2011). *Make better beverage choices.* Retrieved from http://www.choosemyplate.gov/foodgroups/downloads/TenTips/DGTipsheet19MakeBetterBeverageChoices.pdf

U.S. Department of Health and Human Services (DHHS). (2011). *Healthy people 2020.* Retrieved from http://www.healthypeople.gov

U.S. Food and Drug Administration (FDA). (2011). *Birth control guide.* Retrieved from http://www.fda.gov/forconsumers/byaudience/forwomen/ucm118465.htm

U.S. Preventive Services Task Force. (2004). *Prevention of dental caries in preschool children: Recommendations and rationale.* Retrieved from http://www.uspreventiveservicestaskforce.org/3rduspstf/dentalchild/dentchrs.htm

U.S. Preventive Services Task Force. (2006). *Screening for elevated blood lead levels in children and pregnant women.* Retrieved from http://www.uspreventiveservicestaskforce.org/uspstf/uspslead.htm

U.S. Preventive Services Task Force. (2007). Screening for high blood pressure: U.S. Preventive Services Task Force reaffirmation recommendation statement. *Annals of Internal Medicine, 147*(11), 783-786.

U.S. Preventive Services Task Force. (2008a). *Behavioral counseling to prevent sexually transmitted infections.* Retrieved from http://www.uspreventiveservicestaskforce.org/uspstf/uspsstds.htm

U.S. Preventive Services Task Force. (2008b). *Screening for lipid disorders in adults: Recommendation statement.* Retrieved from http://www.uspreventiveservicestaskforce.org/uspstf08/lipid/lipidrs.htm

U.S. Preventive Services Task Force. (2008c). *Universal screening for hearing loss in newborns: Recommendation statement.* Retrieved from http://www.uspreventiveservicestaskforce.org/uspstf08/newbornhear/newbhearrs.htm

U.S. Preventive Services Task Force. (2009a). *Aspirin for the prevention of cardiovascular disease.* Retrieved from http://www.uspreventiveservicestaskforce.org/uspstf/uspsasmi.htm

U.S. Preventive Services Task Force. (2009b). *Screening and treatment for major depressive disorder in children and adolescents: Recommendation statement.* Retrieved from http://www.uspreventiveservicestaskforce.org/uspstf09/depression/chdeprrs.htm

U.S. Preventive Services Task Force. (2009c). *Screening for colorectal cancer.* Retrieved from http://www.uspreventiveservicestaskforce.org/uspstf/uspscolo.htm

U.S. Preventive Services Task Force. (2009d). *Screening for impaired visual acuity in older adults: Recommendation statement.* Retrieved from http://www.uspreventiveservicestaskforce.org/uspstf09/visualscr/viseldrs.htm

U.S. Preventive Services Task Force. (2010a). *Screening for breast cancer.* Retrieved from http://www.uspreventiveservicestaskforce.org/uspstf/uspsbrca.htm

U.S. Preventive Services Task Force. (2010b). *Screening for obesity in children and adolescents.* Retrieved from http://www.uspreventiveservicestaskforce.org/uspstf10/childobes/chobesrs.htm

U.S. Preventive Services Task Force. (2011a). *Recommendations for adults.* Retrieved from http://www.uspreventiveservicestaskforce.org/adultrec.htm

U.S. Preventive Services Task Force. (2011b). *Screening for bladder cancer in adults.* Retrieved from http://www.uspreventiveservicestaskforce.org/uspstf/uspsblad.htm

U.S. Preventive Services Task Force. (2011c). *Screening for visual impairment in children ages 1 to 5: Recommendation statement.* Retrieved from http://www.uspreventiveservicestaskforce.org/uspstf11/vischildren/vischildrs.htm

U.S. Preventive Services Task Force. (2012). *Screening for cervical cancer.* Retrieved from http://www.uspreventiveservicestaskforce.org/uspstf/uspscerv.htm

University of Washington. (2011). *Manage your weight: What is your desirable body weight?* Retrieved from http://www.washington.edu/admin/hr/benefits/wellness/weight.html

Additional Readings

Agency for Healthcare Research and Quality (AHRQ). (n.d.). *U.S. Preventive Services Task Force: Introduction.* Retrieved from http://www.ahrq.gov/clinic/uspstfix.htm

Buchwald, H. (2004). *Bariatric surgery for morbid obesity: Health implications for patients, health professionals, and third-party payers.* Retrieved from http://s3.amazonaws.com/publicASMBS/GuidelinesStatements/Guidelines/2004_ASBS_Consensus_Conference_Statement.pdf

Centers for Disease Control and Prevention (CDC). (n.d.). *Can lifestyle modifications using therapeutic lifestyle changes reduce weight and the risk of chronic disease?* Retrieved from http://www.cdc.gov/nutrition/downloads/R2P_life_change.pdf

Grundy, S.M., Cleeman, J.I., Merz, C.N., Brewer, H.B., Jr., Clark, L.T., Hunninghake, D.B., ... American Heart Association. (2004). Implications of recent clinical trials for the National Cholesterol Education Program Adult Treatment Panel III Guidelines. *Circulation, 110*(2), 227-239.

Hill, N.H., & Sullivan, L.M. (2004). *Management guidelines for nurse practitioners working with children and adolescents* (2nd ed.). Philadelphia: F.A. Davis.

National Eye Institute (NEI). (2008). *Causes and prevalence of visual impairment among adults in the United States.* Retrieved from http://www.nei.nih.gov/eyedata/pbdl.asp

National Heart, Lung, and Blood Institute (NHLBI). (2001). *Third report of the National Cholesterol Education Program Expert Panel on Detection, Evaluation, and Treatment of High Blood Cholesterol in Adults (Adult Treatment Panel III) executive summary.* Retrieved from http://www.nhlbi.nih.gov/guidelines/cholesterol/atp3xsum.pdf

National Heart, Lung, and Blood Institute (NHLBI). (2005). *Your guide to lowering your cholesterol with TLC.* Retrieved from http://www.nhlbi.nih.gov/health/public/heart/chol/chol_tlc.pdf

National Heart, Lung, and Blood Institute (NHLBI). (2010). *Diseases and conditions index: Overweight and obesity.* Retrieved from http://www.nhlbi.nih.gov/health/dci/Diseases/obe/obe_diagnosis.html

U.S. Department of Agriculture (USDA). (2011a). *Choose my plate.* Retrieved from http://www.choosemyplate.gov

U.S. Department of Agriculture (USDA). (2011b). *Dietary guidelines for Americans 2010.* Retrieved from http://www.cnpp.usda.gov/dietaryguidelines.htm

U.S. Department of Agriculture (USDA). (2011c). *Dietary reference intakes: Electrolytes and water.* Retrieved from http://www.iom.edu/Global/News%20Announcements/~/media/442A08B899F44DF9AAD083D86164C75B.ashx

Chapter 18

Care of the Acutely Ill Patient

Kristene K. Grayem, MSN, CNP, RN
Annette S. Hamlin, BSN, RN
Jane Holloway, BSN, RN

Jennifer Allen, MSQSM, RN, CPAN
Candia Baker Laughlin, MS, RN-BC
CAPT Wanda C. Richards, MSM, MPA, BSN

PATIENT PROTOTYPES

Medical Emergencies
Loss of Consciousness • Cardiac and Respiratory Arrest • Seizure • Acute Hypoglycemia and Hypoglycemic Shock
Anaphylactic Shock • Tuberculosis (TB) Skin Test Conversion • Depression and Suicide • Domestic Violence

Adult Acute Illnesses
Headache • Low Back Pain • Sinusitis • Sexually Transmitted Diseases • Abdominal Pain

Adolescent Acute Illnesses
Headache • Sexually Transmitted Diseases

Pediatric Acute Illnesses
Upper Respiratory Infection • Nausea, Vomiting, and Diarrhea • Fever • Ear Pain

OBJECTIVES – *Study of the information in this chapter will enable the learner to:*	KEY POINTS – *The major points in this chapter include:*
1. Describe the incidence, pathophysiology, assessment, and care of life-threatening conditions in ambulatory care. 2. Describe the incidence, pathophysiology, assessment, and care of acute conditions commonly seen in ambulatory care. 3. Discuss patient and family education and preventive care counseling for acute illnesses.	1. It is important for nurses in ambulatory care to maintain a current knowledge base of emergency procedures based on the latest evidence. 2. Patients with common acute illnesses may present at almost any ambulatory care setting or via a telehealth encounter, requiring timely and knowledgeable assessment and care.

Ambulatory health care has seen a paradigm shift in the last decade. Procedures once requiring hospital stays are now being performed in outpatient settings. The general population is aging as the "baby boomers" reach retirement age. Technology has aided our population to live longer and manage chronic disease better than ever before. A shift to outpatient status has also been fueled by rising health care costs to both patients and health care institutions. Nurses in ambulatory care are not only providing care to patients, but also supervising employees, delegating nursing tasks, and delivering telehealth care, requiring that they possess astute assessment skills and the ability to respond to the unexpected. It is important in ambulatory care to maintain one's knowledge base of acute illness care and emergency procedures through continuing education and review of evidence-based guidelines. Routinely updated written policies and protocols will help the nurse remain current on developing technology and nursing practice. Such measures will allow the nurse to implement condition-specific care in a timely and confident manner.

MEDICAL EMERGENCIES

Emergency conditions are an ever-present risk in ambulatory care. However, because they do not routinely occur, it is imperative that health care workers routinely practice emergency procedures to remain comfortable with processes and be able to respond in a timely manner.

Loss of Consciousness

Patient Population: Adult and Pediatric

I. Overview

Management of a patient who has lost consciousness requires careful and rapid assessment, both to determine the probable etiology and to provide supportive care.

II. Pathophysiology

The most common causes for sustained loss of consciousness are uncontrolled diabetes (hyper or hypoglycemia), stroke, head injury, alcohol or drug overdose, bleeding, myocardial infarction (MI), or cardiac dysrhythmias. While head trauma and drug or alcohol overdoses are not usually experienced in ambulatory care settings, other chronic illnesses are inherent to primary and specialty care areas. Knowledge of the disease process and patient education may decrease the risk of loss of consciousness. Other conditions that may cause unconsciousness in ambulatory care include vasovagal response (such as fainting when receiving an injection) or dehydration (hypovolemia). Each situation requires a keen assessment by the nurse and timely action by protocol or in conjunction with a physician.

III. Assessment and Triage

The initial assessment is the key to identifying the appropriate steps to initiate in an emergency. The assessment is divided into two phases – primary and secondary.

A. Primary assessment.
1. Assess airway.
   a. Head-tilt, chin-lift.
   b. Look, listen, and feel for respirations.
2. Assess breathing.
   a. Spontaneous breathing.
   b. Rate and pattern.
   c. Symmetrical rise and fall of chest wall.
   d. Increased work of breathing.
   e. Use of accessory muscles.
   f. If breathing is not present, refer to the *Cardiac and Respiratory Arrest* section later in this chapter.
3. Assess circulation.
   a. Capillary refill.
   b. Skin temperature, color, and moistness.
   c. Palpate central and peripheral pulses – Assess rate and quality.
   d. If no carotid pulse is present, initiate basic life support according to American Heart Association (AHA) 2010 guidelines.
4. Assess level of consciousness.
   a. Awake.
   b. Alert.
   c. Responsive to command.
   d. Responsive to verbal/voice.
   e. Responsive to pain.
   f. Unresponsive to voice or pain.
   g. Pupil assessment.
B. Secondary assessment.
1. Assess vital signs.
2. Initiate telemetry monitoring, if available.
3. Assess blood glucose level.
4. If possible, obtain history from patient or accompanying family/friends.
   a. Onset of symptoms.
   b. Activity before onset of symptoms.
   c. Recent complaints.
   d. Recent injuries.
   e. Medication and medical history.
   f. Alcohol and/or recreational drug consumption.

IV. Indication for Emergency Care or Urgent Consultation

A. Notify provider immediately. In some settings or situations, it may be necessary to activate EMS, such as by calling 9-1-1.

B. Protect the airway.

C. Obtain IV access.

D. Assess for bleeding or signs of trauma.

E. Assess neurological function.

F. Monitor blood pressure and heart rate at least every 15 minutes.

G. Obtain laboratory specimens per protocol or provider's order.

H. Obtain an electrocardiogram, as ordered.

V. Plan of Care

A. Primary/secondary/tertiary prevention.

   1. Decreasing risk for an unconscious episode due to diabetes.

      a. Perform regular blood glucose checks.

      b. Follow the prescribed diabetes diet plan.

      c. Follow prescribed medication regimen.

   2. Preventing hypoglycemic shock by good glycemic control (discussed later in this chapter and in the *Diabetes* section of Chapter 21, "Care of the Chronically Ill Patient").

   3. Decreasing risk of stroke.

      a. Regularly check blood pressure readings, even if feeling well.

      b. Follow prescribed diet, such as a low-salt, low-fat diet.

      c. Follow prescribed medication regimen.

      d. Follow prescribed exercise plan.

      e. Abstain from smoking.

   4. Decreasing risk of seizure (discussed later in this chapter and in the *Diabetes* section of Chapter 21, "Care of the Chronically Ill Patient").

B. Goals of plan of care.

   1. Client regained consciousness.

   2. Client safely transferred to tertiary care.

   3. Family accepting of situation.

   4. Coordination of care was accomplished.

C. Education of patient and family.

   1. Client discharge teaching on chronic disease management, if applicable.

   2. Client instruction on medication management, if applicable.

   3. Client instruction on following prescribed exercise plan.

   4. Client instruction on smoking abstinence.

   5. Client instruction on performing foot inspections daily and observing for signs of open wounds and infections.

   6. Support the patient and family utilizing therapeutic communication skills.

D. Collaboration and referrals.

   1. Convey assessment information to a provider.

   2. Refer for tertiary care, as indicated.

   3. Coordinate care with EMS and tertiary care.

   4. Refer to social services or chaplain services, as indicated.

E. Telehealth nursing considerations.

   1. Recognize emergency situations.

   2. Avoid delay in assessing and directing patients in emergencies.

   3. Procedure and protocols need to assure that office staff do not take messages, but keep the patient with a potentially life-threatening emergency on the line until a nurse or other health professional can assess and determine the appropriate course of action.

   4. Refer to EMS, such as by calling 9-1-1.

F. Protocol/algorithms/guidelines.

   1. Emergency care protocols should reflect latest evidence-based and expert agency guidelines (such as the American Heart Association [AHA]).

   2. Documentation tools.

   3. Communication/documentation.

      a. Time of onset.

      b. Course of treatment.

      c. Response to treatment including vital signs.

      d. Report to EMS/tertiary health care workers.

Cardiac and Respiratory Arrest

Patient Population: Adult and Pediatric

I. Overview

According to Howard and Steinmann (2010), "More than 700,000 American adults die annually from cardiovascular disease; of these, approximately 850 die every day from sudden cardiac arrest" (p. 414). Without initiation of life-saving techniques, permanent cellular damage occurs within 4–6 minutes. Survival is less than 10% after 9 minutes (AHA, 2010). The AHA has developed the chain of survival in basic life support (BLS) training to increase survival rates from sudden cardiac arrest. The chain of survival consists of rapid EMS activation, initiation of cardiopulmonary resuscitation (CPR), rapid defibrillation with an emphasis on chest compression, effective advanced cardiac life support (ACLS) or pediatric advanced life support (PALS) protocols, and integrated post-cardiac arrest care (AHA, 2010). The key to successful outcomes for sudden cardiac arrest due to ventricular tachycardia is timely defibrillation. In the ambulatory care setting, this step is most efficiently reached by use of the automated external defibrillator (AED). In the pediatric population, cardiac arrest is usually secondary to respiratory arrest, such as those caused by infectious processes (e.g., croup), foreign body blockage of the airway, or drowning.

In October 2010, the AHA released recommendations for changes in BLS designed to simplify the guidelines, with more similarities across age groups (Hazinski, 2010). Changes include the BLS sequence steps from A-B-C (Airway, Breathing, Chest Compression) to C-A-B (Chest Compression, Airway, Breathing) for adults, children, and infants (AHA, 2010).

A. Definitions.
1. Advanced cardiac life support (ACLS) – Protocols and algorithms created through the AHA to provide guidelines for medical management of cardiac arrest and/or arrhythmia, respiratory arrest and/or respiratory support, and stroke.
2. Automated external defibrillator (AED) – Device delivering electrical joules in response to shockable cardiac arrhythmias utilizing ACLS protocol.

3. Basic life support (BLS) – Process of providing circulation and respiration through artificial means (such as chest compressions and rescue breathing) in an organized, scientifically proven way in an effort to sustain life until advanced care can be provided.
4. Pediatric advanced life support (PALS) – Protocols and algorithms created through the AHA to provide guidelines for medical management of potentially fatal health conditions in the pediatric population, as well as to provide guidelines for medical management of cardiac arrest and/or arrhythmia and respiratory arrest and/or respiratory support.
5. Perfusion – Tissues in the body exchanging metabolic waste (carbon dioxide) and receiving oxygen through arterial/venous circulation.
6. Respiratory arrest – Lung tissue is not able to receive carbon dioxide or give oxygen to circulating blood.
7. Ventilation – Mechanism by which the blood gives off carbon dioxide and takes on oxygen in the lungs.
8. Ventricular tachycardia – Fatal heart arrhythmia with wide QRS complexes. Not necessarily resulting in pulselessness initially. The rapid rate of ventricular contraction inhibits adequate blood filling and decreased cardiac output.
9. Ventricular fibrillation – Fatal heart arrhythmia that results in pulselessness. The ventricles contract in an unorganized manner resembling a quiver and produce no cardiac output.

II. Assessment and Triage

A. Assess CABs of BLS (see Table 18-1).
1. Gently shake and call, "Are you OK?"
2. Assure open airway and check to see if the victim is breathing utilizing the head-tilt, chin-lift.
3. If unresponsive, call for help and activate EMS according to facility's protocols (e.g., call 9-1-1) and get the AED.

Table 18-1.
2010 Health Care Provider Adult
BLS Recommendations

Action	Recommendation
Recognition	No breathing, or abnormal breathing No pulse
CPR sequence	C-A-B (chest compression-airway-breathing)
Compression rate	At least 100/minute
Compression depth	At least 2 inches (5 cm)
Chest wall recoil	Allow complete chest recoil Rotate compressors every 2 minutes
Compression interruptions	Minimize interruptions Limit interruptions to less than 10 seconds
Airway	Head-tilt, chin-lift Jaw thrust in suspected trauma
Compression to ventilation ratio	30:2
Ventilation with untrained or non-proficient rescuer	Compressions only
Ventilations with advanced airway	1 breath every 6–8 seconds (8–10 breaths per minute) Asynchronous 1 second/breath Visible chest rise
Defibrillation	Attach and use AED as soon as possible Minimize interruptions in compressions Resume compressions immediately after shock

Source: Developed by CAPT Wanda C. Richards. Adapted from Hazinski, 2010.

4. Check pulse (at least 5, but no more than 10 seconds).
5. If no pulse, begin chest compressions and breaths, utilizing BLS protocol.
6. If unable to ventilate, check inside mouth for foreign object. Remove object, if visible.

7. If unable to visualize object, unblock airway utilizing BLS protocol for foreign body airway obstruction.
8. Once airway is unblocked, begin supportive breathing.

B. When EMS providers arrive, direct them to the location of the emergency.
C. An AED should be available beside the patient within 3–4 minutes. Studies have shown increased survivability with fast intervention of cardiac arrhythmia with external defibrillation (AHA, 2010). Use of AEDs in the pediatric population requires adaptive pads to decrease the number of joules delivered. The user of the AED must be familiar with pediatric protocols and equipment before use.
   1. Turn AED on.
   2. Place one AED pad on the victim's upper right chest (directly below the collarbone) and the other pad to the side of the left nipple. Illustrations on the pads will aid in placement.
   3. Follow AED prompts. The nurse should be familiar with how to operate the model of AED in use.
   4. Announce "clear" loudly so no individual is touching the patient before delivering the shock.
   5. Follow AED prompts for discharging joules.
   6. Quality checks should be performed on AED at least weekly to ensure battery is functional, and that pads are present and have not reached their expiration date.

III. **Indication for Emergency Care or Urgent Consultation**
A. All staff involved in direct patient care should complete a BLS course. High-risk areas may have protocols for ACLS/PALS course completion. Follow facility guidelines.
   1. Appropriate equipment is available to meet the requirements of the patient population (e.g., bag-valve-mask, airways).
   2. One-way valve/masks should be available throughout the facility to provide mouth protection of the rescuer while waiting for AED and bag-valve-mask to arrive.

3. Emergency carts or kits should be checked and ready at all times.
B. In the ambulatory setting, sustained critical care is often not available in the same facility. Initiate EMS and transport to tertiary care.
C. Cardiac arrest is not a frequent scenario in most ambulatory care areas, and periodic review of protocol and practice with peers is highly recommended.
D. During the incident, crowds may gather, especially if it occurs in a public area. Assign a staff member to crowd control.
E. Protect the patient's privacy as much as possible.
F. Support for family/friends is essential. Utilize social services or chaplain services, if available.
G. Provide assessment and treatment course information to EMS personnel as care is transferred.
H. Coordinate transfer to tertiary care.

IV. Plan of Care
A. Primary/secondary/tertiary prevention.
   1. Teach parents about the importance of toddler-proofing the home.
      a. Small objects can become lodged in pediatric airways and cause respiratory arrest, leading to death.
      b. Household cleaners and other poisons should be stored above child level.
      c. The poison control phone number should be posted near a telephone for easy access.
   2. Coronary risk factors should be controlled or eliminated, including smoking, hypertension, hyperlipidemia, diabetes, and a sedentary lifestyle.
   3. Patients and families should recognize early warning signs of cardiac or respiratory distress and seek immediate care.
   4. Refer patients and families to a post-cardiac rehabilitation program.
B. Goals of plan of care.
   1. Successful resuscitation efforts.
   2. Coordination of care to appropriate tertiary care setting.

3. Family members' understanding of cardiac or respiratory arrest incident.
C. Education of patient/family.
   1. Once acute respiratory distress is resolved, educate the patient/parent regarding early signs and management of respiratory distress.
   2. Teach parents the signs of increased work of breathing in the pediatric population.
      a. Sternal notch sinking.
      b. Intercostal retractions.
      c. Audible wheezing.
   3. Teach clients how to best control active airway disease including:
      a. Use of metered dose inhalers.
      b. Medication management.
      c. Peak flow meters to measure airflow and implement treatment, if indicated.
      d. Pursed-lip breathing.
      e. Postural drainage.
      f. Disease process and progression.
      g. Triggers for exacerbation of symptoms.
      h. Smoking cessation.
D. Telehealth nursing considerations.
   1. Recognize emergency situations. Avoid delay in assessing and directing patients in emergencies.
   2. Procedure and protocols need to assure that office staff does not take messages, but keep the patient with a potentially life-threatening emergency on the line.
   3. Refer to EMS, such as by calling 9-1-1.
E. Protocol/algorithms/guidelines.
   1. Facility-specific code announcements and ACLS/BLS guidelines.
   2. Documentation tool.
   3. Post-incident guidelines.
   4. Communication/documentation.
      a. Careful documentation of event.
         (1) Time of onset.
         (2) Treatment course including tracings or memory disc from AED.
         (3) Responses from treatment.
      b. Communication.
         (1) Report of sequencing of events, assessment data, and interventions to EMS personnel.

(2) Report of incident to receiving tertiary care unit, if possible.

(3) Use effective communication skills in conveying information to family.

(4) Coordinate with social services or chaplain services, as available.

Seizure

Patient Population: Adult and Pediatric

I.   Overview

In the U.S., approximately 2.3 million Americans are diagnosed with a seizure disorder yearly. A seizure, which may occur at any age, is usually a symptom of an underlying problem instead of a diagnosis. Seizures are classified as partial, generalized, or unclassified. Seizures are often described in phases, such as pre-ictal, prodromal, aura, post-ictal, tonic-clonic, and atonic (Brown & King, 2010).

A. Definitions.

1. Atonic – Loss of muscle tone (drop attacks).

2. Absence seizure (petit mal) – Type of seizure resulting in brief loss of consciousness, usually 10 seconds or less, with the absence of hypertonicity or muscular contracture. Presentation is predominantly in children.

3. Aura – Subjective indication of oncoming seizure. Clients may describe a change in vision, taste, or smell pursuant to the onset of seizure activity.

4. Focal seizure – Seizure activity initiating from one side of the brain. Presentation of seizure activity is seen on the opposite side of the body. The seizure may or may not generalize to include both sides of the body.

5. Epilepsy – Diagnosis for congenital or acquired brain disease resulting in seizure activity.

6. Tonic-clonic seizure (grand mal) – Increased neuronal activity in the brain with presenting loss of consciousness, muscle rigidity, involuntary muscular twitching, and incontinence.

7. Post-ictal period – Time after a seizure during which the patient may present with confusion and lethargy.

8. Seizure – Increased neuronal activity in the brain caused by disease process or trauma leading to hypertonicity and muscular contracture.

9. Status epilepticus – Increased neuronal activity in the brain resulting in seizure activity that continues for more than 10 minutes. Status epilepticus is considered a medical emergency.

II. Pathophysiology

There are three types of causes for seizure activity: Physiological, iatrogenic, and idiopathic. Physiological causes include, but are not limited to: Central nervous system infections, congenital malformations, acquired metabolic disorders, stroke, trauma, and tumors. Iatrogenic causes include, but are not limited to: New medications, withdrawal from medications, alcoholism, and drug usage or withdrawal. Idiopathic causes include, but are not limited to: Fevers, menstrual cycles, flashing lights, fatigue, and loud music.

III. Assessment and Triage

A. Active seizure activity.

1. Ensure patient safety from injury.

a. If the patient is sitting or standing at onset, lay him or her on floor.

b. If the patient is lying on a bed, protect him or her from fall.

c. Protect airway by rolling onto side.

d. Protect the patient's head by cradling in lap or placing head on a pillow.

e. Loosen clothing.

f. Do not place a bite stick or other object in the patient's mouth.

g. Do not give the patient water, pills, or food until fully alert.

2. Objective assessment.

a. Time of onset.

b. Location(s) of initial muscle activity.

c. Progression of muscle activity, if any.

d. Patency of airway.

e. Time of resolution.

f. Presence and extent of fever in pediatric patients.

B. History of seizure prior to current seizure activity.
1. Sequence of events, if known.
2. Type of aura, if present.
3. Frequency and length of seizures, including time of last seizure.
4. Medications taken and consistency of use.

C. Clinical procedures.
1. Neurological assessment.
2. Blood tests, such as medication levels.
3. Lumbar puncture.
4. Electroencephalogram (EEG).

IV. Indications for Emergency Care or Urgent Consultation

A. Obtain and utilize suction equipment, as indicated.
B. Obtain IV access.
C. Monitor heart rate and respirations.
D. Monitor for subsequent seizure activity following acute seizure symptoms.
E. Activate EMS, if appropriate, according to facility's protocol.

V. Plan of Care

A. Pharmacotherapeutics.
Pharmacological intervention is the most common treatment for seizure activity. The most common medications include, but are not limited to:
1. Phenytoin (Dilantin®).
2. Carbamazepine (Tegretol®).
3. Topiramate (Topamax®).
4. Gabapentin (Neurontin®).
5. Phenobarbital (Luminal®).

B. Primary/secondary/tertiary prevention.
1. Protect against head injury.
    a. Wear headgear during contact sports or bike riding.
    b. Wear seatbelts while riding in automobiles.

C. Goals of plan of care.
1. The patient remains injury-free.
2. Seizure activity controlled.
3. Return demonstration and verbalization of safety measures to use during seizure activity.
4. Self-esteem intact.

D. Psychosocial considerations.
1. During period of adjustment, may experience personal relationship issues.
    a. Work.
    b. Home.
    c. Fear of discrimination.
    d. Social isolation.

E. Education of patient/family.
1. Identify barriers to communication.
2. Use effective communication skills.
3. Discuss the disease process including stages of seizure activity (i.e., aura, unconsciousness, seizure activity, post-ictal phase, possible incontinence).
4. Identify learning needs related to seizure activity and safety measures.
    a. If the patient experiences aura, lay down flat and make sure no objects are close by.
    b. Instruct family/friends not to place anything in the patient's mouth, but to protect the patient's head.
    c. The patient should not drive a car.
    d. Recommend seizure disorder support groups.
    e. Refer to library and Internet information resources.

F. Collaboration and referrals.
1. Neurology or neurosurgery consults.
2. Electrode implant.

G. Community resources and education.
1. Epilepsy Foundation of America (EFA).
2. National Institutes of Health (NIH) (www.nih.gov).
3. American Epilepsy Foundation (AEF) (www.aesnet.org).
4. National Society for Epilepsy (www.epilepsynse.org.uk).
5. Epilepsy Foundation (www.epilepsyfoundation.org).

H. Telehealth nursing considerations.
1. Information resource.
2. Triage/referrals.
3. Provide instruction for seizure management when necessary.
4. Support timely prescription renewals for anti-convulsants.

I. Protocols/algorithms/guidelines.
   1. Provide for patient privacy.
   2. Discuss the episode and answer any questions.
   3. Communication/documentation.
      a. Patient record.
      b. Telephone advice documentation.
   4. Protocol development.
      a. Emergent treatment guidelines or care maps.
      b. Increase understanding of interventions and outcomes.
      c. Decrease anxiety of the patient and family in home management of seizure disorder.

Acute Hypoglycemia and Hypoglycemic Shock

Patient Population: Adult and Pediatric

I. **Overview**

   Hypoglycemia occurs when there is a significant decrease in circulating blood glucose. For diabetics, the most common cause is injection of insulin, followed by inadequate intake of calories. Hypoglycemic shock is an emergent situation that requires fast response. Symptoms rapidly progress from confusion and lethargy to unconsciousness and possible death.

II. **Pathophysiology**

   There are two known types of diabetes mellitus. Type 1 diabetes usually occurs in early childhood or adulthood and was formally known as "insulin-dependent" diabetes. It results from little or no insulin production (hypoglycemia) due to the destruction of the beta cells of the pancreas (Daniels & Nicoll, 2012). Type 2 diabetes was formally known as "non-insulin-dependent" or "adult onset" diabetes. In this type, there is a defect in the beta cell production, which results in the liver overproducing glucose. There is more glucose circulating in the blood (hyperglycemia) two hours post-prandially (Daniels & Nicoll, 2012). Hypoglycemia occurs in both Type 1 and Type 2 diabetes as a result of an imbalance in food, activity, and insulin and/or oral anti-diabetic agents.

III. **Assessment and Triage**
   A. Assess for skin temperature and color.
   B. Other symptoms such as:
      1. Headache.
      2. Nausea.
      3. Tremors.
      4. Hunger.
      5. Lethargy.
      6. Confusion.
      7. Slurred speech.
      8. Anxiety.
   C. Assess blood glucose level.
   D. Vital signs.
   E. Look for causes of level of consciousness changes.
      1. Trauma.
      2. Blood glucose abnormality.
      3. Toxins.
      4. Stroke.
   F. Breathing/respirations.
      1. Rapid, deep, Kussmaul respirations indicate diabetic ketoacidosis; an arterial blood gas is required to diagnose.

IV. **Indications for Emergency Care or Urgent Consultation**
   A. Blood glucose level measurement of less than 70 mg/dl.

V. **Plan of Care**
   A. Pharmacotherapeutics.
      1. Rapid glucose replacement.
         a. If responsive and able to eat:
            (1) Oral carbohydrates should be consumed, such as 1/2 cup or 4 ounces of fruit juice or regular soda, 8 ounces of skim milk, hard candies (3–5 pieces), glucose tablets, or a tablespoon of sugar, jelly, or honey.
         b. If unresponsive and/or unable to eat:
            (1) Obtain IV access and an order to administer dextrose, 50% IV push.
            (2) If no IV access, obtain order and administer glucagon 1 mg IM or SQ.

    c. Recheck capillary blood glucose 15 minutes after glucose replacement. If blood glucose remains below 70 mg/dl, repeat treatment, until desired level is reached (above 70 mg/dl).

B. Primary/secondary/tertiary prevention.
1. Diabetic education and good glycemic control.
2. Nutritional counseling.
3. Jewelry identifying patient as a diabetic.
4. Foot care.

C. Goals of plan of care.
1. Hypoglycemic episode resolved.
2. Patient free from injury.
3. Patient verbalizes understanding of causes and prevention of hypoglycemia.

D. Education of patient/family.
1. Self-administration of insulin injection.
2. Initial signs and symptoms of low blood glucose levels.
    a. Mild symptoms: Dizziness, irritability, hunger but no thirst, clumsiness, numbness, tingling in extremities, shakiness, diaphoresis, tachycardia.
    b. Moderate symptoms: Confusion, headache, poor coordination.
    c. Severe symptoms: Unconsciousness, seizures, coma.
3. Treatment measures for self or family members to manage low blood glucose levels.
    a. Do not drive when blood sugar is low.
    b. Drink or eat some form of carbohydrate as soon as possible:
      (1) Orange juice.
      (2) Candy.
      (3) Soda pop.
      (4) Glucose tablets.
    c. Self-monitoring of capillary blood glucose (Daniels & Nicoll, 2012).
      (1) If glucose level is less than 70 mg/dl, administer 10–15 grams of a simple, fast-acting carbohydrate.
      (2) If glucose level remains below 70 mg/dl after 15 minutes of the above treatment, the patient should repeat the treatment and repeat the blood glucose measurement in 15 minutes.

      (3) The treatment and blood glucose measurements should continue every 15 minutes until the blood glucose level is above 70 mg/dl.
      (4) The patient should eat a regular meal or snack and recheck the blood glucose in 45 minutes.
    d. If severe, call for EMS support, such as by calling 9-1-1.
    e. Self-inspections of lower extremities.

E. Collaboration and referrals.
1. Tertiary care, if needed.
2. Nutritional counseling.
3. Group training classes.
4. Podiatry.

F. Community resources and education.
1. Recommend community support groups.
2. Refer to library and Internet information resources.
    a. National Institute of Diabetes and Digestive and Kidney Disease (www.niddk.nih.gov).
    b. American Diabetes Association (www.diabetes.org).
    c. Specialty groups.

G. Telehealth nursing considerations.
1. Information resource.
2. Recognize emergent situations.
3. Refer when necessary.

H. Protocols/algorithms/guidelines.
1. Communication/documentation.
    a. Patient record.
    b. Telephone advice documentation.

Anaphylactic Shock

Patient Population: Adult

I. **Overview**

Anaphylaxis is a rare, but severe, systemic allergic reaction. Roughly 30 out of 100,000 people will experience anaphylaxis in their lifetime. In addition to anaphylaxis due to an exposure in the community, it may occur in the ambulatory setting related to the administration of a vaccine or other medication.

A. Anaphylactoid reaction – This type of reaction is not caused by immune globulins (IgE), but mimics the IgE-mediated anaphylactic reaction.

It may be induced by aspirin, nonsteroidal anti-inflammatory drugs (NSAIDs), radiopague contrast media, fluorescein, dextran, and opiates.

B. Anaphylaxis – A severe, whole-body allergic reaction to a chemical that has become an allergen (A.D.A.M., 2010). This can be fatal if not immediately treated.

II. Pathophysiology

"Anaphylactic shock is caused by an exaggerated widespread antibody response following a previous exposure to the antigen" (Daniels & Nicoll, 2012, p. 1862). As the tissues of the body release histamine and other substances, the airways constrict. Blood vessels dilate, lowering blood pressure severely and causing lightheadedness. Fluid leaks from the bloodstream into the tissues, including the bronchioles, resulting in pulmonary edema, lowering blood pressure, and if left unchecked, shock and cardiovascular collapse.

III. Assessment and Triage

A. Subjective assessment.
  1. Assess for sensations of burning and itching of the skin.
  2. Determine any related symptoms, such as abdominal pain, vomiting, or diarrhea.
  3. Assess for insect bites.
  4. Assess for history of allergies. Allergies to food items such as nuts and fish have a high risk of anaphylactic-type reactions (Krause, 2011).
B. Objective assessment.
  1. Ensure patent airway.
    a. Position appropriately to facilitate breathing.
    b. Assess for dyspnea, hoarseness, wheezing, and/or stridor.
    c. Perform pulse oximetry.
  2. Monitor vital signs.
    a. Pulse rate and quality.
    b. Blood pressure, including orthostatics, if possible.
  3. Observe for:
    a. Skin rash/hives.
    b. Swelling of eyes, lips, and/or tongue.
    c. Nausea/vomiting.
    d. Diarrhea.

IV. Indications for Emergency Care or Urgent Consultation

A. CABs of BLS, as indicated.
B. Notify provider immediately. Symptoms that may not be immediately life-threatening might progress rapidly unless treated promptly. Treatment recommendations are subject to provider discretion, and variations in sequence and performance rely on provider judgment.

V. Plan of Care

A. Administer oxygen.
B. Establish IV access.
C. Pharmacotherapeutics.
  1. Nebulizer treatments with bronchodilators.
  2. Medication administration per protocol or provider's order.
    a. Aqueous epinephrine 1:1000 dilution (1 mg/mL) – Administer 0.3–0.5 mL in adolescent and adult intramuscularly or subcutaneously every 5 minutes, as necessary, should be used to control symptoms and increase blood pressure (Nettina, 2010).
    b. Other medications and fluids – Administer per provider order in response to assessed needs, such as bronchodilators, dopamine, corticosteroids, diphenhydramine, or ranitidine. Note: Diphenhydramine and other H1 antihistamines are considered secondary, and should never be administered alone in anaphylaxis (Joint Council of Allergy, Asthma and Immunology [JCAAI], 2005).
D. Primary/secondary/tertiary prevention.
  1. Patient education on allergy condition.
  2. Insect or allergen control measures in the home.
  3. Medication administration.
E. Goals of plan of care.
  1. Patient's airway is patent, and respirations are even and non-labored.
  2. Patient understands triggers that caused anaphylaxis.
  3. Patient recognizes and can verbalize symptoms of emergent disease process.

4. Patient verbalizes and demonstrates correct technique for medication administration.

F. Education of patient/family.
 1. Information on allergen and how to protect against exposure.
 2. Self-injections with epinephrine (such as EpiPen®), as indicated.
 3. Signs and symptoms that indicate an emergency situation.
 4. Family and patient aware of how to activate EMS and when to call.
 5. Advise patient to obtain and wear a medical ID tag, if known to have serious allergic reaction.

G. Collaboration and referrals.
 1. Allergist for screening and possible desensitization therapy.
 2. Refer to tertiary care, as indicated.

H. Community resources and education.
 1. The Food Allergy & Anaphylaxis Network (www.foodallergy.org).
 2. American Latex Allergy Association (www.latexallergyresources.org).
 3. Asthma and Allergy Foundation of America (www.aafa.org).

I. Telehealth nursing considerations.
 1. Identify emergent situations and refer to EMS (9-1-1).
 2. Stay on the phone with the patient until EMS personnel arrive.

J. Protocols/algorithms/guidelines.
 1. Personnel administering radiographic contrast, immunizations, IV infusions (chemotherapy, antibiotic, biologics, and other drugs) or other parenteral medications should have protocols for independent and immediate recognition and response to systemic allergic reactions.
 2. Communication/documentation.
    a. Patient record.
    b. EMS personnel, as indicated.
    c. Collaboration with allergist, as indicated.

Tuberculosis (TB) Skin Test Conversion

Patient Population: Adult and Pediatric

I. **Overview**

Dugdale, Hadjiliadis, and Zieve (2010) stated that pulmonary tuberculosis (TB) is a contagious bacterial infection that involves the lungs, but may spread to other organs. It is a communicable disease spreading from person to person by droplet nuclei. If exposed, the bacteria, *Mycobacterium tuberculosis*, implants in lung tissue. Health care workers must be knowledgeable and mindful of active TB disease and take appropriate steps to protect themselves and those around them from exposure.

II. **Pathophysiology**

Mycobacterium tuberculosis is able to gain entrance into the body through droplets that are inhaled into the alveoli, and the bacterium becomes implanted. Once implanted, the body is able to encapsulate the bacteria. The bacteria can then reside in the lungs for the lifetime of the individual and not develop into active TB. This condition is known as latent TB infection (LTBI). The individual with LTBI is at a greater risk for developing active TB disease if the body's immune system is weak, especially in those with human immunodeficiency virus (HIV) infection, substance abuse, diabetes mellitus, prolonged corticosteroid use, cancer of the head or neck, or end stage renal disease (Daniels & Nicoll, 2012). If the person has LTBI, the screening tuberculin Purified Protein Derivative (PPD) test will become positive, although the individual is not infectious. Current focus within the United States is to find and treat LTBI with oral antibiotics. The first line of choice is isoniazid (INH) (Centers for Disease Control and Prevention [CDC], 2010a).

III. **Assessment and Triage**
A. PPD screening (see Chapter 14, "Application of the Nursing Process in Ambulatory Care," for PPD administration information). The test interpretation depends on the size of the skin reaction and other factors in the health of the person being tested.
 1. A small reaction of 5 mm induration is considered positive in:

a. Those who are HIV positive.
b. Recipients of an organ transplant.
c. People with suppressed immune systems or who are taking steroid therapy (about 15 mg of prednisone per day for one month).
d. Those in close contact with a person who has active TB.
e. Patients demonstrating changes on a chest X-ray consistent with past TB.

2. Larger reactions of 10 mm or greater induration are considered positive in:
   a. People with a known negative test in the past two years.
   b. Health care workers.
   c. People with diabetes, kidney failure, or other conditions that increase their chance of acquiring active TB.
   d. Injection drug users.
   e. Immigrants who have moved from a country with a high TB rate in the past five years.
   f. Children under the age of 4.
   g. Infants, children, or adolescents who are exposed to high-risk adults.
   h. Students and employees of certain group living settings, such as prisons, nursing homes, and homeless shelters.

3. In people with no known risks for TB, a 15 mm or more induration at the site indicates a positive reaction (Dugdale, Vyas, & Zieve, 2010).

B. Assess for signs or symptoms of active TB disease.
   1. Hemoptysis.
   2. Fatigue.
   3. Unintentional weight loss.
   4. Night sweats.
   5. Chronic cough.
   6. Fever.
   7. Clubbing of the fingers or toes (advanced disease).
   8. Enlarged or tender lymph nodes in neck or other areas.
   9. Pleural effusion.
   10. Abnormal breath sounds: Wheezing, rales, and rhonchi (Dugdale, Hadjiliadis, & Zieve, 2010).

C. If signs or symptoms of active disease exist, place client in respiratory isolation.
   1. Negative pressure room with door closed. If a negative pressure room is not available, place the patient in a single occupancy room and keep the door closed.
   2. All staff involved in direct patient care should don an N–95 or greater respirator.
   3. Place respiratory isolation signage on door of client room. Follow Infection Control policies after use regarding turnover of the room.
   4. The patient should don a surgical mask when leaving the room.

D. If signs or symptoms of active disease do not exist, document history of exposure to TB.

E. Diagnostic tests.
   1. Chest X-ray.
   2. Bronchoscopy.
   3. Chest CT scan.
   4. Interferon-gamma blood test such as the QFT-Gold test (Dugdale, Hadjiliadis, & Zieve, 2010).
   5. Sputum cultures and gram stains.
   6. Thoracentesis.
   7. Tuberculin skin test.
   8. Screening PPDs for family members to rule out exposure source.

IV. **Plan of Care**
A. Pharmacotherapeutics.
   1. Treatment depends on the cause and epidemiology. Four medications are used together for the immediate treatment of active TB. These include: isoniazid (INH), pyridoxine, rifampin (RIF), and ethambutol (EMB). Treatment may be individualized (Daniels & Nicoll, 2012).

B. Primary/secondary/tertiary prevention.
   1. Primary prevention of active TB.
      a. Annual TB screening for health care workers and residents of long-term care facilities.
      b. Education regarding prevention of disease transmission.

c. INH for nine months for PPD conversions (LTBI) for patients without contraindications.

d. Education regarding signs of hepatotoxicity due to INH.
   (1) Anorexia.
   (2) Nausea.
   (3) Aches.
   (4) Upper abdominal pain.
   (5) Increased ALT levels (3–5 times higher than normal).

e. Risks of INH hepatotoxicity increased by:
   (1) Over 50 years of age.
   (2) Alcoholism or other active liver disease.
   (3) Postpartum (three months post-delivery or less).

f. Risk of peripheral neuropathy due to INH increased by:
   (1) Individuals with diet deficient in B6.
   (2) History of alcohol abuse.
   (3) History of diabetes.

g. Possible fever or rash from INH.

2. Secondary prevention.

a. Detection of active TB development.

b. Completion of treatment course. Treatment is at risk due to extended treatment time frame.
   (1) Medication regimen may consist of several drugs being taken for 6–12 months.
   (2) If medication is not finished, it may result in the patient becoming sick again.
   (3) If the medication is not taken as prescribed, the germs that are still alive may become resistant to that specific medication(s).
   (4) Resistant TB germs are more difficult and expensive to treat.
   (5) Patients may be required to participate in directly observed therapy, such as when the local health department meet regularly with the patient and observe the medication being taken.

c. Education on importance of completion is imperative.

C. Goals of plan of care.
   1. The patient understands disease process.
   2. The patient understands importance of completion of treatment.
   3. Health department follows the patient to ensure completion of treatment.
   4. The patient is accepting of condition.

D. Education of patient/family.
   1. Process of tuberculosis infection and infection control measures.
   2. Medication management and length of treatment.
   3. Signs and symptoms of treatment complications (as stated in the *Assessment and Triage* section, above).

E. Collaboration and referrals.
   1. Health department notified for disease reporting and contact follow-up.
   2. Infectious disease and/or pulmonary medicine specialty care, if active disease.
   3. Infection control services.

F. Community resources and education.
   1. Centers for Disease Control and Prevention (CDC) (www.cdc.gov).
   2. National Institutes of Health (NIH) (www.nih.gov).

G. Telehealth nursing considerations.
   1. Information resource for the recognition of signs and symptoms for active TB disease.
   2. Information resource for recognition of signs and symptoms for hepatotoxicity from INH therapy.
   3. Refer as necessary.

H. Protocols/algorithms/guidelines.
   1. Protocols may guide independent nursing care for:
      a. Management and referral of a reactive PPD.
      b. Monitoring and managing compliance with INH prophylaxis.
   2. Communication/documentation in patient record.
   3. Coordinate with the community health department reporting structure.

Depression and Suicide

Patient Population: Adult and Adolescent

I. Overview

In 2007, suicide was considered the tenth leading cause of death in the United States. It accounted for 34,598 deaths with the overall rate being 11.3 suicide deaths per 100,000 people. An estimated 11 attempted suicides occur per every suicide death (National Institute of Mental Health [NIMH], 2010). Most individuals who die from suicide have some or all of the following risk factors: Prior suicide attempt, family history of mental disorder or substance abuse, family history of suicide, family violence, and firearms in the home. Usually the attempt at suicide is staged for the possibility for rescue and is seen as a desperate cry for help. The health care provider needs to take the threat of suicide seriously and coordinate care to provide for the mental health services necessary to achieve emotional stability.

A. Major depression – Five or more symptoms of depression (see the *Assessment and Triage* section, below).

B. Dysthymia – Depression that is chronic in nature; milder than major depression, lasting up to two years.

C. Atypical (psychotic) depression – Occurs when there is a severe depressive illness that is accompanied by some form of psychosis, such as hallucinations or delusions.

D. Postpartum depression – Feeling of sadness or "blue mood" after delivery; usually induced by hormonal changes.

E. Premenstrual dysphoric disorder (PMDD) – Feeling of depression with onset one week prior to menses. After onset of menstruation, symptoms resolve.

F. Seasonal affective disorder (SAD) – Feeling of depression that ensues during the autumn and winter months due to decreased length of sunlight (NIMH, 2009).

G. Suicide – The act or an instance of taking one's own life voluntarily and intentionally, especially by a person of years of discretion and of sound mind (Merriam-Webster, 2010).

II. Assessment and Triage

A. Assess for common complaints of depression.
   1. Insomnia.
   2. Excessive sleeping.
   3. Change in appetite leading to weight gain or loss.
   4. Fatigue.
   5. Feelings of hopelessness, helplessness, worthlessness, self-hate, and inappropriate guilt.
   6. Inability to concentrate.
   7. Withdrawal from social or usual activities.
   8. Recurring thoughts of death or suicide.
   9. Lack of pleasure.
   10. Low self-esteem.
   11. Sudden bursts of anger.

B. Subjective assessment.
   1. Conduct interviews in private.
   2. Psychological review/history.
   3. Description of moods.
   4. Stressors.
   5. Thoughts of suicide or self-harm.
   6. If there are thoughts of suicide, is there a plan?
   7. The means to implement plan (such as poison or a gun).
   8. Recreational drug or alcohol use.
   9. Medications.

C. Have patient complete the Patient Health Questionnaire-2 (PHQ-2).
   1. If positive, proceed to the Patient Health Questionnaire-9 (PHQ-9).
   2. For adolescents, use the Patient Health Questionnaire-A (PHQ-A).

III. Indications for Emergency Care or Urgent Consultation

A. Threat of suicide during interview.

IV. Plan of Care

A. Pharmacotherapeutics.
   1. Antidepressant therapy.
      a. Selective serotonin reuptake inhibitors (SSRIs).
         (1) Selectively inhibits the reuptake of serotonin.

(2) Receptor-mediated side effects are affected by: The dosage and type of SSRI, age, other medical conditions, and other medications being taken.

(3) Side effects may include, but are not limited to:

    (a) Nausea.

    (b) Sleep disturbances.

    (c) Sexual dysfunction.

    (d) Agitation.

    (e) Headache.

b. Secondary amine tricyclics.

(1) Nonselectively inhibits the reuptake of serotonin, norepinephrine, and dopamine into presynaptic storage vesicles in the brain.

(2) Receptor-mediated side effects may include, but are not limited to:

    (a) Dry mouth.

    (b) Blurred vision.

    (c) Constipation.

    (d) Drowsiness.

    (e) Bladder problems.

    (f) Sexual dysfunction.

2. Monoamine oxidase inhibitors (MAOIs).

a. Prescribed when found unresponsive to other treatments.

b. Use caution with the food and medication taken.

c. Food and medicine which contain high levels of tyramine should be avoided if taking an MAOI.

(1) Tyramine is found in wine, cheeses, pickles, and some over-the-counter cold medicines.

(2) Mixing MAOIs and tyramine can cause an increase in blood pressure, which could result in a stroke.

(3) Patients should be given a complete list of food, medicines, and other products to avoid when taking an MAOI.

d. Side effects may include, but are not limited to: Dry mouth, dizziness, lightheadedness, orthostatic hypotension, constipation, and sexual dysfunction (NIMH, 2008).

B. Complementary and alternative therapies.

1. The herbal supplement St. John's Wort has been used for centuries for treatment of mild to moderate depression.

2. It has been shown to help some; however, this herb reacts with other medications such as antidepressants, birth control pills, protease inhibitors, theophylline, warfarin, and digoxin. The patient should counsel with a health care provider before adding St. John's Wort or any herbal remedy to daily regimen (NIMH, 2008).

C. Primary/secondary/tertiary prevention.

1. Always take threats of suicide seriously.

2. Education on self-care.

a. Get enough sleep.

b. Eat a healthy diet.

(1) Adding supplements to daily nutritional intake may be helpful.

    (a) Omega-3 fatty acids.

    (b) Folate (B9) in MVI: 400 to 800 micrograms.

c. Exercise regularly.

d. Avoid alcohol or recreational drugs.

e. Participate in social events that bring joy.

f. Seek out faith-based and/or secular support.

g. Mental health evaluation is necessary.

h. Utilize effective communication skills, especially empathetic listening. Many people who attempt suicide will talk about it first. Talking may be enough to prevent action.

i. Sudden changes in behavior from anxiety to calmness in one who has history of suicide threat can be a sign that a decision to commit suicide has been made.

D. Goals of plan of care.

1. The patient remains free from harm.

2. The patient and family are involved in co-ordinated mental health care.

3. The patient verbalizes self-help measures.

4. The patient verbalizes information on community resources.

E. Education of patient/family.
   1. Signs and symptoms of worsening depression.
   2. Importance of medication compliance.
   3. Dangers of alcohol consumption while taking antidepressants.
F. Collaboration and referrals.
   1. For depression and suicidal ideation, mental health providers will need to be involved.
   2. For major depression and suicide attempt, consider hospitalization.
   3. Family members often feel responsible and will require mental health support.
G. Community resources and education.
   1. National Institute of Mental Health (NIMH) (www. nimh.nih.gov).
   2. American Academy of Child and Adolescent Psychiatry (AACAP) (www.aacap.org).
   3. National Suicide Prevention Lifeline (1-800-273-8255).
H. Telehealth nursing considerations.
   1. Recognize signs and symptoms, and refer to a crisis center, police, and/or EMS (such as by calling 9-1-1) if necessary for management of suicide threat or attempt.
   2. Information resource.
   3. Therapeutic communication.
   4. Referral to community support.
I. Protocols/algorithms/guidelines.
   1. Communication/documentation.
      a. Patient record.
      b. Maintain confidentiality.
      c. Collaborate with tertiary care, if necessary.
   2. Depression support groups provided by community services.
   3. Collaboration with mental health services.
   4. Ongoing medication management.
   5. Family/significant other support system.

Domestic Violence

Patient Population: Adult and Adolescent

I. **Overview**

Domestic violence (also known as domestic abuse and intimate partner violence) is a significant health care problem that is found among people of every gender, age, ethnicity, economic, and social group. Domestic violence is defined as emotional, physical, sexual, psychological, or economic abuse of power and the exercise of control by another individual (or individuals) on a family member, partner, or ex-partner regardless of gender, age, or sexual orientation (Soria, 2011). Domestic violence has widespread and devastating effects for patients, their children, families, and communities. Each year, women in the U.S. experience about 4.8 million partner-related physical assaults and rapes. Men are the victims of about 2.9 million intimate-related physical assaults (CDC, 2011). Domestic violence is the cause of more than 1,300 deaths and more than 2 million injuries annually. The annual cost of domestic violence has been calculated at more than $5.8 billion, with $4.1 billion for direct medical and mental health expenditures (Jagim, 2009). The CDC has identified four behaviors for intimate partner violence and six behaviors for elder violence (CDC, 2010b, 2011).

A. Behavior: Intimate partner violence.
   1. Physical abuse – Occurs when a partner is hurt by physical force; this could be by hitting, kicking, or burning.
   2. Sexual abuse – Involves forcing a partner to take part in a sexual act when the partner does not consent.
   3. Threats of physical or sexual abuse – The use of intimidation, words, gestures, or weapons to communicate the intent to cause harm.
   4. Emotional abuse – Refers to tactics that are used to demean a person's self-worth or emotional well-being. Examples are stalking, name-calling, intimidation, embarrassing on purpose, or not letting a partner see friends and family.
B. Behavior: Elder maltreatment (affecting those 60 years of age and older).
   1. Physical – Occurs when an elder is hurt through the use of physical force such as hitting, kicking, or pushing.
   2. Sexual – Occurs when an elder is forced to take part in a sexual act when the elder does not consent.

3. Emotional – Occurs when the elder's sense of self-worth and emotional well-being is harmed.
4. Neglect – Refers to when the elder's basic needs (such as feeding, housing, clothing, and medical care) are not met.
5. Abandonment – Occurs when the caregiver leaves an elder alone and no longer provides care for him or her.
6. Financial – Occurs when an elder's money, property, or assets are illegally taken advantage of.

C. Risk factors.
1. Prior history of intimate partner violence.
2. Family history or witnessing/experiencing violence as a child.
3. Individuals with low self-esteem.
4. Using drugs or alcohol.
5. Loss of or not having a job or other life events that cause stress.

II. Assessment and Triage
A. Subjective data.
1. Loss of appetite.
2. Difficulty passing urine.
3. Fainting.
4. Increased anxiety.
5. Reluctance to talk about an injury.
6. Explanations that are inconsistent with type of injury.
7. Symptoms of posttraumatic disorder such as nightmares, difficulty concentrating, depressed mood, and change in sleeping pattern.

B. Objective data.
1. Examine and interview patient in privacy.
2. Vital signs.
3. Repeated emergency or office visits for physical injuries, or delayed treatment for injuries or illnesses.
4. Complete a head-to-toe assessment. Pay close attention to:
   a. Injuries to the head, face, and neck.
   b. Upper extremity and breast, buttock, and back injuries.
   c. Bruises and cuts.
   d. Sprains and broken bones.
   e. Various pains (chest, abdomen, pelvic, and genital).
   f. Injuries at various stages of healing.

C. Diagnostic tests.
1. Depending on the subjective, objective, and clinical assessment.
2. Appropriate tests should be ordered for assessing the injuries.

III. Indications for Emergency Care or Urgent Consultation
A. Treatment of immediate injuries.
B. Immediate crisis management – Arrange for advocacy appointment.
C. Report to legal authorities.

IV. Plan of Care
A. Goals of plan of care.
1. Immediate injuries treated and facilitate a safe environment.
2. Patient aware of resources available.
3. Maintain the safety of patient and any family victims.

B. Psychosocial considerations.
1. During period of adjustment.
2. May experience personal relationship issues:
   a. Work.
   b. Home.
   c. Fear of discrimination.
   d. Social isolation.

C. Education of patient/family.
1. Verbal and written instruction regarding any diagnostic test given.
2. Given verbal and written instructions on advocacy, social work, and support programs.
3. Verbal and written instruction on any follow-up appointments and counseling.
4. Reassure patient that he or she is not to blame.

D. Collaboration and referrals.
1. Give patient resources, such as a phone number, that he or she can utilize 24 hours a day.

E. Community resources and education.
1. National Coalition Against Domestic Violence (NCADV) (www.ncadv.org).

2. National Center on Elder Abuse (NCEA) (www. ncea.aoa.gov).
3. National Institute on Aging (NIA) (www. nia.nih. gov).
4. Dating Matters: Understanding Teen Dating Violence Prevention (www.veto violence.org/datingmatters).
5. National Domestic Violence Hotline (NDVH) (1-800-799-SAFE [7233], 1-800-787-3224 [TTY], or www.ndvh.org).

F. Telehealth nursing considerations.
   1. Information resource.
   2. Triage/referral.
   3. Provide reassurance when indicated.
   4. Maintain confidentiality.

G. Protocols/algorithms/guidelines.
   1. Documentation of screening and suspected abuse; include an assessment of patient's safety at present.
   2. Evidence collected.
   3. Collaborate with law enforcement regarding evidence collection and appropriate chain of custody.

ACUTE ILLNESSES

Like medical emergencies, patients may present with acute illnesses in any ambulatory care setting, either in-person or via telecommunications. Characteristics may include (but are not limited to): rapid onset, short duration, or severe symptoms that impair normal function. An acute illness may be medical and/or surgical related. Some acute illnesses may require emergency care, while others may be readily assessed and managed in the ambulatory setting, or managed effectively at home by the patient and/or family (given education and reassurance).

Headache

Patient Population: Adult and Adolescent

I. Overview

Headache is one of the most common health complaints worldwide. "Headache is defined as pain in the head that is located above the eyes or the ears, behind the head, or in the back of the upper neck" (Lee, 2011). Muscular contraction and vascular abnormalities account for approximately 90% of headaches; up to 10% of Americans are affected by throbbing, vascular, and migraine headaches (Pellico, 2008). Migraine headaches tend to start in childhood or adolescence and may occur throughout adulthood. These headaches are more prevalent in women than in men. Some common causes of headaches are emotional stress or fatigue, menstruation, environmental stimuli, glaucoma, vasodilators, hypertension, and head trauma.

II. Pathophysiology

Headaches are classified as primary or secondary. There are three types of headaches: Tension, migraine, and cluster. Primary headaches account for 90–98%; of that, tension headaches account for 90%, whereas secondary headaches have an underlying cause, usually aneurysm or tumors (Daniels & Nicoll, 2012).

A. Definitions.
   1. Tension headache – Headache typically starting in the back of the head, radiating forward. Caused by tight, contracted muscles in shoulders, neck, scalp, and jaw. Brought on by stress, depression, anxiety, overwork, lack of sleep, not eating properly, or alcohol or drug use.
   2. Migraine headache – Severe, recurrent headache with other symptoms, including visual changes, nausea and vomiting, and photophobia. Starts on one side of the head and may spread to both sides. Some may have an aura before onset. Pain described as throbbing, pounding, or pulsating.
   3. Cluster headaches – Sharp, extremely painful headaches that tend to occur several times a day for months, then go away for a similar period of time. These occur more often in men. They can occur after the patient has fallen asleep, are located near or above the eye, and are associated with nasal congestion.

III. Assessment and Triage

A. Subjective data.
   1. History of headaches.
      a. Age of onset.
      b. Frequency and duration.
   2. Accompanying symptoms.
   3. Pain level on a scale of 0–10 (see Chapter 14, "Application of the Nursing Process in Ambulatory Care").
   4. History of onset (sudden vs. gradual), association with activity, trauma, change in method of birth control, or other hormonal changes.
   5. Location of onset.
   6. Visual changes.
   7. Precipitating, aggravating, and alleviating factors.
B. Objective data.
   1. Neurological assessment.
   2. Vital signs.
C. Emergent situations with presentation of headache.
   1. Sudden, severe onset with neurological symptoms including mental status changes or paralysis.
   2. Headache with accompanying fever and neck stiffness may indicate meningitis.
   3. "Worst headache in my life" may indicate a medical emergency (e.g., cerebral aneurysm).
   4. Headache with accompanying loss of memory.
   5. Headache that gets progressively worse over 24 hours.
   6. First time the patient has ever had a severe headache.
D. Diagnostic tests.
   1. Radiography including:
      a. Head CT.
      b. Head MRI.
      c. Sinus X-ray.
   2. Lumbar puncture.

IV. Indications for Emergency Care or Urgent Consultation

A. Complaint of the worst headache ever.
B. Treat any injuries immediately.
C. Complaint of slurred speech, visual changes, problems moving extremities, loss of balance, confusion, and/or memory loss with headache.
D. Over age 50 and headaches just began, associated with visual problems and pain while chewing.
E. Close monitoring of vital signs and neurological status in emergent situations.
F. Close monitoring of pain management.
G. Place the patient in a darkened, quiet room, reclining with head supported and eyes closed. May apply warm or cool compresses to face/neck, depending upon facility protocol.

V. Plan of Care

A. Pharmacotherapeutics.
   1. Prophylactic: To prevent migraine or tension headaches.
      a. Calcium channel blockers.
      b. Sumatriptan (Imitrex®).
      c. Midrin.
      d. Beta blockers.
      e. Serotonin antagonists.
      f. Anticonvulsants.
      g. Ergot derivatives.
   2. Acute treatment: For migraine headaches, prompt treatment is important to a good response.
      a. Simple analgesics: Acetaminophen, NSAIDs, aspirin.
      b. Ergot alkaloids.
      c. Triptans (such as Imitrex®).
      d. Combination analgesics (such as caffeine and analgesics).
      e. Narcotic analgesics.
      f. Nasal spray: Dihydrogotomine (DHE-45), butorphanol, or sumatriptan.
      g. Parenteral medication: Dihydrogotomine (DHE-45) or sumatriptan.
B. Complementary and alternative therapies.
   1. Provider may refer for physical therapy, manipulation, or acupuncture.
      a. Application of heat or cold.
      b. Biofeedback.
      c. Acupressure.
   2. Hypnosis.
   3. Exercise program.
      a. Walking, swimming, bicycle riding.

b. Yoga.

c. Tai chi.

C. Primary/secondary/tertiary prevention.

1. Adequate sleep.

2. Eat a healthy diet.

3. Exercise regularly.

4. Relaxation techniques such as, meditation, deep breathing, and yoga.

5. Stretch at least once an hour if the patient spends the day working at a desk/computer.

6. Correct posture.

7. Abstain from smoking or proximity to secondhand smoke.

8. Avoid known personal triggers (such as chocolate).

9. Perform stretching neck and upper body exercises periodically if you are using a computer for extended periods of time.

10. Wear proper eyeglasses.

D. Goals of plan of care.

1. Pain diminished on pain scale.

2. Client verbalizes understanding of etiology.

3. Client verbalizes preventive and treatment self-care interventions.

4. Number of acute or chronic headaches reduced or eliminated.

E. Education of patient/family.

1. Identification of triggers. Client should keep a headache diary to help determine cause.

2. Measures to ease discomfort, including non-pharmacological management.

3. Relaxation techniques and other behavioral therapies.

4. Medication management.

F. Collaboration and referrals.

1. Neurology consult.

2. Ophthalmology consult.

3. Pain clinic referral.

4. Stress management classes.

G. Community resources and education.

1. National Migraine Association (www. migraines.org)

2. National Institutes of Health (NIH) (www. nih.gov).

H. Telehealth nursing considerations.

1. Triage for severity of illness.

2. Information resource on pain management.

3. Referral, if necessary.

4. Telephone advice documentation.

I. Protocols/algorithms/guidelines.

1. Transfer to tertiary care in emergent situations.

2. Communication/documentation.

a. Patient record.

b. Telephone advice documentation.

Low Back Pain

Patient Population: Adult

I. **Overview**

Low back pain can range from mild to severe and can last from one day to years. At some point, most people will experience low back pain. It is reported that up to 90% of adults will have low back pain during their lifetime. According to Pasero and McCaffery (2011), "next to upper respiratory infection, it is the most common reason for lost work" (p. 222). Americans spend at least $50 billion each year on low back pain, the most common cause of job-related disability and a leading contributor to missed work (National Institute of Neurologic Disorders and Stroke [NINDS], 2011). The pain can be caused by trauma, sprain, strain, or spasm, or may be referred pain and an indication of an underlying disease process. Pain may also be caused by degenerative conditions, such as arthritis or disc disease, osteoporosis, or other bone diseases, viral infections, irritation to joints and discs, or congenital abnormalities in the spine. Obesity, smoking, weight gain during pregnancy, stress, poor physical condition, posture inappropriate for the activity being performed, and poor sleeping position also may contribute to low back pain (NINDS, 2011).

A. Definitions.

1. Acute or short-term back pain – Sudden onset of pain that is temporary, lasting a few days to a few weeks.

2. Chronic back pain – Pain that is persistent and disabling, for more than three months. It may be progressive in nature and the cause is difficult to determine.

II. Pathophysiology

There are four mechanisms involved in the pain experience. They have been identified as transduction, transmission, modulation, and perception. During *transduction*, an electrical activity is initiated due to the impact of noxious, painful, or unpleasant stimuli. *Transmission* is the process of carrying the pain information to a sensory nerve, the spinal cord, and brain centers via the axon. *Modulation* is the alteration of the pain sensation and ultimately affects the perception of the pain. The individual's recognition or appreciation of the pain is *perception* (Daniels & Nicoll, 2012).

III. Assessment and Triage

A. Onset of pain.
B. Pain description (sharp, dull, aching, stabbing, limited flexibility, unable to stand straight).
C. Pain level on a scale of 0–10.
D. Associated symptoms.
   1. Weakness, numbness, or paresthesias.
   2. Urinary retention or incontinence.
   3. Constipation or loss of bowel control.
   4. Hematuria.
   5. Associated fever.
   6. Difficulty walking.
   7. Foot drop.
   8. Headache.
E. Medical history.
   1. Weight loss.
   2. Fever.
   3. Injuries.
   4. Osteoporosis.
   5. Steroid use.
   6. Cancer.
F. Diagnostic tests commonly performed.
   1. Radiography.
   2. Intravenous pyelography (IVP) if necessary for suspected kidney pathology.
   3. Ultrasound, CT scan or MRI, and electromyelogram (EMG) for radicular pain.

IV. Indications for Emergency Care or Urgent Consultation

A. Indication of sensory or motor nerve damage.
B. Complaint of problems moving extremities, loss of balance, or foot drop.

V. Plan of Care

A. Pharmacotherapeutics.
   1. Muscle relaxants.
   2. Over-the-counter analgesics:
      a. Tylenol®, because of its favorable safety profile.
      b. Nonsteroidal anti-inflammatory drugs (NSAIDs).
      c. Topical analgesics.
      d. Counter irritants (Ben Gay®, Icy Hot®, etc.).
   3. More research is indicated to support the use of combination pain management to include opioid and non-opioid formulations (Pasero & McCaffery, 2011).
   4. Antidepressants (NINDS, 2011).
      a. Tricyclic antidepressants have been used to relieve pain and assist with sleep.
         (1) Amitriptyline.
         (2) Desipramine.
      b. Selective serotonin reuptake inhibitors (SSRIs) are being studied for their effectiveness in pain relief.
B. Complementary and alternative therapies.
   1. Alternate heat and ice on the affected area every 20 minutes.
   2. Physical therapy.
C. Primary/secondary/tertiary prevention.
   1. Relaxation techniques.
   2. Weight loss, if necessary.
   3. Education on proper body mechanics.
   4. Education on back strengthening exercises.
   5. Back-healthy exercises including:
      a. Stretching (may include yoga).
      b. Swimming.
      c. Walking.
   6. Healthy lifestyle.
   7. Women: Do not wear high heels.
D. Goals of plan of care.
   1. Resolution of acute pain.
   2. Motor function intact.
   3. Sensory function intact.
   4. Patient accepting of treatment plan.
   5. Resumption of activities of daily living and return to work, as relevant.

E. Education of patient/family.
1. Proper body mechanics.
2. Medication usage.
3. Maintain activities of daily living as pain allows. Bed rest is *not* recommended.
4. Alternate heat and ice on the affected area every 20 minutes.
F. Collaboration and referrals.
1. Pain management to keep the patient comfortable enough to remain as active as possible.
2. Physical therapy.
G. Community resources and education.
1. American Chronic Pain Association (ACPA) (www.theacpa.org).
2. American Pain Foundation (www.painfoundation.org).
3. National Institute of Arthritis and Musculoskeletal and Skin Diseases (NIAMS) (www.niams.nih.gov).
4. National Institutes of Health (NIH) (www.nih.gov).
5. National Chronic Pain Outreach Association (www.chronicpain.org).
H. Telehealth nursing considerations.
1. Triage for severity of illness.
2. Information resource.
3. Referral as necessary.
4. Telehealth advice documentation.
I. Protocols/algorithms/guidelines.
1. Transfer to tertiary care in emergent situations.
2. Communication/documentation.
a. Patient record.
b. Telephone advice documentation.

Sinusitis

Patient Population: Adult

I. Overview

Sinusitis is an infection or inflammation of the sinus cavities. Sinuses are air-filled chambers located around the nasal passages, the eyes, and head. There are four sets of sinus cavities in the human body: Ethmoid, sphenoid, frontal, and maxillary. Mucous membranes in the sinuses are connected to nasal passages. Bacteria or allergens causing nasal irritation can travel along mucous membranes and settle in the sinus cavities. As mucus thickens and plugs the passageways to the sinus, pressure causes pain that is palpable over the sinus area. The National Institute of Allergy and Infectious Diseases (NIAID, 2011) reported that in 2009, nearly 39 million adults were diagnosed with sinusitis. Almost twice as many women than men are diagnosed. Also, more cases are reported in the southern United States than elsewhere in the country (NIAID, 2011).

II. Pathophysiology

Most sinus infections result from unresolved upper respiratory tract infections of seven or more days' duration. The sinuses become obstructed with an overproduction of secretions, and the mucus is trapped within the sinus cavities. The infection may be viral or bacterial. According to Daniels and Nicoll (2012), the most common bacterial organisms that cause sinusitis are *Streptococcus pneumonia, Haemophilus influenza*, and *Moraxella catarrhalis*.

III. Assessment and Triage
A. Subjective data.
1. Date of onset.
2. Drainage color and amount.
3. History of sinus infections.
4. Lack of improvement on decongestants.
5. Other accompanying symptoms, such as facial tightness, pressure or pain, nasal obstruction, headache, decreased sense of smell, sore throat, fever, post nasal drip, ear pain, dental pain, nasal speech, cough, and halitosis.
6. Evidence of periorbital cellulitis and excessive tearing, which may result from with ethmoid sinusitis.
B. Objective data.
1. Palpate or percuss sinuses for tenderness.
2. Vital signs.
3. Inflammation of the nasal mucosa.
C. Risk factors for sinusitis.
1. Asthma.
2. Recent upper respiratory infection.
3. Overusing nasal decongestants.
4. Deviated nasal septum.
5. Frequent swimming and diving.
6. Dental work.

7. Air pollution or smoke.
8. Gastroesophageal reflux disease (GERD).
9. Allergic rhinitis.
D. Diagnostic tests.
   1. Radiography of sinus (X-ray, CT, or MRI) for persistent, recurring, or chronic sinusitis.
   2. Transillumination.
   3. Endoscopy.
   4. Nasal smear.
   5. Sinus puncture for treatment failures, suspected intracranial extension, and nosocomial sinusitis.

IV. **Indications for Emergency Care or Urgent Consultation**
A. Presence of any of the following: Periorbital cellulitis, subperiosteal abscess, cavernous sinus thrombosis, dental abscess, meningitis, and encephalitis (Daniels & Nicoll, 2012).

V. **Plan of Care**
A. Pharmacotherapeutics.
   1. Antibiotics for bacterial infection.
      a. First-line choice is amoxicillin (Amoxil®), trimethoprim/sulfamethoxazole (Bactrim®), or erythromycin (E-mycin®) (Daniels & Nicoll, 2012).
      b. Second-line choice is the second-generation cephalosporins, which include cefprozil (Cefzil®), cefuroxime (Ceftin®) and cefpodoxime (Vantin®), or amoxicillin/clvulanic acid (Augmentin®) (Daniels & Nicoll, 2012).
      c. Newer, broad-spectrum antibiotics that have been effective include azithromycin (Zithromax®) and clarithromycin (Biaxin®) (Daniels & Nicoll, 2012).
      d. Quinolones, such as ciproflaoxacin (Cipro®) and levofloxacin (Levaquin®), can be used in individuals allergic to penicillin or in those patients who have not been responsive to first-line treatment (Daniels & Nicoll, 2012).
   2. Nasal vasoconstrictors.
   3. Topical decongestants.
   4. Systemic decongestants.
   5. Nasal or systemic corticosteroids.

6. Nasal irrigations with hypertonic or normal saline.
7. Pain management with acetaminophen or ibuprofen.
B. Complementary and alternative therapies.
   1. Air humidification with vaporizers or humidifiers.
   2. Application of hot, wet towel over the face.
   3. Sipping hot beverages and hydration.
C. Goals of plan of care.
   1. Resolution of acute infection.
   2. Decreased incidence of recurring infection.
   3. Adequate relief of pain; ability to cope with the pain if not completely relieved.
   4. Maintains adequate airway by managing secretions.
   5. Maintains adequate fluid intake.
D. Patient education.
   1. Humidifier.
   2. Nasal saline drops.
   3. Increase fluid intake.
   4. Warm compresses to face.
   5. Avoid temperature extremes.
   6. Avoid flying during upper respiratory infection.
   7. Over-the-counter decongestants (e.g., pseudoephedrine) and anticholinergics (e.g., chlorpheniramine and diphenhydramine).
E. Collaboration and referrals.
   1. Referral to otolaryngologist for unresolved or chronically recurring infection.
   2. Surgical procedure for fungal infection or threatened intraorbital or intracranial complications.
   3. Surgical procedure for polyps or deviated septum with accompanying infections.
F. Community resources and education.
   1. National Institute of Allergy and Infectious Diseases (NIAID) (www.niaid.nih.gov).
   2. National Institutes of Health (NIH) (www.nih.gov).
G. Telehealth nursing considerations.
   1. Triage for severity of illness.
   2. Information resource on comfort measures.
   3. Referral as necessary.

H. Protocols/algorithms/guidelines.
1. Transfer to tertiary care in emergent situations.
2. Communication/documentation.
   a. Patient record.
   b. Telephone advice documentation.

Sexually Transmitted Diseases

Patient Population: Adult and Adolescent

I. **Overview**

Sexually transmitted diseases (STDs), also known as sexually transmitted infections (STIs), are very common. The term *STD* includes diseases caused by more than 25 infectious organisms that are transmitted by sexual activity. In the United States, the most common STDs include Chlamydia, gonorrhea, syphilis, genital herpes, human papillomavirus (HPV), and hepatitis B (Green, 2008). STDs affect people of all social and income levels. Women are at greater risk of being infected than men, and younger women are at greater risk than those who are older. Idso (2009) reported that studies have shown an increase in STDs in newly single, older women; this group has been identified as a vulnerable population in need of safe sex education, strategies, and interventions. Women may develop additional health problems associated with STDs, such as infections spreading to the uterus and fallopian tubes leading to pelvic inflammatory disease (PID), a major cause of female infertility and ectopic pregnancy. HPV infections increase the risk of cervical cancer. HIV (human immunodeficiency virus) can be sexually transmitted, and upon progression to AIDS (acquired immunodeficiency syndrome), may cause numerous debilitating symptoms and death (CDC, 2010d) (see HIV described in Chapter 21, "Care of the Chronically Ill Patient"). Prevention of STDs is a major nursing focus when caring for any sexually active female. Communication between sexual partners about sexual history and STDs is of primary importance. Counseling about testing for HIV and other STDs is one way that a professional nurse can make a difference in the long-term health status of patients. Providing reassurance about the confidential nature of the patient's treatment/testing is critical in gaining the trust of the patient and allowing him or her to share information necessary to develop a plan of care.

II. **Pathophysiology**
A. Gonorrhea is a bacterial infection caused by *N. gonorrhoeae*. It typically infects the cervix, but also may be found in the anus and/or pharynx.
B. Chlamydia is caused by *C. trachomatis* and infects the cervix, urethra, anus, and/or pharynx.
C. Hepatitis B may be spread by contact with infected blood or sexual contact.
D. Syphilis is caused by *Treponema pallidum* and is contracted by direct contact with a syphilitic lesion or by contact with syphilis-infected blood.

III. **Assessment and Triage**
A. Determine factors.
1. Number of sexual partners.
2. Partner history of STDs.
3. Personal history of STDs.
4. History of abnormal Pap smears.
5. Condom use.
B. Determine presence of partner violence.
C. Signs and symptoms of STDs.
1. Many STDs have no symptoms.
2. Vaginal burning, itching.
3. Urethral burning, itching, discharge.
4. Unusual vaginal discharge.
5. Chancre, or vaginal, perianal, or penile lesions.
6. Rash.
7. Acute discomfort/pain.
8. Foul-smelling discharge.
9. Pain during intercourse.
10. Irritation or pain around the anus.
11. Infection also possible in the oropharynx, conjunctiva, or disseminated gonococcal meningitis and endocarditis.
12. Neonatal infection of eyes, scalp, or other areas.
D. Diagnosis.
1. Vaginal/pelvic exam.
2. Intraurethral swab (men).
3. Culture.
4. Slide prep for wet mount or gram stain.
5. Pap smear.
6. Colposcopy.
7. Biopsy.
8. Blood tests.

IV. Indications for Emergency Care or Urgent Consultation

A. Signs and symptoms of systemic disease not appropriate for outpatient treatment.
B. Ineffective outpatient treatment.
C. Complications related to an STD.
D. Pregnancy.
E. Tubo-ovarian abscess.
F. Referral to an infectious disease specialist may be indicated.

V. Plan of Care

A. Pharmacotherapeutics.

Treatment depends on the causative agent. Bacterial infections (such as gonorrhea, Chlamydia, and syphilis) can be cured with antibiotics. Viral infections (such as HPV, herpes, and HIV) cannot be cured. Medications can be taken to control the symptoms, but there is no way to completely remove the virus from the body.
  1. Appropriate antibiotic(s) for causative agent.
  2. Antivirals.
  3. Antifungals.
  4. Ensure simultaneous treatment of all partners.
B. Clinical procedures.
  1. Pelvic/penile exam for patient and partner.
  2. Blood tests.
  3. Biopsy.
  4. Microscopy, including gram stain and wet prep for Trichomonas, yeast, and WBCs.
C. Primary/secondary/tertiary prevention.

Prevention counseling should be offered in all health care facilities that treat patients at high risk for HIV/STDs.
  1. Primary prevention.
    a. Annual health checks.
      (1) Pelvic exam.
      (2) Pap smear.
      (3) Screening of pregnant women.
      (4) Other tests, as indicated.
    b. Patient education.
      (1) Communication with sexual partner(s).
      (2) Abstinence.
      (3) Monogamy.
      (4) Barrier protection using condoms and/or female condoms.
      (5) Signs and symptoms (and prevalence of infections with no symptoms).
  2. Secondary prevention.
    a. Education.
    b. Detection of asymptomatically infected persons.
    c. Identification of symptomatic persons unlikely to seek diagnosis and treatment.
    d. Effective diagnosis and treatment, as well as counseling to complete treatment.
    e. Evaluation, testing, treatment, and counseling of sex partners.
    f. Pre-exposure vaccination if at risk for:
      (1) Hepatitis B.
      (2) Hepatitis A.
      (3) Human papillomavirus (HPV).
      (4) Herpes simplex virus (HSV) vaccines are currently undergoing trials.
    g. Reporting requirements.
      (1) According to state law.
      (2) Reports are maintained in strictest confidentiality.
      (3) Most states require public health officials to verify diagnosis and treatment, and to notify contacts for screening and treatment.
  3. Tertiary prevention.
    a. Assisted lifestyle changes.
    b. Reinfection prevention education.
    c. Long-term effects.
      (1) Infertility or ectopic pregnancy.
      (2) Fetal risk.
      (3) Death.
    d. Support groups for people with herpes and/or HIV.
D. Goals of plan of care.
  1. Early detection and treatment.
  2. Risk-reducing behavior changes.
  3. Improvement in health status.
  4. Patient satisfaction.

E. Psychosocial considerations.
   1. Examine and interview patient in privacy.
   2. Stigma may delay seeking treatment.
   3. Need support to comply with complete course of treatment.
F. Education of patient/family.
   1. Individualized teaching tailored to the patient.
   2. Include specific actions the patient can take.
   3. Use effective communication skills.
   4. Use all opportunities for proactive interviewing.
   5. Provide with information on local support groups.
G. Collaboration and referrals.
   1. Provide resources and referrals when appropriate.
      a. Personal provider.
         (1) Physician.
         (2) Nurse practitioner.
         (3) Certified nurse midwife.
         (4) Staff nurse.
      b. Planned Parenthood clinics and public health clinics.
      c. Family/social services/community services.
      d. Recommend specialty groups.
      e. Refer to library and Internet information resources.
   2. Provide education.
   3. Support patient decision-making.
H. Community resources and education.
   1. Centers for Disease Control and Prevention (CDC): Division of STD Prevention (www.cdc.gov/std).
   2. American Social Health Association (ASHA) (www.ashastd.org).
I. Telehealth nursing considerations.
   1. Information resource.
   2. Triage/referrals.
   3. Provide reassurance when indicated.
   4. Maintain confidentiality.
J. Protocols/algorithms/guidelines.
   1. The CDC is a resource for protocol development (www.cdc.gov).
   2. Areas for protocol development include:
      a. Contact mechanisms for informing patients of test results.
      b. Reporting of positive STD test protocols (usually based on government requirements). Partner identification may also be required.
      c. Diagnosis/treatment protocols for patients and partners.
      d. Domestic violence, substance abuse screening.
   3. Number system (for confidentiality purposes) versus names, often used for STD/HIV testing.
   4. Transfer to tertiary care in emergent situations.
   5. Communication/documentation.
      a. Patient record.
      b. Telephone advice documentation.

Abdominal Pain

Patient Population: Adult

I. Overview

Abdominal pain is a common complaint. It accounts for up to 10% of emergency department visits (Prather, 2007). The causes are myriad, and often the patient's description is vague (Buttaro, 2008). It may be continuous, episodic, or associated with eating. Abdominal pain may be reported as heartburn, indigestion, or stomach ache. Characteristics may include sudden and severe, colicky, rebound tenderness, steady with episodes of severe and extreme pain, sharp, progressively severe, deep, boring, and steady (Monahan, 2008).

II. Pathophysiology

There are two types of abdominal pain: Chronic and acute. Acute abdominal pain, also known as acute abdomen, may be life-threatening. There are nerve fibers that innervate the abdominal viscera and parietal peritoneum. Pain results when these fibers are either mechanically (due to stretching or spasm) or chemically (due to inflammation, irritation, or ischemia) stimulated (Daniels & Nicoll, 2012). Pain is noted in the solid organs of the abdomen when the capsule is stretched or invaded. This may be from obstruction, congestion, or a space-occupying lesion (Daniels & Nicoll, 2012).

III. Assessment and Triage

A. Subjective data.
  1. History of abdominal pain.
     a. Onset.
     b. Frequency and duration.
     c. Character.
     d. Location.
     e. Relationship to meals, stressful events, or activity.
     f. Past and current medication usage (prescription and over-the-counter).
     g. Previous surgery.
     h. Family history.
     i. Female patient:
        (1) Date of last menses.
        (2) Menstruation pattern.
        (3) Number of pregnancies.
        (4) Obtain a sexual history.
  2. Accompanying symptoms.
     a. Fatigue.
     b. Elimination patterns.
     c. Difficulty swallowing.
     d. Nausea and vomiting.
     e. Fever.
  3. Pain level on a scale of 0–10.

B. Objective data.
  1. Vital signs.
  2. Abdominal assessment to determine presence or absence of:
     a. Tenderness.
     b. Organ enlargement.
     c. Masses.
     d. Status of abdominal muscles.
        (1) Spasms.
        (2) Rigidity.
     e. Fluid or air in abdominal cavity.
  3. Perform assessment in the following order:
     a. Inspection.
     b. Auscultation.
     c. Percussion.
     d. Palpation.
  4. When assessing the abdomen, the surface is anatomically divided into quadrants and the location may indicate the source of discomfort.
     a. Right upper quadrant:
        (1) Liver.
        (2) Gallbladder.
        (3) Duodenum.
        (4) Right kidney.
        (5) Hepatic flexure of the colon.
     b. Left upper quadrant:
        (1) Stomach.
        (2) Spleen.
        (3) Left kidney.
        (4) Pancreas.
        (5) Splenic flexure of the colon.
     c. Right lower quadrant:
        (1) Cecum.
        (2) Appendix.
        (3) Right ovary and tube.
     d. Left lower quadrant:
        (1) Sigmoid colon.
        (2) Left ovary and tube.

C. Diagnostic tests.
  1. Laboratory tests.
     a. Blood tests.
        (1) Electrolytes.
        (2) Complete blood count.
        (3) Blood urea nitrogen.
        (4) Osmolality.
        (5) Serum amylase.
        (6) Alkaline phosphatase.
        (7) Creatine kinase.
        (8) *H.pylori* testing.
     b. Stool specimen.
        (1) Culture.
        (2) Fat content.
        (3) Presence of ova and parasites.
        (4) Fresh and occult blood.
        (5) Bacteria.
  2. Radiological tests.
     a. Abdominal films: Upright, supine, and lateral decubitus.
     b. Chest film.
     c. Barium swallow.
     d. Upper GI series.
     e. Barium enema.
     f. Ultrasonography.
     g. Computed tomography (CT).
     h. Cholecystography.
     i. Cholangiography.
  3. Special tests.
     a. Electrocardiogram to rule out cardiac origin of pain.
     b. Gastric function.
     c. Biopsy.

d. Endoscopy.
e. Esophagogastroduodenoscopy (EGD).
f. Endoscopic retrograde cholangiopan-creatography (ERCP).
g. Colonoscopy.

IV. Indications for Emergency Care or Urgent Consultation

A. Suspected appendicitis.
B. Suspected bowel obstruction.
C. Signs and symptoms of ruptured abdominal aortic aneurysm (AAA).
D. Suspected ruptured ectopic pregnancy.
E. Evidence of cardiac origin.

V. Plan of Care

A. Pharmacotherapeutics – Dependant on final diagnosis.
B. Complementary and alternative therapies.
1. Nutritional counseling.
2. Dietary management.
3. Restrict or limit use of irritating agents:
a. Caffeine.
b. Nicotine.
c. Nonsteroidal anti-inflammatory drugs (NSAIDs).
C. Goals of plan of care.
1. Disease-specific; definitive management of the underlying problem.
2. Supportive care, which may range from aggressive symptom care to emergent care.
3. Surgical intervention, if indicated.
4. Resolution of pain.
5. Patient acceptance of treatment plan.
D. Psychosocial – Fear in response to the diagnosis.
E. Education of patient/family.
1. Verbal and written instructions regarding diagnostic tests.
2. Dietary restrictions.
3. Bowel preparation.
4. Medication instructions.
5. Answer questions regarding procedures, rationale for use, and specific preparation.
6. Assure patient is physically and mentally prepared for tests to avoid repetition of time-consuming and expensive procedures.

F. Collaboration and referrals.
1. Primary care management for routine care.
2. Referral to specialist/surgeon for secondary/tertiary care.
3. Coordinate transfer to tertiary care.
4. Pain management.
G. Community resources and education.
1. Provide referrals as necessary.
2. Education.
H. Telehealth nursing considerations.
1. Triage for severity of illness.
2. Information resource on pain management.
3. Referral if necessary.
4. Telephone advice documentation.
I. Protocols/algorithms/guidelines.
1. Transfer to tertiary care in emergent situations.
2. Communication/documentation.
a. Patient record.
b. Telephone advice documentation.

Upper Respiratory Infection

Patient Population: Pediatric

I. Overview

An upper respiratory infection (URI) is a non-specific term describing acute infections of the nose, throat, and upper respiratory structure. URIs are the most common acute illness in infancy and childhood. Bacterial (*Streptococcus pneumoniae, Microplasma pneumoniae, Haemophilus influenzae, Chlamydophila pneumoniae, Legionella species*) and viral upper respiratory infections affect the nasal passages, throat, bronchioles, and lungs. The most frequent URI is the common cold. Healthy children have an average of six colds per year (Hockenberry & Wilson, 2011). For children under the age of 3, viral infections (usually rhinoviruses, respiratory syncytial virus [RSV], adenovirus, influenza virus, parainfluenza virus, human metapneumovirus, and coronavirus) are the greatest cause of upper respiratory illness, while school-age children are at a higher risk of bacterial infection. URIs are generally mild, but in rare cases may be fatal.

II. Pathophysiology

Invading organisms initiate an inflammatory process in the epithelial cells of the mucous membrane layers of the nasopharynx and oropharynx (Muscari, 2005).

III. Assessment and Triage

A. Subjective data.
1. Onset and duration of normal cold symptoms:
   a. Fever up to three days.
   b. Sore throat up to five days.
   c. Nasal discharge and congestion up to two weeks.
   d. Cough up to three weeks.
2. Secondary symptoms:
   a. Earache, ear discharge.
   b. Sinus pain.
   c. Fever longer than three days.
   d. Difficult/rapid respirations.
   e. Fever that subsides for 24 hours and then returns.
   f. Sore throat longer than five days.
   g. Nasal discharge lasting longer than two weeks.
   h. Cough lasting greater than three weeks.
3. Medication history.
4. Description of symptoms.
5. Identifiable exposure.
6. Functional status:
   a. Level of activity.
   b. Change in dietary or fluid intake.
B. Objective data.
1. Vital signs, weight, plus pulse oximetry.
2. Physical assessment.
   a. Color.
   b. Work of breathing and use of accessory muscles.
      (1) Intercostal or sternal retractions.
      (2) Nasal flaring.
      (3) Grunting.
      (4) Stridor.
   c. Pattern of breathing.
      (1) Rate.
      (2) Depth.
      (3) Ease.
      (4) Rhythm.

d. Child's energy/activity level (eye contact, ability to answer questions, etc.), behavior changes, and changes in level of consciousness.
e. Auscultate lung sounds for:
   (1) Air movement.
   (2) Wheezes.
   (3) Rales/rhonchi.
   (4) Crackles.
   (5) Diminished breath sounds.
3. Diagnostic tests as indicated by disease process: Throat culture, nasal culture, nasal wash, X-ray.

IV. Indications for Emergency Care or Urgent Consultation

A. Signs of moderate to severe respiratory distress: Accessory muscle use, tachypnea, tachycardia, retractions, nasal flaring, grunting, cold and clammy skin, wheezing, restlessness, refusal to eat, listlessness, agitation, labored breathing, and/or cyanosis.
B. Altered level of consciousness.
C. Newborns under 3 months of age with fever greater than 100.4 °F (38.0 °C).

V. Plan of Care

A. Pharmacotherapeutics (see Table 18-2).
B. Complementary and alternative therapies – There is no conclusive evidence that complementary and alternative therapies prevent or substantially reduce the duration or severity in children (National Center for Complementary and Alternative Medicine, 2011).
C. Primary/secondary/tertiary prevention.
1. Patient/parent education on respiratory etiquette, "Cover Your Cough" (CDC, 2010c).
   a. Infected individuals should sneeze or cough by covering their mouths and noses with a tissue, or by coughing into their elbows.
   b. Throw the tissue away and wash hands with soap and water or use hand sanitizer.
2. Administer appropriate vaccines: Pneumococcal, influenza, and hemophilus influenzae B.
3. Wash hands and toys frequently.

Table 18-2.
Recommendations Related to Medications of URIs in Children

Age	Recommendation
Younger than 4 years	Do not give over-the-counter cough and cold medications. Administration of cough and cold medications can produce serious side effects. May administer acetaminophen or ibuprofen for fever and pain per fever protocol. Do not use aspirin. All children less than 12 weeks of age with fever need to be evaluated by a provider.
From 4–6 years	Cough and cold medications are not recommended at this age because they do not have proven efficacy. If a parent insists on giving medication, advise him or her of the proper dose to administer. May administer acetaminophen or ibuprofen for fever and pain per fever protocol. Do not use aspirin.
Older than 6 years	Advise the best treatment for cough is honey or cough drops, and the best treatment for nasal congestion is nasal washes. If the parent insists on giving medication, advise him or her of the proper dose to administer. May administer acetaminophen or ibuprofen for fever and pain per fever protocol. Do not use aspirin.

Source: Schmitt, 2011. Used with permission.

4. Avoid overusing antibiotics.
5. Humidify air.
6. Minimize risk factors: Pollution and secondhand smoke.
D. Goals/plan of care (outcomes desired).
  1. Parent verbalizes understanding and is supportive of home treatment and avoidance of risk factors.
  2. Completes entire course of antibiotics, if prescribed.
  3. Infection resolves.
E. Psychosocial considerations.
  1. Return to school or childcare provider after the fever has subsided and the child feels well enough to join in normal activities.
  2. Parent reassurance.
F. Education of patient/family.
  1. Disease process.
    a. Fever up to three days.
    b. Sore throat up to five days.
    c. Nasal congestion up to two weeks.
    d. Cough up to three weeks.
  2. Medication management and administration.
    a. Antipyretics, per fever protocol. Do not use aspirin.
    b. Antibiotic for bacterial infections.
    c. No antibiotic use for viral infection.

3. Exacerbations, signs, and symptoms of ineffective breathing:
    a. Severe difficulty breathing.
    b. Rapid breathing.
    c. Breathing with a grunting noise.
    d. Slow, shallow, weak breathing.
    e. Retractions.
    f. Inconsolable or lethargic.
    g. Inability to eat/drink.
G. Clinical procedures and treatments, as indicated.
  1. Nebulizer.
  2. Peak flow.
  3. Blood samples, such as complete blood count.
  4. Cultures (throat, sputum, etc.).
  5. X-ray of chest, if indicated.
  6. Medications.
H. Self-care of primary and secondary problems.
  1. Nasal washes with warm water or saline nose drops and suctioning with a bulb syringe, as needed. Saline nose drops can be purchased or made by mixing 1/2 teaspoon of salt to one cup of lukewarm water (Schmitt, 2011).
  2. Suction prior to feeding infants.
  3. Warm shower for the older child, to loosen mucus.

4. Increase intake of fluids.
5. Humidify air.
6. Increase rest.
I. Telehealth practice.
    1. Information resource.
    2. Triage/assessment.
    3. Referral as necessary.
    4. Instruct patient to call back if:
        a. Signs of respiratory distress.
        b. Fever greater than three days.
        c. Fever for infant less than 12 weeks.
        d. Cough greater than three weeks.
        e. Symptoms worsen.
        f. Difficulty swallowing.
J. Protocols/algorithms/guidelines.
    1. Institution-specific guidelines about which patients to triage to emergency department versus seen by a provider or advised on home care.
    2. Other appropriate protocols specifically for fever, cough, and respiratory distress.

Nausea, Vomiting, and Diarrhea

Patient Population: Pediatric

I. **Overview**

Just as sneezing is the body's defense against allergens and pathogens, nausea, vomiting, and diarrhea are the body's way of eliminating irritants from the gastrointestinal tract. Nausea, vomiting, and diarrhea are common in childhood and leading causes of illness in children less than five years of age. In the United States, pediatric dehydration contributes to approximately 200,000 hospitalizations and 300 deaths per year (Takayesu & Lozner, 2010). Typically, the symptoms related to the gastrointestinal tract are self-limiting, with vomiting usually resolving within 24–48 hours and diarrhea resolving within 14 days (Hockenberry & Wilson, 2011). However, when not managed correctly, vomiting and diarrhea pose a risk for dehydration and electrolyte loss.

II. **Pathophysiology**

Nausea, vomiting, and diarrhea in pediatrics arise from the inflammation of the stomach and small and large intestines. Rotovirus is the most common cause of severe gastroenteritis in infants and children under five years old. Most common viruses affecting older children and adolescents are adenoviruses, astroviruses, and noroviruses.

III. **Assessment and Triage**
A. Subjective data.
    1. Onset of symptoms.
    2. Color, frequency, amount, consistency of stool/emesis.
    3. Location, nature, and pattern of pain.
    4. Recent contact with animals, birds, or reptiles.
    5. Recent illness within the household.
    6. School/daycare center attendance.
    7. Medication history.
    8. Intake of untreated water sources.
    9. Recent travel outside the U.S. (evaluation for parasites).
    10. Chronic conditions that may exacerbate risks from dehydration, such as immunosuppressive illnesses or therapies.
    11. Functional status.
    12. Urinary output.
    13. Recent oral intake.
    14. Recent dietary changes.
    15. Signs of lethargy.
    16. Signs of dehydration.
B. Objective data.
    1. Vital signs, including weight.
    2. Physical examination.
        a. Delayed capillary refill.
        b. Sunken fontanel and/or eyes.
        c. Skin turgor.
        d. Bowel sounds.
        e. Gastric distention and tenderness.
        f. Level of activity.
    3. Diagnostic – Tests are rarely used and are not indicated in uncomplicated vomiting and diarrhea without evidence of dehydration.

IV. Indications for Emergency Care or Urgent Consultation
(Schmitt, 2011)
A. Signs of severe dehydration.
   1. No urine output for eight hours.
   2. No tears.
   3. Very dry mouth.
   4. Sunken eyes, fontanels.
B. Blood in vomit or stool.
C. Projectile vomiting followed by currant jelly stool.
D. Altered level of consciousness.
E. Fever greater than 100.4 °F (38.0 °C) in infants less than 3 months old.
F. Right lower quadrant pain lasting more than two hours.
G. Head or abdominal injury within the past three days.
H. Bile in vomit in infants less than 6 months old.
I. Signs of hypovolemic shock.
   1. Tachypnea.
   2. Tachycardia.
   3. Decreased peripheral pulses.
   4. Decreased capillary refill.
   5. Cool to cold, pale, mottled diaphoretic skin.
   6. Dusky, pale distal extremities.
   7. Change in level of consciousness.
   8. Oliguria.

V. Plan of Care
A. Pharmacotherapeutics – The Centers for Disease Control and Prevention (2010c) and the American Academy of Pediatrics (Schmitt, 2011) do not recommend the use of medications for treatment of nausea, vomiting, or diarrhea.
B. Complementary and alternative therapies.
   1. Lactobacilli (probiotics) may shorten the course of diarrhea.
C. Primary/secondary/tertiary prevention.
   1. Hand hygiene.
   2. Disinfection of contaminated surfaces, Including toys.
   3. Proper food handling.
   4. Rotovirus vaccine administration.
D. Goals/plan of care (outcomes desired).
   1. Parent verbalizes understanding of home treatment for rehydration.
   2. Parent understands and is supportive of treatment plan.
   3. Electrolyte and fluid balance intact.
   4. Illness resolved.
E. Psychosocial considerations.
   1. Anxiety of parents about unknown origin of vomiting or diarrhea, possibility of serious illness.
   2. Child needs care and needs to be off from school until vomiting and diarrhea resolve and the child feels well enough to return to normal daily activities.
F. Education of patient/family.
   1. Disease process.
      a. Is mostly of viral origin, but may be bacterial or parasitic.
      b. Is usually self-limiting and resolve with supportive care.
   2. Rehydration management (see Table 18-3). Wash diaper area after each stool and apply diaper ointment.
   3. Exacerbations – When to seek health care attention.
      a. Vomiting longer than 48 hours.
      b. Diarrhea more than 14 days.
      c. Signs and symptoms of dehydration.
         (1) Very dry mucous membranes.
         (2) No urine output for 8 hours or 12 hours in older children.
         (3) No tears with crying.
         (4) Sunken eyes, fontanels.
         (5) Irritable, restless, increased sleep, or difficult to awake.
G. Clinical procedures.
   1. Specimens: Blood, stool, and urine, as required.
   2. Fluid replacement including IV hydration, if indicated.
H. Collaboration and referrals.
   1. Triage for emergency care, as indicated.
   2. Appointment with child's primary care provider, as indicated.
I. Telehealth practice.
   1. Information resource.
   2. Triage/assessment.
   3. Referral as necessary.
J. Protocols/algorithms/guidelines.

Table 18-3.
Guidelines for Rehydration Therapy

	Vomiting	Diarrhea
Infant less than 1 year	Avoid water, fruit juice, and soda due to potential osmotic properties. Oral rehydration solutions (ORS) like Pedialyte® and store brands may be given.	
Breastfed infant	Reduce the amount of time at breast, but increase the frequency of feedings. If continues to vomit, change to ORS. Return to breastfeeding after 4 hours without vomiting.	Increase breastfeeding. Continue regular diet, including solids. For frequent, watery stools, offer 2–4 ounces ORS after each stool.
Bottle-fed infant	Stop formula and offer ORS for 8 hours in increasing amounts as tolerated. Return to normal diet within 24 hours.	Increase formula feeding. Continue regular diet. For frequent, watery stools, initially stop formula and offer unlimited ORS for 4–6 hours. Restart formula after 6 hours.
Older than 1 year	Initially offer small amounts of water or ice chips and gradually progress over 4–8 hours. If vomits water, use ORS. If patient refuses ORS, use half-strength Gatorade™ or other sports drink. Other options: Half-strength flat lemon-lime soda or popsicles. After 8 hours without vomiting, add solids. Starchy foods are easiest to digest. Return to normal diet within 24 hours.	Continue regular diet; encourage starchy foods (cereal, crackers, rice). Drink more fluids. If taking solids, give water or half-strength sports drinks. If not taking solids, give milk or formula. Give probiotics (yogurt) twice daily.

Source: Schmitt, 2011. Used with permission.

1. Institution-specific guidelines about which patients to triage to emergency department versus seen by a provider or advised on home care.
2. Other appropriate protocols specifically for fever and abdominal pain.

Fever

Patient Population: Pediatric

I. Overview

Fever is a temporary, abnormal elevation in body temperature in response to an illness or disease. Fever is a common reason given for pediatric visits in ambulatory care, accounting for nearly one-third (Allen, 2011). Fever is of greater clinical importance in younger children because of their limited immunologic development and incomplete vaccinations. Normal core body temperature measured rectally ranges from 97–100 °F (36.1–37.8 °C), but there is great individual variation. Also, body temperature fluctuates during the day, with the lowest temperature in the morning and the highest in the late afternoon, including during a febrile condition. Fever is usually defined as a rectal temperature of 100.4 °F (38 °C) or higher (Smitherman & Macias, 2010). Lethargy with fever may be a sign of meningitis, and children with fever and lethargy need immediate evaluation.

II. Pathophysiology

A. Fevers may be the sign of one of several problems.
  1. Most often, fevers are caused by a viral illness.
    a. Generally follow a benign course and are self-limited.

b. Viral infections commonly seen are upper respiratory infections, bronchiolitis, croup, viral gastroenteritis, roseola, mononucleosis, and varicella (CDC, 2010e).

c. More serious viral infections are also seen, such as infection with herpes simplex virus (HSV) at any age, or respiratory syncytial virus (RSV).

2. Bacterial infections are also an important cause of fevers in children.

a. Bacterial infections in children may include, but are not limited to: Streptococcal pharyngitis, urinary tract infection (UTI), bacteremia, meningitis, osteomyelitis, bacterial gastroenteritis, or bacterial pneumonia.

b. Bacterial infections may arise secondary to a viral illness.

3. Although less common, fever may be the presenting symptom of autoimmune diseases such as rheumatoid arthritis or Kawasaki syndrome.

B. Fever is a normal physiologic response, not an illness (Sullivan & Farrar, 2011).

1. Hypothalamus increases the set point in response to a stimulus.

2. Fever increases production of neutrophils and t-lymphocytes.

3. A fever fights the growth and reproduction of bacteria.

III. Assessment and Triage

A. Subjective data.

1. History of fever.

a. Length of time the fever has been present.

b. Onset gradual or sudden.

c. Exposure to an antigen 4–6 hours prior.

d. Severity and pattern of fever.

e. Response to antipyretics.

f. Associated with frequent crying, which means the child is in pain in addition to having the fever.

g. Other symptoms present, such as rash, rhinorrhea, cough, vomiting, or diarrhea.

2. Functional status.

a. Lethargy.

b. Fluid intake and output.

c. Mobility of limbs.

d. Mental alertness.

e. Irritability.

f. Change in dietary intake and/or bowel habits.

B. Objective data.

1. Age of patient.

2. Vital signs – Temperature, pulse, respirations. Blood pressure if suspicious of dehydration or other complications.

3. Weight, compared to previous weight, and graphed on growth chart.

4. Physical assessment.

a. General appearance, such as limp, weak, not moving, unresponsive.

b. Respiratory effort.

c. Fontanel.

d. Mobility of neck.

e. Skin color and appearance (e.g., any rashes or cyanotic discoloration).

5. Diagnostic tests, which may be indicated.

a. Complete blood count to screen for elevated white count or shift in differential.

b. Lumbar puncture.

c. Urinalysis.

d. Cultures of blood, urine, cerebrospinal fluid, throat (may also do Strep screen), sputum, or other suspected sources of infection.

e. X-rays.

IV. Indications for Emergency Care or Urgent Consultations

A. Emergent symptomology, if associated with a fever, indicate need for immediate transport to an emergency department, such as by EMS (Schmitt, 2010).

1. Limp, weak, or not moving.

2. Unresponsive or difficult to arouse.

3. Purplish rash.

4. Severe difficulty breathing.

5. Cyanosis of lips or face.

6. Seizure lasting more than five minutes.

B. Caregiver should take child to emergency department.
1. Confusion, in speech or behavior.
2. Newborn less than 4 weeks old with fever greater than 100.4 °F (38.0 °C) rectally.
3. Infant with sickle cell disease.

C. Child needs to see a provider urgently, in office, urgent care, or emergency department.
1. Stiff neck (child unable to touch chin to chest).
2. Bulging fontanel.
3. Seizure with a fever.
4. Weakened immune system (e.g., sickle cell disease, transplant, immunosuppressive drugs, HIV).
5. Newborn less than 4 weeks old with abnormal behavior.
6. Signs of dehydration (such as dry mouth, no urine output for more than 12 hours).
7. Burning or painful urination.
8. Lethargy.
9. Temperature greater than 105 °F (40.6 °C).
10. Chills with shaking for more than 30 minutes.
11. Limited mobility of a limb (R/O septic arthritis).
12. Difficulty breathing.
13. Inconsolable crying and cries when touched or moved.
14. Accompanying earache, throat pain, or cough.

V. Plan of Care

A. Pharmacotherapeutics.
1. Only treat fevers with antipyretics if the fever is causing discomfort.
2. Use over-the-counter antipyretics, such as acetaminophen or ibuprofen, for fever over 102 °F (39 °C).
   a. Do not use ibuprofen for children under the age of 6 months (not FDA approved).
   b. Do not recommend use of acetaminophen by caretakers of children younger than 12 weeks. Infant's fever needs to be evaluated in a medical setting.
3. Alternating acetaminophen and ibuprofen is **not** recommended unless fever is over 104 °F (40 °C) and the child is unresponsive to one medication alone (American Academy of Pediatrics, 2011).
   a. Risk of dosing error and even poisoning.
   b. Increases parents' fears about fever.
4. Do not use multi-ingredient preparations in children under 6 years. Most cold preparations are contraindicated.
5. Do not give aspirin to children for treatment in fever because of the risk of Reye's Syndrome.
6. Dosages are based on the child's weight and the form of the antipyretic preparation.

B. Complementary and alternative therapies.
1. Homeopathic, herbal, and other alternative therapies do not have support of scientific evidence, but parents/patients may be using them.
2. Herbal remedies for fever.
   a. Many herbal teas are believed to enhance the action of a fever on the metabolism and strengthen the immune system.
   b. Some induce sweating (e.g., yarrow, black elder, linden flowers, cayenne).
3. Hydrotherapy (Consumer Guide, 2007).
   a. Treatment with hot or cold water or alternating to stimulate the immune system.
   b. Bathing in warm water to induce sweating.
   c. Sponging the body with tepid water to slightly reduce a fever, but avoid chilling the patient.

C. Primary/secondary/tertiary prevention.
1. Immunizations for prevention of many viral and bacterial illnesses.
2. Early identification and treatment of possible sepsis or meningitis using assessment and triage guidelines, as stated above.

D. Goals of plan of care.
1. Control discomfort associated with fever.
2. Prevent dehydration.
3. Use antibiotics only for bacterial infections and not for viral infections.

4. Parent understands and supports treatment plan.
E. Psychosocial considerations.
1. Anxiety of parent about unknown origin of fever, possibility of serious illness.
2. Fever phobia of some parents with unwarranted fears that fevers are harmful to children.
3. Child needs care and should be off from school until fever resolves and child feels well enough to return to normal activities.
F. Education of parent/patient.
1. Reassure parents that a fever is a normal response to help a child's body fight infection. Low-grade to moderate fevers are generally beneficial.
2. Dress in lightweight clothing, and avoid bundling with blankets (Hockenberry & Wilson, 2011).
3. Provide cold fluid in unlimited amounts.
4. Antipyretics are only indicated if the fever causes discomfort, which usually occurs over 102 °F (39 °C).
5. Antipyretics are intended to lower the temperature to a comfortable level, usually 2–3 °F (1–2 °C).
6. Contraindications to antipyretics.
   a. Acetaminophen contraindicated for infants younger than 12 weeks, unless ordered by a provider.
   b. Ibuprofen is contraindicated in infants younger than 6 months.
   c. Aspirin should be avoided unless specifically ordered by a provider (risk of Reye's Syndrome).
7. Do not alternate acetaminophen and ibuprofen.
8. Sponging may be used for a fever over 104 °F (40 °C) that does not respond to antipyretics. Use lukewarm water (85–90 °F) (29.4–32.2 °C). Do not use cold baths or alcohol rub. Doing so will cool the skin, causing shivering and raising core temperature (Schmitt, 2011).
9. Most fevers last 2–3 days.
10. Contact the child's primary care provider if symptoms get worse, the fever persists for three days, or if the fever goes above 105 °F (40.6 °C).

G. Collaboration and referrals.
1. Triage for emergency care, as indicated.
2. Appointment with child's primary care provider, as indicated.
H. Community resources and education.
1. Health departments often provide immunizations at no charge or reduced charge for primary prevention.
2. Information resources for parents for fever control.
I. Telehealth nursing considerations.
1. Recognize emergent situations and refer for emergent care or appointment, as necessary.
2. Instruct patient to call back.
   a. Fever over 105 °F (40.6 °C).
   b. Fever persists over three days.
   c. Symptoms become worse.
J. Protocols/algorithms/guidelines.
1. Institution-specific guidelines about which patients to triage to emergency department versus seen by a provider or advised on home care.
2. Dosing guidelines for acetaminophen and ibuprofen.
3. Other appropriate protocols specifically for colds, cough, sore throat, influenza, earache, sinus pain, rash, vomiting, or diarrhea.

Ear Pain

Patient Population: Pediatric

I. **Overview**

Approximately 80% of children have at least one episode of acute otitis media (AOM) and 80–90% will experience at least one episode of otitis media with effusion by age 3. However, there is great variability in diagnostic criteria and approaches to therapy.

Acute otitis externa occurs in 4 of every 1,000 people annually, and the chronic form affects 3-5% of the population. The condition is most common in swimmers, divers, and those whose ears are regularly exposed to or submerged in water.

Acute otitis media (AOM) is defined as middle ear effusion with evidence of acute inflammation (purulent effusion and/or erythematous tympanic membrane) accompanied by symptoms of ear pain or fever. *Otitis media with effusion* (OME) is a middle ear effusion without symptoms of acute otitis media with or without evidence of inflammation. *Otitis externa* is the term for infection of the external auditory canal. It is considered chronic when it lasts over four weeks or the patient has four episodes in a year.

II. Pathophysiology

A. Acute otitis media (AOM).
  1. Inflammation and fluid collection in the middle ear usually a complication of an upper respiratory infection.
  2. Not exclusively caused by bacterial infections.
  3. Multiple bacteria pathogens have been associated: *Streptococcus pneumonia, Haemophilus influenza, Moraxella catarrhalis and Staphylococcus aureus* (Linsk, Blackwood, Cooke, Harrison, & Passamani, 2007).
  4. Infants and toddlers are more often affected than older children.
B. Otitis media with effusion (OME).
  1. Fluid collects in the middle ear without inflammation.
  2. May be associated with bacteria or not, the same as acute otitis media.
  3. May be spontaneous result of poor Eustachian tube function (American Academy of Family Physicians [AAFP], 2004).
C. Otitis externa.
  1. Protective cerumen is reduced, allowing collection of water and debris, facilitating bacteria or fungal growth in the canal.
  2. Localized trauma from foreign objects placed in canal may also allow bacteria invasion.
  3. Most common organisms are *Pseudomonas, Staphylococcus,* and *Streptococcus* species. Fungi are less common (Waitzman, 2010).
  4. Rarely, the infection may invade underlying structures of soft tissue and temporal bone. This malignant otitis externa is a complication seen in immunocompromised persons.

III. Assessment and Triage

A. Subjective data.
  1. Symptoms to screen.
    a. Severity of pain.
    b. Presence of drainage.
    c. Fever.
    d. Upper respiratory infection symptoms, such as rhinorrhea, sore throat, or cough.
    e. Foreign body in the ear.
    f. Stiff neck (R/O meningitis).
    g. Itching.
  2. Functional status.
    a. Weakness.
    b. Malaise.
B. Objective data.
  1. Physical assessment.
    a. Vital signs, including temperature.
    b. Examination and manipulation of the external ear. Assess for pain, erythema, and discharge (Hockenberry & Wilson, 2011).
    c. Otoscopy.
    d. Pneumatic otoscopy recommended for diagnosis of AOM and OME.
  2. Diagnostic procedures.
    a. Cerumen removal, if necessary.
    b. Tympanometry/acoustic reflectometry to assess middle ear pressures and the presence of fluid.
    c. Audiogram to assess hearing, if indicated.

IV. Indications for Emergency Care or Urgent Consultation

A. Signs of sepsis.
B. Signs of meningitis (see previous section on *Fever*).
C. Clear or bloody drainage from ear following head trauma (R/O cerebrospinal fluid leak from skull fracture (Schmitt, 2011).
D. Fever over 105 °F (40.6 °C).

V. Plan of Care

A. Pharmacotherapeutics.
  1. Acute otitis media (AOM).
    a. Analgesics for symptoms of ear pain, irritability, and fever.

b. Antibiotics, if moderate to severe symptoms (Linsk et al., 2007).
  (1) Many guidelines recommend observation for minor symptoms.
  (2) Antibiotic of choice is amoxicillin. If sensitivity occurs, azithromycin is an alternative.
  (3) If suspect coexistent disease, ceftriaxone.

2. Otitis media with effusion (OME).
  a. No antibiotic indicated.
  b. Anti-histamines and decongestants are not recommended (AAFP, 2004).

3. Otitis externa.
  a. Ear wick may be necessary to allow delivery of medication into a swollen, narrow auditory canal.
  b. Acetic acid and drying agents were often formerly recommended, but can be very irritating to inflamed tissue.
  c. Aminoglycosides with a second antibiotic and a topical steroid, such as neomycin-polymyxin B-hydrocortisone are often used, but aminoglycosides are ototoxic. This should never be used if the tympanic membrane is not known to be intact.
  d. Ciprofloxacin 0.3%/dexamethasone 0.1% otic suspension is another option.
  e. Fluoroquinolones are not associated with ototoxicity.
  f. Mild fungal infections can usually be treated with an acetic acid solution.

B. Complementary and alternative therapies.
  1. Often used in European countries for the prevention of recurrent otitis media, but there is insufficient scientific evidence of the safety and efficacy to recommend it (Marchisio et al., 2011).
  2. American Academy of Family Physicians (2004) states "no recommendation" for the use of CAM in the treatment or prevention of otitis media with effusion because of the lack of evidence.

C. Primary/secondary/tertiary prevention.
  1. Primary prevention of otitis media.
    a. Pneumoccocal conjugate vaccine administration.

b. Annual influenza vaccine administration.
c. In children, Eustachian tubes become blocked easily. Educate parent on home prevention.
  (1) Wash hands and toys frequently.
  (2) For the child who is not breastfed, hold the child upright while bottle-feeding.
  (3) Place child in daycare that has six children or fewer in the area.
  (4) Avoid pacifier use.
  (5) Do not use antibiotics leftover from an unused prescription.
  (6) Keep child away from second-hand smoke.
  (7) Older children can chew gum containing the sugar "xylitol."

2. Secondary prevention – Parent education regarding common causes of ear infections.
  a. Colds.
  b. Allergies.
  c. Secondhand smoke.
  d. Infected or overgrown adenoids.
  e. Excess mucus and saliva during teething.
  f. Drinking from a sippy cup or bottle while lying down.

3. Prevention of otitis externa (Schmitt, 2011).
  a. Limit number of hours the child spends in water.
  b. Do not insert cotton swabs into the ear canal.
  c. Dry the opening of the canal carefully after bathing or swimming.
  d. For recurrences, may prevent (but not treat acutely) by rinsing the ear canal with rubbing alcohol or 50% white vinegar solution after swimming.

D. Goals of plan of care.
  1. Limit acute symptoms and complications of infection.
  2. Maximize hearing and language development.
  3. Limit complications of antibiotic therapy.
  4. Educate parent about prevention and early recognition.

E. Psychosocial considerations.
1. Anxious parents may need reassurance, particularly when child is crying in pain or has discharge from his or her ear.
2. Reassure parent that ear pain without signs of more serious illness (see *Indications for Emergency Care or Urgent Consultation* section above) can be examined safely within 24 hours (Schmitt, 2011).
3. Parent may be frustrated with recurrent infections and want treatment without being seen, or will restart a prescription that was not completed previously. Encourage parent to have the child examined each time.

F. Education of parent/patient.
1. Home treatment and risk factors.
2. How to administer antibiotics, if prescribed, and to complete the course of treatment.
3. May apply warm compresses to outer ear.
4. Use over-the-counter pain preparations.
   a. Acetaminophen.
   b. Ibuprofen; do not use ibuprofen in children 6 months old or less.
   c. Do not use aspirin to treat pain in children.
5. Return for ear check, if ordered.
6. How to administer ear drops, if prescribed.
7. Call back if:
   a. Fever lasts more than two days after antibiotic started.
   b. Earache and/or ear discharge does not improve within three days on antibiotics.
   c. Child becomes worse.
8. Fluid in the ear may cause a temporary hearing loss, which will improve with treatment. It may not resolve as quickly as the infection. Parent may be required to speak in a louder voice and face the child closely for the child to hear.

G. Collaboration and referrals.
1. Patient's primary care provider for acute management as indicated in triage, above.
2. Otolaryngologist for chronic otitis media for possible myringotomy and tubes.
3. Otolaryngologist for signs of sustained hearing loss.

H. Community resources and education.
1. Health departments often provide immunizations at no charge or reduced charge for primary prevention.
2. Information resources online for parents for otitis media, "swimmer's ear," and hearing and/or speech impairment.

I. Telehealth nursing considerations.
1. Reassure parent and schedule to see a provider within 24 hours of reporting symptoms of AOM.
2. Instruct patient to call back if:
   a. Fever over 105 °F (40.6 °C).
   b. Fever persists over three days.
   c. Symptoms become worse.

J. Protocols/algorithms/guidelines.
1. Institution-specific guidelines related to ear pain.
2. Dosing guidelines for acetaminophen and ibuprofen.
3. Other appropriate protocols specifically for fever, colds, cough, sore throat, influenza, and sinus pain.
4. Guidelines for cerumen removal.
5. Staff competencies for audiograms and tympanograms.

References

A.D.A.M. (2010). *Anaphylaxis.* Retrieved from http://www.ncbi.nlm.nih.gov/pubmedhealth/PMH0001847/

Allen, C.H. (2011). *Fever without a source in children 3 to 36 months of age.* Retrieved from http://www.uptodate.com/contents/fever-without-a-source-in-children-3-to-36-months-of-age

American Academy of Family Physicians (AAFP). (2004). *Clinical practice guideline: Otitis media with effusion.* Retrieved from http://www.aafp.org/online/en/home/clinical/clinicalrecs/children/otitismedia.html

American Academy of Pediatrics. (2011). Clinical report: Fever and antipyretic use in children. *Pediatrics, 127*(3), 580-587.

American Heart Association (AHA). (2010). CPR priorities for the healthcare provider. *Currents in Emergency Cardiovascular Care, 16*(4), 12-15.

Brown, A., & King, D. (2010). Neurologic emergencies: Seizures. In P.K. Howard & R.A. Steinmann (Eds.), *Sheehy's emergency nursing: Principles and practice* (6th ed., pp. 457-466). St. Louis, MO: Mosby Elsevier.

Buttaro, T.M. (2008). Abdominal pain and infections. In T.M. Buttaro, J. Trybulski, P.P. Bailey, & J. Sandberg-Cook (Eds.), *Primary care: A collaborative practice* (3rd ed., pp. 624-626). Philadelphia: Mosby Elsevier.

Centers for Disease Control and Prevention (CDC). (2010a). *Basic TB facts.* Retrieved from http://www.cdc.gov/tb/publications/factsheets/general/LTBIandActiveTB.htm

Centers for Disease Control and Prevention (CDC). (2010b). *Elder maltreatment.* Retrieved from http://www.cdc.gov/violenceprevention

Centers for Disease Control and Prevention (CDC). (2010c). *Seasonal flu: Cover your cough.* Retrieved from http://www.cdc.gov/flu/protect/covercough.htm

Centers for Disease Control and Prevention (CDC). (2010d). Sexually transmitted diseases treatment guidelines, 2010. *MMWR, 59*(RR-12), 1-116. Retrieved from http://www.cdc.gov/std/treatment/2010/STD-Treatment-2010-RR5912.pdf

Centers for Disease Control and Prevention (CDC). (2010e). *Viral gastroenteritis.* Retrieved from http://www.cdc.gov/ncidod/ dvrd/revb/gastro/faq.htm

Centers for Disease Control and Prevention (CDC). (2011). *Understanding intimate partner violence.* Retrieved from http://cdc.gov/violenceprevention/intimatepartnerviolence/index.html

Consumer Guide. (2007). *Alternative medicines for fever.* Retrieved from http://health.howstuffworks.com/wellness/natural-medicine/alternative/alternative-medicines-for-fever.htm

Daniels, R., & Nicoll, L. (2012). *Contemporary medical-surgical nursing* (2nd ed.). Clifton Park, NY: Delmar, Cengage Learning.

Dugdale, D.C., Hadjiliadis, D., & Zieve, D. (2010). *Pulmonary tuberculosis.* Retrieved from http://www.ncbi.nlm.nih.gov/pubmedhealth/PMH0001141/

Dugdale, D.C., Vyas, J.M., & Zieve, D. (2010). *PPD skin test.* Retrieved from http://www.ncbi.nlm.nih.gov/pubmedhealth/PMH0004294/

Green, M.B. (2008). Screening for sexually transmitted diseases. In T.M. Buttaro, J. Trybulski, P.P. Bailey, & J. Sandberg-Cook (Eds.), *Primary care: A collaborative practice* (3rd ed., pp. 108-111). Philadelphia: Mosby Elsevier.

Hazinski, M.F. (Ed.). (2010). *BLS for healthcare providers.* Dallas: American Heart Association.

Hockenberry, M.J., & Wilson, D. (2011). *Wong's nursing care of infants and children* (9th ed.). St. Louis, MO: Elsevier Mosby.

Howard, P.K., & Steinmann, R.A. (2010). *Sheehy's emergency nursing: Principles and practice* (6th ed.). St. Louis, MO: Mosby Elsevier.

Idso, C. (2009). Sexually transmitted infection prevention in newly single older women. *The Journal for Nurse Practitioners, 5*(6), 440-446.

Jagim, M. (2009). Intimate partner violence. In *Sheehy's emergency nursing e-book* (6th ed.). Philadelphia: Mosby Elsevier.

Joint Council of Allergy, Asthma and Immunology (JCAAI). (2005). The diagnosis and management of anaphylaxis: An updated practice parameter. *Journal of Allergy and Clinical Immunology, 115*(3 Suppl), S483-523.

Krause, R.S. (2011). *Anaphylaxis.* Retrieved from http://www.emedicine.com/emerg/topic25.htm

Lee, D. (2011). *Headache.* Retrieved from http://www.medicinenet.com/headache/article.htm

Linsk, R., Blackwood, R., Cooke, J., Harrison, R., & Passamani, P.P. (2007). *Guideline for clinical care: Otitis media.* Retrieved from http://www.guideline.gov/content.aspx?id=11685&search=otitis+media

Marchisio, P., Bianchini, S., Galeone, C., Baggi, E., Rossi, E., Albertario, G., ... Principi, N. (2011). Use of complementary and alternative medicine in children with recurrent otitis media in Italy. *International Journal of Immunopathology &*

Pharmacology, 24(2), 411-419.

Merriam-Webster. (2010). *Suicide.* Retrieved from http://www.m-w.com/dictionary/suicide

Monahan, F.D. (2008). Examining the abdominal region. In *Mosby's expert physical exam handbook* (3rd ed., pp. 246-273). St. Louis, MO: Mosby.

Muscari, M.E. (2005). *Lippincott's review series: Pediatric review* (4th ed.). Philadelphia: Lippincott, Williams & Wilkins.

National Center for Complementary and Alternative Medicine (NCCAM). (2011). *The flu, the common cold, and complementary health practices.* Retrieved from http://nccam.nih.gov/health/flu/ataglance.htm#refs

National Institute of Allergy and Infectious Diseases (NIAID). (2011). *Sinusitis.* Retrieved from http://www.niaid.nih.gov/topics/sinusitis/Pages/sinusitis.aspx

National Institute of Mental Health (NIMH). (2008). *Mental health medications.* Retrieved from http://www.nimh.nih.gov/health/publications/mental-health-medications/complete-index.shtml

National Institute of Mental Health (NIMH). (2009). *What are the different forms of depression?* Retrieved from http://www.nimh.nih.gov/health/publications/women-and-depression-discovering-hope/what-are-the-different-forms-of-depression.shtml

National Institute of Mental Health (NIMH). (2010). *Suicide in the U.S.: Statistics and prevention.* Retrieved from http://www.nimh.nih.gov/health/publications/suicide-in-the-us-statistics-and-prevention/index.shtml

National Institute of Neurologic Disorders and Stroke (NINDS). (2011). *Low back pain fact sheet.* Retrieved from http://www.ninds.nih.gov/disorders/backpain/detail_backpain.htm

Nettina, S.M. (2010). *Lippincott manual of nursing practice* (9th ed.). Ambler, PA: Wolters Kluwer Health/Lippincott, Williams & Wilkins.

Pasero, C., & McCaffery, M. (2011). Low back pain. In *Pain assessment and pharmacologic management* (p. 222). St. Louis, MO: Mosby Elsevier.

Pellico, L.H. (2008). *Medical-surgical nursing: Made incredibly easy* (2nd ed.). Philadelphia: Lippincott, Williams & Wilkins.

Prather, C. (2007). Inflammatory and anatomic diseases of the intestine, peritoneum, mesentery, and omentum. In L. Goldman (Ed.), *Cecil medicine* (23rd ed., pp. 1042-1050). Philadelphia: Saunders Elsevier.

Schmitt, B.D. (2010). *Pediatric telephone protocols, office version* (13th ed.). Littleton, CO: American Academy of Pediatrics.

Schmitt, B.D. (2011). *Pediatric telephone protocols* (13th ed.). Littleton, CO: American Academy of Pediatrics.

Smitherman, H.F., & Macias, C.G. (2010). *Definition and etiology of fever in neonates and infants (less than three months of age).* Retrieved from http://www.uptodate.com/contents/definition-and-etiology-of-fever-in-neonates-and-infants-less-than-three-months-of-age

Soria, S. (2011). Intimate partner violence in the ambulatory care setting. *ViewPoint, 33*(3), 1, 8-10.

Sullivan, J.E., & Farrar, H.C. (2011). Fever and antipyretic use in children. *Pediatrics, 127*(3), 580-587.

Takayesu, J.K., & Lozner, A.W. (2010). *Pediatric dehydration.* Retrieved from http://emedicine.medscape.com/article/801012-overview#a0199

Waitzman, A. (2010). *Pediatric otitis externa.* Retrieved from http://emedicine.medscape.com/article/994550-overview

Chapter 19

Care of the Perioperative Patient In Ambulatory Care

Jennifer Mills, LCDR, NC, USN, MSN, CNS-BC

OBJECTIVES – *Study of the information in this chapter will enable the learner to:*

1. Describe the key elements of the preoperative, intraoperative, and postoperative phases of care and their applications to ambulatory care nursing.
2. Identify the assessment and care of patients throughout the perioperative continuum.
3. Explain how to manage common postoperative problems and complications related to moderate sedation and anesthesia.
4. Discuss patient and family education for preoperative and postoperative patient teaching.

KEY POINTS – *The major points in this chapter include:*

1. Patients undergoing operative procedures in the ambulatory environment require special considerations for education, safety measures, monitoring, and discharge care.
2. Nurses play a critical role in all aspects of the perioperative continuum.
3. Effective preoperative and postoperative patient and family education and preparation are instrumental in positive surgical outcomes.

Government Disclaimer: The views expressed in this chapter are those of the author and do not necessarily reflect the official policy or position of the Department of the Navy, Army, or Air Force, the Department of Defense, nor the U.S. Government.

Ambulatory care of the surgical patient has seen incredible change in the last decade. Increasingly, procedures requiring hospital stays are being performed in outpatient settings or with a very short inpatient stay. Nurses in ambulatory care are not only providing care to preoperative, intraoperative, and postoperative patients, but also coordinating the care of these patients and their transitions across venues. The ambulatory care surgical nurse must maintain knowledge of surgical patient needs and changes in technology and science through review of evidence-based guidelines. Nurse leaders and other professionals must collaboratively and routinely update written policies and protocols and facility guidelines to support nurses remaining current on developing technology and nursing practice.

The first freestanding ambulatory surgery practices were established in the late 1960s. In 1971, the American Medical Association endorsed the use of surgicenters. The American Society for Outpatient Surgeons (now known as American Association of Ambulatory Surgery Centers) was formed in 1978, beginning the process for surgery to be performed in doctors' offices. During the 1980s, a shortage of inpatient beds existed, leading to a proliferation in ambulatory surgery. Cost control has been a primary force in the development of ambulatory surgery. Third-party payers now require many procedures to be performed in an ambulatory setting to avoid the cost of hospitalization. Patients recovering in 23-hour units are considered outpatient for purposes of reimbursement by Medicare and third-party payers. The 1989 Omnibus Budget Reconciliation Act increased the reimbursement rates for surgical procedures in ambulatory centers.

I. Care of the Perioperative Patient

A. Goals of surgery.
1. Surgery is performed for multiple reasons.
   a. Diagnostic reasons, such as biopsies or visualization of tissue through a scope.
   b. Ablative (e.g., removal of a diseased body part).
   c. Constructive, to restore function or appearance.
   d. Palliative, to reduce pain and/or make patient more comfortable.
   e. Transplant, to replace malfunctioning organs.
2. Surgery may be emergent, urgent, required, elective, or optional.
3. Setting selection – Depends on patient risks and severity of surgical procedure.
   a. Inpatient.
      (1) Patient is admitted to hospital to undergo surgical procedure.
      (2) Patient recovers inpatient for one or more days.
      (3) Patient usually requires higher-level care postoperatively than ambulatory surgical patients.
   b. Ambulatory setting.
      (1) Outpatient basis.
      (2) Arrives, undergoes procedure, and discharges on same day.
B. Surgical approaches.
1. Open.
   a. A wide incision is made into a body part to expose the underlying structures and the diseased anatomical structure.
   b. Very invasive; usually requires longer recovery period.
2. Laparoscopic (also referred to as "minimally invasive").
   a. Video-assisted approach.
   b. Commonly used in abdominal, gynecological, urologic, and orthopedic procedures.
   c. Advantages include: Reduced postoperative pain, early mobilization, reduced infection rates, and shorter length of hospital stay.
3. Robotic surgery.
   a. Form of laparoscopic surgery that employs surgeon's console, robotic arms, and video tower.
   b. Three-dimensional views allow for better visualization.
   c. Advantages include greater surgical precision due to better visual perception, shorter hospital stay, quicker recovery time, and reduced postoperative pain.

II. Sedation and Anesthesia Types

A. Minimal sedation (anxiolysis).
1. Patient responds normally to verbal commands.
2. Cognitive function and coordination may be impaired.
3. Ventilatory and cardiac functions remain unaffected.
B. Moderate sedation.
1. Use of medication resulting in amnesia and/or analgesia.
2. Patient responds purposefully to verbal commands.
3. Patient independently maintains patent airway.
4. Cardiovascular function usually maintained.
C. Deep sedation and analgesia.
1. Drug-induced depression of consciousness.
2. Patient cannot be immediately aroused.
3. Responds purposely after repeated or painful stimulation.
4. Ability to independently maintain ventilator function may be impaired.
5. May require assistance to maintain patent airway.
6. Cardiovascular function usually maintained.

D. Anesthesia is a state of narcosis, analgesia, relaxation, and reflex loss.
E. General anesthesia.
   1. Loss of all sensation and consciousness.
   2. Protective reflexes temporarily lost.
   3. Assistance to maintain a patent airway often required.
   4. Positive pressure ventilation may be required due to depressed spontaneous ventilation or drug-induced depression of neuromuscular function.
   5. Cardiovascular function may be impaired.
F. Regional anesthesia.
   1. Temporary interruption of nerve impulse transmission to a specific area or region of the body.
      a. Topical – Applied to skin to produce localized dermal anesthetic.
      b. Local.
         (1) Surgical site is injected with anesthetic agent into tissues.
         (2) Induces temporary numbness at site.
      c. Nerve block.
         (1) Local anesthetics are injected into a specific nerve or nerve group.
         (2) Allows for intraoperative anesthesia and postoperative analgesia.
      d. Intravenous block or Bier block.
         (1) Local anesthesia is injected into an extremity following mechanical exsanguinations with a compression bandage and a tourniquet.
         (2) Allows for a bloodless work field.
      e. Spinal or subarachnoid block – Agent is injected into cerebrospinal fluid, resulting in block of nerve transmission.
      f. Epidural block – Local anesthetic is injected into epidural space via thoracic or lumbar space.

III. Preoperative Care

The preoperative care begins with the decision to have surgery and ends when the patient is transferred to the operating or procedure table.
A. Preoperative evaluation.
   1. Preoperative nurse is primary educator on the perioperative process. Responsible to:
      a. Assess learning needs to determine patient's educational needs.
      b. Promote patient safety.
      c. Provide patient and family opportunity for questions.
      d. Clarify patient's understanding of:
         (1) Procedure.
         (2) Informed consent.
         (3) Expected outcomes.
         (4) Patient responsibilities.
         (5) Postoperative care and follow-up.
      e. Identify any postoperative care needs.
         (1) Determine need for equipment and supplies and arrange.
         (2) Arrange for home care services.
         (3) Review transportation plan for outpatient surgery.
      f. Assure responsible adult available to assist for the first 24 hours after procedure.
   2. Preoperative instructions.
      a. Instrumental in minimizing patient's anxiety level.
         (1) Use non-medical terms with plenty of time for questions.
         (2) Reinforce verbal instructions with written information.
      b. Review plan for day of procedure, including anticipated time line.
         (1) Scheduled arrival time.
         (2) What to bring and not to bring.
         (3) Removal of all jewelry, body piercings, contact lenses, dentures, and dental appliances.
         (4) Fasting guidelines (American Society of Anesthesiologists [ASA], 2011).
            (a) Clear liquids – Two hours minimum fasting period.
            (b) Breast milk – Four hours minimum fasting period.
            (c) Infant formula – Six hours minimum fasting period.
            (d) Nonhuman milk – Six hours minimum fasting period.
            (e) Light meal – Consists of toast and clear liquids, and may be at discretion of surgeon; six hours minimum fasting period.

(5) Smoking restrictions: Recommend quitting prior to surgery due to increased surgical risks. No smoking day of surgery.

(6) Use of GI preps if needed for abdominal/gynecological procedures.

   (a) Allows satisfactory visualization of the lower GI tract.

   (b) Prevents trauma to intestine or contamination of peritoneum by feces.

   (c) Should be initiated well before bedtime.

(7) Medication plans prior to surgery.

   (a) Review prescribed medications with patient.

   (b) Critical to identify plan for diabetic, hypertension, and beta blocker medications.

   (c) Hold anticoagulants and thrombolytics as ordered to prevent excess blood loss.

(8) Review complication-preventing activities.

   (a) Exercises to prevent respiratory complications.

      i. Use of incentive spirometer.

      ii. Turn, cough, and deep breathing.

      iii. Splinting of incisions during exercises.

   (b) Exercises to facilitate venous return.

      i. Simple leg exercises while in bed.

      ii. Ambulating as soon as possible.

      iii. Compression devices/support stockings.

      iv. Review postoperative physical limitations.

(9) Postoperative pain management.

   (a) Importance of utilizing pain medication as often as needed.

   (b) Use of PCA pump, if anticipated.

(10) Designated family waiting areas.

(11) Review how information is relayed to waiting family.

(12) Length of time in recovery areas, as well as facility visitation policy.

3. Obtain a comprehensive medical and health history.

   a. Obtained within 30 days and updated within 24 hours of surgery.

   b. Should include:

      (1) Patient diagnosis.

      (2) Medical history, including use of alcohol, tobacco, and illicit drugs.

      (3) Comprehensive allergy list.

      (4) Prior surgical procedures and any untoward reactions.

      (5) Comprehensive pain history.

      (6) Any complementary medicines or therapies utilized.

      (7) Medication reconciling to include prescription, over-the-counter medications, and dietary supplements per Joint Commission's National Patient Safety Goals (see Chapter 7, "Regulatory Compliance and Patient Safety").

4. Preadmission testing may include (ASA, 2008b):

   a. Laboratory tests, such as complete blood count, electrolyte panel, coagulation studies, blood typing, and cross matching.

   b. Urinalysis.

   c. Pregnancy test for women between ages 10 and 55.

   d. Chest X-ray may be done for patients with respiratory symptoms, history of cardiac and/or respiratory issues, smokers, cancer patients, and elderly patients.

   e. EKG is usually performed for those over 40 years of age or with a cardiac history.

5. American Society of Anesthesiologists physical status classified (ASA, n.d.).

   a. ASA 1 or (P1): Healthy patient.

   b. ASA 2 or (P2): Healthy patient with mild systemic disease.

(1) Diet controlled diabetes.
(2) Moderate obesity.
(3) Mild hypertension.
(4) Well controlled chronic bronchitis.

  c. ASA 3 or (P3): Severe systemic disease that limits activity, but is not incapacitating.

(1) Coronary artery disease with angina.
(2) Morbid obesity.
(3) Moderate to severe pulmonary insufficiency.

  d. ASA 4 or (P4): Patient with severe systemic disease that is a constant threat to life.

(1) Heart disease with marked cardiac insufficiency.
(2) Intractable dysrhythmia.
(3) Advanced pulmonary, hepatic, renal, or endocrine insufficiency.

  e. ASA 5 or (P5): Moribund patient who is not expected to survive 24 hours without surgical intervention.

(1) Ruptured aneurysm.
(2) Head trauma with increasing intracranial pressure.
(3) Major multi-system trauma.

  f. ASA 6 or (P6): Patient is declared brain dead and organs are being harvested for donation.

  g. E: The E suffix denotes an emergency surgery and can be added to patient classification ASA 1–5.

B. Locations of preoperative evaluations.
  1. Hospitals or ambulatory surgery centers (ASCs).
    a. Allows for preoperative instructions and diagnostic testing at same time.
    b. Permits interviewer to clearly ascertain level of patient's knowledge.
    c. Allows patient opportunity to visualize facility and meet staff.
  2. Surgeon's office.
    a. Saves patient time.
    b. Allows preoperative interview to be done at time of history and physical.
    c. Prevents patient from visiting place of surgery or meeting staff.

  3. Phone interview.
    a. May be done at patient's convenience; saves inconvenience of in-person visit.
    b. Still requires a visit for necessary testing.
    c. May be difficult to ascertain patient's level of understanding.
  4. Computer-based assessment and teaching programs.
    a. Patient accesses a secure Web site to complete medical history.
    b. RN reviews and assesses if follow-up is needed.
    c. Patient may find this most convenient.
    d. Some patients may not have computer access.
    e. Patient unable to visualize surgery facility and meet staff.
    f. Unable to assess if patient has transportation issues or surgery-precluding illnesses, such as upper respiratory infections.

C. Ethical and legal considerations.
  1. Surgical and anesthesia consent.
    a. Protects patient from undergoing procedures he or she does not want or understand.
    b. Protects the hospital and staff from claims that permission was not granted by patient.
    c. Patient must be fully informed by the physician about the risks and benefits of the procedure, alternatives, and consequences of no treatment.
    d. Need to ensure patient has legal and mental capacity to sign.
    e. Staff who sign as witnesses are only witnessing the signature of individual signing consent form.
    f. Interpreter must be used if patient is not proficient in English.

D. Day of surgery preoperative care.
  1. Patient's psychological and spiritual needs must be met.
    a. Anticipate anxiety and fear, which are common.
    b. Assess patient's desire for pastoral care.

c. Allow time for significant others to be alone with patient.

d. Ensure privacy and allow for emotional support.

2. Complete patient assessment.
   a. Assess for changes since preoperative evaluation.
      (1) Some changes may result in cancellation of procedure.
         (a) Abnormal vital signs.
         (b) Upper respiratory infections or fever.
         (c) Abnormal EKG.
   b. Assess for compliance with preoperative regimen.
      (1) NPO status.
      (2) Smoking status.
      (3) Medications taken.
      (4) Availability of responsible adult and transportation.
      (5) Removal of all jewelry and body piercings.
      (6) Assess need for infection control, airborne, droplet, or contact precaution.

3. Clarify patient's understanding.
   a. Procedure.
   b. Anesthesia.
   c. Postoperative needs.
   d. If patient has questions regarding procedure or anesthesia, contact the physician.

4. Review documentation.
   a. Use of preoperative checklist.
   b. Day of surgery assessment complete and accurate.
   c. History and physical complete within 24 hours of procedure.
   d. Consent forms accurate, up-to-date, signed, and dated by all parties.

5. Prepare patient for the operating room.
   a. Hospital gowns usually required.
   b. Undergarments usually removed.
   c. Facility-specific requirements in regards to removal of dentures, partials, eyeglasses, and hearing aids. Some facilities allow these items in the OR holding area.
   d. All jewelry and body piercings removed.
   e. Clothing and personal items secured.
   f. Obtain IV access per facility instructions. May be completed in OR holding area.
   g. Administer preoperative medications as ordered.
      (1) May be used to reduce risk for nausea, vomiting, and gastric acidity.
      (2) May be used to reduce anxiety.
      (3) Antibiotic prophylaxis as needed.
   h. Have patient void; verify whether sample needed for pregnancy test.

6. Ensure patient has ample time to have all questions answered.

7. Turn over care of patient to anesthesia, holding area, or operating room staff.
   a. Follow The Joint Commission's National Patient Safety Goal (NPSG) 2 on patient handoff.
      (1) NPSG 2 is to improve effectiveness of communication among caregivers.
      (2) The goal further states facilities should "implement a standardized approach to handoff communications including an opportunity to ask and respond to questions" (The Joint Commission, 2012b).
   b. Method determined by facility.
      (1) Face-to-face.
      (2) Phone.
      (3) Written report.
      (4) Combination of above.

IV. Intraoperative Care

Intraoperative care begins when the patient is transferred to the operating room table and ends when the patient arrives in the recovery area. The goal of the ambulatory nurse in the operating room is to maintain safety and physiologic integrity of the patient. In ambulatory care procedures performed outside of operating rooms, the ambulatory care nurse is crucial in the administration of moderate sedation.

A. Moderate sedation is the use of medication resulting in amnesia and/or analgesia to sufficiently blunt, but not remove, a patient's protective reflexes to allow the performance of a procedure.
   1. Overall goal is to reduce patient's fear and anxiety with minimum medication.
   2. Benefits include:
      a. Enhanced patient cooperation.
      b. Elevation of pain threshold.
      c. Intact protective reflexes.
      d. Rapid recovery.
      e. Minimal risk as compared to other anesthesia types.
B. Intraoperative care under moderate sedation.
   1. Legal scope of practice.
      a. Nurses must understand the differing levels of sedation.
      b. Nurses must comply with scope of practice issues as delineated by state boards of nursing.
      c. Nurses must be aware of their state board of nursing's formal position or policy statement on moderate sedation administration.
   2. Regulatory standards of the Joint Commission (2012b).
      a. Operative or other procedures and/or the administration of moderate sedation is planned.
      b. Sufficient numbers of qualified personnel are present during moderate sedation procedures.
      c. Pre-sedation assessment is performed before beginning.
      d. Patient's physiological status is monitored during sedation.
      e. Patient is monitored immediately after the administration of sedation.
   3. Sources of authoritative statements and standards for the provision of moderate sedation in the ambulatory setting.
      a. American Nurses Association (ANA).
      b. Association of periOperative Registered Nurses (AORN).
      c. American Society of PeriAnesthesia Nurses (ASPAN).
      d. Emergency Nurses Association (ENA).
      e. Local standards per medical policy and procedure committees.
      f. American Society of Anesthesiologists Task Force on Sedation and Analgesia by Non-Anesthesiologists (2002) *Practice Guidelines for Sedation and Analgesia by Non-Anesthesiologists.*
   4. Professional organization guidelines, The Joint Commission standards, and statutory regulations require policy development for administration of sedation. Moderate sedation training programs are standardized, competency-based, have established baseline educational requirements, and ensure comparable training throughout an institution. Key components of a moderate sedation education program include (Kost, 2004):
      a. Current basic life support (BLS) course completion and advanced cardiac life support (ACLS) or pediatric advanced life support (PALS) course completion.
      b. Anatomy, physiology, cardiac dysrhythmias, and complications that may occur during the administration of moderate sedation.
      c. Sedation assessment and monitoring of:
         (1) Ventilatory function and oxygen status.
         (2) Blood pressure.
         (3) Cardiac rate and rhythm.
         (4) Level of consciousness.
      d. Pre-procedural sedation assessment, ASA (n.d.) physical status classifications, and patient selection criteria.
      e. Recognition of moderate sedation versus deep sedation, general anesthesia, and local anesthesia
      f. Medications, dosages, administration rates, onset/duration/peak, adverse effects, contraindications, and reversal agents.
      g. Management and monitoring of patients before, during, and after moderate sedation.

h. Competency in operating and troubleshooting essential equipment.
i. Critical thinking skills to manage emergency situations.
j. Patient education.
k. Discharge criteria.
l. Documentation and medico-legal issues.
m. Pre- and post-testing, preceptorship to practice newly acquired skills, and regularly scheduled recertification.

5. Prior to the procedure to ensure patient safety, the Universal Protocol is exercised: All documents and studies are available and have been reviewed, and the patient's expectations and team's understanding of the intended procedure are in concert (The Joint Commission, 2012a).
   a. Verify the correct person, procedure, and site.
      (1) When the procedure is scheduled.
      (2) On entry into the facility.
      (3) At points in which care responsibility is transferred to another caregiver.
      (4) With the patient's involvement, if possible.
      (5) When the patient is transferred from the pre-procedure area to the procedure room.
      (6) Relevant documentation (such as consent, history, and physical), images, and special equipment is available.
   b. The operative site is marked.
      (1) Mark is unambiguous. No marks are used to indicate the non-operative site.
      (2) Mark is visible after the patient is positioned and draped.
      (3) Marking methodology is consistent throughout the institution.
      (4) Marking involved the patient, awake and aware.
      (5) Marking is performed in all cases involving laterality, multiple structures (e.g., fingers), or multiple levels (e.g., spine).
      (6) Marking is performed by the person performing the procedure.
   c. A "time out" is performed immediately before starting the procedure.
      (1) Entire team in the procedure room use active communication and document on the patient record.
      (2) Team agrees to correct patient, correct side/site, correct procedure, correct position, and implants or special equipment are available.

6. Monitoring consists of vital signs, including.
   a. Heart rate.
   b. Oxygenation using pulse oximetry.
   c. Respiratory rate.
   d. Adequacy of ventilation.
   e. Cardiac monitoring.
   f. Blood pressure.

7. Essential monitoring and support equipment and supplies available:
   a. Intravenous fluid and drug administration equipment and supplies, with capability of administering blood or blood products for operative procedures.
   b. Functional source of oxygen (and a back-up source).
   c. Positive-pressure ventilation (bag-valve-mask).
   d. Suction equipment and appropriately sized suction catheters.
   e. Sufficient electrical outlets and clearly labeled emergency power.
   f. Adequate illumination with backup battery-powered equipment.
   g. Emergency cart with equipment appropriate for the patient's age and size (defibrillator, emergency drugs, airway equipment, and IV solutions and supplies).
   h. Equipment to monitor cardiac rate and rhythm, blood pressure, pulse rate, respiratory rate, oxygen saturation (pulse oximetry).
   i. All pre-filled syringes labeled.

8. Communication/documentation.

a. Sedation scale to describe the spectrum of consciousness (McCaffery & Pasero, 1999).
 (1) S = Sleep.
 (2) 1 = Awake and alert.
 (3) 2 = Slightly drowsy, easily aroused.
 (4) 3 = Frequently drowsy, arousable, drifts off to sleep during conversation.
 (5) 4 = Somnolent, minimal or no response to physical stimulation.
b. Ramsey scale is also used, facility dependent (Ramsey, Savege, Simpson, & Goodwin, 1974).
 (1) 1 = Patient is anxious and agitated or restless, or both.
 (2) 2 = Patient is cooperative, oriented, and tranquil.
 (3) 3 = Patient responds to commands only.
 (4) 4 = Patient exhibits brisk response to light glabellar tap or loud auditory stimulus.
 (5) 5 = Patient exhibits a sluggish response to light glabellar tap or loud auditory stimulus.
 (6) 6 = Patient exhibits no response.
c. Documentation of monitoring data on a time-based record.
 (1) Cardiac rate and rhythm.
 (2) Blood pressure, pulse rate, respiratory rate (taken every 1–2 minutes during onset of sedation and every 5–10 minutes during the procedure).
 (3) Oxygen delivery route (nasal cannula, facemask) and flow rate, oxygen saturation.
 (4) Level of consciousness.
 (5) Verbal response.
 (6) Medication administered – Dosage, time, route, patient response, name of ordering physician or anesthesia provider.
 (7) Type and amounts of IV fluids and blood components administered.
 (8) Pre- and post-procedural temperatures.
 (9) Any interventions and the patient's response.
 (10) Any significant events or untoward reactions and their resolution.

9. Pharmacological agents commonly used during moderate sedation.
a. Sedation and analgesia medications.
 (1) Benzodiazepines.
 (a) No analgesic properties.
 (b) Amnesic, anxiolytic, hypnotic, and sedative properties.
 (c) Monitor respiratory rate closely, may cause respiratory depression.
 (d) Midazolam (Versed®).
 i. Dosing guidelines individualized and titrated to effect.
 ii. Must be administered slowly.
 iii. Reversal agent is flumazenil (Romazicon®).
 (2) Opioids.
 (a) Used for analgesic and sedative effects.
 (b) Rapid onset.
 (c) Side effects include bradycardia, hypotension, and nausea.
 (d) Fentanyl, meperidine, and morphine commonly used.
 (3) Anesthetic induction agents.
 (a) Most commonly used in moderate sedation is propofol.
 (b) Administration by registered nurses depends on statutory, regulatory, and recommended standards of care.
 (c) Very specific educational components required to administer.
 (d) Disadvantages of propofol include:
 i. Unpredictable action.
 ii. Demanding airway requirements.
 iii. No known reversal.

V. Postoperative Care

The postoperative period begins when the patient enters the post-anesthesia care unit (PACU) and ends when healing is complete. Phase I recovery starts when the patient enters the PACU and ends when the patient is physiologically stable, free from anesthetic/surgical complications, adequately recovered from anesthesia, and responds to external stimuli. Phase II begins when the patient moves to an extended observation unit or is admitted to an inpatient floor. Ambulatory surgery patients may be "fast tracked" and bypass Phase I recovery by meeting Phase I discharge criteria prior to leaving the operating room.

A. Phase I of postoperative care.
1. Nurses must be acutely aware of the patient's status in the postoperative phase in order to ensure return of physiological function. Basic life-sustaining needs are the highest priority (ASPAN, 2010).
2. Monitoring procedures.
   a. Assess patient and readiness for discharge.
   b. Treat any complications that arise.
   c. Must assess objective parameters:
      (1) Respiration.
      (2) Circulation.
      (3) Level of consciousness.
      (4) Oxygenation.
      (5) Activity.
      (6) Intake and output.
      (7) Temperature.
3. Emergency airway complications may arise after anesthesia.
   a. Airway obstruction.
      (1) Patient very sedated, may blunt airway reflexes.
      (2) Soft tissue obstruction, oropharynx blocked.
      (3) Reposition, insert oral airway, side lying, jaw support.
   b. Hypoxia.
      (1) Defined as oxygen saturation less than 90%.
      (2) Manifested as reduced respiratory rate, rhythm, effort.
      (3) Caused by over sedation, which may reduce stimulus to breathe.

c. Laryngospasm, bronchospasm, and airway edema.
   (1) May be precipitated by irritants or allergy.
   (2) May be related to history of asthma, smoking, or COPD.
   (3) May be caused by airway trauma.
d. Aspiration pneumonia.
   (1) Caused by inhalation of gastric contents.
   (2) Prevented by reducing risk.
4. Cardiovascular complications may arise after anesthesia.
   a. Hypotension.
      (1) Consider causes, such as opioids or hypovolemia.
      (2) Often transient and mild.
      (3) Be prepared to respond quickly to profound low pressure.
      (4) May require fluid resuscitation.
   b. Hypertension.
      (1) May be pre-existing.
      (2) May be due to fluid overload, uncontrolled pain, hypothermia, and shivering.
      (3) Treat causes.
   c. Cardiac dysrhythmias.
      (1) Sinus bradycardia.
      (2) Atrial fibrillation or flutter.
      (3) Premature ventricular contractions.
      (4) Supraventricular tachycardia.
5. Thermoregulation issues may arise after anesthesia.
   a. Hypothermia (core body temperature below 37 °C).
      (1) May be due to vasodilating anesthetics, open body cavities during procedure, or cold temperatures in the operating room.
      (2) Increased shivering may lead to increased oxygen consumption.
      (3) Interventions include rewarming measures and supplemental oxygen if shivering.
      (4) May cause patient discomfort, morbidity and mortality.

b. Hyperthermia.
   (1) Normal response to infection.
   (2) May be prelude to sepsis.
c. Malignant hyperthermia.
   (1) Emergency.
   (2) Rare, genetically determined skeletal muscle response.
   (3) Triggered by succinylcholine and volatile inhalation agents.
   (4) Occurs most often in young and healthy patients.
   (5) Goal is prevention: Identify those at risk.
   (6) Every facility should have a malignant hyperthermia protocol and maintain an easily accessible cart with equipment.
   (7) Symptoms.
       (a) Sudden unexplained tachycardia.
       (b) Profound muscle rigidity.
       (c) Metabolic and respiratory acidosis.
       (d) Cyanosis.
       (e) Fever a late sign.
   (8) Interventions.
       (a) Aggressive immediate cooling.
       (b) Massive doses of IV dantrolene sodium (Dantrium®), skeletal muscle relaxant.
       (c) Oxygenate.
       (d) Correct severe metabolic acidosis.
6. Treating postoperative nausea and vomiting.
   a. Occurs in 1/3 patients undergoing anesthesia.
   b. Costly as each vomiting episode causes prolonged postoperative stay and may lead to unanticipated admissions.
   c. Assess patient routinely for nausea; patient may decline to tell staff.
   d. Diverse therapy options.
       (1) Increasing IV hydration.
       (2) Implementing risk-reducing interventions.
           (a) Cool cloths.

(b) Deep breathing.
(c) Repositioning.
(3) Pharmacological therapy.
   (a) Serotonin receptor antagonists.
       i. Prophylactically given 30 minutes prior to end of surgery.
       ii. Ondansetron (Zofran®).
       iii. Dolasetron (Anzemet®).
   (b) Antidopaminergics.
       i. Droperidol (Inapsine®).
       ii. Metoclopramide (Reglan®).
   (c) Phenothiazines.
       i. Promethazine (Phenergan®).
       ii. Prochlorperazine (Compazine®).
(4) Complementary therapy.
   (a) Ginger.
       i. Possible anti-emetic effect.
       ii. Not recommended for patients taking warfarin.
   (b) Aromatherapy – Use of essential oils.
   (c) P6 stimulation.
       i. Acupuncture, acupressure, transcutaneous electrical stimulation.
       ii. May reduce nausea; little effect on vomiting.
7. Treating pain and discomfort.
   a. Pain is whatever the patient says it is. Goal is adequate pain management as perceived by the patient. Continuous multi-modal approach is best.
   b. A combined analgesic regimen reduces the risk of side effects from a single agent.
   c. Around-the-clock dosing.
       (1) Critical in the immediate 12–24 hours postoperative period.
       (2) Prevents pain and allows patient a satisfactory pain rating.
       (3) Should be accompanied by measures for breakthrough pain.

d. As needed (PRN) dosing.
    (1) Patient request dosing.
    (2) Educate patient on importance of asking for pain medication prior to pain worsening.
e. Patient controlled analgesia (PCA).
    (1) Method that allows patients to control their pain management by self-administering doses.
    (2) Initiation of PCA in PACU is recommended to prevent any delays in receiving analgesia on inpatient floor.
    (3) Most commonly routed through an IV.
    (4) Education of patient.
        (a) Stress to patient importance of self-dosing.
        (b) Do not allow family members access to button ("PCA by proxy").
        (c) Review that patients cannot "overdose" themselves.
    (5) Monitor closely for sedation and respiratory depression. Have naloxone (Narcan®) readily available.
f. Pharmacological pain management.
    (1) Non-opioids.
        (a) Acetaminophen.
        (b) Cox-2 inhibitors.
        (c) NSAIDs.
    (2) Opioids.
        (a) Morphine.
        (b) Hydromorphone.
        (c) Fentanyl.
    (3) Adjuvants include:
        (a) Anticonvulsants.
        (b) Tricyclic antidepressants.
        (c) Anti-anxiety drugs.
        (d) Local anesthetics.
g. Provide for comfort measures as desired.
    (1) Physical.
        (a) Positioning.
        (b) Extra blankets and pillows.
        (c) Heat and cold therapies.
    (2) Provide for education.
        (a) Music.
        (b) Guided imagery.
        (c) Biofeedback.
        (d) Distraction.

B. Phase II of post-anesthesia care.
    Phase II patients generally require less acute level of care. Ongoing assessment occurs in this phase with a focus on preparing the patient for discharge. The goal is to facilitate adequate recovery from anesthesia/sedation rather than the procedure.
    1. Complete initial assessment occurs upon transfer to the unit.
    2. Ongoing reassessments will occur per departmental policy until the patient is discharged.
    3. Allow visitors in as soon as patient is stable and privacy needs are addressed, per facility policy.
    4. Ongoing care focuses on:
        a. Vital signs monitoring.
        b. Level of consciousness.
        c. Pain and comfort level.
        d. Assessment and care of surgical site.
        e. Increasing patient's level of activity.
        f. Intake and output.

C. Discharge from the post-anesthesia care unit – Nurses are responsible for evaluating a patient's readiness for discharge from the PACU. A criteria-based scoring system is widely used.
    1. Must meet established criteria developed in conjunction with statutory, regulatory, and professional organization standards.
    2. Scoring criteria should:
        a. Allow patient to be scored by different providers simultaneously.
        b. Be simple to administer.
        c. Be applicable to all patients.
        d. Be easy to remember.
        e. Ensure a standard of care is met for all patients.
        f. Allow nurses to act on behalf of anesthesia personnel.
    3. ASA (2008a) standards for post-anesthesia care note that in absence of anesthesia provider, the PACU nurse shall determine discharge eligibility.

4. Discharge criteria are used frequently throughout postoperative period.
   a. Prior to leaving OR.
   b. On admission to PACU.
   c. Every 15–30 minutes, dependent upon facility policy.
   d. Support providers' critical judgment of discharge readiness.
5. The post-anesthetic recovery, also called Modified Aldrete, score is a widely used, effective, reliable, and safe assessment and documentation tool that incorporates the trend in ambulatory surgery (Aldrete, 1995). Discharge criteria should be developed in consultation with anesthesiology department.
   a. Ten items are assessed.
      (1) Activity: Ability/inability to move extremities.
      (2) Respiration: Airway patency.
      (3) Circulation: Blood pressure readings within pre-anesthetic level, as well as skin color and condition.
      (4) Consciousness: Awake or arousable.
      (5) Oxygenation: On room air or with oxygen supplement.
      (6) Pain: None, mild, or severe.
      (7) Ambulation: Dizziness/vertigo, able to walk.
      (8) Feeding: Nauseated/vomiting, able to drink.
      (9) Urinary status: Voiding/unable to void.
      (10) Dressing: Clean and intact, soaked.
   b. Maximum score of 20.
      (1) PACU Phase I discharge requires minimum score of 8–10.
      (2) Home discharge requires minimum score of 18.
6. Discharge education begins as soon as nurse determines readiness. Discharge instructions should include:
   a. Self-care/family-care of operative site(s), to include any wound care.
      (1) Instructions for appropriate care.
      (2) Dressing changes.
      (3) Any bathing limitations.
      (4) Ice and elevation, if ordered.
   b. Activity level and limitations.
      (1) Minor discomforts that may occur (sore throat, muscle aches, etc.).
      (2) Advise to rest the remainder of the day.
      (3) Fatigue and dizziness are to be expected.
      (4) Specifics about heavy lifting.
   c. Symptoms to expect following procedure.
   d. Symptoms that need to be brought to the health care professional's attention.
      (1) Fever greater than 101 °F.
      (2) Breathing problems.
      (3) Bleeding problems.
      (4) Urinary retention issues.
      (5) Pain not relived by pain medications.
      (6) Continued nausea and vomiting.
      (7) Swelling or redness around wound, leaking pus.
   e. Dietary restrictions.
      (1) Should start with clear liquids, then progress as tolerated or as directed by physician.
      (2) Avoid heavy, fried, or spicy foods the day of surgery.
   f. Medication instructions.
      (1) Purpose and limitations of pain medications.
      (2) Resume medications prescribed before procedure.
      (3) Patient should be aware that it is nearly impossible to alleviate all postoperative pain.
      (4) Review possibility of medication interactions and side effects.
      (5) The nurse should write the next time the patient is due for a dose of pain medication on discharge instructions.
   g. Avoidance of operating motor vehicles, electric equipment, or heavy equipment as advised by the health care provider, but at least 24 hours.

h. Avoidance of alcohol consumption, tobacco, and making important decisions for 24 hours following the procedure.
i. Follow-up care (time, place, and date).
j. Information regarding who to call if any issues arise once home.
k. Must be in care of responsible adult for 24 hours.
7. Determine whether patient meets discharge criteria of facility.
  a. Patient's condition is stable.
  b. Patient will be accompanied by a responsible adult.
  c. Patient meeting all criteria may be discharged from the Phase II PACU.
8. Discharge process.
  a. Return all patient's valuables and belongings.
  b. Verify safe ride home with responsible adult.
  c. Ensure patient has written copy of instructions, and patient and escort verbalize understanding.
  d. Complete discharge assessment and vital signs.
  e. Patient may require wheelchair to exit per facility protocol.

VI. Pediatric Population
A. It is essential that both child and family or caregiver receive adequate education prior to and during the process to alleviate feelings of separation and general anxiety.
B. Stressors common to this population include:
  1. Fear of separation.
    a. Optimize parental visiting and involvement.
    b. Consider parents' presence during induction.
  2. Fear of procedure.
    a. Provide simple age-appropriate explanations.
    b. Encourage hands-on practice with equipment.
    c. Allow liberal access to comfort items.
      (1) Wrap child in his/her own blanket.
      (2) Allow a favorite stuffed toy to accompany them during the surgical process.

d. Expect and accept developmental regression.
3. Pain.
  a. Adequately assess and meet patient pain needs.
  b. Use "Faces" scale or other age-appropriate tools to properly assess pain.
  c. Important to obtain adequate pain control in immediate postoperative period to decrease subsequent level of anxiety.
C. Practice family-centered care, acknowledging parents as partners in care.
  1. Collaboration between family and health care team.
  2. Allows for parents' feelings of security and trust.
    a. Parents have control over what happens to their child.
    b. Parents tend to be more amenable when accepted as members of team.
  3. Child Life Specialists at many facilities are available throughout the process to explain the perioperative process and serve as partners/resources in the continuum of care.
D. Pediatric accommodations for the preoperative phase.
  1. Allow for pediatric tours so child has understanding of what will occur.
  2. Involve child in education process.
    a. Provide easy to understand instructions about what is going to happen.
    b. Use visual aids (e.g., dolls, books, video) to explain process to child.
    c. Introduce family to Child Life Specialist, if available.
  3. Pediatric-specific assessment.
    a. Provide painful procedures last.
    b. Consider premedication prior to surgery.
      (1) Allows easier transition from family to OR team.
      (2) Decreases fear, emotional trauma.
E. Pediatric accommodations for the postoperative phase.
  1. Ensure pediatric-specific equipment is available.

2. Provide for comfort measures.
    a. Pillows, bed rail padding.
    b. Chair for parent at bedside.
3. Airway problems are most common in the immediate postoperative phase.
    a. Observe for respiratory distress.
        (1) Increased respiratory rate.
        (2) Oxygen desaturation.
        (3) Tachycardia.
        (4) Nasal flaring and retractions.
        (5) Apnea, grunting, wheezing, stridor.
    b. Interventions.
        (1) Stimulate and reposition airway.
        (2) Administer oxygen; blow by tolerated best by infants and toddlers when alert.
        (3) Notify provider, immediately in pediatric populations.
4. Hypothermia occurs rapidly in pediatric population.
    a. Due to high ratio of body surface area to weight and decreased mass.
    b. Observe for hypothermia.
        (1) Temperature less than 98.6 °F.
        (2) May observe shivering.
    c. Interventions.
        (1) Maintain warm room.
        (2) Apply warming blankets as needed.
        (3) Monitor temperature closely until returns to normal range.
5. Postoperative agitation common.
    a. May be due to pain, emergence of delirium, and anxiety.
    b. Consider causes.
    c. Protect from injury, and reunite with parent as soon as possible.
    d. Administer pain medication.

VII. Geriatric Population

A. Physical changes of aging make this population more at risk for adverse events.
    1. Cardiovascular alterations.
        a. Narrow vessel lumens lead to a subsequent increase in blood pressure.
        b. Heart valves are thicker and more rigid.
        c. Decreased cardiac output.
    2. Respiratory alterations.
        a. Less compliant chest wall.
        b. Decreased lung elasticity and vital capacity.
        c. Decreased gag reflex.
    3. Gastrointestinal alterations.
        a. Reduced peristalsis.
        b. Decreased liver enzyme production.
        c. May have bowel incontinence.
    4. Genitourinary alterations.
        a. Decreased kidney efficiency.
        b. Weaker bladder muscles.
    5. Hearing and vision loss/reduction common.
    6. Skin thinner, more fragile.
B. Geriatric considerations in the preoperative period.
    1. Focused preoperative assessment.
        a. Coexisting diseases increase with age.
        b. Poor nutrition hinders healing process.
        c. Assess adequate support system.
        d. Identify any special needs.
            (1) Communication barriers.
            (2) Mobility aids.
            (3) Hearing aids, glasses.
    2. Assess for compatibility with ambulatory surgery.
C. Geriatric consideration in the postoperative period.
    1. Respiratory considerations.
        a. At high risk for atelectasis.
            (1) Promote optimal gas exchange.
            (2) Encourage deep breathing, raise head of bed.
            (3) Protect from aspiration.
    2. Fluid balance considerations.
        a. Carefully monitor intake to avoid fluid overload.
        b. Closely monitor breath sounds and intake and output.
        c. Monitor urine output – High risk for urinary retention.
    3. Comfort considerations.
        a. Carefully titrate pain medications.
        b. Turn frequently and protect bony prominences.
        c. Reorient and avoid sensory overload.
        d. Return glasses, hearing aids, and dentures as soon as possible.

4. Ensure physical safety.
    a. Assistance when ambulating first time.
    b. Ensure plan for safety at home.
    c. Provide clear instructions to patient and responsible adult.

VIII. Obese Populations

A. Risk of co-existing disease places obese patient at higher risk.
    1. Hypertension, coronary artery disease, diabetes, congestive heart failure.
    2. Decreased lung capacity, increased work of breathing, obstructive sleep apnea (OSA).
B. Considerations in the operative process.
    1. Provide for privacy and ensure proper equipment.
        a. Appropriately sized patient gowns.
        b. Special beds and chairs to accommodate obese patients.
        c. Properly sized blood pressure cuffs, etc.
        d. Lifting/transfer equipment available.
    2. Consider increased risk of aspiration.
    3. Maintain adequate respiratory status.
        a. Ensure usage of positive airway pressure machine, if patient utilizes one at home.
        b. Closely monitor respiratory status.
            (1) Elevate head of bed to maximize lung expansion.
            (2) Encourage incentive spirometry, coughing, and deep breathing.
    4. Increased risk of deep vein thrombosis.
        a. Encourage ambulation.
        b. Utilize compression devices while in bed.

IX. Patients with Substance Abuse or Addiction

A. Staff often fear feeding a patient's addiction.
    1. May lead to inadequate pain control in postoperative period.
    2. Important to accept patient self-evaluation of pain and treat as necessary.
    3. Nurse has ethical responsibility to patient, regardless of addiction.

4. Patient has right to be free of pain post-operatively.
B. May have cross-tolerance to other drugs; will usually have increased need for anesthetics and analgesia.

References

Aldrete, J.A. (1995). The post-anesthesia recovery score revisited. *Journal of Clinical Anesthesia, 7*(1), 89-91.

American Society of Anesthesiologists (ASA). (n.d.). *ASA physical status classification system.* Retrieved from http://www.asahq.org/clinical/physicalstatus.htm

American Society of Anesthesiologists (ASA). (2008a). *Guidelines for ambulatory anesthesia and surgery.* Retrieved from http://www.asahq.org/~/media/For%20Members/documents/Standards%20Guidelines%20Stmts/Ambulatory%20Anesthesia%20and%20Surgery.ashx

American Society of Anesthesiologists (ASA). (2008b). *Statement on routine preoperative laboratory and diagnostic screening.* Retrieved from http://www.asahq.org/~/media/For%20Members/documents/Standards%20Guidelines%20Stmts/Routine%20Preoperative%20Laboratory%20and%20Diagnostic%20Screening.ashx

American Society of Anesthesiologists (ASA). (2011). Practice guidelines for preoperative fasting and the use of pharmacology agents to reduce the risk of pulmonary aspiration: Application to healthy patients undergoing elective procedures. *Anesthesiology, 114*(3), 495-511.

American Society of Anesthesiologists (ASA) Task Force on Sedation and Analgesia by Non-Anesthesiologists. (2002). Practice guidelines for sedation and analgesia by non-anesthesiologists. *Anesthesiology, 96*(4), 1004-1017.

American Society of PeriAnesthesia Nurses (ASPAN). (2010). *Perianesthesia nursing standards and practice recommendations 2010-2012.* Cherry Hill, NJ: Author.

Joint Commission, The. (2012a). *Comprehensive accreditation manual for hospitals.* Oakbrook Terrace, IL: Author.

Joint Commission, The. (2012b). *National patient safety goals.* Retrieved from http://www.jointcommision.org/assets/1/6/NPSG_Chapter_Jan2012_AHC.pdf

Kost, M. (2004). *Moderate sedation/analgesia: Core competencies for practice* (2nd ed.). Philadelphia: Saunders.

McCaffery, M., & Pasero, C. (1999). *Pain: Clinical manual* (2nd ed.). St. Louis, MO: Mosby.

Ramsey, M.A., Savege, T.M., Simpson, B.R., & Goodwin, R. (1974). Controlled sedation with alphaxalone-alphadolone. *British Medical Journal, 22*(2), 656-659.

Additional Readings

Association of periOperative Registered Nurses (AORN). (2007). *Standards, recommended practice and guidelines 2007.* Denver, CO: Author.

Drain, C., & Odom-Forren, J. (2009). *Perianesthesia nursing: A critical care approach* (5th ed.). Philadelphia: Author.

Odom-Forren, J., & Watson, D. (2005). *Practical guide to moderate sedation/analgesia.* Philadelphia: Saunders.

Chapter 20

Ambulatory Nursing Role in Chronic Illness Care

Marie Beisel, MSN, RN, CPHQ
Mary Anne Bord-Hoffman, MN, RN-BC
Barbara Pacca, BSN, RN, CPN, HTP

OBJECTIVES – *Study of the information in this chapter will enable the learner to:*

1. Explain deficiencies in the current health system related to the management of chronic disease.
2. Describe how the six elements of the chronic care model address the management of chronic illness.
3. Define the role of the RN in a patient-centered medical home (PCMH) practice.
4. Identify key characteristics of collaborative interactions between the health care team and the patient.
5. Define the role of the RN in transitional care.
6. Identify issues related to polypharmacy and methods for managing this.
7. Discuss the goals, methods, and issues of complementary, alternative, and integrative therapies.

KEY POINTS – *The major points in this chapter include:*

1. The current health care system is not set up well to handle chronic disease.
2. The chronic care model provides a framework for managing chronic illness within primary care.
3. The patient-centered medical home (PCMH) is one model that incorporates the chronic care model to care for patients with chronic illnesses.
4. The role of the ambulatory care nurse in the PCMH model focuses on the health care team.
5. Self-management support is the care and encouragement provided to people with chronic conditions to help them understand their central role in managing their illness, making informed decisions about their care, and engaging in healthy behavior.
6. Transitional care services and programs have been developed and implemented in an effort to improve quality and reduce the cost of health care related to the movement of the patient between level of care or settings.
7. Patients with chronic illnesses, particularly the elderly, are susceptible to complex medication regimens and polypharmacy.
8. Nurses are in a unique position to facilitate the integration of complementary and alternative medicine therapies into the conventional health care environment.

While there are many ways to define chronic illness, the MacColl Center for Health Care Innovation defines *chronic condition* as "any condition that requires ongoing adjustments by the affected person and interactions with the health care system" (Improving Chronic Illness Care, 2012a). More than 100 million people in the United States have at least one chronic condition (Improving Chronic Illness Care, 2012d). That number is projected to increase by more than 1% each year through 2030, resulting in an estimated chronically ill population of 171 million. Chronic conditions (such as heart disease, hypertension, diabetes, asthma, and depression) have been rapidly replacing acute and infectious diseases as the major causes of death, disease, and disability in the United States. However, the prevailing health care system is based on the diagnosis and treatment of acute illness, and it, therefore, is not well suited for the effective care of patients with chronic illness (Improving Chronic Illness Care, 2012d; Wagner et al., 2001).

This chapter reviews approaches, tools, and trends in addressing chronic illness care and the role of the ambulatory care nurse related to the care of patients with these conditions.

I. Chronic Condition Care

A. Current health care system not optimal for delivering chronic disease management (Homer & Baron, 2010).
1. Deficiencies in the current management of chronic disease:
   a. Rushed practitioners not following evidence-based established practice guidelines.
   b. Lack of care coordination.
   c. Lack of follow-up to ensure the best outcomes.
   d. Patients inadequately trained to manage their illnesses.
2. The current system is reactive and based on illness, not proactive, with goal of keeping people as healthy as possible.

B. Chronic care model (Bodenheimer, Lorig, Holman, & Grumbach, 2002; Fiandt, 2007; Wagner et al., 2001).
1. Developed as an organized framework designed to improve chronic illness care.
2. Provides a tool for improving care at both the individual and population levels.
3. Addresses practice strategies and patient-centered/self-managed care.

C. Six elements of the chronic care model.
1. Organizational support: Addresses culture of the practice, as well as system leadership.
   a. Key values:
      (1) Optimal management of chronic conditions.
      (2) Physician practice improvement.
   b. Leadership:
      (1) Is committed and visibly involved.
      (2) Supports change.
      (3) Supports quality improvement.
      (4) Creates incentives for physicians and patients to improve care.
      (5) Creates incentives for physicians to adhere to evidence-based practice.

2. Clinical information systems (Improving Chronic Illness Care, 2012a) – Provide organized patient and population data to facilitate efficient and effective care by:
   a. Using an electronic medical record (EMR).
   b. Providing timely reminders for providers and patients.
   c. Identifying relevant subpopulations for proactive care.
   d. Facilitating individual patient care planning.
   e. Sharing information with patients and providers to coordinate care.
   f. Monitoring performance of the team and care system.

3. Delivery system design: Emphasizes several innovative delivery system interventions (Fiandt, 2007; Improving Chronic Illness Care, 2012b):
   a. Defining roles and distributing tasks among team members.
   b. Using planned interactions to support evidence-based care (such as phone and group visits).
   c. Providing case management services for complex patients.
   d. Ensuring regular follow-up by the care team; may or may not be face-to-face.
   e. Providing care that patients understand and that fits with their cultural background (health literacy and cultural sensitivity).

4. Decision support: Enables treatment decisions to be based on explicit, proven guidelines supported by clinical research and includes:
   a. Embedding evidence-based guidelines into daily clinical practice, including:
      (1) Real-time practice guideline reminders.
      (2) Protocols and standing orders.
   b. Sharing evidence-based guidelines and information with patients to encourage their participation.
   c. Using proven provider education methods.

d. Integrating expertise of specialists with primary care, such that specialty experts are readily available to primary care providers for consultation at the time patients are being seen by the primary care provider.

5. Self-management (Improving Chronic Illness Care, 2012c): Decisions and behaviors of patients with chronic illness that affect their health – Emphasizing the patients' central role in managing their own health.
   a. Using effective self-management strategies.
   b. Organizing resources to provide ongoing support to patients.

6. Community support: Includes mobilization of community resources to meet needs of patients. Care is enhanced without duplicating efforts when the health care system looks outside itself.
   a. Encouraging patients to participate in effective community programs.
   b. Forming partnerships between the health system and community organizations to support and develop interventions to fill gaps in services needed.
   c. Using free health departments' and other agencies' materials. Using national patient organizations to promote self-management strategies (such as the American Diabetes Association and American Cancer Society).
   d. Advocating through medical organizations with local and state governments, insurers, and others on behalf of patients to improve their care.

D. Select models of care based on the chronic care model.
   1. Patient-centered medical home (PCMH), sometimes called the primary care medical home, advanced primary care, or the health care home (further described below).
   2. Patient Aligned Care Teams (PACT): The Veterans Administration PCMH model (Love, 2011).

3. Guided care (Boult, Karm, & Groves, 2008): Developed by researchers at Johns Hopkins University and focuses on older adults with chronic conditions/complex health needs.
4. Care Management Plus (n.d.).
   a. Cooperative project between the Oregon Health and Science University and The John A. Hartford Foundation.
   b. Focused on improving the quality of care for seniors and patients with chronic illnesses.

II. Patient-Centered Medical Home (PCMH)

As mentioned above, the PCMH is a model of care designed to facilitate care delivery consistent with the chronic care model. Historically, complex care was defined based on number and complexity of medical diagnoses. Care was often not adequately delivered based on rushed practitioners, lack of coordination, focus on illness rather than disease prevention, and patient self-management. In the PCMH model, patients may have only one medical diagnosis, but their social and other needs are complex and affect their health; therefore, these patients are more closely managed. Payers are developing payment structures that take into consideration the labor intensiveness of the model on the premise the care model results in less costly care later.

A. PCMH:
   1. Facilitates partnerships between individual patients, their health care team, and when appropriate, the patient's family (Patient-Centered Primary Care Collaborative, n.d.).
   2. Can be implemented in various ways.
   3. Has been developed to identify a system where chronic disease can be better managed through the primary care team.

B. PCMH attributes and functions (Laughlin & Beisel, 2010).
   1. Patient-centered.
      a. Primary care is relationship-based and oriented toward the whole person.
      b. Health care is based on understanding and respecting each patient's unique needs, culture, values, and preferences.

c. Patients and families are recognized as core members of the care team and are fully informed partners in establishing care plans.

d. Team members support patients in learning to manage and organize their own care at the level patients choose.

2. Comprehensive.

a. The team is accountable for meeting the majority of patients' physical and mental health care needs, including:
   (1) Illness and injury prevention.
   (2) Wellness and health promotion.
   (3) Acute care.
   (4) Chronic care.

b. The team of care providers is required to provide comprehensive care and might include:
   (1) Physicians.
   (2) Advanced practice nurses.
   (3) Physician assistants.
   (4) Nurses.
   (5) Pharmacists.
   (6) Nutritionists.
   (7) Social workers.
   (8) Educators.
   (9) Care coordinators.

c. Some PCMH practices bring together large and diverse teams of care providers; many others, including smaller practices, build virtual teams, linking themselves and their patients to providers and services in their communities.

3. Coordinated.

a. Care is coordinated across all elements of the broader health care system, including specialty care, hospitals, home health care, and community services and supports.

b. Coordination is particularly critical during transitions between sites of care, such as when patients are being discharged from the hospital.

4. Accessible.

a. Services are accessible and delivered with:

(1) Short waiting times for urgent needs.
(2) Enhanced, extended hours.
(3) Around-the-clock telephone or electronic access to a member of the care team.
(4) Alternative methods of communication, such as email and telephone care.

b. The team is responsive to patients' preferences regarding access.

5. Continuously improved through a systems-based approach to quality and safety. Approach:

a. Uses evidence-based medicine and clinical decision-support tools to guide shared decision-making with patients and families.

b. Engages in performance measurement and improvement.

c. Measures and responds to patient experiences and patient satisfaction.

d. Practices population health management.

e. Shares quality and safety data and improvement activities publicly.

C. Tools and resources used to implement medical home.

1. Secure messaging.

2. Telephone appointments.
   a. Transition care discharge phone calls.
   b. Coordination between primary and specialty care.
   c. In-hospital/nursing home visits.

3. Use of technology.
   a. Electronic medical record (EMR).
   b. Telehealth monitoring (such as blood pressure, blood sugar, weight).
   c. Virtual appointments.
   d. Virtual care by specialists.
   e. Electronic disease registries.
   f. Personal health record.
   g. Health information exchange (HIE).

D. Team: Composition of the PCMH team varies depending on how the PCMH has been defined and what resources are available. In general:

1. Core team consists of:
   a. Provider (physician, nurse practitioner) team leader.
   b. RN care coordinator.
   c. MA/LPN/LVN/clerk.
2. Roles are clearly defined.
3. Scopes of practice are clearly understood and maximized through the use of standard orders and protocols.

E. Role of the RN care manager in the PCMH: Historically there have been few professional RNs in primary care settings. Those nurses were nurse practitioners or specialists dealing with disease-related populations (e.g., patients with diabetes, asthma). Their roles reflected the emphasis on disease rather than on wellness and chronic disease management. In the PCMH, the RN is generally responsible for (Laughlin & Beisel, 2010):
1. Coordination of care as patients navigate a complex health system.
2. Assessment of symptoms/identification of triggers.
3. Patient/family education.
4. Assistance with establishing patient self-management goals.
5. Medication reconciliation/education.
6. Linkage with community resources.
7. Panel management/population management.

F. PCMH reimbursement: Many models have been developed by payers to evaluate the PCMH and determine payment schedules. In some cases, recognition, designation, or credentialing as a PCMH by the National Committee for Quality Assurance (NCQA) is considered in deciding partnerships and payments. In general, the criteria for measurement include:
1. Improved quality of patient care.
2. Improved outcomes.
3. Improved results.
4. Evidence of coordinated care.
5. Reduction in cost.

III. **Self-Management and Self-Management Support**

A. Self-management: "The ability of the patient to deal with all that a chronic illness entails" (Coleman & Newton, 2005, p. 1503).
1. Symptoms.
2. Treatment.
3. Physical consequences.
4. Social consequences.
5. Lifestyle changes.

B. Self-management support – Care and encouragement provided to people with chronic conditions to help them understand their central role in:
1. Managing their illness.
2. Making informed decisions about care.
3. Engaging in healthy behaviors.

C. Self-management support is based on a collaborative model and cannot be optimally achieved using the traditional health care model. Self-management support involves both patient education and collaborative decision-making. The patient's interest drives the focus of the education. Bodenheimer and colleagues (2002) identified key characteristics that demonstrate the shift in the patient and health care provider interaction from traditional to collaborative.
1. Traditional interactions:
   a. Information and skills are taught based on the health care provider's agenda.
   b. There is an assumption that knowledge creates behavior change.
   c. The goal is compliance with the health care provider's agenda.
   d. Decisions are made by the health care provider.
2. Collaborative interactions:
   a. Information and skills are taught based on the patient's agenda.
   b. There is a belief that one's confidence in the ability to change, together with knowledge, creates behavior change.
   c. The goal is increased confidence in the ability to change, rather than compliance with a health care provider's advice.
   d. Decisions are made as a patient-health care provider partnership.

D. Tasks in chronic disease self-management (Lorig & Holman, 2003).
   1. Patients' perspectives about their diseases will change over time and depend on many factors, including the severity of current symptoms.
   2. Three sets of tasks are faced by patients with chronic illness throughout their lives.
      a. Learning and acting upon the knowledge and skills essential to effectively manage their conditions.
      b. Adapting usual activities and roles to the condition.
      c. Dealing with emotions resulting from the realities of having a chronic illness:
         (1) Fear.
         (2) Anger.
         (3) Frustration.
         (4) Sadness.
         (5) Depression.
E. Core self-management skills – Lorig and Holman (2003) described self-management as being problem-based. Patients are taught problem-solving skills, not solutions to the problem. Core self-management skill involves:
   1. Forming a patient/health care provider partnership.
   2. Problem-solving.
   3. Decision-making.
   4. Taking action.
   5. Resource utilization.
   6. Tools to guide goal setting and action planning.
F. Motivational interviewing (MI) – The chronic care model, medical home, and self-management concepts are all based on the premise that the patient is at the center of care. In promoting self-care, professionals must embrace new ways of interacting with patients. Motivational interviewing (MI) is a collaborative, person-centered form of guiding patients to elicit and strengthen motivation for behavioral change (Miller & Rollnick, 2009). MI takes into consideration theory of stages of readiness to change and seeks to capitalize on where the patient is at the time.
   1. MI is:
      a. Psychotherapeutic method.
      b. Evidence-based.
      c. Relatively brief.
      d. Applicable across a wide variety of problem areas.
      e. Complementary to other active treatment methods.
      f. Learned by a broad range of helping professionals.
   2. MI theory emphasizes two components (Miller & Rose, 2009).
      a. Relational: Focuses on empathy and spirit of MI.
      b. Technical: Uses specific skills to differentially evoke and reinforce client change talk.
   3. Change talk: Refers to statements made by a patient that reveals consideration of change, motivation to change, or commitment to change.
      a. Commitment ("I will make changes").
      b. Activation ("I am ready, prepared, willing to change").
      c. Taking steps ("I am taking specific actions to change").
   4. Actions that increase the likelihood the patient will take action and implement a change:
      a. Helping the patient verbalize the arguments for change.
      b. Helping the patient, when ready, to develop a specific change plan.
   5. Four MI processes (Miller & Rollnick, 2010):
      a. Engaging: Person-centered style, listening to understand dilemma and values.
      b. Guiding: Setting an agenda; finding a focus, information, and advice.
      c. Evoking: Eliciting, responding, summarizing.
      d. Planning: The bridge to change.
   6. Guiding principles of motivational interviewing (Rollnick, Miller, & Butler, 2008)
      a. Resist the "Righting Reflex," which is a reflex to offer advice to correct whatever is "wrong."
      b. Understand and explore the patient's own motivations.

c. Listen with empathy and empower the patient.
d. Encourage hope and optimism.

G. Empowerment – A patient-centered collaborative approach and defined as "helping patients discover and develop the inherent capacity to be responsible for one's own life" (Funnell & Anderson, 2004, p. 124).
   1. Empowerment was developed specifically for diabetes care, and as yet, has not been widely adapted to other chronic diseases.
   2. Motivational interviewing and empowerment share similarities and differences.
      a. Both acknowledge and respect the rights of patients to freely make decisions about how to manage their disease (e.g., diabetes).
      b. One difference in the empowerment philosophy is that it incorporates interactive teaching strategies designed to actively involve patients in problem-solving and to address both cultural and psychological needs of patients.
   3. Empowerment approach goal setting is a 5-step process:
      a. Explore the problem or issue (past).
      b. Clarify the feelings and meaning (present).
      c. Develop a plan (future).
      d. Commit to action (future).
      e. Experience and evaluate the plan (future).

IV. Transitional Care

Transitional care refers to care directed at making a smooth transition between levels of care and/or care settings. Transitional care programs and services have been developed and implemented in an effort to improve quality and reduce the cost of health care.

A. Coleman's Transition Model (Coleman et al., 2004): Combines patient activation and development of a patient coach The coach's role is to teach patients and families to coordinate care for themselves. This model is based on Four Pillars of Care Transition:

1. Medication self-management:
   a. Patient and caregiver understand medications so medications are taken correctly.
   b. Patient has a medication self-management system.
2. Patient-centered record: Personal health record is used by patient, and brought to every health care encounter.
3. Follow-up: Visit with primary care provider or specialist is scheduled and completed.
4. Red flags: Patient is aware of the list of symptoms indicative of a worsening condition and knows how to respond to them.

B. Transitional Care Model (TCM) (Naylor et al., 1999): Focuses on assisting patients who have complex chronic conditions to safely transfer from one type of care setting to another or from one level of care to another.
   1. Heart of model is the transitional care nurse who follows patients from the hospital into their homes and provides services designed to:
      a. Streamline plans of care.
      b. Interrupt patterns of frequent hospital and emergency use.
      c. Prevent health status decline.
   2. TCM is nurse-led; it is a multidisciplinary model that includes:
      a. Physicians.
      b. Other nurses.
      c. Social workers.
      d. Discharge planners.
      e. Pharmacists.
   3. The health care team implements tested protocols focused on increasing the ability of patients and their caregivers to manage their care.
   4. Compared with other transitional care interventions that limit their focus to "hand-offs" of patients from hospital to home, the TCM:
      a. Focuses on all the health problems and risks that contribute to re-hospitalizations.
      b. Addresses the "root causes" of poor outcomes to assure longer-term positive outcomes.

V. Polypharmacy

Polypharmacy is the use of multiple medications and/or the administration of more medications than are clinically indicated, representing unnecessary drug use. Patients who have more than one chronic illness may take multiple medications. Polypharmacy is common among the elderly. For the elderly population, the complexity increases because the potential for multiple diagnoses exists, and physiological changes may affect how medications are absorbed, distributed, metabolized, and excreted. It is a particular concern because older adults make up 13% of the population, but account for almost 30% of all prescribed drugs (Bushardt, Massey, Simpson, Ariail, & Simpson, 2008).

A. Various definitions of polypharmacy (Bushardt et al., 2008):
   1. Increased number of medications:
      a. Prescription medications.
      b. Nonprescription medications – Over-the-counter (OTC) medications and herbal/supplementary agents.
   2. Potentially inappropriate medication: May not be appropriate for a given patient because of age or a concurrent illness.
   3. Medication underuse: Medications with a clear benefit for a given illness/condition that a patient is not taking or taking a lower dose.
   4. Medication duplication: The same or a similar drug class or therapeutic effect concurrently being used that may not be beneficial.
B. Factors that may contribute to polypharmacy include:
   1. Self-medication practices (Curry, Walker, Hogstel, & Burns, 2005):
      a. Discontinuing or reducing medications because of lack of funds or fears of side effects or dependency.
      b. Failing to follow food- or alcohol-related recommendations when taking certain medications.
      c. Failing to keep track of medications as they are taken, resulting in missed doses or added doses.

   d. Taking OTC medications and/or herbal products in addition to prescribed drugs for the same problem.
   e. Adding doses when symptoms are not relieved or skipping doses when symptoms are not present.
   f. Taking the wrong doses or using the wrong technique with inhalers, eye drops, suppositories, or injections. Poor ability to understand health information due to health literacy and physical impairments, such as poor eyesight; poor hearing of instructions may lead to the wrong dose/technique.
   2. Patient seeks care from various health care providers, and there is no coordination among these providers in terms of their treatment plans.
   3. Direct-to-consumer drug marketing.
   4. Increased pressure on provider visit time; it is often easier for providers to write a prescription than take the time to fully assess the patient's situation and provide the education necessary to have the patient try a different mode of treatment.

C. Strategies for decreasing negative effects of polypharmacy.
   1. Medication reconciliation: Identified as one of the National Patient Safety Goals (The Joint Commission, 2011).
      a. Obtain and document a current medication list or other usable format every time a patient is seen in any setting.
      b. Medication list should contain name of drug, dose, route, frequency, and purpose.
      c. Update the information when medications are discontinued, doses are changed, or new medications are added (including OTC medications).
      d. Identify and resolve discrepancies.
      e. Provide the patient (or family as needed) with written information on the medication that the patient should be taking at the end of the outpatient encounter.
      f. Advise the patient of the importance of carrying medication information to every health care encounter.

2. Having the patient bring all medications, including vitamins, OTC products, and herbal remedies, periodically to outpatient visits.
3. Electronic prescribing: The process of prescribing medications using a computerized provider order entry system that electronically exchanges prescriptions directly with the pharmacy and/or the pharmacy benefits manager (Brooks & Sonnenschein, 2010).
   a. Makes medication prescribing process more efficient:
      (1) Helps eliminate errors.
      (2) Improves patient safety.
      (3) Reduces costs.
   b. Prevents medication errors caused by difficulties in reading or understanding handwritten prescriptions.
   c. Reduces adverse drug events by making information, such as drug interactions and contraindications, available at time the prescriber is ordering.
   d. Decreases out-of-pocket cost when formulary coverage and co-payment information is available and referenced electronically.
4. Obtaining hospital medical records for patients after they are hospitalized.
5. Post-discharge calls to review and reconcile medications.
6. Use of medication management assistive devices.
   a. Alarm watches, clocks, timers, pagers to prompt patients to take medications.
   b. Pill dispensers that organize medications according to time and day, day only, week, month.
7. Use of the Beers Criteria – A list of medications (American Geriatrics Society, 2012; Beers, 1997).
   a. Drug or drug classes considered inappropriate for the elderly.
   b. Drugs that may be inappropriate for use in elderly based on presence of diseases or conditions.
8. Use of the Zahn Criteria of medications inappropriate for elderly (Zahn et al., 2001).

   a. Zahn Criteria is streamlined.
   b. Identifies fewer at-risk medications deemed inappropriate by expert consensus.

VI. **Complementary, Alternative, and Integrative Therapies (CAM)**
   The 2007 National Health Interview Survey documented that approximately 38% of adults and 12% of children use complementary and alternative medicine (CAM) (National Center for Complementary and Alternative Medicine [NCCAM], 2007). Knowledge and use of CAM therapies among health care consumers have been growing steadily over the past few years. Nurses are in a unique position to facilitate the integration of CAM therapies into the conventional health care environment and should be prepared to assist patients in making safe, knowledgeable decisions.
   A. Definitions by NCCAM (2011).
      1. *Complementary medicine* refers to non-traditional therapies used together with conventional medicine.
      2. *Alternative medicine* refers to the use of non-traditional therapies in place of conventional medicine.
      3. *Integrative medicine* refers to a practice that combines conventional medicine with non-traditional therapies.
      4. *CAM* refers to complementary and alternative medicine.
      5. *NCCAM* is a division of the National Institute for Health.
   B. Goals of CAM therapies.
      1. Reduce or eliminate pain.
      2. Enhance the effectiveness of other treatments.
      3. Improve mood and affect.
      4. Enhance a sense of well-being.
      5. Reduce stress.
      6. Improve functionality and the ability to perform activities of daily living.
      7. Provide the patient with a better sense of control over his or her life (Hart, 2008).
   C. Categories and examples of CAM modalities – CAM practices are sometimes grouped into categories based on the type of techniques in practice. These categories are not formally de-

fined, and some practices are consistent with more than one category. Categories most often used and some examples of each are as follows:

1. Natural products: This would include some dietary supplements, probiotics, some vitamins and minerals, and botanicals, including herbal preparations.
2. Mind-body interventions: These would include acupuncture, meditation, yoga, Tai Chi, guided imagery, biofeedback, and relaxation techniques, along with numerous other techniques.
3. Manipulative and body-based practices: These refer to chiropractic care, cranial sacral therapy, massage, and effleurage.
4. Energy medicine: This group of techniques refers to Healing Touch, Qi Gong, Reiki, and Therapeutic Touch, along with many others.
5. Medical systems, such as Ayurveda, traditional Chinese medicine, and homeopathy, which have developed over time in different cultures, can be considered CAM.
6. Other: There are other practices considered to be CAM that do not fit into any particular group or category. Some examples would be Pilates, Rolfing structural integration, and some traditional healers, such as Native American Healers and Shamans.
7. The techniques listed are examples representative of each category noted, although there are many other types of CAM practice not specifically noted here.
   a. More thorough explanations and descriptions are available on the NCCAM Web site (www.nccam.nih.gov).
   b. There are also information sheets available for specific techniques that can be downloaded or printed from the site.
   c. There is information regarding additional CAM resources and government regulation, as well as links to related sites (e.g., the Food and Drug Administration [FDA] Center for Food Safety and Applied Nutrition).

d. Research results and information about ongoing studies in CAM therapies are also available.

D. Criteria for selecting providers.
1. Licensure: Not all modalities require licensure. State law determines licensing requirements, and these vary state to state.
2. Experience and training: Most CAM therapies require some type of training. More formal education programs often provide certification if licensing is not required.
3. Experience working with other providers, including conventional practitioners, to ensure coordination of care.
4. Some educational programs or professional organizations maintain a database of approved/credentialed providers by location/provider name on their Web site (Healing Touch Program, 2012).

E. It is important to note that there is no standardized, national system for credentialing CAM practitioners.
1. Nurses should gain and maintain the appropriate knowledge and skills to practice and/or recommend CAM therapies.
2. Knowledge of available resources to provide reliable, evidence-based research is an appropriate foundation for practice.
3. There is ongoing research available regarding the safety and efficacy of CAM practice; many CAM professions as well as NCCAM and the American Holistic Nurses' Association (AHNA) support research and practice of CAM therapies, and share this information on their Web sites or in publications.

F. Nursing scope of practice in CAM.
1. A study conducted for the White House Commission on Complementary and Alternative Medicine Policy in 2001 found that 47% of state boards of nursing had taken positions that allowed for nurses to practice CAM (Sparber, 2001).
2. In most states, the RN is held accountable to hold the proper credentials – License, certificate, or registration to safely engage in any specific practice, including CAM modalities (Sparber, 2001).

3. Implications:
   a. Nurses should be familiar with the nurse practice act in their state, with specific reference to the position on CAM.
   b. Nurses should know their resources.
   c. Published research supporting evidence-based practice reliable resources include:
      (1) American Botanical Council (http://abc.herbalgram.org).
      (2) American Holistic Nurses' Association (AHNA) (http://www.ahna.org/research).
      (3) Healing Touch Program (www.healingtouchresearch.com).
      (4) NCCAM (http://nccam.nih.gov/research).
      (5) Professional organizations supporting CAM professionals.
   d. One should become familiar with CAM credentialing and education/training in the state for the modalities that patients will be using.
   e. Web sites, such as those of NCCAM and AHNA, support ongoing CAM research and education of health care providers and consumers.
   f. Nurses should be aware of the potential effects of CAM therapies and their potential interactions with other modalities, including the physiological, emotional, and spiritual aspects.
   g. CAM interventions and patient responses should be documented in the patient record.
   h. Nursing professionals should develop and maintain policies and procedures for safe and effective CAM practice within their organization, as well as guidelines for referrals to other providers.
G. Insurance reimbursement.
   1. According to the 2007 National Health Interview Survey, out-of-pocket expenditures on CAM treatments accounted for approximately 1.5% of total health care expenditures and 11.2% of the total out of pocket health care expenditures in the United States (NCCAM, 2007).
   2. Insurance coverage of CAM therapies is very limited. Some private insurance plans offer coverage of certain therapies, such as acupuncture, massage, and chiropractic.
   3. The Healing Touch Program is an ANCC-approved provider of continuing nursing education and has applied to the National Commission for Certifying Agencies (NCCA) for accreditation of the program as a specialty practice. Accreditation establishes recognized standards of education and practice and communicates transparency of practice to consumers and other providers. Healing Touch is the first energy medicine discipline to apply for accreditation, which could, if successful, make their services eligible for insurance reimbursement.
   4. Patients should be familiar with their insurance coverage and verify exactly what services are eligible for reimbursement before beginning treatment. Deductibles and co-pays should also be verified because these may be higher for CAM therapies than for conventional therapies.
   5. Patients should also check with the CAM provider being considered regarding services, cost per visit, and number of visits that may be needed for treatment of the patient's particular health condition. Additional fees for supplies or equipment should also be clarified prior to beginning treatment. Payment options should be discussed with the provider as well, because some CAM providers are willing to work with patients to develop an individual plan to make their services affordable.
H. As consumer interest in CAM therapies grows and research outcomes provide more evidence to the safety and effectiveness of CAM therapies in the promotion of health, insurance companies and managed care organizations may consider improving coverage of these services.

References

American Geriatrics Society 2012 Beers Criteria Update Expert Panel. (2012). American Geriatrics Society updated Beers Criteria for potentially inappropriate medication use in older adults. *Journal of the American Geriatrics Society, 60*(4), 616-631.

Beers, M.H. (1997). Explicit criteria for determining potentially inappropriate medication use by the elderly. An update. *Archives of Internal Medicine, 157,* 1531-1536.

Bodenheimer, T., Lorig, K., Holman, H., & Grumbach, K. (2002). Patient self-management of chronic disease in primary care. *Journal of the American Medical Association, 288*(19), 2469-2475.

Boult, C., Karm, L., & Groves, C. (2008). Improving chronic care: The "guided care" model. *The Permanente Journal, 2*(1), 50-54.

Brooks, P., & Sonnenschein, C. (2010). E-prescribing: Where health information and patient care intersect. *Journal of Healthcare Information Management, 24*(2), 53-59.

Bushardt, R.S., Massey, E., Simpson, T., Ariail, J., & Simpson, K. (2008). Polypharmacy: Misleading but manageable. *Clinical Interventions in Aging, 3*(2), 383-389.

Care Management Plus (CMP). (n.d.). *Home page.* Retrieved from http://caremanagementplus.org

Coleman, E.A., Smith, J.D., Frank, J.C., Min, S.J., Parry, C., & Kramer, A.M. (2004). Preparing patients and caregivers to participate in care delivered across settings: The care transitions intervention. *Journal of American Geriatrics Society, 52,* 1817-1825.

Coleman, M.T., & Newton, K.S. (2005). Self-management support for patients with chronic illness. *American Family Physician, 72*(8), 1503-1510.

Curry, L.C., Walker, C., Hogstel, M.O., & Burns, P. (2005). Teaching older adults to self-manage medications: Preventing adverse drug reactions. *Journal of Gerontological Nursing, 31*(4), 32-42.

Fiandt, K. (2007, January 5). The chronic care model: Description and application for practice. *Topics in Advanced Practice Nursing, 6*(4).

Funnell, M.M., & Anderson, R.M. (2004). Empowerment and self-management of diabetes. *Clinical Diabetes, 22*(3), 123-137.

Hart, J. (2008). Complementary therapies for chronic pain management. *Alternative and Complementary Therapies, 14*(2), 64-68.

Healing Touch Program. (2012). *Home page.* Retrieved from www.healingtouchprogram.com

Homer, C.J., & Baron, R. (2010). How to scale up primary care transformation: What we know and what we need to know? *Journal of General Internal Medicine, 25*(6), 625-629.

Improving Chronic Illness Care. (2012a). *Clinical information systems.* Retrieved from http://www.improvingchronic care.org/index.php?p=Clinical-Information-Systems&s=25

Improving Chronic Illness Care. (2012b). *Delivery system design.* Retrieved from http://www.improvingchroniccare.org/index.php?p=Delivery_System_Design&s=21

Improving Chronic Illness Care. (2012c). *Self-management support.* Retrieved from http://www.improvingchroniccare.org/index.php?p=Self-Management_Support&s=22

Improving Chronic Illness Care. (2012d). *The chronic care model.* Retrieved from http://www.improvingchroniccare.org/index.php?p=The_Chronic_Care_Model&s=2

Joint Commission, The. (2011). *National Patient Safety Goals 2011: Ambulatory health care accreditation program.* http://www.jointcommission.org/assets/1/6/NPSG_EPs_Scoring_AHC_20110707.pdf

Laughlin, C., & Beisel, M. (2010). Evolution of the chronic care role of the registered nurse in primary care. *Nursing Economic$, 28*(6), 409-414.

Lorig, K.R., & Holman, H.R. (2003). Self-management education: History, definition, outcomes, and mechanisms. *Annals of Behvioral Medicine, 26*(1), 1-7.

Love, W.B. (2011). *PACT: A plus for veterans.* Retrieved from http://muskogeephoenix.com/features/x234219833/PACT-A-plus-for-veterans

Miller, W.R., & Rollnick, S. (2009). Ten things that motivational interviewing is not. *Behavioral and Cognitive Psychotherapy, 37,* 129-140.

Miller, W.R., & Rollnick, S. (2010). *What makes it motivational interviewing?* Retrieved from http://www.motivational interview.org/Documents/Miller-june7-plenary.pdf

Miller, W.R., & Rose, G.S. (2009). Toward a theory of motivational interviewing. *American Psychologist, 64*(6), 527-537.

National Center for Complementary and Alternative Medicine (NCCAM). (2007). *Statistics on complementary and alternative medicine: National health interview survey.* Retrieved from http://nccam.nih.gov/news/camstats/NHIS.htm

National Center for Complementary and Alternative Medicine (NCCAM). (2011). *CAM basics: What is complementary and alternative medicine?* Retrieved from http://nccam.nih.gov/health/whatiscam

Naylor, M., Brooten, D., Campbell, R., Jacobsen, B., Mezey, M., Pauly, M., & Schwartz, S. (1999). Comprehensive discharge planning and home follow-up of hospitalized elders: A randomized clinical trial. *Journal of the American Medical Association, 281,* 613-620.

Patient-Centered Primary Care Collaborative. (n.d.). *Joint principles of the patient-centered medical home.* Retrieved from http://www.pcpcc.net/content/joint-principles-patient-centered-medical-home

Rollnick, S., Miller, W.R., & Butler, C.C. (2008). *Motivational interviewing in health care – Helping patients change behavior.* New York: Guilford Press.

Sparber, A. (2001). State boards of nursing and scope of practice of registered nurses performing complementary therapies. *Online Journal of Issues in Nursing, 6*(3), 10.

Wagner, E.H., Austin, B.T., Davis, C., Hindmarsh, M., Schaefer, J., & Bonomi, A. (2001). Improving chronic illness care: Translating evidence into action. *Health Affairs, 20*(6), 64-78.

Zhan, C., Sangle, J., Bierman, A.S., Miller, M.R., Friedman, B., Wickizer, S.W., & Meyer, G.S. (2001). Potentially inappropriate medication use in the community dwelling elderly: Findings from the 1996 Medical Expenditure Panel Survey. *Journal of the American Medical Association, 286*(22), 2819-2823.

Additional Readings

American Botanical Council. (n.d.). *Home page.* Retrieved from http://abc.herbalgram.org

American Holistic Nurses' Association (AHNA). (2012). *Home page.* Retrieved from http://www.ahna.org

Barnes, P.M., Bloom, B., Nahin, R. (2008). Complementary and alternative medicine use among adults and children: United States, 2007. *CDC National Health Statistics Report, 12,* 1-24. Hyattsville, MD: National Center for Health Statistics.

Benson, J. (2009). Healing Touch program pursues accreditation. *Energy Magazine, 37,* 19-21.

Bilyeu, K.M., Gumm, C.J., Fitzgerald, J.M., Fox, S.W., & Selig, P. (2011). Reducing the use of potentially inappropriate medications in older adult. *American Journal of Nursing 111*(1), 47-52.

Blue Cross Blue Shield of Michigan. (2011). *Fact sheet: What is a patient-centered medical home?* Retrieved from http://www.valuepartnerships.com/pcmh/pcmh_factsheet.pdf

Bodenheimer, T. (2008). Coordinating care – A perilous journey through the health care system. *New England Journal of Medicine, 358*(10), 1064-1071.

Bodenheimer, T., & Abramowitz, S. (2010). *Helping patients help themselves: How to implement self-management support.* Retrieved from http://www.chcf.org/publications/2010/12/helping-patients-help-themselves

Bodenheimer, T., Wagner, E.H., & Grumbach K. (2002). Improving primary care for patients with chronic illness: Part I. *Journal of the American Medical Association, 288*(14), 1775-1779.

Boult, C., Giddens, J., Frey, K., Reider, L., & Novak, T. (2009). *Guided care: A new nurse-physician partnership in chronic care.* New York: Springer Publishing Company, LLC.

Brewer-Lowery, A.N., Arcury, T., Bell, R.A., & Quandt, S.A. (2010). Differentiating approaches to diabetes self-management of multi-ethnic rural older adults at the extremes of glycemic control. *The Gerontologist, 50*(5), 657-667.

Centers for Disease Control and Prevention (CDC). (2012). *National health interview survey.* Retrieved from http://www.cdc.gov/nchs/nhis.htm

Centers for Medicare & Medicaid Services/Center for Medicare and Medicaid Innovations. (n.d.). *Home page.* Retrieved from http://innovations.cms.gov/index.html

Coleman, E.A., Parry, C., Chalmers, S., & Min, S.J. (2006). The care transitions intervention results of a randomized controlled trial. *Archives of Internal Medicine, 166,* 1822-1828.

"Definition of motivational interviewing." (n.d.) Retrieved from http://www.motivationalinterview.org/Documents/1%20A%20MI%20Definition%20Principles%20&%20Approach%20V4%20012911.pdf

Guided Care. (2012). *Home page.* Retrieved from http://www.guidedcare.org

Haggerty, J., Pineault, R., Beaulieu, M.D., Brunelle, Y., Bauthier, J., Coulet, F., & Rodiquez, J. (2008). Practice features associated with patient-reported accessibility, continuity, and coordination of primary health care, *Annals of Family Medicine, 6*(2), 116-123.

Levine, C., Halper, D., Peist, A., & Gould, D. (2010). Bridging troubled waters: Family caregivers, transitions, and long-term care. *Health Affairs, 29,* 116-124.

Maggiore, R., Gross, C.P., & Hurria, A. (2010). Polypharmacy in older adults with cancer. *The Oncologist, 15,* 507-522.

Mor, V., Intrator, O., Feng, Z., & Grabowski, D. (2010). The revolving door of rehospitalization from skilled nursing facilities. *Heatlh Affairs, 29,* 57-64.

Nahin, R., Barnes, P.M., Stussman, B.J., & Bloom, B. (2009). Costs of complementary and alternative medicine (CAM) and frequency of visits to CAM practitioners: United States, 2007. *CDC National Health Statistics Report, 18,* 1-14. Hyattsville, MD: National Center for Health Statistics.

National Center for Complementary and Alternative Medicine (NCCAM). (n.d.). *Home page.* Retrieved from http://nccam.nih.gov/

National Committee for Quality Assurance. (2011). *Information for media and medical practices.* Retrieved from http://www.ncqa.org/tabid/1302/Default.aspx

National Priorities Partnership. (2010). *Input to the Secretary of Health and Human Services on priorities for the 2011 National Quality Strategy, convened by the National Quality Forum.* Retrieved from http://www.nationalpriorities partnership.org

Naylor, M., Aiken, L., Kurtzman, E., Olds, D., & Hirschman, K. (2011). The importance of transitional care in achieving health reform. *Health Affairs, 30*(4), 746-754.

Naylor, M., Hollander Feldman, P., Keathing, S., Koren, M., Kurtzman, E., Maccoy, M., & Krakauer, R. (2009). Translating research into practice: Transitional care for older adults. *Journal of Evaluation in Clinical Practice, 15,* 1164-1170.

Piekes, D., Chen, A., Schore, J., & Brown, R. (2009). Effects of care coordination on hospitalization, quality of care, and health care expenditures among Medicare beneficiaries: 15 randomized trials. *Journal of the American Medical Association, 301*(6), 603-618.

Russell, S. (2004). The dangers of polypharmacy: Nurses should be on high alert when caring for elderly patients on multiple medications. *ViewPoint, 26,* 8-10.

Springhouse Corporation. (2001). *Nurse's handbook of alternative & complementary therapies* (2nd ed.). Philadelphia: Lippincott, Williams & Wilkins.

Chapter 21

Care of the Chronically Ill Patient

Nancy M. Albert, PhD, CCNS, CHFN, CCRN, NE-BC
Diana Anderson, BSN, RN, CPN
Catherine M. Besthoff, RN, MHA, CPHQ
Deborah Byrne-Barta, BSN, RN-BC, CPN
Renée Y. Cecil, MSN, RN

Mark Cichocki, RN
Pamela Del Monte, MS, RN-BC
Roslyn C. Kelly, MSN, RN-BC, CDE
Patricia Lucarelli, MSN, RN-BC, CPNP, APN

PATIENT PROTOTYPES

Adult Chronic Illnesses
Hypertension • Diabetes • Coronary Artery Disease/Coronary Heart Disease (CAD/CHD) • Chronic Heart Failure
Chronic Obstructive Pulmonary Disease (COPD) • Human Immunodeficiency Virus (HIV) • Peptic Ulcer Disease

Adolescent Chronic Illnesses
Human Immunodeficiency Virus (HIV)

Pediatric Chronic Illnesses
Asthma • Sickle Cell Disease • Developmental Delays • Autism Spectrum Disorder

OBJECTIVES – *Study of the information in this chapter will enable the learner to:*	KEY POINTS – *The major points in this chapter include:*
1. Describe the chronic illnesses common in the ambulatory care setting, including the prevalence of the disease in the population and the pathophysiology. 2. Identify the essential elements of the nursing process for the care of patients with chronic illnesses, including assessment and triage, indications for emergent or urgent care, preventive measures, and the plan of care.	1. Patients with chronic illnesses present in every ambulatory care setting and in telehealth encounters. 2. Ambulatory care nurses need to understand the key aspects of these illnesses and their treatments to competently assess and manage the patient's care, whether it is the primary reason for the encounter or secondary to the other aspects of assessment and care of that encounter.

Hypertension

Patient Population: Adult

I. Overview

Hypertension in adults is defined as blood pressure greater than or equal to 140/90. It can be diagnosed at any age. See Table 21-1 for classifications of blood pressure. Nearly 68 million (one out of three) adults in the United States (31.3%) has high blood pressure, including nearly 19% of adults ages 24–32 (Centers for Disease Control and Prevention [CDC], 2012). This is a significant increase in a younger, healthier population, which may be related to an increase in overweight/obesity rates and physical inactivity. *Healthy People 2020* (U.S. Department of Health and Human Services [DHHS], 2012) set a goal to decrease the incidence of hypertension in adults by 10% in the current decade.

Hypertension is the most common primary diagnosis with greater than 46.3 million ambulatory care (CDC, 2011) visits in the U.S. annually. Awareness, treatment, and control rates have been

Table 21-1.
Classifications of Blood Pressure for Adults
Ages 18 and Older

BP Classification	SBP mm Hg	DBP mm Hg
Normal	< 120	and < 80
Prehypertension	120–139	or 80–89
Stage 1 hypertension	140–159	or 90–99
Stage 2 hypertension	≥ 160	or ≥ 100

Note: Based on the average of 2 or more properly measured, seated BP readings on 2 or more office visits.

Source: National Heart, Lung, and Blood Institute, 2004. Used with permission.

steadily increasing over the past several decades. In the time frame 1976–1980 compared to 2003–2006, the percentage of people who were aware they had hypertension increased from 51% to 78%. Treatment rates increased from 31% to 67% and control rates showed an increase from 10% to 45%. Only 70% of adults with hypertension who took medication had their high blood pressure controlled. Hypertension, combined with complicating conditions, such as diabetes and chronic kidney disease, should be treated to achieve blood pressure levels of 130/80 or below. Hypertension is a significant risk factor for adverse cardiac events and stroke and is a primary or contributing cause of death for 326,000 Americans each year. It was estimated that health care costs of hypertension in 2010 in the U.S., including care services, medications, and missed days of work, totaled $76.6 billion (National Institutes of Health [NIH], 2011).

Men under the age of 45 are affected by hypertension at a higher rate than women. That rate changes for adults over the age of 65, with women developing hypertension at a higher rate than men. African Americans develop hypertension at a higher rate and at an earlier age than Whites and Mexican Americans. Adults 55-years-old and older have a 90% lifetime chance of developing hypertension, and nearly one in four American adults has prehypertension and is more apt to develop hypertension than those not diagnosed with prehypertension (CDC, 2011).

Complications of hypertension can be prevented or delayed with screening, early detection, and early and adequate blood pressure control. Lifestyle modifications, including healthy eating, being physically active, maintaining a healthy weight, and stopping tobacco use, are paramount in the management of hypertension and prehypertension. The treatment of hypertension can decrease the incidence of cardiovascular disease to a large extent. The ambulatory care nurse is positioned to increase awareness in these patients (given that they often present feeling well without obvious symptoms), promote a healthy lifestyle, coach lifestyle changes, and promote adherence to medication regimes.

II. **Pathophysiology**
A. Normal blood pressure is a balance between cardiac output and total peripheral resistance by the vascular system. Any increase to either of those factors changes that balance, and will increase blood pressure.
B. The renin-angiotensin system affects the control of blood pressure.
   1. Renin is secreted from the kidney in response to decreased renal perfusion or a reduced salt intake.
   2. Renin increases cardiac output by spurring the release of aldosterone, which causes sodium and water retention, increasing blood volume.
   3. Renin is also responsible for converting renin substrate (angiotensinogen) to angiotensin I, which is then converted to angiotensin II, a potent vasoconstrictor, resulting in an increase in blood pressure.
C. Sympathetic nervous system stimulation, in response to stress and physical activity, causes vasoconstriction and an increase in total peripheral resistance, increasing blood pressure.
D. Arterial thickening by genetic factors increases resistance, which in turn increases blood pressure.

III. **Assessment and Triage**
A. Evaluation and risk factors.
   1. Assess lifestyle; identify other cardiovascular risk factors and associated disorders.
   2. Assess for identifiable causes of high blood pressure.

3. Assess for presence/absence of target organ damage and cardiovascular disease.
4. Family history of hypertension, cardiovascular disease, coronary artery disease, renal disease.
5. Patient history of diabetes, elevated lipid levels, renal disease; medication history to include prescription, over-the-counter, and herbal supplements.
6. Patient demographics: Age, race, gender, weight, body mass index (BMI).

B. Functional status.
1. Excess body weight.
2. Excess dietary sodium intake.
3. Inadequate intake of fruits, vegetables, and potassium.
4. Excess alcohol intake.
5. Excessive caffeine intake.
6. Tobacco use.
7. Inadequate physical activity.

C. Physical assessment.
1. Blood pressure measurement.
   a. Assess for the need for alternative sites for blood pressure measurement (e.g., status post axillary node dissection, presence of dialysis fistula or shunt, and/or status post-radical mastectomy).
   b. Auscultatory blood pressure readings with patient seated for at least 5 minutes in a chair, feet on floor, and arm supported at heart level, with an appropriately sized cuff, cuff bladder, and cuff placement. See Chapter 14, "Application of the Nursing Process in Ambulatory Care," for detail about blood pressure measurement.
   c. No caffeine, smoking, or exercise for 30 minutes prior to reading.
   d. Take at least two measurements and average the readings.
   e. Verify blood pressure readings in contralateral arm.
   f. Assess standing blood pressure readings, especially with risk of postural hypertension, before starting medications and when changing dosing.

2. Examine optic fundi.
3. Calculate BMI and measure waist circumference.
4. Palpate thyroid.
5. Perform thorough examination of heart and lungs and heart sounds.
6. Auscultate for carotid, abdomen, and femoral bruits.
7. Examine abdomen.
8. Palpate for enlarged kidneys, masses, distended urinary bladder, and abnormal aortic pulsations.
9. Palpate lower extremities for edema and pulses.
10. Perform neurological assessment.

D. Diagnostic tests.
1. Routine labs, including urinalysis, blood chemistries, glucose, serum potassium, serum creatinine, hematocrit, lipoprotein panel.
2. 12-lead electrocardiogram.

IV. **Indications for Emergency Care or Urgent Consultation**

A. Hypertensive emergency.
1. Severe elevation of BP (greater than 180/120 mm Hg) complicated by evidence of impending or progressive target organ dysfunction.
2. Goal of therapy includes:
   a. Continuous monitoring of blood pressure and administration of appropriate parenteral antihypertensive agents.
   b. Immediate mean arterial blood pressure reduction of no more than 25% within minutes to 1 hour. Further decrease, if stable, to 160/100–110 mm Hg within 2–6 hours. Further gradual decrease of blood pressure over next 24–48 hours.
   c. Minimization and prevention of target organ damage for either maintained elevations or from too rapid and vast a decrease in blood pressure.
   d. Determine organic and treatable cause(s) of elevated blood pressure.

B. Hypertensive urgencies.
1. Severe elevation of BP without progressive target organ dysfunction.
2. Goal of therapy includes:
    a. Pharmacological intervention with short-acting oral agents.
    b. Blood pressure reduction within a few hours, followed by several hours of observation.
    c. Confirmed follow-up appointment, within one to a few days, prior to discharge from emergency department.

V. Plan of Care
A. Pharmacological management.
1. Diuretics.
2. Beta blockers.
3. ACE inhibitors.
4. Angiotensin II antagonists.
5. Calcium channel blockers.
6. Alpha blockers.
7. Central alpha-2 agonists.
8. Direct vasodilators.
9. Renin inhibitors.
10. Alpha beta blockers.
B. Primary/secondary/tertiary prevention.
1. Annual screening for hypertension, as blood pressure rises with increasing age.
2. Identify those at risk and educate to risk factors and lifestyle modifications.
3. Self-blood pressure monitoring.
    a. Check equipment for accuracy.
    b. Have patient demonstrate technique.
    c. Review patient log of blood pressure readings.
    d. Validate self-blood pressure measurements.
4. Ambulatory blood pressure monitoring.
    a. Provides blood pressure information during activities of daily living and sleep.
    b. Detects levels that may correlate with target organ injury.
5. Weight appropriate to height.
6. Physical activity of two hours and 30 minutes (150 minutes) of moderate-intensity aerobic activity (e.g., brisk walking) every week.

7. Dietary modifications; DASH (Dietary Approaches to Stop Hypertension) eating plan (NHLBI, 2006).
    a. An evidence-based eating plan that is low in saturated fat, cholesterol, and total fat; reduced consumption of red meats, sweets, and sugar-containing beverages.
    b. Concomitant emphasis on fruits, vegetables, and low fat dairy products.
    c. Rich in magnesium, calcium, protein, and fiber.
    d. Sodium consumption limited to 1500–2400 mg/day.
8. Encourage those with prehypertension to engage in lifestyle changes to reduce the risk of developing hypertension (see Table 21-2).
9. Identify patients where lifestyle modifications have not achieved blood pressure control (adequate antihypertensive medication and dose).
10. Minimize target organ damage (heart, brain, eyes, and kidneys).
11. Additional laboratory and diagnostic tests/procedures to monitor therapy and target organ function.
12. Potential for non-adherence/reasons for non-adherence.
    a. Note missed appointments.
    b. Note missed medication refills.
    c. Have goals for therapy been mutually set?
    d. Integration of medication administration into daily routines.
C. Goals of care.
1. Maintain blood pressure within desired range.
2. Minimize and/or prevent target organ damage to heart, brain, kidneys, eyes.
3. Adherence to medication and lifestyle plans.
4. Manage co-morbidities.
    a. Compelling indications require lower blood pressure targets.
    b. Co-morbidities may benefit or be adversely affected, and may require medication adjustments.

Table 21-2.
Impact of Lifestyle Therapies on BP in Hypertensive Adults

Intervention	Lifestyle Modification or Change	Systolic BP Reduction (Range)
Daily Sodium Intake	Maximum of 2.4 g sodium or 6 mg sodium chloride.	2–8 mm Hg
Weight Loss	Reduce to and/or maintain BMI of 18.5–24.9.	5–20 mm Hg/10 kg wt loss
Alcohol Consumption	Limit of no more than 2 drinks per day for men and no more than 1 drink per day for women and lightweight persons.	2–4 mm Hg
Exercise	Aerobic exercise for at least 30 minutes, most days of the week.	4–9 mm Hg
DASH Diet	Dietary Approaches to Stop Hypertension (DASH) diet rich in fruits, vegetables, and low-fat dairy products, with overall reduced saturated and total fat content.	8–14 mm Hg

Source: Adapted from U.S. Department of Veterans Affairs, 2005.

D. Psychosocial considerations.
  1. Lack of healthy food choices in workplace, schools, restaurants, and home.
  2. Cost of healthier food products.
  3. Amounts of sodium in packaged/prepared/restaurant foods.
  4. Cost for medications and services (clinical and education).
  5. Integrating physical activity into daily lifestyle.
  6. Target organ damage from uncontrolled hypertension may result in cardiovascular disease, vascular disease, renal disease, and retinopathy.
E. Patient education.
  1. Goal setting.
  2. Lifestyle modifications.
    a. Dietary modifications.
      (1) DASH eating plan.
      (2) Limit alcohol intake.
    b. Activity modifications.
      (1) Increasing activity safely.
      (2) Integrating activity into daily lfe.
  3. Risk factor modification.
    a. Weight appropriate to height.
    b. Tobacco use cessation.
  4. Adherence to regimen.
    a. Medication administration.
    b. Adherence with prescription.
    c. Side effects.

    d. Nonprescription medications.
    e. Herbal supplements.
  5. Typical lack of overt symptoms.
  6. When to access health care.
    a. Routine follow-up for monitoring of blood pressure control.
    b. Signs and symptoms of untoward events. These can include:
      (1) Onset of severe headache.
      (2) New onset of mental status changes.
      (3) New onset of vision changes.
      (4) Numbness and weakness.
      (5) Chest pain.
      (6) Palpitations.
      (7) Shortness of breath.
  7. Self-monitoring/remote monitoring of blood pressure.
  8. Follow-up care.
    a. Scheduled visits, monthly or less, until blood pressure goal is reached. Include blood pressure monitoring discussion and re-emphasis on lifestyle modifications.
    b. Home telehealth/remote blood pressure monitoring to electronically transmit vital signs information to care team.
  9. Disease self-management.
    a. Self-blood pressure monitoring.

    b. Adherence to medication regime.

    c. Limit alcohol intake.

    d. Limit salt intake.

    e. Quit tobacco use.

    f. Physical activity.

    g. Weight appropriate to height.

F. Collaboration and referrals.

   1. Utilization of services including, but not limited to: Pharmacy, nurse case managers, registered dietitians, licensed nutritionists, and health educators.

   2. Reinforce patient education with patient and significant other(s).

   3. Manage co-morbidities.

   4. Utilization of specialty services as needed.

    a. Cardiology.

    b. Nephrology.

    c. Ophthalmology.

    d. Neurology.

    e. Nutrition counseling.

G. Community resources and advocacy.

   1. The National Heart, Lung, and Blood Institute (NHLBI) provides leadership for research, training, and education programs to promote the prevention and treatment of heart, lung, and blood diseases, including hypertension.

   2. American Heart Association provides information for health professionals and lay public on hypertension.

   3. The CDC monitors health, conducts research, promotes healthy behaviors, and provides information to health professionals and the lay public.

H. Telehealth practice.

   1. Assessment and triage.

    a. Onset of symptoms.

    b. Pertinent history.

    c. Current blood pressure readings.

    d. Associated symptoms: Severe headache, visual changes, weakness, numbness, and chest pain.

    e. Signs and symptoms of stroke – Call 9-1-1.

    f. Nurse recommended changes or follow-up.

   2. Remote blood pressure monitoring and disease management to provide case management and improve access to care.

VI. Protocols/Algorithms/Guidelines

A. Agency for Healthcare Research and Quality (AHRQ) National Guideline Clearinghouse (2009) – *Nursing Management of Hypertension.*

B. Institute for Clinical Systems Improvement (2010) – *Health Care Guideline: Hypertension Diagnosis and Treatment.*

C. U.S. Department of Veterans Affairs (2005) – *Clinical Practice Guidelines: Management of Hypertension in Primary Care.*

Diabetes

Patient Population: Adult

Diabetes is a group of diseases marked by high levels of blood glucose resulting from defects in insulin production, insulin action, or both. Diabetes is a chronic metabolic disorder in which the body cannot metabolize carbohydrates, fats, and proteins because of defects in insulin secretion and/or action. Diabetes can lead to serious complications and premature death. However, people with diabetes can take steps to control the disease and lower the risk of complications by working together with their health care providers and support network. Diabetes affects 8.3% of the U.S. population, 25.8 million people: 18.8 million people diagnosed, 7.0 million people undiagnosed (CDC, 2011).

Diabetes was the seventh leading cause of death in 2007. This ranking is based on the 71,382 death certificates in 2007 on which diabetes was the underlying cause of death. Diabetes was a contributing cause of death on an additional 160,022 death certificates for a total of 231,404 certificates in 2007 in which diabetes appeared as any-listed cause of death (CDC, 2011). Overall, the risk of death among people with diabetes is about twice that of people of similar age but without diabetes.

Table 21-3.
Estimated Costs Related to
Diabetes in the United States

Indirect Costs	$58 billion (disability, work loss, premature mortality)
Direct Medical Costs	$116 billion After adjusting for population age and sex differences, average medical expenditures among people with diagnosed diabetes were 2.3 times higher than what expenditures would be in the absence of diabetes.
Total (Direct and Indirect)	$174 billion

Source: Adapted from CDC, 2011.

I. Diabetes Overview

Diabetes is the source of a high volume of health care costs in the U.S. (see Table 21-3).

A. Classification of diabetes mellitus.
1. Type 1.
2. Type 2.
3. Gestational diabetes mellitus (GDM).
4. Diabetes associated with certain conditions of syndromes.
5. Prediabetes.
   a. Impaired fasting glucose.
   b. Impaired glucose tolerance.
B. Type 1 diabetes – Develops when the body's immune system destroys pancreatic beta cells, the only cells in the body that make the hormone insulin, which regulates blood glucose.
1. To survive, people with Type 1 diabetes must have insulin delivered by injection or a pump.
2. This form of diabetes usually strikes children and young adults, although disease onset can occur at any age, even in the eighth and ninth decade.
3. In adults, Type 1 diabetes accounts for approximately 5% of all diagnosed cases of diabetes.
4. Risk factors for Type 1 diabetes may be autoimmune, genetic, or environmental.
5. There is no known way to prevent Type 1 diabetes.

C. Type 2 diabetes – Previously called non-insulin-dependent diabetes mellitus (NIDDM) or adult-onset diabetes.
1. In adults, Type 2 diabetes accounts for about 90–95% of all diagnosed cases of diabetes.
2. It usually begins as insulin resistance, a disorder in which the cells do not use insulin properly. As the need for insulin rises, the pancreas gradually loses its ability to produce it.
3. Type 2 diabetes is associated with older age, obesity, family history of diabetes, history of gestational diabetes, impaired glucose metabolism, physical inactivity, and race/ethnicity.
4. African Americans, Hispanic/Latino Americans, Native Americans, and some Asian Americans and Native Hawaiians or other Pacific Islanders are at particularly high risk for Type 2 diabetes and its complications.
5. Type 2 diabetes in children and adolescents, although still rare, is being diagnosed more frequently among American Indians, African Americans, Hispanic/Latino Americans, and Asians/Pacific Islanders.
D. Gestational diabetes – A form of glucose intolerance diagnosed during pregnancy.
1. Gestational diabetes occurs more frequently among African Americans, Hispanic/Latino Americans, and American Indians.
2. It is also more common among obese women and women with a family history of diabetes.
3. During pregnancy, gestational diabetes requires treatment to optimize maternal blood glucose levels to lessen the risk of complications in the infant.
4. Women who have had gestational diabetes have a 35–60% chance of developing diabetes in the next 10–20 years (CDC, 2011).
E. Diabetes associated with certain conditions or syndromes.

1. *Latent autoimmune diabetes of adulthood* (LADA) is the most common term describing patients with a Type 2 diabetic phenotype combined with islet antibodies and slowly progressive beta cell failure.

    a. LADA is a genetically linked, hereditary autoimmune disorder that results in the body mistaking the pancreas as foreign and responding by attacking and destroying the insulin-producing beta islet cells of the pancreas.

    b. In its early stages, LADA typically presents as Type 2 diabetes and is often misdiagnosed as such. However, LADA more closely resembles juvenile (Type 1) diabetes and shares common physiological characteristics of Type 1 for metabolic dysfunction, genetics, and autoimmune features.

    c. LADA accounts for roughly 10% of people with diabetes, making it probably more widespread than Type 1.

2. Other types of diabetes result from specific genetic conditions (such as maturity-onset diabetes of youth), surgery, medications, infections, pancreatic disease, and other illnesses. Such types of diabetes account for 1–5% of all diagnosed cases.

F. Prediabetes – A condition in which individuals have blood glucose or A1c levels higher than normal, but not high enough to be classified as diabetes.

1. People with prediabetes have an increased risk of developing Type 2 diabetes, heart disease, and stroke.

2. Studies have shown that people with prediabetes who lose weight and increase their physical activity can prevent or delay Type 2 diabetes and in some cases return their blood glucose levels to normal (CDC, 2011).

II. Pathophysiology

A. Autoimmune (Type 1) diabetes mellitus.

1. The body attacks its own insulin-producing tissue, the beta cells of the islets of Langerhans in the pancreas. When so many of these cells are destroyed that there are no longer enough to meet the body's need for insulin, the patient becomes diabetic and must take insulin injections.

2. In Type 1 diabetes, an inability to metabolize carbohydrates is caused by an absolute insulin deficiency.

B. Type 2 diabetes mellitus.

1. Type 2 diabetes usually occurs due to a metabolic failure at the cellular level; usually prompted by poor diet, obesity, environmental factors, and genetics (American Diabetes Association [ADA], 2011a).

2. Body tissues, such as cell receptor sites, lose their sensitivity. As insulin attempts to deliver glucose into the cell, the "key no longer fits the lock." Blood glucose, blocked from the cell, accumulates in the bloodstream.

III. Assessment, Screening, and Triage

A. Risk factors.

1. Obesity (body mass index [BMI] greater than 25).

2. First degree relative with diabetes.

3. Race: High-risk populations include Non-Hispanic Blacks, Hispanic/Latino Americans, Asian Americans and Pacific Islanders, and American Indians and Alaska Natives.

4. Previous gestational diabetes, baby over 9 pounds, or history of glucose intolerance.

5. History of insulin-resistant syndrome or polycystic ovarian syndrome (PCOS).

6. Impaired glucose tolerance (IGT) and/or impaired fasting glucose.

7. Over the age of 45.

8. Physical inactivity.

9. Hypertension, defined as greater than 140/90.

10. HDL cholesterol less than 35 or triglycerides greater than 250.

11. History of vascular disease.

12. Other: Hypothyroidism, HIV/AIDS, bipolar/schizophrenia (ADA, 2011a).

B. Diagnosis.

1. Criteria for the diagnosis of diabetes. One of the following must exist:

Table 21-4.
Laboratory Diagnostic Criteria for Diabetes

Status	Fasting	Non-Fasting	A1c
Prediabetes	≥ 100 mg/dL and < 126 mg/dL (on two occasions)	> 140 mg/dl but < 200 mg/dL	≥ 5.7% but < 6.5%
Diabetes	≥126 mg/dL (on two occasions)	> 200 mg/dL	≥ 6.5%
Normal	< 100 mg/dL		< 5.7%

a. A1c 6.5% or greater. The test should be performed in a laboratory using a method that is National Glycohemoglobin Standardization Program (NGSP) certified and standardized to the Diabetes Control and Complications Trial (DCCT) assay.

b. Fasting Plasma Glucose (FPG) greater than 126 mg/dl (7.0 mmol/l). Fasting is defined as no caloric intake for at least 8 hours.

c. 2-h plasma glucose 200 mg/dl (11.1 mmol/l) or greater during an Oral Glucose Tolerance Test (OGTT). The test should be performed as described by the World Health Organization (WHO), using a glucose load containing the equivalent of 75 g anhydrous glucose dissolved in water.

d. Classic symptoms of hyperglycemia or hyperglycemic crisis, a random plasma glucose of 200 mg/dl (11.1 mmol/l) or greater.

2. In the absence of unequivocal hyperglycemia, result should be confirmed by repeat testing (ADA, 2011a).

3. Laboratory diagnostic criteria for diabetes (see Table 21-4).

4. FPG is the preferred test for diagnosis, but either of the other two listed (hemoglobin A1c and non-fasting) is acceptable. In the absence of unequivocal hyperglycemia with acute metabolic decompensation, one of these two tests should be done on different days.

5. Use a clinical laboratory (not a point of care test) methodology standardized to the NGSP.

6. "Random" means any time of day without regard to time since the last meal.

7. "Classic symptoms" include polyuria, polydipsia, and unexplained weight loss.

8. OGTT is no longer recommended in routine clinical practice because it is an imprecise test with poor reproducibility. The WHO suggests continued use of the OGTT for patients with blood glucose values in the "uncertain range." Also, the OGTT does seem to better predict macrovascular complications.

C. Type 1 diabetes assessment.

1. Onset: Usually acute with pronounced symptoms of increased hyperglycemia (e.g., thirst and hunger, frequent urination, weight loss, and fatigue).

2. Presenting symptoms (see Table 21-5).

Table 21-5.
Symptoms of Type 1 Diabetes

Polyuria
Polyphagia
Polydipsia
Unexplained weight loss
Bed-wetting
Yeast infection that does not respond to treatment or frequent yeast infections
Flushed skin
Fruity breath
Severe abdominal pain
Lethargy
Nausea and/or vomiting

D. Type 2 diabetes assessment.
1. Onset usually gradual; may or may not have hyperglycemia symptoms.
2. Insulin production at onset may be normal or elevated, but insulin resistance, elevated liver production of glucose, and other factors may prevent insulin from functioning normally.

E. History.
1. Age and characteristics of onset of diabetes (e.g., diabetic ketoacidosis [DKA], asymptomatic laboratory finding).
2. Review of previous treatment regimens and response to therapy (A1c records).
3. Current status: Home blood glucose pattern and use of data in self-treatment, episodes of hypoglycemia, acute complications, presenting problem(s), symptoms.
4. Co-morbidities: Hypertension, dyslipidemia, cardiovascular disease, peripheral vascular disease, cerebral vascular disease.
5. Presence of diabetes complications: Neuropathy, nephropathy, retinopathy, foot disease (Charcot's foot).
6. Other: Psychosocial problems, dental disease.

F. Physical examination.
1. Height, weight, BMI.
2. Blood pressure determination, including orthostatic measurements when indicated.
3. Fundoscopic examination.
4. Thyroid palpation.
5. Skin examination (for acanthosis nigricans and insulin injection sites).
6. Comprehensive foot examination:
   a. Inspection.
   b. Palpation of dorsalis pedis and posterior tibial pulses.
   c. Presence/absence of patellar and Achilles reflexes.
   d. Determination of proprioception, vibration, and monofilament sensation.

G. Laboratory evaluation.
1. A1c, if results not available within past 2–3 months.

2. If not performed/available within past year:
   a. Fasting lipid profile, including total LDL and HDL cholesterol and triglycerides.
   b. Liver function tests.
   c. Test for urine albumin excretion with spot urine albumin-to-creatinine ratio.
   d. Serum creatinine and calculated glomerular filtration rate (GFR).
   e. Thyroid-stimulating hormone in Type 1 diabetes, dyslipidemia, or women over age 50.
   f. Testosterone.

H. Lifestyle, health behaviors, and functional status.
1. Current weight; weight changes.
2. Eating patterns: Skip meals, meal/snack time, portion sizes, usual foods, meal log (food diary).
3. Exercise (type, frequency, location).
4. Smoking (type and amount).
5. Alcohol usage (type and amount).
6. Stress; coping skills, stress management.
7. Occupation (e.g., type, shift worker, commercial driver's license, heavy machinery operator).
8. Support system.
9. Type of income (e.g., disability, welfare).
10. Type of insurance (e.g., self-pay, insurance, Medicaid, Medicare).

I. Laboratory parameters.
1. Diagnostic – See Table 21-4.
2. C-peptide – Newly diagnosed diabetes patients often get their C-peptide levels measured as a means of distinguishing Type 1 diabetes and Type 2 diabetes. Persons with LADA typically have low, although sometimes moderate, levels of C-peptide as the disease progresses. Patients with insulin resistance or Type 2 diabetes are more likely to, but will not always, have high levels of C-peptide due to an over production of insulin.
3. Blood glucose control: Hemoglobin A1c, fasting glucose, fructosamine.
4. Fasting lipid panel.
5. Kidney function: Urine microalbumin and serum creatinine.
6. Thyroid function test.

J. Diabetes assessment schedule.
1. At each regular diabetes visit: Every 3–4 months.
    a. Weight and blood pressure.
    b. Inspection of feet.
    c. Review self-monitoring glucose record.
    d. Review/adjust medications to control glucose, blood pressure, and lipids.
    e. Review self-management skills; use of blood glucose monitor and techniques, insulin administration techniques, dietary habits, and physical activity.
    f. Assess for depression or other mood disorder.
    g. Counsel on smoking cessation and alcohol use.
2. Quarterly – Obtain hemoglobin A1c in patients whose therapy has changed or who are not meeting glycemic goals (twice a year if at goal with stable glycemia). Use of point-of-care testing of hemoglobin A1c allows for timely decisions on therapy changes.
3. Annually.
    a. Fasting lipid profile.
    b. Serum creatinine to estimate glomerular filtration rate and stage the level of chronic kidney disease.
    c. Urine test for albumin-to-creatinine ratio in patients with Type 1 diabetes more than 5-years-old and in all patients with Type 2 diabetes.
    d. Refer for dilated eye examination.
    e. Comprehensive foot exam: Evaluation of skin integrity, circulation, sensitivity using monofilament, and deformities.
    f. Refer for dental/oral examination.
    g. Administer influenza vaccine.
    h. Review need for other preventive care or treatment.
4. Lifetime: Pneumococcal vaccine; repeat dose after age 65 if 5 years since first dose.
K. Referrals.
1. Annual dilated eye examination.
2. Family planning for women of reproductive age.
3. Registered dietitian for Medical Nutrition Therapy (MNT).
4. Diabetes Self-Management Education (DSME).
5. Dental examination.
6. Mental health professional, if needed.

IV. **Plan of Care**
A. Pharmacologic therapy.
1. Oral diabetes medications (see Table 21-6).
    a. Biguanides decrease hepatic glucose output.
    b. Sulfonylureas stimulate insulin secretion (may cause hypoglycemia).
    c. Thiazolidinediones increase insulin sensitivity.
    d. Glinides stimulate insulin secretion.
    e. Alpha-glucosidase inhibitors reduce the rate of digestion of polysaccharides in the proximal small intestine, lowers postprandial glucose.
    f. Dipeptidyl peptidase – IV inhibitors (DPP-4) stimulate insulin secretion while inhibiting glucagon.
    g. Glucogon-like peptide-1 agonists (subcutaneous injection) incretin hormone analog, which reduces postprandial glucose excursions.
    h. Amylin analogues (subcutaneous injection) – Amylin analog that reduces postprandial glucose excursions.
2. Insulin (see Table 21-7) – Short-acting, rapid-acting analog, intermediate-acting, long-acting analog, and pre-mixed.
B. Complementary and alternative medicine (some of the most commonly used).
1. Alpha-Lipoic Acid – Lowers blood glucose and insulin levels, reduces insulin resistance, and improves insulin sensitivity.
2. Bilberry – Reduces blood glucose levels.
3. Biotin – Aids in metabolism of macronutrients and glucose utilization and is beneficial in diabetic retinopathy.
4. L-Carnitine – Improves blood glucose and A1c levels, increases insulin sensitivity and glucose storage, and optimizes fat and lcarbohydrate metabolism; deficiencies ap-

Table 21-6.
Oral Diabetes Medications

Generic Name	Brand Name	Dosing	Other Considerations
Biguanides			Contraindicated: Elevated creatinine **Caution: History of CHF**
Metformin Metformin Extended Release	Glucophage® Glucophage® XR	500 mg, 850 mg, 1000 mg 500 mg, 750 mg	Increases insulin sensitivity to decrease blood glucose levels: • Decreases liver glucose production. • Increases insulin sensitivity.
Sulfonylureas			All in this class can cause hypoglycemia.
Glimepiride Glipizide Glipizide Extended Release Glyburide Glyburide Micronase	Amaryl® Glipizide Glucotrol® XL Diabeta® Glynase Pres™ Tab	1 mg, 2 mg, 4 mg 5 mg, 10 mg 5 mg, 10 mg 1.25 mg, 2.5 mg, 5 mg 1 mg, 5 mg, 3 mg, 6 mg	Increases insulin secretion in people with capacity to produce insulin, to decrease blood glucose.
Thiazolidinediones			Contraindicated in those with impaired liver function, CHF.
Pioglitizone Rosiglitizone	Actos® Avandia®	15 mg, 30 mg, 45 mg 2 mg, 4 mg, 8 mg	Increase insulin sensitivity to increase glucose uptake and reduce blood glucose levels. May cause edema, headache, weight gain.
Meglitinides			May cause hypoglycemia.
Nateglinide Repaglinide	Starlix® Prandin®	60 mg, 120 mg 0.5 mg, 1 mg, 2 mg	Short-acting agents that increase insulin secretion and decrease blood glucose in people with capacity to produce insulin.
Alpha-Glucosidase Inhibitors			
Acarbose Miglitol	Precose® Glyset®	25 mg, 50 mg, 100 mg 25 mg, 50 mg, 100 mg	Inhibit carbohydrate digestion to delay and lessen the rise in post-meal glucose levels.
DPP-4 Inhibitors (Dipeptidyl Peptidase-4 Inhibitors)			
Sitagliptin Phosphate Linagliptin Saxagliptin	Januvia® Tradjenta® Onglyza™	50 mg, 100 mg 5 mg 2.5 mg, 5 mg	Enhances function of both alpha and beta cells to improve glucose uptake and decrease glucose production.

continued on next page

Table 21-6. (continued)
Oral Diabetes Medications

Generic Name	Brand Name	Dosing	Other Considerations
Peptide Analogs **Incretin Mimetics** **DPP-4 Inhibitors** **Amylin Analogs**			
Incretin Mimetics Injection			Act like (mimic) the natural hormones in the body that lower blood sugar. These hormones are called incretins. Allows the pancreas to release insulin. This drug lowers blood sugar levels only when they rise too high. Prevents the pancreas from giving out glucagon. Helps to slow the rate at which your stomach empties after eating. This may make you feel less hungry and more satisfied after a meal.
GLP-1 Agonist			
Exenatide	Byetta®	Initiate at 5 mcg per dose twice daily; increase to 10 mcg twice daily after 1 month based on clinical response.	Stimulates post-meal insulin secretion, restores first phase insulin production.
Exenatide Extended Release (GLP-1 Receptor Agonist)	Bydureon®	2 mg once every 7 days	Stimulates post-meal insulin secretion, restores first phase insulin production.
Amylin Mimetic			
Pramlintide Injection	Symlin™	In patients with insulin-using **Type 2 diabetes**, Symlin should be initiated at a dose of 60 mcg and increased to a dose of 120 mcg as tolerated. In patients with **Type 1 diabetes**, Symlin should be initiated at a dose of 15 mcg and titrated at 15-mcg increments to a maintenance dose of 30 mcg or 60 mcg as tolerated.	Synthetic analog of human amylin, a naturally occurring neuroendocrine hormone synthesized by pancreatic beta cells that contributes to glucose control during the postprandial period (Amylin Pharmaceuticals, Inc., 2011).

continued on next page

Table 21-6. (continued)
Oral Diabetes Medications

Generic Name	Brand Name	Dosing	Comments
GLP-1			
Liraglutide	Victoza®	Initiate at 0.6 mg per day for one week. This dose is intended to reduce gastrointestinal symptoms during initial titration, and is not effective for glycemic control. After one week, increase the dose to 1.2 mg. If the 1.2 mg dose does not result in acceptable glycemic control, the dose can be increased to 1.8 mg.	**Risk Of Thyroid C-Cell Tumors** Glucagon-like peptide-1 (GLP-1) receptor agonist indicated as an adjunct to diet and exercise to improve glycemic control in adults with Type 2 diabetes mellitus.

pear allied to cardiomyopathy and diabetic neuropathy.

5. Chromium – Modulates blood glucose levels, fights insulin resistance, lowers A1c levels, aids weight loss, and inhibits glycation.
6. Coenzyme Q_{10} (CoQ_{10}) – Has antioxidant value and may enhance beta cell function and glycemic control.
7. Conjugated linoleic acid (CLA) aids in weight management, improves insulin sensitivity, and reduces blood glucose levels.
8. DHEA (dehydroepiandrosterone) – Is beneficial to diabetic and obese individuals; helps with insulin resistance.
9. Fiber lowers blood glucose levels.
10. Magnesium lowers blood glucose levels, increases insulin sensitivity, and calms the sympathetic nervous system.

C. Primary/secondary/tertiary prevention.
1. There is no known primary prevention strategy to prevent Type 1 diabetes.
2. The Diabetes Prevention Program Trials showed that people with prediabetes could significantly delay or even prevent the onset of Type 2 diabetes by lifestyle modification (weight loss of 7% of body weight and 150 min/week of moderate activity, such as walking) (Segala, 2003).

a. Prediabetes education; medical nutrient therapy, exercise.
b. Metformin therapy for prevention of Type 2 diabetes may be considered in those at the highest risk for developing diabetes. These include those with multiple risk factors, especially if they demonstrate progression of hyperglycemia (e.g., hemoglobin A1c ≥ 6%) despite lifestyle intervention (ADA, 2011a).
c. The U.S. Preventive Services Task Force recommends screening for Type 2 diabetes in asymptomatic adults with sustained blood pressure (either treated or untreated) greater than 135/80 mm Hg, but evidence is insufficient to recommend screening of normotensive, asymptomatic adults (Agency for Healthcare Research and Quality [AHRQ], 2011).
3. Secondary prevention: Preventing/delaying diabetes and related long-term complications through the achievement of blood glucose control (without hypoglycemia), as well as blood pressure and lipid management.
a. Achieve individualized A1c target through diet, exercise, medications, and patient self-management education.

Table 21-7.
Types of Insulin

Type of Insulin and Brand Names	Onset	Peak	Duration	Role in Blood Sugar Management
Rapid-Acting				
Humalog or lispro	15–30 minutes	30–90 minutes	3–5 hours	Rapid-acting insulin covers insulin needs for meals eaten at the same time as the injection. This type of insulin is used with longer-acting insulin.
Novolog or aspart	10–20 minutes	40–50 minutes	3–5 hours	
Apidra or glulisine	20–30 minutes	30–90 minutes	1–2.5 hours	
Short-Acting				
Regular (R) humulin or novolin	30 minutes– 1 hour	2–5 hours	5–8 hours	Short-acting insulin covers insulin needs for meals eaten within 30–60 minutes.
Velosulin (for use in the insulin pump)	30 minutes– 1 hour	2–3 hours	2–3 hours	
Intermediate-Acting				
NPH (N)	1–2 hours	4–12 hours	18–24 hours	Intermediate-acting insulin covers insulin needs for about half the day or overnight. This type of insulin is often combined with rapid- or short-acting insulin.
Lente (L)	1–2.5 hours	3–10 hours	18–24 hours	
Long-Acting				
Ultralente (U)	30 minutes– 3 hours	10–20 hours	20–36 hours	Long-acting insulin covers insulin needs for about one full day. This type of insulin is often combined, when needed, with rapid- or short-acting insulin.
Lantus	1–1.5 hours	No peak time; insulin is delivered at a steady level	20–24 hours	
Levemir or detemir	1–2 hours	6–8 hours	Up to 24 hours	
Pre-Mixed*				
Humulin 70/30	30 minutes	2–4 hours	14–24 hours	These products are generally taken twice a day before mealtime.
Novolin 70/30	3 minutes	2–12 hours	Up to 24 hours	
Novolog 70/30	10–20 minutes	1–4 hours	Up to 24 hours	
Humulin 50/50	30 minutes	2–5 hours	18–24 hours	
Humalog mix 75/25	15 minutes	30 minutes–2.5 hours	16–20 hours	

*Pre-mixed insulins are a combination of specific proportions of intermediate-acting and short-acting insulin in one bottle or insulin pen (the numbers following the brand name indicate the percentage of each type of insulin).

Source: WebMD, 2012. Used with permission.

b. Control blood pressure to improve quality and length of life, and to prevent micro and macrovascular complications.

c. Control cholesterol to reduce risk for cardiovascular disease.

4. Tertiary prevention: Management of the complications of diabetes – Retinopathy, neuropathy, nephropathy, and cardiovascular complications.

    a. Screen annually for kidney disease (urine microalbumin and serum creatinine).

    b. Screen for retinopathy every 12–24 months based upon ophthmalogic and clinical findings. Primary care providers are providing Digital Retinal Screening in their office for early detection of diabetic eye disease.

    c. Screen annually for lower extremity complications (such as calluses, ulcers, skin irritations, abrasions, or neuropathy).

5. General health promotion measures.

    a. Consider aspirin therapy to reduce the risk of fatal cardiovascular events.

    b. Advise about tobacco use cessation.

    c. Provide influenza vaccination annually in season.

    d. Provide pneumonia vaccine (see adult immunizations described in Chapter 17, "Care of the Well Client").

D. Goals of plan of care.

1. Improved clinical outcomes, risk reduction, reduced cost, appropriate resource utilization.

2. Goals for glycemic control for non-pregnant adults with diabetes.

    a. A1c less than 7.0%. (See d & e, below.)

    b. Pre-prandial capillary plasma glucose 70–130 mg/dl* (3.9–7.2 mmol/l). (See d & e, below.)

    c. Peak postprandial capillary plasma glucose less than 180 mg/dl (10.0 mmol/l). (See f & g, below.)

    d. Goals should be individualized based on:

        (1) Duration of diabetes.

        (2) Age/life expectancy.

        (3) Co-morbid conditions.

        (4) Known cardiovascular disease or advanced microvascular complications.

        (5) Hypoglycemia unawareness.

        (6) Individual patient considerations.

    e. More or less stringent glycemic goals may be appropriate for individual patients.

    f. Postprandial glucose may be targeted if A1c goals are not met despite reaching pre-prandial glucose goals.

    g. Postprandial glucose measurements should be made 1–2 hours after the beginning of the meal, generally peak levels in patients with diabetes.

V. Psychosocial Considerations

A. Education of patient/family.

1. According to national standards, people with diabetes should receive diabetes self-management education (DSME) when their diabetes is diagnosed and as needed thereafter.

2. Education in core competencies, also known as "survival skills," should be provided to all patients newly diagnosed with diabetes. Core competency education includes response to acute complications (hyperglycemia and hypoglycemia); how and when to take medication(s); self-monitoring of blood glucose, basic diet guidelines; sick day management; and guidance on when and how to seek further treatment or medical advice.

3. Comprehensive education on self-management and diet should be provided to all patients newly diagnosed with diabetes. Education should be individualized and tailored to the patient's needs. Education can be provided through an in-house comprehensive diet consultation for medical nutrition therapy (MNT), or a comprehensive DSME program recognized by the Ameri-

can Diabetes Association (ADA). If neither of these options is available, comprehensive DSME should be provided at the provider's facility.

4. Safety measures: Management of hypoglycemia.
   a. Assess for signs and symptoms of inadequate glucose control or end-organ damage at every encounter/visit.
   b. Evaluate blood glucose patterns for wide fluctuations, which include below normal blood glucose.
   c. Determine causes, whether clinical management or patient behavior, and implement intervention to reduce possibility of future episodes.
   d. Establish plan to be followed until blood glucose is stable.
   e. Patient education on proper treatment of hypoglycemia.
      (1) Oral glucose (15–20 g) is the preferred treatment for the conscious individual with hypoglycemia, although any form of carbohydrate that contains glucose may be used.
      (2) If self-monitoring of blood glucose (SMBG) shows continued hypoglycemia 15 minutes after treatment, the treatment should be repeated.
      (3) Once SMBG result returns to normal, the individual should consume a meal or snack to prevent recurrence of hypoglycemia.

5. Exacerbations and when to seek medical attention: Acute hyperglycemia.
   a. Blood glucose over 240 mg/dL or presence of infection, gastroenteritis, other acute illness including fever, nausea, diarrhea.
   b. High-risk for severe hyperglycemia, dehydration, ketoacidosis. Requires hospitalization if treatment delayed or inadequate.
   c. Requires immediate intervention: Provide guidance for the patient to maintain hydration and short-term, frequent

advice about insulin adjustments, and blood glucose and urine ketone monitoring.
   d. Arrange or provide outpatient intravenous fluid administration if patient unable to maintain hydration.
   e. Medical nutrition therapy (MNT): Individual meal plan by a Registered Dietitian (RD), preferably Certified Diabetes Educator (CDE).

6. Clinical procedures and treatments.
   a. Blood glucose monitoring: Frequency of routine laboratory testing, proper use of home blood glucose monitor, proper fingerstick technique, discuss individual goals of blood sugars, additional testing to determine causes of blood glucose problems (e.g., hypoglycemia or hyperglycemia).
   b. Hemoglobin A1c – A laboratory test that reflects a 3-month blood glucose average and risk for microvascular disease.
   c. Self-monitoring of blood glucose (SMBG) recommendations.
      (1) Allows patients to evaluate their individual response to therapy and assess whether glycemic targets are being achieved.
      (2) Results of self-management blood glucose monitoring can be useful in preventing hypoglycemia and adjusting medications, diet, and physical activity.
      (3) A blood glucose monitor is an instrument that is user-dependent; patients should be taught proper technique on obtaining blood samples and use of their personal blood glucose monitors.
      (4) Patients should be taught how to use the data to adjust food intake, exercise, or pharmacological therapy to achieve specific glycemic goals, and these skills should be reevaluated periodically.

(5) SMBG should be carried out three or more times daily for patients using multiple insulin injections or insulin pump therapy.

(6) For patients using less-frequent insulin injections, noninsulin therapies, or MNT alone, SMBG may be useful as a guide to the success of therapy.

(7) To achieve postprandial glucose targets, postprandial SMBG may be appropriate.

d. SMBG – Evaluate each patient's monitoring technique, initially and at regular intervals, to achieve specific glycemic goals.

(1) Proper interpretation of the data.

(2) Use the data to adjust food intake.

(3) Exercise.

(4) Pharmacological therapy.

7. Self-care of primary and secondary problems.

a. Physical activity (exercise) – Recommended for all patients with diabetes for health benefits and weight loss.

(1) Regular physical activity reduces insulin resistance and prevents Type 2 diabetes in high-risk individuals.

(2) Patient should be advised to perform at least 150 minutes per week of moderate-intensity aerobic physical activity (50–70% of maximum heart rate).

(3) In the absence of contraindications, people with Type 2 diabetes should be encouraged to perform resistance training three times per week.

(4) The nurse should regularly discuss level of activity, including type of exercise, intensity, frequency, and timing in relation to meals and medications.

b. Blood pressure management.

(1) Target for blood pressure control in a diabetic: <130/80 mmHg.

(2) Low sodium diet: Dietary Approaches to Stop Hypertension (DASH) diet, <1500 mg of sodium a day (CDC, 2011).

(3) Physical activity: 150 minutes a week.

(4) Ace-inhibitors: Drug of choice for managing hypertension in people with diabetes, because has additional renal protection.

(5) Additional medications may be needed to reach blood pressure goal.

c. Lipid management.

(1) Target for men older than the age of 40 and women older than age 50: LDL cholesterol less than 100, triglycerides less than 150.

(2) Lifestyle management; reduction of saturated fat, trans fat, and cholesterol intake; increase of omega-3 fatty acids, viscous fiber, and plant stanols/sterols; weight loss; and increased physical activity.

(3) Statin therapy and other lipid-lowering agents may be considered.

B. Collaboration, resource identification, and referral.

1. Endocrinology.

a. Recommended for all patients with Type 1 diabetes, those with multiple endocrinopathies, and those with other complex management issues.

b. Provide ongoing support and education to primary care providers.

2. Certified diabetes educators (CDEs): RNs, RDs, and other professionals with diabetes education experience who have passed the CDE examination.

a. Diabetes educators are health care professionals who focus on educating people with and at risk for diabetes and related conditions to achieve behavior change goals that, in turn, lead to better clinical outcomes and improved health status.

b. Diabetes educators apply in-depth knowledge and skills in the biological and social sciences, communication, counseling, and education to provide self-management education/self-management training (American Association of Diabetes Educators, 2010).

3. Nutritionists – May provide individualized medical nutrition therapy (MNT) to individuals who have prediabetes or diabetes, as needed, to achieve treatment goals. A registered dietitian familiar with the components of diabetes MNT is preferred.

4. Resources supporting appropriate routine care:
   a. Pharmacy.
   b. Ophthalmology.
   c. Podiatry.
   d. Exercise specialist, physical therapist.
   e. Mental health professionals.

5. Resources to manage diabetes complications/special needs.
   a. Cardiology.
   b. Nephrology.
   c. Neurology.
   d. Ophthalmology.
   e. Podiatry.
   f. Others as needed: Gastroenterology, obstetrics and gynecology, urology, and home care.

C. Community resources and advocacy.
1. Community support groups.
   a. Usually offered at faith-based organizations, hospitals, clinics by ADA local chapters (www.diabetes.org).
   b. May be facilitated by organizations providing care for patients with unique or similar needs (e.g., Korean, Spanish, teens with Type 1 diabetes, insulin pump patients).
2. Special needs education – Additional education may be needed for individuals experiencing unique needs (e.g., visual impairments, behavioral health problems, stroke rehabilitation).
3. Advocacy.
   a. Facilitate appropriate communication between patient and physician.

b. Facilitate access to appropriate resources.
c. Provide patient-centered, flexible support and interventions.
d. Promote positive, pro-active expectations with the patient, provider, and other providers.

D. Telehealth nursing considerations.
1. Support day-to-day blood glucose management.
2. Facilitate patient access for acute situations.
3. Provide reminders: Annual lab tests, vaccinations, and eye and foot examinations.

VI. Protocols/Algorithms/Guidelines

A. ADA standards (2011b): Criteria by which regulatory bodies (such as CMS and The Joint Commission) evaluate quality of care provided by health care organizations and by managed care organizations.

B. Diabetes treatment algorithms or guidelines.
1. Promote consistent level of care throughout an organization.
2. Guide provider through steps to advance therapy to help patients achieve diabetes control goals in an efficient and appropriate manner per the ADA (2011a) and/or American College of Physicians (2007).

C. Medical home model – The patient-centered medical home concept (see Chapter 20, "Ambulatory Nursing Role in Chronic Illness Care") aims to provide accessible, continuous, coordinated, and comprehensive, patient-centered care. The registered nurse is the care coordinator for the patient (i.e., across specialists, hospitals, home health agencies, and nursing homes).

Coronary Artery Disease/Coronary Heart Disease (CAD/CHD)

Patient Population: Adult

I. Overview

Coronary artery disease/coronary heart disease (CAD/CHD) is a chronic disease process that begins as early as adolescence, slowly progressing as people age. CAD/CHD is the most common type of heart disease that can lead to myocardial infarction, causes approximately 26% of deaths in U.S., and is the leading cause of death in both men and women (Centers for Disease Control and Prevention [CDC], 2012b). Men account for more than one-half of all cardiac deaths.

For those with a primary diagnosis of ischemic heart disease, the total cost for the U.S. population is about $316.4 billion, nearly one of every six health care dollars (CDC, 2012a), which includes health care services, medications, and lost productivity. In a 2011 policy statement, the American Heart Association (AHA) cited costs for all cardiovascular diseases together at $444.2 billion in 2010.

The most common symptom of CAD/CHD is angina, resulting from damage and narrowing of the coronary arteries. Should the coronary artery completely occlude or a piece of plaque rupture, myocardial infarction can occur. Each year, about 785,000 Americans will have a first heart attack and nearly 470,000 will have a recurrent attack (Libby & Theroux, 2005). It is estimated that 195,000 Americans will have a silent first myocardial infarction. Over time, CAD/CHD can cause the heart muscle to weaken, leading to heart failure or an arrhythmia.

In 2010, there were an estimated 13.9 million visits to physician offices and hospital outpatient and emergency department visits. The number of hospital discharges with heart disease as the first listed diagnosis totaled 4 million with an average length of stay of 4.4 days (CDC, 2012c).

II. Risk Factors for CAD/CHD

A. Age – The risk of developing CAD/CHD increases with age.
B. Gender – Men are at greater risk than women until the age of 65. Risk for men increases after age 45. Risk for women increases ten years after menopause.
C. Family history – Include family history, presence of risk factors, and any symptoms. Risk increases if a primary relative (i.e., parent, sibling, first cousin) developed heart disease at an early age.
   1. Risk is highest if first-degree male relative is diagnosed with heart disease before the age of 55.

   2. Risk increases if first-degree female relative is diagnosed with heart disease before the age of 65.
D. Tobacco – Tobacco exposure, whether due to direct or indirect exposure, increases the risk of heart disease and heart attack.
   1. Nicotine causes damage to the arterial wall.
   2. Nicotine causes vasoconstriction, which can cause elevations in blood pressure.
   3. Carbon monoxide, a by-product of tobacco smoke, reduces the level of oxygen in the blood.
   4. Cigarette smokers are 2–4 times more likely to develop coronary heart disease than non-smokers (CDC, 2010).
   5. The risk of heart attack is 2 times greater for people who smoke a pack of cigarettes a day as compared to people who have never smoked (AHA, 2012).
   6. Secondhand smoke can increase the risk of heart disease in non-smokers.
E. Hypertension – Blood pressures of greater than 140/80, and blood pressures of greater than 130/80 in persons with diabetes, can lead to thickening of the coronary arteries.
F. Hyperlipidemia – Elevated cholesterol levels can increase the risk of plaque development.
G. Diabetes – Increased blood sugar is associated with increased risk of coronary heart disease.
H. Obesity – Excess weight can worsen other risk factors.
   1. Obesity is linked to the development of diabetes, elevated LDL levels and elevated triglycerides, elevated blood pressure, and decreased levels of HDL.
I. Physical inactivity – Increasing daily activity can decrease one's risk related to developing CAD/CHD.
J. Diet.
   1. Foods high in refined carbohydrates, saturated fats, and cholesterol can promote atherosclerosis.
   2. High dietary intake of salt/sodium can increase blood pressure.
K. Alcohol – Excessive alcohol intake increases risk of heart disease, can elevate blood pressure, and increases triglyceride levels.

1. In men, "risky" or "hazardous" drinking has been defined as greater than 14 drinks per week or more than four drinks per occasion.
2. In women, "risky" or "hazardous" drinking has been defined as greater than seven drinks per week or more than three drinks per occasion (National Institute on Alcohol Abuse and Alcoholism [NIAAA], 2012).

III. Pathophysiology

CAD/CHD is the result of plaque (fat, cholesterol, calcium, cellular debris, and other substances that build up inside the coronary arteries), inflammation, and endothelial dysfunction, resulting in atherosclerosis. Normal endothelial cells secrete enzymes that control dilation and contraction, clotting, immune function, and platelet adhesion. Endothelial dysfunction results in the inability of the vessel to dilate fully, inhibiting blood flow. Inflammation of the endothelium results in plaque formation and leukocyte infiltration. Platelets aggregate and accumulate at the site of injury, forming clots and further narrowing the artery (Mohler, 2012).

IV. Assessment and Triage

A. Acute symptoms will need immediate medical intervention up to and including reperfusion.
   1. Acute signs and symptoms include:
      a. Chest discomfort/heaviness/squeezing/pain (something is sitting on the chest).
      b. Pain in one or both arms, back, neck, shoulders, jaw, and/or upper abdomen.
      c. Chest pain unrelieved by nitroglycerine.
      d. Nausea, indigestion, diaphoresis, fatigue.
      e. Shortness of breath.
      f. Light-headedness/sudden dizziness.
      g. Arrhythmia.
      h. Abnormal vital signs.
      i. EKG changes.
   2. Women are more likely to have atypical symptoms, including feeling unusual fatigue; indigestion-like pain; nausea and vomiting; pain in the back, shoulders, and jaw; and a sense of impending doom.

a. Assess risk factors, including family history and co-morbidities (history of diabetes, hypertension, and hyperlipidemia).
b. Functional status.
   (1) Tobacco use.
   (2) Excess body weight.
   (3) Excess alcohol intake.
   (4) Inadequate physical activity.
   (5) Diet high in fat and cholesterol.
c. Physical assessment.
   (1) Vital signs.
   (2) Heart sounds.
   (3) Breath sounds.
   (4) Peripheral pulses/edema.
   (5) Pain assessment with alleviating and aggravating factors.
d. Diagnostic studies.
   (1) Laboratory studies.
      (a) Elevated cardiac markers, including positive troponin levels.
      (b) Fasting lipid levels (total cholesterol) high-density lipoprotein (HDL) cholesterol, triglycerides, calculated low-density lipoprotein (LDL) cholesterol levels.
      (c) High sensitivity C-reactive protein (hsCRP).
      (d) Electrocardiogram (ECG).
   3. Echocardiography.
   4. Exercise stress testing.
      a. Dobutamine nuclear.
      b. Adenosine nuclear.
      c. Stress echocardiogram.
   5. Pharmacologic nuclear stress testing.
   6. CT angiography.

V. Indications for Emergency Care or Urgent Consultation

A. Heart attack symptoms – Chest discomfort/pain; pain in one or both arms, back, neck, shoulders, jaw, and/or upper abdomen and unrelieved by nitroglycerine; nausea; indigestion; diaphoresis; shortness of breath; light-headedness/sudden dizziness.
B. EKG changes/arrhythmia.
C. Abnormal vital signs.

VI. Plan of Care

A. Pharmacotherapeutics.
1. Anti-platelet therapy, which may include aspirin, Plavix®, Effient®, Persantine®, or Heparin®.
2. Anti-anginal agents, including beta blockers, calcium channel blockers, and nitrates.
3. Lipid-lowering medications.
4. Morphine may be indicated for severe chest pain (see Table 21-8).

B. Procedures for reperfusion: Interventions for reperfusion do not negate the need for lifestyle changes and medication adherence.
1. Angioplasty or percutaneous coronary intervention.
2. Coronary artery bypass surgery.

C. Primary/secondary/tertiary prevention.
1. Primary prevention: Lifestyle changes (also see Chapter 17, "Care of the Well Client: Screening and Preventive Care," regarding preventive cardiac health practices, such as smoking cessation and exercise).

Table 21-8.
Oral Antihypertensive Medications for Treatment and Management of Hypertension and Coronary Artery Disease

Medication	Dosing	Peak Effect	Other Considerations
Diuretics (Thiazide)			
Hydrochlorothiazide (Hydrodiuril®)	12.5–50 mg 1x/day	1.5 hours	Pediatric dosing.
Chlorothiazide (Diuril®)	0.5–1g 1x/day	Half-life = 45–120 minutes	Pediatric dosing.
Diuretics (Thiazide-like)			
Metolazone (Zaroxolyn®)	2.5–5 mg 1x/day	8 hours	Start at low end of dosing range for elderly.
Diuretics (Loop®)			
Furosemide (Lasix®)	40 mg 2x/day	1.5–2 hours	Reduce dose of other antihypertensive meds by 50%.
Bumetanide (Bumex®)	0.5–2 mg daily	1–2 hours	Dosing can be every other day or every 3–4 days.
K+ Sparing Diuretics			
Spironolactone (Aldactone®)	50–100 mg 1x/day	2.6 hours	Avoid K+ supplements, K+ rich diet.
Triamterene (Dyrenium®)	100 mg 2x/day	3 hours	Take after meals. Decrease dose if with other diuretics or antihypertensives.

continued on next page

Table 21-8. (continued)
Oral Antihypertensive Medications for Treatment and Management of
Hypertension and Coronary Artery Disease

Medication	Dosing	Peak Effect	Other Considerations
ACE Inhibitors			
Captopril (Capoten®)	25–50 mg 2–3x/day	1 hour	Take 1 hour before meals.
Enalapril (Vasotec®)	10–40 mg 1x/day	1 hour	Lower dose if on diuretic.
Lisinopril (Prinivil®, Zestril®)	10–40 mg 1x/day	7 hours	Max dose is 80 mg/day.
Benazepril (Lotensin®)	10–40 mg 1x/day	0.5–1 hour (fasting) 2–4 hours (non-fasting)	
Fosinopril (Monopril®)	10–40 mg 1x/day	3 hours	Max dose is 80 mg/day. Decreased absorption with antacids.
Ramipril (Altace®)	2.5–20 mg 1–2x/day	1 hour	Titrate for blood pressure control after 2–4 weeks. Single dose or in 2 equally divided doses.
Angiotensin II Antagonists (ARB)			
Candesartan (Atacand®)	8–32 mg 1x/day	3–4 hours	
Irbesartan (Avapro®)	150–300 mg 1x/day	1.5–2 hours	
Olmesartan (Benicar®)	20 mg 1x/day	1–2 hours	Titrate to 40 mg/day after 2 weeks of therapy if needed. Pediatric dosing.
Losartan (Cozaar®)	50 mg 1x/day	1 hour	Avoid K+ supplements or salt substitutes containing K+. Pediatric dosing.
Valsartan (Diovan®)	80–160 mg 1x/day	2–4 hours	Titrate up to 320 mg daily. Avoid K+ supplements or salt substitutes containing K+. Pediatric dosing.
Telmisartan (Micardis®)	20–80 mg 1x/day	0.5–1 hour	
Eprosartan (Teveten®)	400–800 mg 1–2x/day	1–2 hours6–12 hours	May need to be on medication 2–3 weeks for ideal blood pressure reduction.
Calcium Channel Blockers			
Amlodipine (Norvasc®)	5–10 mg 1x/day	2.5–5 hours	Titrate in 7–14 day time frame. Pediatric dosing.
Felodipine (Plendll®)	5–10 mg 1x/day	1.5 hours	Take with food. Do not crush or chew; swallow whole.
Isradipine (DynaCirc CR®)	2.5–10 mg 2x/day		Titrate in 2–4 week intervals.

continued on next page

Table 21-8. (continued)
Oral Antihypertensive Medications for Treatment and Management of
Hypertension and Coronary Artery Disease

Medication	Dosing	Peak Effect	Other Considerations
Calcium Channel Blockers *(continued)*			
Nicardipine (Cardene SR®)	30–60 mg 2x/day	1–4 hours	Titrate per blood pressure response.
Nifedipine (Procardia XL®)	10–30 mg 3–4x/day	30 minutes	Do not chew, crush, or divide tablet. Titrate over 7–14 days.
Diltiazem (Cardizem®)	180–360 mg 4x/day	2–4 hours	Administer before meals and at bedtime.
Nisoldipine (Sular®)	17–34 mg 1x/day	9.2 hours	Take on an empty stomach. Do not chew, crush, or divide tablet.
Verapamil (Calan®)	80–160 mg 3x/day	1–2 hours	
Verapamil (Calan SR®)	180–240 mg 1x/day	7.71 hours	Add evening dose if needed.
Alpha Blockers			
Doxazosin (Cardura®)	1–16 mg 1x/day	2–3 hours	Administer in a.m. or p.m.
Prazosin (Minipress®)	1–40 mg 2–3x/day	3 hours	Administer in divided doses; 2–3x/day.
Terazosin (Hytrin®)	1–5 mg 2x/day	1 hour	Slowly increase dose; use 2x/day dosing schedule. Max dose is 40 mg/day.
Central Alpha-2 Agonists			
Clonidine (Catapres®)	0.2–0.6 mg 2x/day	3.5 hours	Administer in divided doses; a.m. and at bedtime.
Clonidine patch (Catapres-TTS®)		Half-life = 12.7 hours	
Methyldopa (Aldomet®)	250–500 mg 2–3x/day	Half-life = 105 minutes	Titrate in greater than 48-hour intervals. Pediatric dosing.
Reserpine	0.5 mg 1x/day (initial dosing)	2.5 hours	Maintenance dose is 0.1–0.25 mg/day. May cause depression.
Guanfacine (Tenex®)	1–3 mg 1x/day	2.6 hours	Administer at bedtime. Tolerance for alcohol and CNS depressants may decrease.
Direct Vasodilators			
Hydralazine (Apresoline® tablets)	10–50 mg 4x/day	1–2 hours	Titrate on a weekly schedule. Use lowest dose needed. Pediatric dosing.
Minoxidil	10–40 mg 1–2x/day	1 hour	Administer in single or divided doses. Max dose is 100 mg/day. Pediatric dosing.

continued on next page

Table 21-8. (continued)
Oral Antihypertensive Medications for Treatment and Management of
Hypertension and Coronary Artery Disease

Medication	Dosing	Peak Effect	Other Considerations
Renin Inhibitors			
Aliskiren (Tekturna®)	150–300 mg 1x/day	1–3 hours	Max dose is 300 mg/day.
Alpha Beta Blockers			
Carvedilol (Coreg®)	6.25–25 mg 2x/day	5 hours	Titrate every 7–14 days as needed. Do not chew, crush, or divide capsule.
Labetalol Hydrochloride (Normodyne®, Trandate®)	100–400 mg 2x/day	1–2 hours	Severe HTN may require doses of 1,200–2,400 mg/day in 2-3 divided doses.
Anti-Platelet Therapy			
Aspirin	75–325 mg daily	1–2 hours	Increased bleeding risk with 3 or more drinks/day.
Clopidogrel Bisulfate (Plavix®)	Loading dose: 300 mg	30–60 minutes	Drug interactions with warfarin and NSAIDs. Maintenance dose is 75 mg/day
Prasugrel (Effient®)	Loading dose: 60 mg	30 minutes	with aspirin.
Dipyridamole (Persantineª)	75–100 mg 4x/day	75 minutes	Maintenance dose is 10 mg/day.
Nitrates			
Nitroglycerin (Nitrostat® tablets)	1 tablet sublingual (SL); repeat every 5 minutes until relief is obtained, for a total of 3 tablets in 15 minutes	6.4 minutes	Do not chew, crush, or swallow.
Nitroglycerin (Nitro-Bid Ointment®)	0.5–2 inches 2x/day	1–4 hours	Should have a 10–12 hour nitrate-free period.
Nitroglycerin (NitroMist®)	1–2 sprays at onset of pain, for a total of 3 sprays in 15 minutes	8 minutes	
Beta Blockers			
Atenolol (Tenormin®)	50 mg 1x/day	2–4 hours	Increase to 100 mg after 1 week.
Propranolol (Inderal LA®)	80–160 mg 1x/day	6 hours	Titrate dose in 3–7 day intervals. Max dose is 320 mg/day.
Metoprolol (Lopressor®)	100–400 mg 1x/day in 2 divided doses	Half-life = 2.8–7.5 hours	Increase weekly until response achieved.
Nadolol (Corgard®)	100–400 mg 1x/day by mouth (PO) in 2 divided doses	3–4 hours	Increase in 3–7 day intervals.

continued on next page

Table 21-8. (continued)
Oral Antihypertensive Medications for Treatment and Management of
Hypertension and Coronary Artery Disease

Medication	Dosing	Peak Effect	Other Considerations
Lipid Lowering Medications			
Atorvastatin (Lipitor®)	10–40 mg 1x/day	1–2 hours	Monitor liver function tests 12 weeks after starting therapy, with increase in doses. Pediatric dosing.
Fluvastatin (Lescol®)	10–40 mg 1x/day	1–2 hours	Titrate at 2–4 week intervals. Max dose is 80 mg/day.
Lovastatin (Mevacor®)	10–80 mg 1–2x/day	2 hours	Administer in single or 2 divided doses. Pediatric dosing.
Pravastatin (Pravachol®)	40–80 mg 1x/day	1–1.5 hours	Pediatric dosing.
Simvastatin (Zocor®)	5–40 mg 1x/day	4 hours	Restricted dosing of 80 mg for chronic use. Change medication if LDL-C goal not reached with 40 mg. Pediatric dosing.
Rosuvastatin (Crestor®)	5–40 mg 1x/day	Peaks 3–5 hours	Use 40 mg dose only if LDL-C goal not reached with 20 mg. Pediatric dosing.
Niacin	500–2,000 mg 1x/day	5 hours	Take at bedtime with low-fat snack. Titrate by 500 mg every 4 weeks. Do not divide, crush, or chew tablet.

Source: Adapted from PDR Network, LLC, 2012.

a. Therapeutic lifestyle changes (TLC) diet.
   (1) Limit total fat intake to 25–35% of total calories.
      (a) Limit saturated fats to less than 7% of total calories.
      (b) Limit cholesterol to 200 mg.
      (c) Eliminate trans fats.
   (2) Six or more servings per day of grains, including whole grains.
   (3) Five or more servings of fruits/vegetables per day.
   (4) Consume meat/poultry/fish up to 6 cooked ounces per day.
   (5) Limit salt/sodium to no more than 2,300 mg daily.
   (6) Limit alcohol: A standard drink is any drink that contains about 14 grams of pure alcohol (about 0.6 fluid ounces or 1.2 tablespoons) and equals 12 ounces of regular beer, 8–9 ounces of malt liquor, 5 ounces of table wine or 1.5 ounces of 80-proof spirits (NIAAA, n.d., 2011).
      (a) Adult men younger than 65, no more than two drinks per day.
      (b) For adult women and men older than 65, no more than one drink per day.
b. Physical activity: At least 2 hours and 30 minutes (150 minutes) of moderate-intensity aerobic activity (i.e., brisk walking) every week.
c. Quit smoking – Can refer to National Quitline at 1-877-44U-QUIT (1-877-448-7848) or www.smokefree.gov.
d. Manage stress.
e. Weight management with weight appropriate to height. BMI between 19–25 kg/m^2 and waist circumference less than 40 inches for men and 35 inches for women (National Heart, Lung, and Blood Institute [NHLBI], 2012).

2. Secondary prevention.
   a. Identification of those where lifestyle changes have not reduced risk factors, and add medication therapy.
   b. Medication therapy to decrease the potential for damage to myocardium.
      (1) Anti-platelet medications.
      (2) Anti-anginal medications.
      (3) Blood pressure management.
      (4) Lipid-lowering medications.
   c. Management of co-morbidities.
      (1) Hypertension.
      (2) Diabetes.
      (3) Hyperlipidemia.
      (4) Obesity.
3. Tertiary prevention.
   a. Minimize damage to heart.
   b. Minimize complications resulting from damage to heart.
   c. Cardiac rehabilitation to include exercise training, ongoing education regarding lifestyle, and counseling/intervention to assist in the management and reduction of stress.
D. Psychological considerations.
   1. Barriers to change.
      a. Cultural norms.
      b. Inadequate attention to health education by clinicians.
      c. Cost for services; clinical and education.
      d. Integrating lifestyle modifications including healthy diet and physical activity into daily lifestyle.
      e. Amounts of sodium and fat in packaged/prepared/restaurant foods.
   2. Potential for non-adherence/reasons for non-adherence.
      a. Note missed appointments.
      b. Note missed medication refills.
      c. Have goals for therapy been mutually set?
      d. Integration of medication administration into daily routines.
E. Education of patient and family.
   1. Progression of disease and potential for complications.

2. When to seek care – New onset chest pain/chest pain-like symptoms.
3. Medication adherence including the importance of refilling medications.
4. Lifestyle changes.
5. Need to continue with lifestyle changes after intervention for reperfusion.
6. Follow-up monitoring, including the importance of keeping scheduled appointments.
F. Collaboration and referrals.
   1. Utilization of services, including (but not limited to): Medical specialists, pharmacy, nurse case managers, registered dietitians, licensed nutritionists, health educators, and counselors.
   2. Reinforce patient education with patient and significant other(s).
   3. Management of co-morbidities.
   4. Utilization of specialty services as needed, including cardiology, endocrinology, physical therapy, clinical pharmacist, and health behavior psychologist.
G. Community resources and advocacy.
   1. The CDC monitors health, conducts research, promotes healthy behaviors, and provides information to health professionals and the lay public.
   2. The National Heart, Lung, and Blood Institute (NHLBI) provides leadership for a research, training, and education program to promote the prevention and treatment of heart, lung, and blood diseases.
   3. American Heart Association (AHA) provides information for health professionals and lay public on heart disease.
   4. Smokefree.gov offers assistance for quitting tobacco use, with additional information for health care professionals, women, and teens, as well as for military personnel and their families.
H. Telehealth practice.
   1. Pertinent history.
   2. Symptoms – New or exacerbation.
   3. Signs and symptoms of myocardial infarction – Call 9-1-1.
   4. Telehealth monitoring.
      a. Ongoing assessment by health care team.

b. Home telehealth monitoring for blood pressure, vital signs, diabetes, and weight to electronically transmit data to health care team.

c. Ongoing education of patient and significant other(s).

d. Health care resources, including Web-based resources.

I. Protocol/algorithms/guidelines.

1. Agency for Healthcare Research and Quality (AHRQ) National Guideline Clearinghouse (2011) – *Effectiveness-Based Guidelines for the Prevention of Cardiovascular Disease in Women – 2011 Update: A Guideline from the American Heart Association.*

2. Agency for Healthcare Research and Quality (AHRQ) National Guideline Clearinghouse (2009) – *Secondary Prevention of Coronary Artery Disease.*

3. Institute for Clinical Systems Improvement (2011) – *Health Care Guideline: Lipid Management in Adults.*

4. U.S. Department of Veterans Affairs (2006) – *Clinical Practice Guidelines: Management of Dyslipidemia (LIPIDS).*

Chronic Heart Failure

Patient Population: Adult

I. Overview

Heart failure (HF) is a complex clinical syndrome in which cardiac myocytes or the contractile apparatus of the heart has impairment in ejecting blood or filling properly and cannot meet the needs of tissues (Hunt et al., 2009). After the age of 65, one person per 100 will develop HF (Roger et al., 2011). Heart failure has been commonly termed *de novo* (new diagnosis), *acute* (refers to exacerbation of an existing [chronic] condition), or *chronic*. Once diagnosed, there is generally no cure for HF without cardiac transplantation or another therapy that fully reverses cardiac hypertrophy and ventricular remodeling. Over time, cardiac dysfunction involves the cardiac ventricles, atria, valves, and other cardiac structures.

One major problem in caring for patients with chronic HF is that the condition has a high morbidity rate. Hospitalization for HF is the leading discharge diagnosis in Medicare patients and rates have not decreased over time, even though cardiovascular diseases, in general, have been on the decline (Roger et al., 2011). Further, hospitalization for HF decompensation has been associated with an increase in mortality (Setoguchi, Stevenson, & Schneeweiss, 2007). Thus, it is important for ambulatory care nurses to assertively manage HF based on current evidence-based guidelines to improve survival, decrease costly hospitalizations, and ultimately improve quality of life.

II. Pathophysiology

A. Cardiac disorders can be structural or functional and may involve the pericardium, myocardium, endocardium, or great vessels; however, the predominant problem is dysfunction of the left ventricle.

B. Altered peripheral perfusion leads to subsequent mechanical, neuroendocrine, and inflammatory responses aimed at improving systemic organ flow.

C. Compensatory mechanisms fail to improve contractility or filling over time and lead to a maladaptive state characterized by "ventricular remodeling" (myocyte hypertrophy, cardiac dilatation, and reshaping of the left ventricle from an elliptical to a spherical or globular shape), neurohormonal activation, and hemodynamic alterations (systemic and venous vasoconstriction, increased afterload and preload, and low cardiac output).

D. Chronic left ventricular myocyte dysfunction may be due to changes in regional myocyte workload that involve abnormal systolic function, generally defined by an ejection fraction below 40% (normal left ventricular ejection fraction is greater than 55% and up to 75%) or due to changes in passive tension that is associated with preserved systolic function (normal ejection fraction) but abnormal diastolic function (Heart Failure Society of America et al., 2010; Hunt et al., 2009).

1. Systolic dysfunction is also known as HF with reduced ejection fraction (HF-REF).

2. Diastolic dysfunction is known as HF with preserved ejection fraction (HF-PEF).

III. Assessment and Triage

A. Signs and symptoms.

1. Most commonly, patient manifestations include dyspnea and fatigue that may be associated with fluid overload (in blood vessels, known as hemodynamic congestion; in tissues, known as clinical congestion and commonly displayed as ascites, edema, or rales) and exercise intolerance (Hunt et al., 2009).

2. Other common manifestations that are also prevalent in other conditions: Dizziness, change in appetite, nausea, daytime sleepiness, palpitations, nocturia, and orthopnea (Albert, Trochelman, Li, & Lin, 2010).

3. Signs and symptoms of new or worsening volume overload. Note: Less than 50% of ambulatory patients have "congestive" signs (rales) or symptoms (edema); therefore, must carefully assess for sub-clinical volume overload, also known as hemodynamic congestion (Albert et al., 2010).

   a. Dyspnea, orthopnea, paroxysmal nocturnal dyspnea.

   b. Edema, ascites, anasarca, acute pulmonary edema.

   c. Cough or rales.

   d. Sudden, unexpected weight gain of more than three pounds above ideal (dry) weight or nocturia.

      (1) Dry weight reflects the patient's weight when in an euvolemic (normal) fluid state.

      (2) Should NOT compare today's weight to yesterday's weight unless the patient has a weight diary and can review and compare trends over time with dry weight.

   e. S3 gallop, neck vein distension, or elevated jugular venous pressure (greater than 10 cm H_2O pressure); positive hepatojugular reflux test.

4. Assess for signs and symptoms of resting hypoperfusion that may occur with or without volume overload (Albert et al., 2010).

   a. Fatigue, decreased exercise tolerance.

   b. Mental obtundation, dizziness, light-headedness.

   c. Nausea, anorexia, change in bowel habits.

   d. Resting tachycardia (greater than 85 BPM), decreased systolic blood pressure, increased intra-cardiac pressures, and pulsus alternans.

   e. Proportional pulse pressure less than 25%. To obtain proportional pulse pressure, subtract diastolic blood pressure from systolic blood pressure, and then divide results by systolic blood pressure.

5. Assess for cardiac rhythm abnormalities.

   a. Palpitations; may be evident or worse when lying on left side.

   b. Slow, rapid, or irregular heart rate (HR) associated with dizziness, lightheadedness, syncope, or near-syncope.

B. Primary causes.

1. Coronary artery disease.
2. Myocardial infarction.
3. Hypertension.
4. Diabetes.
5. Cardiac valve disease.
6. Anemia.
7. Thyroid disease.
8. Virus.
9. Chemotherapy agents, illicit substances, alcohol use.
10. Age (prevalence increases with age).

C. Secondary causes.

1. Lack of proper intervention or non-adherence of medical management of precipitating disease processes can prompt de novo (new onset) HF or worsen the severity.

   a. Failure to have surgical or interventional cardiac revascularization or valve repair for coronary artery disease and valve disease, respectively.

   b. Non-control of diabetes.

   c. Failure to prevent or not treat anemia.

   d. Failure to optimize blood pressure to within the normal range based on national guideline recommendations.

   e. Failure to monitor and optimize renal function.

f. Failure to prevent or limit atrial tachycardia or fibrillation, or failure to decrease heart rate in persistent or permanent atrial fibrillation.

g. Failure to promote reversal of coronary artery plaque progression with lipid-lowering therapies, or failure to maintain low-density cholesterol at 70 mg/dL or less.

h. Failure to assess and optimize thyroid function.

i. Failure to assess and treat sleep-disordered breathing.

2. Lifestyle can exacerbate HF symptoms and worsen condition, leading to decompensation.

a. Alcohol use/substance abuse.

b. Tobacco use.

c. Fluid indiscretion when HF is advanced, patient has hyponatremia due to fluid overload, or history of frequent rehospitalizations due to HF decompensation.

d. Excess sodium content in diet.

e. Inactivity or passive activity; lack of regular exercise.

f. Anxiety, depression, personality type D, vital exhaustion, or poor stress management.

g. Medication non-adherence based on the medical treatment plan.

h. Social isolation or lack of social support or caregiver, as needed.

i. Economic constraints related to purchase of food and medications; transportation to health care providers.

j. Non-adherence to daily monitoring of signs and symptoms of worsening HF.

k. Failure to notify health care provider of changes in medical condition reflecting worsening HF condition.

D. Problems related to treatment (Heart Failure Society of America et al., 2010; Hunt et al., 2009).

1. Non-adherence to the medical plan of care (including medication therapies, diet, and other lifestyle change recommendations).

2. Failure to receive regular, ongoing medical care or seek early treatment when the medical status changes.

3. Poor communication between the HF health care provider and patient related to specific needs and ability to understand and follow the plan of care.

4. Customs, rituals, and social, psychological (depression and anxiety), and economic issues and constraints.

5. Failure to follow primary, secondary, and tertiary care prevention strategies (see VI C).

E. Functional status: Evaluate patients with HF using two complementary systems.

1. New York Heart Association (NYHA) (Hunt et al., 2009) functional status assessment or classification (NYHA-FC) provides a subjective degree of functional limitations experienced by patients at one point in time (see Table 21-9).

a. Functional status based on symptoms may change over time and with treatments, and does not reflect the overall stage of heart failure.

b. Objective assessment of functional status using valid and reliable measures:

(1) Minnesota Living with Heart Failure Questionnaire (20-item, Likert-type survey).

(2) Kansas City Cardiomyopathy Questionnaire (23-item Likert-type survey).

(3) Specific Activity Scale (5-item tool that objectively measures NYHA-functional class).

(4) Six-Minute Walk Test (American Thoracic Society [ATS], 2002).

2. Stages of HF reflect an objective and reliable system of identifying overall status and treatment expectations for patients with suspected or known systolic dysfunction (see Table 21-10).

a. Stages of HF are a complement to the NYHA-function classification system because current functional status helps gauge the severity of symptoms in pa-

Table 21-9.
New York Heart Association Functional Classifications

Class	Definition	Examples
I	Can carry out ordinary exercise *without physical activity limitation* due to symptoms of fatigue, dyspnea, chest pain, or palpitations.	Can play sports; walk up multiple flights of steps without stopping; carry out all activities of daily living, including strenuous activities such as lifting furniture, vacuuming, and walking uphill.
II	Comfortable at rest, but has symptoms (fatigue, dyspnea, chest pain, or palpitations) with ordinary exercise, which causes a *slight limitation of physical activity.*	Can walk up one flight of steps before stopping to rest; fox trot or walk on level terrain; cannot carry out strenuous sports or walk uphill.
III	Less than ordinary activity results in symptoms (fatigue, dyspnea, chest pain, or palpitations); therefore, the patient has a *marked limitation of physical activity.*	Takes a break before completing a walk up one flight of 12 steps; must take breaks (stop to rest or catch breath) in usual daily activities such as walking small distances, dressing, bathing, changing sheets, or washing clothes.
IV	Has *discomfort with any physical activity* or has *symptoms at rest.*	Fatigue, dyspnea, chest pain, or palpitations with simple activity such as moving from bed to chair.

tients with Stage C and D HF. It is important to assess the patient's HF stage and functional status with every visit because spontaneous reversal of HF is unusual, even though optimal medical management may halt progression.

    b. The ultimate goal of therapy at any stage of HF is to prevent or reverse progression of left ventricular remodeling (Heart Failure Society of America et al., 2010; Hunt et al., 2009).

F. Physical assessment (Heart Failure Society of America et al., 2010; Hunt et al., 2009).

    1. Assessment of volume overload:

        a. Presence of peripheral edema in legs, fingers, or abdomen; ascites in abdomen; anasarca, scrotal, or presacral area edema.

        b. Sitting and standing blood pressure to determine level of jugular venous distension.

        c. Positive hepatojugular reflux test; presence and severity of organ distension (pulmonary congestion and hepatomegaly).

        d. Presence of elevated jugular venous pressure (most reliable sign of fluid overload).

        e. Short-term elevation in body weight.

        f. New onset or worsening of S3 heart sound or systolic murmur.

        g. Subjective assessment of new or worsening orthopnea, paroxysmal nocturnal dyspnea, nocturia, dyspnea with activity or at rest, exercise intolerance, or sleep-disordered breathing (central sleep apnea) are most common.

    2. Assessment of hypovolemia.

        a. Flat neck veins.

        b. Dry mucous membranes/mouth.

        c. Clear lung fields, absence of edema.

    3. Assessment of perfusion.

        a. Blood pressure and orthostatic blood pressure changes.

        b. Narrow pulse pressure may indicate hypoperfusion.

        c. Audible S4 may indicate hypertension.

        d. Subjective complaints of short-lived dizziness, lightheadedness, or presyncope, especially with sudden movement or moving from a lying to sitting or standing position, may reflect temporary hypotension due to HF medications reaching their peak effects at/near the same time.

Table 21-10.
Stages of Heart Failure

Stage	Definition	Description
A	At *high risk* for developing heart failure; do not have heart failure currently (pre-heart failure).	Conditions such as hypertension, diabetes mellitus, coronary artery disease, and family history of cardiomyopathy increase risk of developing heart failure, as does smoking history. Primary prevention strategies are the focus of care (lifestyle modification and drugs).
B	Asymptomatic *left ventricular dysfunction, hypertrophy,* or *geometric chamber distortion;* do not have heart failure currently (pre-heart failure).	Have structural heart disease (for example, valve dysfunction, previous myocardial infarction and left ventricular remodeling, including left ventricular hypertrophy and low ejection fraction), but have not experienced symptoms associated with heart failure. Primary prevention strategies are the focus of care (lifestyle modification, drugs, and ICD, when indicated).
C	Developed the clinical syndrome of heart failure and currently have signs and symptoms or have a history of symptoms.	NYHA-FC can span from I to IV (see Table 21-9). Treatments (drugs and devices) that revise or attenuate left ventricular remodeling and neurohormonal activation predominate as well as secondary prevention strategies, lifestyle modification, and symptom management.
D	End-stage heart failure; management strategies no longer relieve symptoms.	Myocyte, neurohormonal, and other changes escalate or are associated with disabling symptoms and poor quality of life. In addition to Stage C strategies, palliation, end-of-life care, cardiac transplantation, ventricular assist or other mechanical circulatory support device, or other advanced care or treatment strategies may be warranted.

Notes: ICD = implantable cardioverter defibrillator; NYHA-FC = New York Heart Association – Functional Class.

e. Audibly distant S2, diminished pulse amplitude, narrowed pulse pressure, pulsus alternans, and/or laterally displaced apical beat may indicate poor cardiac function and poor perfusion.

f. Cool, mottled skin; cognitive dysfunction or altered mentation; and change in bowel habits may indicate poor perfusion.

g. Tachycardia and/or frequent premature ventricular beats could decrease perfusion.

4. Height, weight, and calculation of body mass index.

5. Heart rate (HR) and oxygen saturation at rest.
   a. Resting HR below 80 beats per minute when on optimal HF medical therapies is associated with improved survival.
   b. Oxygen saturation greater than 92% reflects adequate cardiac output.

6. Cardiovascular assessment.
   a. Normal and abnormal or extra heart sounds in aortic, pulmonary, tricuspid, and mitral regions and apex if point of maximal impulse is not near the mitral region due to cardiac enlargement; murmurs.

b. Palpate apex for visible pulsations, thrills (if mitral stenosis, roll patient to left side to hear thrill), and heaves (at apex).

c. General color, temperature (cool extremities may indicate hypoperfusion), peripheral pulses, presence of peripheral vascular disease, ulceration, edema (pitting versus non-pitting).

7. Neck and pulmonary assessment: Glaring breathing problems.

a. Using accessory muscles of respiration may be due to pulmonary edema, asthma, fulminant pneumonia, chronic obstructive pulmonary disease (COPD); pursed lip breathing may be due to emphysema; audible noises while breathing; ability to speak and breathe at same time.

b. Dyspnea plus wheezing (or whistling) may be due to asthma, COPD, or worsening HF.

c. Cheyne-Stokes breathing may be due to stroke, worsening HF, sedation, or uremia.

d. Cough may be due to worsening HF, pneumonia, angiotensin converting enzyme inhibitor therapy, common cold, or flu.

e. Muffled sounds may be due to pleural effusion; scratchy sound (similar to rubbing strands of hair together) may be due to rales (crackles). Note: Rales are rare in chronic HF.

f. Cyanosis in nailbeds.

g. Obstructive sleep apnea may cause sleep disturbances.

8. Palpate abdomen in liver area for tricuspid regurgitation/hepatojugular reflux.

9. Chest inspection of pacemaker device under left clavicle.

G. Diagnostic tests – Routine.

1. Assess serum laboratory results for electrolyte balance (basic metabolic panel, calcium, magnesium), renal function (blood urea nitrogen, creatinine, or glomerular filtration rate), thyroid function (thyroid-stimulating hormone), fasting blood glucose, lipid profile, liver function tests, and complete blood count (Heart Failure Society of America et al., 2010; Hunt et al., 2009).

a. Initial assessment.

b. Yearly, as needed, based on signs and symptoms and medical history.

2. Ventricular function (B-type natriuretic peptide [BNP] or N-terminal pro-brain BNP [NT-proBNP]) in an urgent care setting when:

a. Clinical diagnosis of HF is uncertain.

b. Diagnosis of HF is known but it is uncertain if current symptoms reflect worsening HF or another medical condition.

3. Assess urinalyses results.

4. Assess 12-lead electrocardiogram for QRS width (ventricular dyssynchrony), intraventricular or other conduction delays, left ventricular hypertrophy, atrial and ventricular dysrhythmias or abnormalities, myocardial ischemia, injury or infarction (prior acute myocardial infarction or new/recent acute coronary syndrome), diffuse myocardial disease, and proper pacemaker or cardiac resynchronization therapy function, when appropriate.

5. Chest radiograph (posterior-anterior and lateral) to detect the presence of cardiac enlargement, pulmonary congestion, or other pulmonary disease.

a. Initial assessment.

b. Pulmonary distress requiring emergency care.

6. Two-dimensional echocardiogram coupled with Doppler flow studies to determine whether abnormalities of myocardium, heart valves, or pericardium are present and which chambers are involved. Evaluates the presence and severity of left ventricular dysfunction and provides a subjective assessment of ejection fraction. Can reveal segmental wall motion abnormalities, chamber size, ventricular thrombus, and degree of cardiac dyssynchrony. Can reveal right ventricular size, right ventricular systolic performance, and right atrial size. Echocardiogram is the most useful diagnostic tool in the evaluation of HF. Echocardiogram is less expensive and

more generally available than radionuclide ventriculography (see H 7, below); it does not require preparation. Numerical data should include:

    a. Estimate of ejection fraction.

    b. Ventricular dimensions and volumes.

    c. Wall thickness and chamber geometry.

    d. Regional wall motion.

    e. Left atrial dimensions and volume.

    f. Anatomic and flow abnormalities in all four valves.

    g. Secondary changes in valve function, with attention to mitral and tricuspid valve insufficiency.

7. Trend data from internal cardiac monitoring features of an implantable cardioverter defibrillator.

    a. Atrial fibrillation prevalence per 24-hour period.

    b. Ventricular heart rate while in atrial fibrillation.

    c. Atrial and ventricular heart rate during the day and at night.

    d. Activity level.

    e. Intrathoracic impedance (reflects intrathoracic fluid volume).

    f. Heart rate variability.

8. Trend data from structured telephone monitoring or telemonitoring devices, used to assess ongoing status.

H. Diagnostic tests – Special studies.

1. Coronary arteriography in patients with chest pain (that may or may not be of cardiac origin) or significant ischemia.

    a. Initial assessment.

    b. Suspected worsening of coronary artery disease or ischemic signs and symptoms in patients without a recent evaluation of coronary anatomy unless the patient is not eligible for revascularization of any kind.

2. Pulmonary function test as necessary for pulmonary dysfunction.

3. 24–48-hour holter monitor, as necessary for cardiac electrophysiology issues; especially in patients with a history of myocardial infarction.

4. Diagnostic right heart catheterization/hemodynamics: Catheter inserted into a vein and guided to the right side of the heart to determine low cardiac output and elevated right ventricular filling pressures. Uses local anesthetics. Does not require preparation.

5. Electrophysiology testing: Heart catheterization that records electrical activity in the heart and can reveal serious rhythm disturbances after electrical stimulation.

6. Maximal cardiopulmonary exercise testing with or without respiratory gas exchange measurement and/or blood oxygen saturation, to determine if HF is the cause of exercise limitation or if patient is a candidate for cardiac transplantation, ventricular assist device therapies, or other advanced treatments. Completed via a graded treadmill or bicycle exercise protocol. Does not require preparation, except to hold medications as necessary.

7. Radionuclide ventriculography: Provides highly accurate measurements of left and right ventricular function and ejection fraction, but no data on valve abnormalities or cardiac hypertrophy is directly assessed.

8. Magnetic resonance imaging or computed tomography: Provides chamber size, ventricular mass, ventricular function, and ejection fraction.

    a. Can detect right ventricular dysplasia or recognize the presence of pericardial disease.

    b. Can identify myocardial viability and scar tissue (useful when making decisions about coronary artery surgical revascularization).

9. Other diagnostic tests, as needed.

    a. Screening for sleep-disordered breathing, hemochromatosis, human immunodeficiency virus (HIV), amyloidosis, rheumatologic diseases, or pheochromocytoma.

    b. Endomyocardial biopsy, if therapy could be influenced by a suspected, specific diagnosis.

IV. **Indications for Emergency Care or Urgent Consultation**
(Heart Failure Society of America et al., 2010; Hunt et al., 2009)

A. New or severe, unexpected chest pain or discomfort that occurs with dyspnea, nausea, sweating, or weakness.

B. If history of chest pain, worsening in status, or lack of relief within 15 minutes of sublingual nitroglycerine spray administration or rest.

C. Sustained heart rate greater than 120 beats per minute, especially if lightheaded, dizzy, or dyspneic.

D. Heart rate greater than 150 beats per minute.

E. New onset or profound worsening of signs and symptoms of low cardiac output state (see III A 3).

F. New onset or profound worsening of fluid overload that are not relieved by rest and additional oral loop diuretic agent (see III A 4).

G. Severe hypovolemia.
1. Physical exam findings (see III F 2).
2. Signs and symptoms of hypoperfusion (see III A 4).
3. Decreased frequency of urination or urine volume; dark urine.
4. Elevated blood urea nitrogen and creatinine.
5. Dizziness/lightheadedness when changing from lying to standing/sitting; lasts more than 15 minutes (sustained orthostatic hypotension).
6. Headache.
7. Blurred vision.
8. Unexplained tachycardia.

H. Sudden onset of severe headache.

I. Syncope or near syncope.

J. Severe electrolyte imbalances.

K. New onset atrial fibrillation, non-sustained ventricular tachycardia, or other cardiac rhythm problem requiring immediate evaluation and treatment.

L. Uncontrolled hypertension requiring immediate evaluation and treatment with intravenous agents.

M. Acute pneumonia concomitant with HF.

N. Advanced renal or hepatic disease with decompensated HF.

V. **Indications for Critical Care Hospitalization Due to Complex Decompensation**
(Heart Failure Society of America et al., 2010; Hunt et al., 2009)

A. Severe or refractory symptoms of volume overload and/or resting hypoperfusion (with metabolic sequelae) requiring intravenous preload and afterload reduction (intravenous vasodilator and diuretic therapies), intravenous inotropic therapies, and/or renal therapies (ultrafiltration).

B. Hemodynamic instability requiring right heart catheterization and continuous or intermittent hemodynamic monitoring to augment management of intravenous vasodilator and/or inotropic therapies.

C. New onset angina or refractory angina, clinical suspicion of myocardial infarction by signs/symptoms, electrocardiogram and cardiac troponin testing.

D. Hypoxemia requiring respiratory support via ventilator.

E. Recent respiratory or cardiac arrest.

F. Shock.

G. Complex cardiac arrhythmias requiring close electrocardiographic monitoring and medication and/or technical therapies.

H. Severe asymptomatic or symptomatic hyponatremia (serum sodium less than 125 mEq/L) requiring intravenous or oral vasopressin antagonist therapy.

I. Requires invasive hemodynamic monitoring (pulmonary artery catheter) to assess:
1. Uncertain fluid status, perfusion, or systemic or pulmonary vascular resistance.
2. Low systolic blood pressure with symptoms despite initial therapy.
3. Worsening renal function with therapy.
4. Consideration of advance device therapy or cardiac transplantation.

VI. **Plan of Care**

A. Pharmacotherapeutics.
1. Core pharmacologic therapies for HF (see Table 21-11) (Hunt et al., 2009):
a. Angiotensin converting enzyme (ACE) inhibitor with efficacy in HF.

Table 21-11.
Core Medication Therapy Drugs and Dosing, by Drug Class, Used in Heart Failure Management

Aldosterone Antagonist Therapy:

Drug Name (Trade)	Increments	Max Dose	Peak Effect
Spironolactone (Aldactone®)	12.5–25 mg daily (use low dose)	25 mg twice daily	2–3 days
Eplerenone (Inspra®)*	25 mg/day x 4 weeks → 50 mg/day	50 mg/day	1.5 hours

*Selectively blocks the mineralocorticoid receptor (not glucocorticoid, progesterone, or androgen receptors); therefore, less sexual dysfunction and gynecomastia.

Beta Blocker Therapy:

Drug Name (Trade)	Increments	Target/Max Dose	Peak Effect
Carvedilol (Coreg®)	3.125 → 6.25 → 12.5 → 25 → 50 mg	25 mg twice daily (<85 kg) 50 mg twice daily (≥85 kg)	1–4 hours
Carvedilol CR (Coreg CR®)	10 → 20 → 40 → 80	80 mg once daily	5–7 hours
Metoprolol succinate (Toprol XL®)	25 → 50 → 100 → 150 → 200	200 mg once daily	6–12 hours
Nebivilol (Bystolic®)	1.25 → 2.5 → 5 → 10	10 mg once daily	0.5–4 hours
Bisoprolol (Zebeta®)	1.2 → 5 2.5 → 5 → 10	10 mg once daily	2–4 hours

Cardiac Glycoside Therapy:

Drug Name (Trade)	Usual Dose **, ***	Max Dose	Peak Effect
Digitalis (Digoxin®)	0.125–0.25 mg day	0.5 mg day	6–8 hours

** Expected digoxin level: 0.6–0.9 ng/dL.
*** If amiodarone initiated, decrease dose by half and assess digoxin level in 2 months.

Diuretic Therapies:

Drug Name (Trade)	Type	IV:PO Conversion	Relative Potency – Oral	Peak Effect
Bumetanide (Bumex®)	Loop	1:1	1 mg	30 minutes– 1 hour
Ethacrynic Acid (Edecrin®)	Loop	1:1	50 mg	2 hours
Furosemide (Lasix®)	Loop	1:2	40 mg	1–2 hours
Torsemide (Demadex®)	Loop	1:1	20–40 mg	1 hour
HCTZ (HydroDIURIL® and others)	Thiazide	00–1000 mg orally	Note: Take with/before loop diuretic	4–6 hours
Chlorthalidone	Thiazide	25–100 mg orally	Used to treat hypertension	4–6 hours
Metolazone (Zaroxolyn®)	Thiazide-like	2.5–5 mg orally	Take with/before loop diuretic	2–4 hours
Triameterene (Dyrenium®)	K+ sparing	Not applicable	Does not inhibit aldosterone	2–3 hours
Amiloride (Midamor®)	K+ sparing	Not applicable	Does not inhibit aldosterone	6–10 hours

continued on next page

Table 21-11. (continued)
Core Medication Therapy Drugs and Dosing, by Drug Class, Used in Heart Failure Management

Vasodilator Therapy: ACEI, angiotensin converting enzyme inhibitor; ARB, angiotensin II receptor blocker; VD, direct acting vasodilator; arterial (a) or venous (v).

Drug Name (Trade)	Type	Starting Dose	Target Dose	Max Dose	Peak Effect
Captopril (Capoten®)	ACEI	6.25 mg 3x/day	50 mg 3x/day	100 mg 3x/day	1–3 hours
Candesartan (Atacand®)	ARB	4–8 mg/day	32 mg/day	32 mg/day	3–4 hours
Enalapril (Vasotec®)	ACEI	2.5 mg 2x/day	10 mg 2x/day	20 mg 2x/day	4–6 hours
Hydralazine (Apresoline®)	VDa†	25 mg 4x/day	–	100 mg 4x/day	1 hour
Isosorbide dinitrate	VDv†	10 mg 3x/day	–	80 mg 3x/day	Less than 1 hour
Isosorbide mononitrate	VDv†	30–60 mg/day	–	240 mg/day	4 hours
Fosinopril (Monopril®)	ACEI	2.5 mg 2x/day	20 mg 2x/day	20 mg 2x/day	3 hours
Lisinopril (Prinivil®; Zestril®)	ACEI	2.5–5 mg/day	20 mg/day	40 mg/day	7 hours
Quinapril (Accupril®)	ACEI	5 mg 2x/day	20 mg 2x/day	20 mg 2x/day	2–4 hours
Ramapril (Altace®)	ACEI‡	1.25–2.5 mg/day	5 mg/day	10 mg/day	3–6 hours
Trandolapril (Mavik®)	ACEI‡	1 mg/day	4 mg/day	4 mg/day	1–2 hours
Valsartan (Diovan®)	ARB	20–40 mg 2x/day	80 mg 2x/day	80 mg 2x/day	2–4 hours

† Titrate dose based on blood pressure and adverse side effects.
‡ Post acute myocardial infarction.
All others: Patients with Stage B, C, or D heart failure with reduced ejection fraction (ejection fraction ≤ 40%).

Source: Copyright © 2011 Nancy M. Albert. Used with permission.

(1) Asymptomatic post myocardial infarction left ventricular systolic dysfunction: Captopril, lisinopril, ramipril, trandopril.

(2) Ischemic or dilated cardiomyopathy: Captopril, enalapril, lisinopril, fosinopril, quinapril.

b. Angiotensin II receptor blocker (ARB) when an ACE inhibitor is contraindicated or as adjunctive therapy.

(1) Asymptomatic post myocardial infarction left ventricular systolic dysfunction (Stage B HF): Valsartan.

(2) Ischemic or dilated cardiomyopathy (Stage C or D HF): Candesartan, valsartan.

c. Beta adrenergic blocker with efficacy in HF.

(1) Asymptomatic post myocardial infarction left ventricular systolic dysfunction (Stage B heart failure): Carvedilol, atenolol, metoprolol tartrate, propranolol, timolol.

(2) Ischemic or dilated cardiomyopathy (Stage B, C or D heart failure): Carvedilol, metoprolol succinate, bisoprolol, and nebivilol.

d. Aldosterone antagonist.

(1) Post myocardial infarction left ventricular systolic dysfunction (Stage B, C, or D HF): Eplerenone.

(2) Ischemic or dilated cardiomyopathy (symptomatic Stage C HF or Stage D HF with REF and meets criteria for serum creatinine and potassium level): Spironolactone.

e. Loop diuretic if signs of volume overload (e.g., furosemide, torsemide, or bumetanide).

f. Digoxin in symptomatic HF-REF or HF-PEF when due to hypertension or ischemic myocardial damage and already on therapeutic levels of ACE inhibitor or ARB and beta blocker therapy.

g. Hydralazine/nitrate combination in self-described African Americans who:
   (1) Remain symptomatic after treatment with an ACE inhibitor (or ARB) and beta blocker.
   (2) As an alternative to ACE inhibitor or ARB when contraindicated due to renal insufficiency/failure, hyperkalemia, angioedema, or bilateral renal artery stenosis.

2. Potentially detrimental medications.
   a. Chronic non-steroidal anti-inflammatory drug use (sodium and water retaining effects).
   b. High dose (greater than 325 mg/day) chronic aspirin use (sodium and water retaining effects).
   c. Decongestant use (vasoconstriction).
   d. Calcium channel blocker therapy, *except* amlodipine or felodipine (cardiodepressant effects).
   e. First generation beta blocker therapy: Propranolol or timolol therapy (cardiodepressant effects).
   f. Class 1a and 1c antiarrhythmic therapy (cardiodepressant and proarrhythmia effects).
   g. Regular sodium-based antacid use.
   h. Thiazolidinedione therapy (sodium and water retaining effects).
   i. Minoxidil therapy (sodium retaining effects).
   j. Dronedarone therapy for atrial fibrillation (worsening HF in patients with NYHA-FC III–IV or with deteriorating HF).

B. Complementary and alternative therapies.
   1. Avoid over-the-counter supplements.
   2. Avoid commonly used alternative therapies.

C. Primary/secondary/tertiary prevention (Heart Failure Society of America et al., 2010; Hunt et al., 2009).
   1. Major modifiable primary and secondary prevention strategies:
      a. Hypertension control.
      b. Hyperlipidemia control.
      c. Cigarette smoking cessation.
      d. Promotion of aerobic exercise and regular activity.
      e. Weight reduction, if overweight.
      f. Prevention of glucose intolerance.
      g. Alcohol cessation; limiting caffeine intake; habitual drug withdrawal.
      h. Low sodium diet of 2,000–3,000 mg/day in Stage C HF.
      i. Low sodium diet of 2,000 mg/day and fluid restriction of 2 liters/day in Stage D HF.
   2. Other secondary prevention strategies:
      a. Self-management education related to fluid management (weight monitoring, fluid intake limitation, and managing thirst).
      b. Adherence to pharmacologic therapies.
      c. Yearly flu vaccine; pneumococcal vaccine once, repeat after age 65 if first dose received before age 65 and it has been at least 5 years.
      d. Regular physical examinations based on clinical status (NYHA-FC and Stage of HF).
      e. Social (family or caregiver) support of lifestyle changes.
      f. Treat depression, anxiety, anemia, renal dysfunction, and other medical conditions that can lead to worsening left ventricular dysfunction.
      g. Routine metabolic status assessment (diabetes, lipids, weight).
   3. Tertiary prevention.
      a. Prompt recognition and treatment of signs and symptoms of worsening condition.
      b. Identification and treatment of exacerbating factors such as: New or worsening stress, atrial arrhythmias (especially

tachyarrhythmias), infection, anemia, COPD or asthma, pulmonary emboli, thyroid disease (hypo- or hyperthyroid), environmental conditions, pregnancy, clinical depression, cardiac valve dysfunction (regurgitation and stenosis), cardiac congenital conditions, or hypertension.

D. Goals of the plan of care.
1. Improve survival and prevent hospitalization by reverse remodeling of HF-REF and prevention of worsening of HF-PEF.
2. Improve and stabilize quality of life by optimizing symptom status and minimizing/preventing worsening of symptoms.
3. Provide evidence-based medical therapies and also maintain a patient-centered care approach that considers the patient's perspective and wishes.
4. Recognize end-of-life and offer palliative care services to prevent undue suffering.

E. Psychosocial considerations.
1. Inability to work/exercise if functional status remains NYHA-FC IV or if activities are strenuous or vigorous and in NYHA-FC III.
2. Change in relationships regarding self-care and need for a caregiver.
3. Financial burden due to the number and cost of core medications and medical follow-up over time.
4. Inability to carry out previous hobbies or usual activities of enjoyment if symptoms worsen or due to environmental limits (too cold/hot, high altitude).
5. Symptoms of clinical depression in HF are common, at 21% (range of 14–38%) and are more likely in patients with worse NYHA-FC (Silver, 2010).

F. Education of patient/family (Heart Failure Society of America et al., 2010; Hunt et al., 2009).
1. Knowledge of heart failure, including prognosis; signs and symptoms of worsening condition; when and where to access health care.
2. Medication management; adherence to prescriptions, side effects; polypharmacy issues.

3. 2000–3000 mg sodium diet; low animal fat diet; limit alcohol intake; limit calories if overweight; promote intake of marine based omega-3 fatty acids.
4. Fluid management: Daily weight monitoring, fluid restriction/monitoring as required in advanced HF, tips to quench thirst.
5. Activity and exercise; increasing activity level safely, including performing warm-up and cool-down exercises when exercising aerobically; prevention of overexertion.
6. Health promotion strategies.
   a. Self-management of symptoms (dyspnea, weight gain, dizziness/lightheadedness).
   b. Risk factor modification (smoking, stress, alcohol, obesity, over-the-counter medications that may worsen HF).
   c. Follow-up management (flu shot, regular check-ups with HF team and other care providers to control other chronic conditions).
   d. Self-monitoring of blood pressure and heart rate; including when to notify provider of changes.
   e. If has an implanted cardiac device with an internal alarm or home monitor that provides alerts, take steps recommended by provider when alarm/alerts signal.
   f. If telemonitoring system that includes devices (blood pressure monitor, weight scale, blood glucose monitor, pulse oximeter, etc.), take steps recommended by health care provider when values exceed usual limits.
7. Prognosis counseling.
   a. Throughout care, discuss typical prognosis based on large multicenter clinical trials and maintain hope by reminding patients that they can control HF via self-care management strategies.
   b. Assess for common variables associated with worsening prognosis to determine timing of initiating end-of-life and palliative care discussions: Decreasing left ventricular ejection fraction, worsening NYHA-FC, degree of

hyponatremia, decreasing peak exercise oxygen uptake, decreasing hematocrit, widened QRS on 12-lead electrocardiogram, chronic hypotension, resting tachycardia, renal insufficiency, intolerance to conventional therapy, and refractory volume overload despite optimal medical therapies.

    c. When in Stage D HF: Discuss options for end-of-life care with patient and family or caregiver, provide information about the option of inactivating an implantable cardioverter defibrillator, or if patient meets criteria, discuss the possibility for a left ventricular assist device as permanent or "destination" therapy.

G. Collaboration and referrals (Heart Failure Society of America et al., 2010).

    1. Ancillary services: Nutrition, social work, pharmacy, cardiac or physical rehabilitation, case manager, home health care provider.

    2. Transition coach or case manager to provide advice and counseling and assist with navigation during care transitions, such as hospital to home, hospital to skilled nursing facility, emergency care to hospital, home health care to independent living at home, and others.

    3. Preventive cardiologist, HF specialist cardiologist, electrophysiologist cardiologist (for cardiac device placement and ongoing monitoring), palliative care medicine, endocrinologist, pulmonologist (for sleep-disordered breathing or pulmonary condition), nephrologist, psychiatrist, or psychologist.

    4. Group therapy programs (smoking cessation, stress management, relaxation, regular group office visits), HF education/social support group.

    5. Cardiothoracic surgeon for hibernating myocardium, congenital conditions requiring surgical treatment, cardiac valve disorders, dyskinesis (with aneurysm) of left ventricle after transmural (ST elevated) myocardial infarction.

H. Community resources and advocacy.

    1. Community resources for the elderly are plentiful, but most, whether led by a parish/church, community center, medical center, or other organization or group may not cater to the needs of patients with HF. For example, Meals on Wheels supplies food, but it may be high in sodium and consumption could worsen HF. Community resources offering the greatest benefit are:

    a. Phase II or III cardiac rehabilitation programs.

    b. Programs encouraging aerobic and flexibility exercises.

    c. Programs that encourage preventive services (flu vaccine, etc.).

    d. Programs that serve sodium-restricted food options.

    e. Programs that provide physical, social, or psychological support and caregiving to patients.

    f. Case management programs specific to HF should provide the following assessment and services (Heart Failure Society of America et al., 2010; Hunt et al., 2009):

        (1) Determine need for changes based on patient signs and symptoms or other objective measures (laboratory results, device or testing results).

        (2) Routine medication up-titration (to target doses based on dosages used in large, randomized clinical trials) as tolerated for ACE inhibitor/ARB and beta blocker therapy.

        (3) Addition of medications if HF is worsening: Loop or thiazide diuretic; aldosterone antagonist, ARB, and/or hydralazine/nitrate (isosorbide dinitrate).

        (4) Addition of digoxin for symptomatic, worsening HF or symptoms due to tachycardia.

        (5) Implantable cardioverter defibrillator and/or cardiac resynchronization therapy, if criteria for use are met.

(6) Regular evaluation of adherence to HF self-care practice expectations.

(7) Regular assessment of understanding of HF condition (signs and symptoms, prognosis, how to control it), therapies used to treat HF, what to monitor to determine a change in status, and the health care provider who should be notified due to a status change.

(8) Surveillance monitoring via telephone or other means (home care visit) within 48 hours following an emergency department visit, inpatient hospitalization, or new report of therapy non-adherence.

(9) In-person visit with an ambulatory health care provider within 7 days of an emergency care visit or discharge following a hospitalization to facilitate care transitions, provide education and further treatment, and develop the plan of ambulatory care.

(10) Assessment of psychosocial and economic issues: Anxiety, depression, social isolation or lack of social support, transportation issues to pharmacy or health care provider office.

(11) Assessment of personal issues related to the senses (sight, hearing) or related to obesity that limits ability to leave the home.

(12) If implantable cardiac device in place (hemodynamic monitor, cardiac resynchronization therapy, and/or implantable cardioverter defibrillator with or without internal monitoring features), regular surveillance of automatically generated data and timely surveillance of data obtained via patient transmission (due to change in status); regular consultation with electrophysiologist cardiologist team to ensure device is operating properly and/or regular consultation with cardiologist to ensure optimal medical management.

2. In ambulatory research reports of a large performance improvement program involving over 15,000 patients treated in over 165-cardiology practice sites, researchers found disparities and gaps in care regarding prescription of HF medications and warfarin for atrial fibrillation, medication dosing, and cardiac device use (Fonarow et al., 2010; Heywood et al., 2010).

3. Documentation of patient education and variables that objectively determine the need for specific HF treatments (e.g., QRS width and NYHA-FC) were missing (Fonarow et al., 2010).

4. Patient adherence to the HF plan of care may vary, creating patient-based gaps in care. A substantial number of HF deaths could potentially be prevented by optimal implementation of evidence-based therapies by health care providers and patients (Fonarow et al., 2011).

5. Managed care initiatives, such as improved quality measures, disease management programs, patient education efforts, hospital discharge checklists, pharmacy-, caregiver-, and home care nurse-led interventions to enhance adherence to medications and other self-care behaviors might be potential solutions.

6. Nurses are being called upon to facilitate the delivery of care, treatments, and services. Nurses:
   a. Can assist with development of standardized health care provider ordering practices that might minimize gaps in care and strengthen collaborative practices.
   b. Must be proactive in clearly communicating patient needs and using their experience and knowledge to coordinate the care of patients.

c.   Are stakeholders in outpatient disease management programs that transition patients from one setting to the next and need to create opportunities to optimize care based on clinical practice guidelines and evidence-based practices (Khan et al., 2008).

d.   Need to intelligently leverage clinical informatics systems to engage patients in self-care and aid health care providers in optimizing care that may decrease patient hospitalizations and improve quality of life (Haglund, 2011).

7.   Nurses have limited knowledge of advanced pathophysiology concepts (ventricular remodeling, neuroendocrine changes, effects on the vascular and end-organ systems).

8.   Nurses have limited knowledge of the hemodynamic goals of therapy.

a.   Optimized systolic blood pressure that maintains mentation, urine output, and does not cause long suffering orthostasis (dizziness and lightheadedness). An adequate systolic blood pressure may be as low as 80 mm Hg in general patients with HF or 90 mm Hg in the frail elderly, but prefer around 120 mg Hg.

b.   Optimized afterload values and definitions if using non-invasive hemodynamic monitoring to guide therapy: 800–1200 dynes/sec/cm^{-5} or use systolic blood pressure value. An ideal afterload is the lowest value that leads to an increase/maintenance of cardiac index and does *not* cause systolic blood pressure and/or renal perfusion to fall, even if cardiac index is increased.

c.   Optimized preload values and definitions if using noninvasive hemodynamic monitoring to guide therapy: Right atrial pressure of 5–8 mm Hg or 6–11 cm H_2O; right internal jugular venous pressure of less than 6–9 cm H_2O; and pulmonary artery wedge pressure of 8–15 mm Hg. An ideal pre-load is the lowest value that can be maintained without a decrease in systolic blood pressure and/or cardiac index.

d.   Optimized preload values and definitions if using invasive hemodynamic monitoring to guide therapy:

(1)   Internal pulmonary artery or left atrial pressure device values; use normal values delineated in the company's product information literature to guide ongoing assessment of status and need for ambulatory therapy changes. Note: Devices may use higher values as the normal range in an ambulatory setting to prevent hypovolemia and subsequent worsening of hemodynamic status.

(2)   Assess waveforms for actual pulmonary artery diastolic or left atrial pressure because mitral regurgitation and other cardiac or pulmonary abnormalities can falsely elevate the hemodynamic value.

9.   Nurses have limited knowledge of the pharmacologic goals of therapy; steps to reach goals, and measures to minimize and/or alleviate side effects and complications.

10.   Nurses have limited understanding and communication of HF non-pharmacologic principles related to cardiac device management and self-care.

11.   Common issues in patient management that can be overcome through advocacy:

a.   Nonaggressive treatment in managing concomitant hypertension.

b.   Nonaggressive treatment in managing hyperlipidemia.

c.   Lack of attention to obesity.

d.   Inadequate patient, family, and caregiver education.

e.   Failure to utilize implantable cardioverter defibrillator and/or cardiac resynchronization therapies, when indicated.

f. Inappropriate or non-effective treatment of HF-PEF.

g. Failure to utilize ACE inhibitor or ARB and aldosterone antagonist therapies in patients with mild renal dysfunction and normal serum potassium level.

h. Weight monitoring goals are not discussed in relation to dry weight; thus patients compare today's weight to yesterday's weight, rather than to expected weight when in an euvolemic state.

i. Lack of understanding or misunderstanding of self-management principles related to self-assessment of worsening condition.

j. Causes of patient non-adherence are unknown or are recognized but not acted on appropriately.

k. In patients with chronic coronary artery disease (three-vessel disease) and systolic dysfunction, revascularization must be considered.

l. In patients with severe mitral regurgitation and HF-REF, mitral valve repair must be considered.

m. In patients with cardiac devices (pacemaker, cardioverter defibrillator, cardiac resynchronization therapy device, or hemodynamic monitor), care coordination between electrophysiology cardiologist and clinical cardiology team is inconsistent or lacking.

n. Heart transplantation referral is delayed and severe decompensation or secondary multi-system organ failure develops.

o. Cardiac rehabilitation program or an exercise prescription is underutilized.

p. Using over-the-counter nutrients and drugs that could interfere with HF medications or worsen HF.

q. Failure to reconcile medications at every office visit, hospital admission, and hospital discharge.

r. Change in HF medical therapies by non-HF care provider without consultation or communication of the change.

s. Home health care specialty program in HF is underused in homebound patients or in patients who meet other criteria for home care.

t. Suboptimal dosing (too low or too high) of ACE inhibitor/ARB, aldosterone inhibitor, digoxin, and/or beta blocker may be based on concerns of possible side or adverse effects rather than on actual issues.

u. Underdosing of diuretics when overt or sub-clinical signs and symptoms of volume overload persist.

v. Overdosing of diuretic therapies that leads to dehydration.

w. Failure to remove medications from the patient's pharmacologic profile that are known to have deleterious effects.

x. Failure to focus on self-management instructions as part of controlling HF. Assuming that telling the patient to "call your doctor or health care provider" is adequate instruction when symptoms develop or worsen in severity.

y. Not providing prompt response and early intervention to patients or home care providers when they phone into the office with complaints or new symptoms.

z. Failure to communicate to patient, family, or caregiver whom to call when symptoms occur or worsen. Patients have multiple care providers, and symptoms of HF are often non-specific. Patients do not know whom to notify for problems.

I. Telehealth nursing considerations.
  1. Rapid response telephone practice:
     a. Priority evaluation protocols that direct the patient to an immediate emergency department visit, when necessary.
     b. Assessment of past medical history and HF history.
     c. Cardiac medication assessment, including recent changes or additions/deletions.

d. Current symptom(s) assessment, including onset and severity.

e. Treatment plans for fluid overload, hypoperfusion, and for symptoms that reflect worsening HF with or without obvious volume overload. These plans need to offer specific treatment options (i.e., additional dose of diuretic, hold ACE inhibitor) rather than just referring the patient to the emergency department or an office visit the following day.

2. Surveillance or vigilance monitoring programs:
   a. Physical and psychosocial status; current symptoms.
   b. Adherence to the pharmacologic and nonpharmacologic plan of care, including diet, fluid management, activity/exercise, and self-monitoring of signs and symptoms.

3. Patient education and counseling programs.

4. Care coordination programs that include optimal care navigation during periods of care transitions.

J. Protocol/algorithms/guidelines (Fonarow et al., 2007; Heart Failure Society of America et al., 2010; Hunt et al., 2009).
   1. Pharmacologic therapy algorithms for ACE inhibitor/ARB, beta blocker, diuretic, digoxin, hydralazine, nitrates, and aldosterone antagonists.
      a. Initiation and up-titration schedules (see Table 21-11).
      b. Serum electrolyte, vital signs, and monitoring of adverse effects.
   2. Decision tree based on clinical severity of symptoms (mild, moderate, or severe).
   3. Device therapy algorithms for cardiac resynchronization therapy, implantable cardioverter defibrillator, and implantable hemodynamic monitor.
   4. How to treat persistent:
      a. Volume overload.
      b. Dyspnea.
      c. Hypertension.
      d. Concomitant angina.
      e. Concomitant atrial fibrillation.

f. Hypotension.

g. Alert values of internal cardiac monitoring or telemonitoring devices.

5. Education.
   a. HF cause, signs/symptoms, chronicity, prognosis, and ways it can be controlled.
   b. Self-care actions.
   c. Who to call for symptoms/issues.
   d. Appointment follow-up expectations.

6. Surveillance/adherence monitoring questionnaire or system.

7. Patient-initiated communication (rapid-response program) algorithm regarding treatment options based on current symptoms or signs.

8. Multidisciplinary consultation and support group expectations (i.e., aggressive home care HF program).

9. When to consult a HF specialist.

10. When a patient should be directly hospitalized; when hospitalized, placement on a routine floor versus intermediate care versus critical care environment.

11. End-of-life issues and guidelines (Goodlin, 2009).

Chronic Obstructive Pulmonary Disease (COPD)

Patient Population: Adult

I. **Overview**

Chronic obstructive pulmonary disease (COPD) is a major cause of morbidity and mortality in the adult patient population. Like many other chronic conditions, it is virtually irreversible and may require frequent office visits for ongoing management as well as hospitalization for acute exacerbations. COPD is the leading cause of morbidity and mortality worldwide and is projected to rank fifth worldwide in terms of disease burden (Global Initiative for Chronic Obstructive Lung Disease [GOLD], 2011). Despite being preventable, an estimated 64 million people worldwide have COPD (World Health Organization [WHO], 2011). While the overall prevalence rates for COPD have not changed considerably from 1998–2009, rates are higher and have grown among women when compared to men. Increased degrees of smoking among women are felt to be contributing to this increased rate. From 2007–2009, approximately 6.1% (7.4 million) of women in the United States had COPD compared to 4.1% (4.4 million) men (Akinbami & Liu, 2011). Chronic Lower Respiratory Disease (CLRD), COPD, and asthma combined was the third leading cause of death in the United States in 2008 (Akinbami & Liu, 2011). The costs of this disease are not only those associated with health care (physician office and emergency department visits and hospitalizations) and premature death, but also indirect costs due to lost working days. In the United States, the direct cost of COPD is $29.5 billion and indirect cost is $20.4 billion (GOLD, 2011).

COPD is a preventable and treatable lung disease characterized by persistent and progressive airflow limitation, chronic inflammation, and structural airway changes resulting in gas exchange abnormalities. Cigarette smoking is the most common risk factor for COPD (GOLD, 2011). Occupational exposures and indoor air pollution such as dust particles, chemical agents, and noxious fumes are additional risk factors for COPD. Asthma may be a risk factor for developing COPD, but evidence is not conclusive (GOLD, 2011). Smoking cessation and prevention efforts, as well as mitigation of occupational exposures through the use of personal protective equipment, must continue to be reinforced across all age groups within our communities. COPD is a major public health concern, greatly affecting large numbers of people. Effective strategies must continue to be implemented to minimize the effects of this chronic disease and aid quality of life.

In 1998, the United States National Heart, Lung, and Blood Institute (NHBLI) and the World Health Organization (WHO) formed the Global Initiative for Chronic Obstructive Lung Disease (GOLD, 2011). With a primary goal of increasing awareness of this chronic disease, in 2001, an expert panel published and widely disseminated a consensus report, *Global Strategy for the Diagnosis, Management, and Prevention of COPD*. Many of the recommendations continue to be implemented by national and international experts. The most recent GOLD report (2011) defines COPD as "a preventable and treatable disease characterized

by persistent airflow limitation, usually progressive in nature and associated with an enhanced chronic inflammatory response in the airways and the lungs to noxious particles or gases" (p. 2).

II. Pathophysiology

The chronic inflammation and structural changes appreciated in COPD are the result of recurring injury and repair in the lungs and airways. Inflammation and structural changes in the airways increase with the severity of the disease (GOLD, 2011). A narrowing of the peripheral airways takes place leading to a decrease in FEV_1. Emphysema, a type of COPD characterized by the abnormal destruction of the alveoli, contributes to airflow limitation, decreased gas exchange, and CO_2 retention (Pauwels & Rabe, 2004). Some patients may experience increased mucus secretion resulting in a chronic cough. Pulmonary hypertension is frequently noted in advanced stages of COPD due to hypoxic vasoconstriction of the small pulmonary arteries (GOLD, 2011). Asthma is the clinical disease that most often mimics COPD. Differences in COPD and asthma are in inflammatory cells and mediators, resultant physiologic response, and symptom response to therapy (GOLD, 2011). The reversibility of the airflow limitation is the key diagnostic criteria. Asthma is further described in another section in this chapter. Co-morbidities of COPD include heart failure, ischemic heart disease, diabetes, metabolic syndrome, osteoporosis, and depression. Individuals with alpha-1 antitrypsin (AAT) deficiency, a genetic abnormality, have a greater predisposition for developing COPD, especially if they smoke.

III. Assessment, Screening, and Triage (GOLD, 2011)
A. Medical history.
   1. Exposure to risk factors.
     a. Smoking history.
     b. Occupational exposures.
     c. Environmental exposures.
   2. Past medical history (GOLD, 2011).
     a. COPD.
     b. Other chronic respiratory diseases.
     c. Symptom development.
       (1) Pattern of symptom development.
       (2) History of exacerbations.

   (3) Previous hospitalizations for respiratory disorders.

   (4) Presence of co-morbidities.

  d. Impact of COPD on quality of life.

   (1) Limitation of activity.

   (2) Missed working days.

   (3) Depression.

   (4) Anxiety.

  e. Social and family support.

  f. Risk factor reduction.

B. Spirometry (GOLD, 2011).

 1. Required to establish a diagnosis of COPD.

 2. Used to measure forced vital capacity (FVC), forced expiratory volume in one second (FEV_1) and FEV_1/FVC ratios (requires calculation).

 3. Frequently used in conjunction with bronchodilators.

  a. Forced vital capacity (FVC).

  b. Forced expiratory volume (FEV_1).

  c. Ratio measurements (FEV_1/FVC).

 4. Presence of a post-bronchodilator FEV_1/FVC less than 0.70 confirms the presence of persistent airflow limitation, evident of COPD.

 5. Considered the gold standard for diagnosis of COPD.

 6. Useful for evaluating the effectiveness of drug interventions, progress of rehabilitation, and health status or stage of COPD.

C. Assessment of symptoms (GOLD, 2011).

 1. Modified British Medical Research Council (mMrc) Questionnaire – Used to assess disability due to breathlessness.

 2. COPD Assessment Test (CAT) – Used to measure health status and disease impact on daily life.

 3. Dyspnea/shortness of breath.

 4. Cough.

 5. Amount of sputum production.

 6. Wheezing and/or chest tightness.

 7. Fatigue.

 8. Weight loss.

 9. Anorexia.

D. GOLD Spirometric COPD Classification by Severity (GOLD, 2011).

 1. COPD may be diagnosed at any stage.

 2. Defined on the basis of airflow limitation; spirometric assessment. In patients with $FEV_1/FVC < 0.70$:

  a. GOLD 1: Mild – FEV_1 80% or greater predicted.

  b. GOLD 2: Moderate – 50% less than or equal to FEV_1 less than 80% predicted.

  c. GOLD 3: Severe – 30% less than or equal to FEV_1 less than 50% predicted.

  d. GOLD 4: Very Severe – Less than or equal to FEV_1 less than 30% predicted.

E. Assessment of co-morbidities (GOLD, 2011).

 1. Cardiovascular disease.

 2. Ischemic heart disease.

 3. Heart failure.

 4. Atrial fibrillation.

 5. Hypertension.

 6. Cor pulmonale with right side heart failure and edema.

 7. Osteoporosis.

 8. Lung cancer.

 9. Infection.

F. Assessment in late stages of COPD (GOLD, 2011).

 1. Increased weight loss.

 2. Poor nutritional status.

 3. Skeletal muscle loss.

 4. Inactivity and/or poor exercise tolerance.

 5. Hypoxia with cyanosis.

 6. Hypercapnia with severe hypoxemia (end stage).

 7. Hemoptysis.

G. Differential diagnosis (GOLD, 2011).

 1. Asthma.

 2. Tuberculosis.

 3. Heart failure, pulmonary edema.

 4. Bronchiectasis.

H. Functional status (American Thoracic Society [ATS], 2002).

 1. Evaluate all aspects of health.

  a. Physical.

  b. Social.

  c. Emotional conditions.

 2. Assess and monitor health-related quality of life (HRQL) and the impact of symptom severity on daily life.

3. Utilize standardized methods and instruments to measure and evaluate functional status.
4. Results are useful for evaluating response to medical intervention; may serve as predictors of morbidity and mortality in COPD.
    a. Six-Minute Walk Distance/Six-Minute Walk Test (6MWD/6MWT) – Measures functional exercise performance status (ATS, 2002).
    b. Functional Performance Inventory (FPI) – 65-item questionnaire to measure 6 subscales: Body care, household maintenance, physical exercise, recreation, spiritual activities, and social activities.
    c. St. George's Respiratory Questionnaire – 76-item questionnaire to measure three domains: Symptoms, activity, and impact of COPD.
    d. Chronic Respiratory Questionnaire (CRQ) – Interview-based instrument to measure physical and emotional aspects of COPD.
    e. COPD Activity Rating Scale (CARS) – Measures life-related activity across four domains: Self-care, domestic, outdoor, and social interaction activities.
    f. Seattle Obstructive Lung Disorder Questionnaire – 29-item questionnaire to measure 4 domains: Physical functioning, emotional functioning, coping skills, and treatment satisfaction.
I. Physical examination (Stephens & Yew, 2008).
    1. Many patients have normal findings with no physical evidence of disease in early stages.
    2. Widened anteroposterior chest diameter.
    3. Hyperresonance on percussion.
    4. Diminished breath sounds.
    5. Cor pulmonale.
        a. Right ventricular failure often seen in later stages of COPD.
        b. Commonly known as right-sided heart failure.
        c. Results from right ventricular hypertrophy caused by progressive pulmonary hypertension and increased pressure in the pulmonary circulation.
            (1) Accentuated second heart sound.
            (2) Peripheral edema.
            (3) Jugular venous distention.
            (4) Hepatomegaly.
    6. Advanced disease.
        a. Use of accessory respiratory muscles; inspiratory retraction of the lower ribs (Hoover's sign).
        b. Paradoxical abdominal movement.
        c. Increased expiratory time.
        d. Pursed lip breathing.
J. Laboratory/radiology (GOLD, 2011; Stephens & Yew, 2008).
    1. Chest radiography, although seldom diagnostic in COPD, may show:
        a. Hyperinflation of the lungs.
        b. Hyperlucency of the lungs.
        c. Rapid tapering of the vascular markings.
    2. Computed tomography (CT), although not routinely recommended, may be performed to assist in differential diagnoses.
    3. Lung volumes and diffusing capacity.
        a. Gas trapping (increased residual volume).
        b. Increased airflow limitation; static hyperinflation (increased total lung capacity).
    4. Oximetry and arterial blood gas measurement.
    5. Electrocardiography/echocardiography for evaluation of pulmonary circulatory pressures, when cor pulmonale is co-morbid.
    6. Alpha-1 antitrypsin deficiency screening.
    7. Exercise testing – Walking tests (6-minute/paced shuttle).

IV. **Indications for Emergency Care or Urgent Consultation**
(GOLD, 2011)
A. Development of sudden resting dyspnea.
B. New onset of cyanosis or peripheral edema.
C. Inability to breathe, acute respiratory failure.

V. Plan of Care

(GOLD, 2011)

A. Reduction of exposure.
   1. Smoking cessation counseling at each encounter, and intervention based on patient readiness and preference.
   2. Smoking cessation nicotine replacement. Nicotine replacement available as:
      a. Gum.
      b. Inhaler.
      c. Nasal spray.
      d. Transdermal patch.
      e. Sublingual tablet.
      f. Lozenge.
   3. Contraindications to nicotine replacement.
      a. Unstable coronary artery disease.
      b. Untreated peptic ulcer disease.
      c. Recent MI.
      d. Stroke.
   4. Reduction in occupational exposure.
   5. Reduction in indoor/outdoor air pollution.
   6. Physical activity.
   7. Pulmonary rehabilitation as indicated based on severity classification.
   8. Influenza and pneumococcal vaccination.
B. Pharmacotherapeutics (GOLD, 2011).
   1. Pharmacologic therapy in stable COPD is used to:
      a. Reduce symptoms.
      b. Reduce frequency and severity of exacerbations.
      c. Improve health status.
      d. Improve exercise tolerance.
   2. Pharmacologic therapy is patient-specific and dependent on:
      a. Symptom severity.
      b. Severity of exacerbations.
      c. Patient's response to therapy.
   3. Bronchodilators.
      a. Increase FEV_1.
      b. Change spirometric variables by altering smooth muscle tone to improve emptying of the lungs.
      c. Given as needed or on a regular basis to prevent or reduce symptoms.
   4. Beta$_2$ agonists (short-acting and long-acting).
      a. Relax smooth muscle airway by stimulating beta$_2$ adrenergic receptors.
      b. Improve FEV_1.
      c. May be available as inhaler, solution for nebulizer, oral.
      d. Short-acting: Wear off within 4–6 hours.
         (1) Fenoterol.
         (2) Levalbuterol.
         (3) Salbutamol (albuterol).
         (4) Terbutaline.
      e. Long-acting: Duration of 12 or more hours.
         (1) Formoterol.
         (2) Arformoterol.
         (3) Indacterol.
         (4) Salmeterol.
         (5) Tulobuterol.
      f. Adverse effects.
         (1) Resting sinus tachycardia.
         (2) Changes in oxygen consumption; decreased PaO_2.
   5. Anticholinergics (short-acting and long-acting).
      a. Blockage of acetylcholine effect on muscarinic receptors.
      b. Short-acting duration of up to 8 hours.
         (1) Ipratropium bromide.
         (2) Oxitropium bromide.
      c. Long-acting duration of more than 24 hours.
         (1) Tiotropium.
      d. Adverse effects.
         (1) Poorly absorbed.
         (2) Mouth dryness.
   6. Methylxanthines.
      a. Effects are controversial; may have non-bronchodilator actions.
      b. Little to no data on duration of action.
      c. Most common is theophylline.
      d. Adverse effects.
         (1) Toxicity.
         (2) Atrial and ventricular arrhythmias.
         (3) Headache.
         (4) Insomnia.
         (5) Nausea.
         (6) Grand mal convulsions.

(7) Drug interactions with digitalis, warfarin.
7. Corticosteroids.
    a. Inhaled corticosteroids.
        (1) Improves symptoms and lung function.
        (2) Reduces frequency of exacerbations in COPD patients with FEV_1 less than 60% predicted.
        (3) Long-term safety in COPD is not known.
        (4) Efficacy and side effects are dependent on dose and type.
        (5) Use in COPD is limited to specific indications.
            (a) Beclomethasone.
            (b) Budesonide.
            (c) Fluticasone.
        (6) May be combined with long-acting $beta_2$ agonist.
            (a) Formeterol/budesonide.
            (b) Salmeterol/fluticasone.
    b. Systemic corticosteroids – Long-term treatment contributes to steroid myopathy and adverse effects.
        (1) Muscle weakness.
        (2) Decreased functionality.
        (3) Respiratory failure.
8. Phosphodiestrase-4 inhibitors.
    a. Reduce inflammation by inhibiting breakdown of intracellular AMP.
    b. Approved for use only in some countries.
9. Vaccines.
    a. Pneumococcal vaccine.
        (1) COPD patients 65 and older.
        (2) Under age 65 with an FEV_1 less than 40% predicted.
    b. Influenza vaccination annually.
10. Antibiotics.
    a. Little to no effect on frequency of COPD exacerbations.
    b. Used to treat infectious bacterial exacerbations of COPD.
11. Mucolytic agents.
    a. Limited benefit.
    b. Widespread use not recommended.

C. Primary/secondary/tertiary prevention.
1. Primary prevention.
    a. Risk factor identification.
        (1) Tobacco smoke.
        (2) Secondhand smoke.
        (3) Air pollution.
        (4) Hyperreactive airway.
        (5) Occupational exposures to industrial pollutants.
        (6) Alpha 1-antitrypsin deficiency.
    b. Education programs.
        (1) American Lung Association.
        (2) National Heart, Lung, and Blood Institute's (NHLBI, n.d.) COPD Awareness and Education Campaign.
        (3) World Health Organization (WHO).
2. Secondary prevention.
    a. Smoking cessation, which may include one or more of the following methods:
        (1) Acupuncture.
        (2) Group programs.
        (3) Pharmacologic therapy (nicotine replacement, antidepressants).
        (4) Hypnosis.
        (5) Herbal therapy.
        (6) Pharmacologic therapy – As described above.
3. Tertiary prevention (Mannino & Buist, 2007).
    a. Prevention of complications in patients with established COPD.
    b. Ongoing monitoring and assessment.
        (1) Level of ongoing exposure to risk factors.
        (2) Disease progression.
        (3) Development of complications.
    c. Pulmonary rehabilitation.
        (1) Patient selection criteria should include: Functional status, severity of dyspnea, motivation, and smoking status.
        (2) Exercise training may improve exercise tolerance and symptoms of dyspnea and fatigue.
        (3) Breathing retraining.
        (4) Nutrition counseling.
        (5) Mobilization of secretions.

D. Surgical treatments.
1. Bullectomy.
2. Lung volume reduction surgery (LVRS).
3. Lung transplantation.
E. Goals of plan of care (outcomes desired).
1. Improved exercise tolerance.
2. Decreased dyspnea.
3. Decreased anxiety/depression.
4. Improved quality of life and functional status.
5. Decreased health care utilization.
6. Longer life.
F. Psychosocial considerations.
1. Progressive debilitation.
2. Loss of functional status.
3. Depression.
4. Inability to perform ADL.
5. Financial burden.
6. Emotional impact on family and personal relationships.
G. Patient/family education.
1. Smoking cessation.
2. Disease process and pathophysiology.
3. Adherence to medication.
4. Mobilization of secretions.
5. Prevention and treatment of infection.
6. Early recognition and seeking of care for acute exacerbation.
7. Advance directives.
8. Self-management and behavior/lifestyle modification.
H. Collaboration/consultation and referrals.
1. Primary care physician/nurse practitioner.
2. Pulmonologist.
3. Cardiologist.
4. Thoracic surgeon.
5. Respiratory therapist.
6. Home care nurse.
7. Nutrition counselor.
8. Home equipment and oxygen supplier.
I. Clinical guidelines/protocol development/usage.
1. Smoking cessation.
2. Pharmacologic therapy.
3. Indications for long-term oxygen therapy.
4. Indications for emergency room evaluation and/or hospitalization for acute exacerbation of COPD.

5. Management of the preoperative patient with COPD – Criteria for lung volume reduction surgery, lung transplantation, and pulmonary rehabilitation.

Human Immunodeficiency Virus (HIV)

Patient Population: Adult and Adolescent

I. **Overview**

Human immunodeficiency virus (HIV) is a retrovirus that uses the body's CD4+ T-lymphocytes to replicate. CD4 T-lymphocytes are specialized cells of the body's immune system. By using CD4 cells to replicate, HIV weakens the body's immune system; making the body more susceptible to a variety of serious and potentially life-threatening illnesses and infections. According to the Centers for Disease Control and Prevention (CDC), by the end of 2008, more than one million people were living with HIV (CDC, 2011). The most current incidence figures from 2009 estimate that more than 48,000 new infections occur each year – a figure that has remained stable since the late 1990s (CDC, 2011).

The case definition of HIV has undergone several revisions since the emergence of the disease in 1981, primarily in response to diagnostic and therapeutic advances. Revisions are necessary to improve standardization and comparability of surveillance data. In 2008, the CDC, in cooperation with the Council of State and Territorial Epidemiologists (CSTE), revised the case definition of HIV, requiring laboratory evidence of HIV infection (Schneider et al., 2008). Prior to 2008, for the purposes of surveillance, diagnostic confirmation of an acquired immune deficiency syndrome (AIDS) defining illness was all that was required to make an HIV diagnosis (Schneider et al., 2008). While the new case definition guidelines require laboratory confirmation to make an HIV diagnosis, the case definition for AIDS, as well as the definition of the stages of illness, has remained unchanged.

One cannot discuss HIV without discussing AIDS. Many people equate HIV with AIDS, when in actuality they are two different things. AIDS is defined as a collection of infections and illnesses that attack an immune system weakened by HIV. In other words, those infections and illnesses said to be "AIDS defining" are considered opportunistic infections, because they take advantage of a weakened immune system. While HIV does weaken the body's immune system, it is the opportunistic infections that make a person sick (Cichocki, 2011).

A. While everyone is potentially at risk for HIV infection, there are certain populations considered to be at higher risk (Kane, 2008).
  1. Men who have sex with men (MSM) – 56% of all new infections.
  2. African American MSM (ages 13–29) – Twice as likely to be infected compared to White and Hispanic MSM of the same age.
  3. African American women – 15 times more likely to be infected compared to White women and 4 times more likely than Hispanic women.
  4. White MSM (ages 29–49) – The population most affected by HIV.
B. According to Dr. Kevin Fenton, Director of the National Center for HIV/AIDS, Viral Hepatitis, STD, and TB Prevention at the CDC, data from the highest risk populations provide experts with three very important pieces of information (Kane, 2008).
  1. The number of new infections among African American MSM ages 13–29 shows the need to provide HIV prevention education earlier in life.
  2. The infection rate among White MSM ages 29–49 shows the need for ongoing HIV prevention education over the course of the entire adult lifetime.
  3. Compared to women of all races, African American women bear the heaviest burden of HIV.
C. The original CDC definition of AIDS was developed in 1986, but was revised to the current definition in 1993.
D. The revised definition categorizes people on the basis of clinical conditions associated with HIV infection and CD4+ T-lymphocyte counts. The system of diagnosing someone with AIDS is based on three ranges of CD4+ T-lymphocytes and three clinical categories:
  1. CD4+ T-lymphocyte Categories (Castro et al., 1992).
    a. Category 1: Greater than or equal to 500 cells per microliter of blood (cells/μL).
    b. Category 2: 200-499 cells/μL.
    c. Category 3: Less than 200 cells/μL (AIDS diagnosis).
  2. Clinical categories (Castro et al., 1992).
    a. Category A – Consists of one or more of the following conditions. Conditions listed in Category B and C must have never occurred.
      (1) Asymptomatic HIV infection.
      (2) Persistent generalized lymphadenopathy.
      (3) Acute HIV infection with accompanying illness or history of acute HIV infection.
    b. Category B – Consists of symptomatic conditions in HIV that are not included in Category C and that meet the following criteria. Note, Category B conditions take precedence over those in Category A. In other words, once a person is treated for a Category B condition, that person is classified in Category B even if they become asymptomatic later.
      (1) Conditions are attributed to HIV or are indicative of a defect of cell-mediated immunity.
      (2) Conditions are considered to have a clinical course or require management that is accompanied by HIV infection.
      (3) Examples of conditions in Category B include:
        (a) Bacillary angiomatosis – The vascular proliferative form of bartonella infection; a bacteria often associated with cat bites and scratches.
        (b) Oral candidiasis (thrush).
        (c) Persistent vaginal candidiasis that responds poorly to treatment.
        (d) Cervical dysplasia (moderate or severe)/cervical carcinoma in situ.
        (e) Fever (38.5 °C and above) or diarrhea lasting greater than 1 month.

(f) Oral hairy leukoplakia (OHL) – A disease of the oral mucosa related to the Epstein-Barr virus. Because of the "fuzzy" appearance of OHL, it is often referred to as "black hairy tongue."

(g) Herpes zoster (shingles), involving at least two distinct episodes or more than one dermatome.

(h) Idiopathic thrombocytopenic purpura (ITP) – A disease of peripheral platelet destruction resulting in a low serum platelet count.

(i) Listeriosis – Infection caused by the bacteria known as *Listeria monocytogenes.*

(j) Pelvic inflammatory disease, particularly if complicated by tubo-ovarian abscess.

(k) Peripheral neuropathy.

c. Category C – Includes those conditions considered to be AIDS defining.

(1) Once a Category C condition occurs, the person remains in Category C regardless of future clinical conditions.

(2) Category C conditions include:

(a) Candidiasis of esophagus, bronchi, trachea, or lungs.

(b) Cervical cancer, invasive.

(c) Coccidioidomycosis, disseminated or extrapulmonary.

(d) Cryptococcosis, extrapulmonary.

(e) Cryptosporidiosis, chronic intestinal (greater than one month's duration).

(f) Cytomegalovirus disease (other than liver, spleen, or nodes).

(g) Cytomegalovirus retinitis (with loss of vision).

(h) Encephalopathy, HIV-related.

(i) Herpes simplex: Chronic ulcer(s) (greater than one month's duration); or resulting in bronchitis, pneumonitis, or esophagitis.

(j) Histoplasmosis, disseminated or extrapulmonary.

(k) Isosporiasis, chronic intestinal (greater than one month's duration).

(l) Kaposi's sarcoma.

(m) Lymphoma, Burkitt's.

(n) Lymphoma, immunoblastic.

(o) Lymphoma, primary, involving the brain.

(p) *Mycobacterium avium* complex (MAC) or *M. kansasii,* disseminated or extrapulmonary mycobacterium tuberculosis, any site (pulmonary or extrapulmonary).

(q) *Mycobacterium,* other species or unidentified species, disseminated or extrapulmonary.

(r) *Pneumocystis jeroveci (carinii)* pneumonia (PCP pneumonia).

(s) Pneumonia, recurrent.

(t) Progressive multifocal leukoencephalopathy (PML).

(u) Salmonella septicemia, recurrent.

(v) Toxoplasmosis of brain.

(w) Wasting syndrome due to HIV.

E. HIV staging/summary.

1. A person is classified or diagnosed with AIDS if he or she is HIV-infected and falls in one of these two groups:

a. Has a CD4+ T-lymphocyte count that is less than 200 cells/μL (or CD4 percentage less than 14%).

b. Has been diagnosed with one of the Category C conditions.

2. Once a person has been AIDS diagnosed, the AIDS diagnosis remains regardless of future medical conditions or CD4+ T-lymphocyte counts.

II. Testing and Early Diagnosis

The keys to slowing the spread of HIV are testing and early diagnosis. These two concepts are important for several reasons (CDC, 2009).

A. Of more than one million people living with HIV, it is estimated that 21% are unaware of their infection. That number is even higher in certain populations. For instance, about 50% of adolescents and 80% of men who have sex with men are unaware of their HIV infection (Rotheram-Borus & Futterman, 2000).

    1. Early identification of HIV infection enables people to get into care sooner; improving health outcomes, which in turn translates to longer, healthier lives.

    2. Studies show that people who are aware of their HIV infection are far less likely to have unprotected sex than those unaware of their infection (Marks, Crepaz, Senterfitt, & Janssen, 2005).

    3. HIV testing provides an opportunity to teach people how to protect themselves and their sexual partners from HIV and sexually transmitted diseases.

B. Diagnosis – HIV antibody tests.

After being infected, the body produces protective antibodies to combat HIV. There are a number of HIV screening tests that detect those HIV antibodies and, in doing so, diagnose an HIV infection (University of California – San Francisco [UCSF] 2011).

    1. The enzyme-linked immunosorbent assay (ELISA), sometimes called the enzyme immunoassay (EIA), detects HIV antibodies produced by the body.

    2. The ELISA test can use three different types of bodily fluids to test for HIV antibodies.

        a. Blood – Acquired by way of venipuncture, blood is the most common testing method.

        b. Oral fluid.

            (1) Specifically, the fluid and cells found on the inner aspect of the cheek are tested; saliva is not a testing medium for HIV antibodies.

            (2) A swab is placed in the mouth, resting between the cheek and the gum. Fluid and cheek cells are absorbed into the Dacron tip of the swab. The swab is then sent to a laboratory for testing.

            (3) This test is slightly less sensitive than testing blood.

        c. Urine – Sample may be stored at room temperature.

    3. The ELISA test is very sensitive to antibodies, assuring no antibodies are missed. However, the increased sensitivity does lead to some false positive tests. For that reason, every positive ELISA test needs a confirmatory test before a diagnosis of HIV infection can be made. While rare, false negative tests can occur during the "window period" of infection when the body has yet to produce enough antibodies to be detected by the ELISA or Western Blot test.

    4. HIV confirmatory tests.

        a. Western Blot.

            (1) Individual HIV proteins are separated by electrophoresis and transferred to nitrocellulose paper.

            (2) Those proteins are then exposed to the test subject's serum.

            (3) Any HIV antibodies present in the serum react with the HIV proteins on the paper, causing a colored band to form.

            (4) The presence of two or more bands (from p24, gp41, gp120, or gp160) confers a positive Western Blot and, therefore, a positive HIV test (Bebell et al., 2010).

        b. Indirect Fluorescent Antibody (IFA) – Detects HIV antibodies and confirms the results of an ELISA test, but is more expensive than a Western Blot test.

        c. HIV viral load measurement.

            (1) Commonly known as a "viral load," a "PCR," or an "RNA" test.

            (2) The viral load measurement detects HIV genetic material (viral RNA) as opposed to HIV antibodies.

(3) The presence of HIV RNA confirms the ELISA and, therefore, a positive HIV test (UCSF, 2011).

III. Assessment/Screening/Triage

A. History.
1. Screen for high-risk behavior.
   a. Unprotected/unsafe sex.
      (1) Men having sex with other men.
      (2) Vaginal intercourse.
      (3) Receptive anal intercourse (male and female).
      (4) Oral sex.
   b. Sex with multiple anonymous partners.
   c. Using drugs and/or alcohol during sex.
   d. Exchanging sex for money or drugs.
   e. Sharing needles.
      (1) Recreational drugs (e.g., heroin).
      (2) Prescription drugs (e.g., insulin, testosterone).
      (3) Homemade/prison tattoos.
   f. The presence of other sexually transmitted diseases:
      (1) Indicates high-risk sexual behavior (Aberg et al., 2009).
      (2) Syphilis/gonorrhea/Chlamydia.
      (3) Increases the risk of HIV infection (Aberg et al., 2009).
2. Acute HIV syndrome/flu-like symptoms.
   a. During this initial period of HIV infection (about 1–4 weeks after exposure), the body's immune system is caught "off guard," allowing HIV replication to go essentially unchecked.
   b. As the amount of active virus rises, symptoms similar to those of influenza or mononucleosis can occur.
      (1) Fever.
      (2) Malaise.
      (3) Fatigue.
      (4) Body aches/muscle stiffness.
      (5) Headache.
      (6) Sore throat.
   c. Because symptoms mimic other viral illnesses, a diagnosis of HIV infection is often missed.
   d. The patient is diagnosed with what he or she believes is a common viral illness, when in actuality it is the beginning phases of an HIV infection (Cichocki, 2011).
   e. Other symptoms of new infection.
      (1) Decreased appetite/weight loss.
      (2) Rash.
      (3) Swollen lymph nodes (lymphadenopathy).
      (4) Ulcers in the mouth and esophagus.
3. Aspects of a detailed sexual history (Cichocki, 2008).
   a. Sexually active?
   b. Sexual partners – Men/women/both.
   c. Number of partners in the past month; six months; lifetime.
   d. Engage in unsafe sex?
   e. Engage in anal sex?
   f. Drug use to enhance sexual pleasure?
   g. Diagnosed with sexually transmitted diseases?
   h. Exchanged sex for money or drugs?
   i. Sexual partners diagnosed with HIV?
   j. Sexual partners who engage in high-risk behavior?

B. Physical examination.
1. History of present illness (Aberg et al., 2009).
   a. Date of diagnosis (date of positive test).
   b. Approximate date of infection (initial exposure).
   c. Last negative HIV test.
   d. Previous HIV medications regimens.
   e. Lowest CD4 count and highest viral load.
   f. Access to old medical records.
2. Past medical history.
   a. Current prescription and over-the-counter medications, including the use of herbal remedies, vitamins, and supplements.
   b. Allergies to food, medicines, or environment.
   c. Current/past alcohol, tobacco, or substance use.

d. Past medical/surgical history.
e. History of current or past mental health issues.
3. Current or recent symptoms.
   a. Cough, dry or productive.
   b. Chest pain/shortness of breath.
   c. Head/nasal/chest congestion.
   d. Fever.
   e. Night sweats.
   f. Weight loss (compare current weight to typical weight).
   g. Headaches/visual changes/worsening vision.
   h. Visual changes.
   i. Oral candida (thrush) or ulceration.
   j. Difficulty swallowing.
   k. Diarrhea.
   l. Skin rashes or lesions.
   m. Changes in mental status and neurological function.
4. Nutritional/dietary assessment.
   a. Problems chewing or swallowing.
   b. Painful mouth/teeth.
   c. Poor appetite.
   d. Ability to obtain, prepare, and store food.
   e. Typical diet and types of food eaten regularly.
   f. Vitamins or supplements used.
5. Women – Menstrual/reproductive history.
   a. Last menstrual period.
   b. Number of pregnancies, live births, miscarriages, and abortions.
   c. Any HIV-positive children.
   d. Any plans for pregnancy.
   e. Prenatal care.
6. Social/family/financial.
   a. Employed.
   b. Insured/drug coverage.
   c. Family structure.
   d. Family awareness of diagnosis.
   e. Support system.
C. Baseline laboratory data.
   1. HIV antibody test.
   2. HIV genotype.
   3. CD4 count and viral load.
   4. CBC.
   5. Electrolytes.

6. Liver function tests (LFTs).
7. Cholesterol panel.
8. Hepatitis A, B, and C status (hepatitis A and B antigen and antibody; hepatitis C antibody).
9. Toxoplasmosis, cytomegalovirus, and varicella titers.
10. Rapid plasma reagin (syphilis test).
D. Other screenings.
   1. Tuberculosis screening – PPD skin test is preferable over QuantiFERON® Gold Blood Test (QFTB).
   2. Colonoscopy.
   3. Men – Rectal exams, prostate exam, prostate-specific antigen (PSA), rectal Paps.
   4. Women – Pap, mammogram.
   5. Annual dental, mental health, and nutritional screenings.
E. Vaccinations/immunizations.
   1. As a general rule, HIV-positive patients should not receive live virus vaccines unless absolutely necessary and unless CD4 T-lymphocyte count ≥ 200 cells/μL. Live virus vaccines include varicella, herpes zoster, and Measles Mumps Rubella (MMR) vaccines, as well as the live attenuated influenza vaccine (nasal mist). HIV-positive patients who are travelling abroad should be aware that Yellow Fever Vaccine is a live vaccine, as is the oral typhoid vaccine. Other live vaccines include the anthrax vaccine and the smallpox vaccine. People with a CD4 count less than 200 cells/mm³ may not have an antibody response adequate enough to confer protection, meaning the vaccine could cause illness (CDC, 2009).
   2. Other vaccinations/immunizations are recommended, unless patient has history of adequate immunization coverage.
      a. Hepatitis A.
         (1) Two injections 6 months to 1 year apart.
         (2) Series can be repeated at double the dose if there is no antibody response.

b. Hepatitis B.
    (1) Three injections: The 1ˢᵗ on day 0, the 2ⁿᵈ one month later, and the 3ʳᵈ five months after dose 2.
    (2) The series can be repeated at double the dose if there is no antibody response.
c. Hepatitis A/hepatitis B combination (Twinrix®).
    (1) Can be used in place of vaccinating for hepatitis A and B separately.
    (2) This vaccine is given on the same schedule as the hepatitis B vaccine.
d. Influenza.
    (1) One dose given each year when the seasonal influenza vaccine is released (can vary from year to year).
    (2) HIV-positive people should only get the injectable influenza vaccine not the nasal mist vaccine.
e. Pneumococcal (Pneumovax®) – Series consists of 2 injections about 5 years apart.
f. Tetanus, diphtheria, and acellular pertussis (Tdap) – Given to patients ages 64 and younger; one adult dose should be given instead of the Tetanus diphtheria (Td) booster vaccine alone in people with HIV.
g. Human papillomavirus (HPV).
    (1) Ideally this vaccine should be given before a person is sexually active, typically around 11- or 12-years-old.
    (2) Catch-up vaccination can be done in females ages 13–26 to reduce the risk of cervical cancer and in males ages 9–26 to prevent genital warts (CDC, 2012).

IV. Indications for Emergency Care or Urgent Referral

A. Notify HIV provider:
    1. Frequent vomiting and/or diarrhea that could lead to dehydration.
    2. Worsening abdominal pain that could signal an intestinal infection, hepatitis, or pancreatitis.
    3. Fever of any duration greater than 100.5 °F orally.
    4. Worsening vision, blurred vision, or changes in vision.
    5. Weight loss and/or poor appetite.
    6. Sore throat and/or difficulty swallowing.
    7. White patches in mouth (on tongue, gums, or inside cheeks).
    8. Chest congestion and/or cough with or without difficulty breathing.
    9. Any rash, but especially after starting a new medication regimen or after starting Bactrim®.
    10. Dark urine and/or yellowing of sclera.
B. Go to emergency room:
    1. Chest, jaw, neck, or left arm pain.
    2. Shortness of breath or difficulty breathing.
    3. Sudden onset headache, weakness, or paralysis on one side of body, speech difficulty, mental status changes, loss of consciousness, or visual changes such as double or loss of vision.
    4. Uncontrolled bleeding from the nose, from the urinary tract, from the vagina, or from the rectum.
    5. Vomiting or coughing up blood.
    6. Seizure activity.

V. Plan of Care

A. Pharmacotherapeutics.
    1. HIV drug regimens – To achieve viral suppression.
        a. Should contain at least two and preferably three active drugs.
        b. Drug regimens should contain medications from two or more drug classes.
        c. Medications for each regimen should be guided by the use of genotyping, phenotyping, tropism assay testing (before starting patient on a CCR5 inhibitor), and HLA-B*5701 (before starting patients on abacavir).

B. Treatment strategies.
   1. Initial regimen – Should be tailored to each patient to enhance adherence and, thus, improve long-term treatment success. Initial regimens will vary according to pill burden, drug interactions, and potential side effects.
   2. Pretreatment drug-resistance testing – Studies show that 6–16% of HIV medication-naïve patients have drug resistance prior to treatment (U.S. Department of Health and Human Services [DHHS], 2012). Because of this, drug resistance testing should be used to guide selection of the most optimal initial therapy regimen.
   3. Improving adherence – Poor adherence may result in reduced treatment response. Therefore, conditions that promote adherence should be maximized prior to and after initiation of an HIV treatment regimen.
   4. When to initiate HIV treatment (DHHS, 2012).
      a. Antiretroviral therapy (ART) should be initiated in all patients with a history of an AIDS defining illness or with a CD4 count less than 350 cells/mm^3.
      b. ART is recommended for patients with CD4 counts between 350 and 500 cells/mm^3.
      c. ART should be initiated regardless of CD4 count in patients with the following conditions:
         (1) HIV-associated neuropathy (HIVAN).
         (2) Hepatitis B (HBV) co-infection when treatment for hepatitis B is indicated.
      d. ARV is recommended for pregnant women regardless of CD4 count in order to prevent perinatal transmission (HIV transmission from mother to unborn child).
      e. For patients with CD4 counts greater than 500 cells/mm^3, members of the DHHS Panel on Antiretroviral Guidelines for Adults and Adolescents are evenly divided:
         (1) 50% are in favor of starting ARV at this stage of HIV disease.
         (2) 50% consider starting ARV at this stage to be optional.
      f. Patients initiating ARV should be willing and able to commit to lifelong treatment and should understand the risks of therapy and the importance of adherence.
      g. Patients may choose to defer treatment; providers, on a case-by-case basis, may elect to defer treatment based on clinical and/or psychosocial factors.
      h. Before initiating therapy, the provider must make certain the patient has a means to obtain his or her medications each month. HIV medications are covered by commercial insurances, Medicaid, Medicare Part D, and Ryan White Care Act state-funded drug assistance programs.
   5. HIV medication classes – HIV is treated with multidrug regimens representing multiple drug classes in order to attack the virus from multiple points within the HIV life cycle.
      a. Nucleoside analog reverse transcriptase inhibitors – These drugs block HIV replication by blocking the reverse transcriptase enzyme. They mimic the building blocks used by reverse transcriptase and interrupt replication.
         (1) Zidovudine (formerly azidothymidine [AZT]) (Retrovir®).
         (2) Zalcitabine (Hivid®), dideoxycytidine (ddC).
         (3) Didanosine (Videx®, Videx® EC), dideoxyinosine (ddI).
         (4) Stavudine (Zerit®, d4T).
         (5) Lamivudine (Epivir®).
         (6) Abacavir (Ziagen®).
         (7) Zidovudine + lamivudine (Combivir®).
         (8) Zidovudine + lamivudine + abacavir (Trizivir®).
         (9) Tenofovir disoproxil fumarate (Viread®).

(10) Emtricitabine (Emtriva®).

(11) Tenofovir disoproxil fumarate + emtricitabine (Truvada®).

(12) Abacavir + lamivudine (Epzicom®).

(13) Hydroxyurea (Hydrea®).

b. Non-nucleoside reverse transcriptase inhibitors – Stop HIV replication by blocking the reverse transcriptase enzyme that changes HIV's genetic material (RNA) to DNA. This step has to occur before HIV's genetic code is combined with the infected cells' genetic code.

(1) Nevirapine (Viramune®).

(2) Efavirenz (Sustiva®).

(3) Delavirdine (Rescriptor®).

(4) Etravirine (Intelence®).

(5) Rilpivirine (Edurant®).

(6) Rilpivirine + emtricitabine + tenofovir (Complera®).

(7) Efavirenz + emtricitabine + tenofovir (Atripla®).

c. Protease inhibitors – These drugs block the protease enzyme. When new viral particles break off from an infected cell, protease cuts long protein strands into the parts needed to assemble a mature virus. When protease is blocked, the new viral particles cannot mature.

(1) Indinavir (Crixivan®).

(2) Ritonavir (Norvir®).

(3) Saquinavir (Invirase®).

(4) Nelfinavir (Viracept®).

(5) Amprenavir (Agenerase®).

(6) Lopinavir + ritonavir (Kaletra®).

(7) Fosamprenavir (Lexiva®).

(8) Tipranavir (Aptivus®).

(9) Darunavir (Prezista®).

d. Attachment and fusion inhibitors – This is a new class of anti-HIV drugs. They are intended to protect cells from infection by HIV by preventing the virus from attaching to a new cell and breaking through the cell membrane.

(1) Enfuvirtide (Fuzeon®).

(2) Maraviroc (Selzentry®).

e. Integrase inhibitor – Interferes with HIV's genetic code, getting integrated into the cell's genetic code.

(1) Raltegravir (Isentress®).

6. Medication adherence – For an HIV regimen to be effective, the regimen must be taken as prescribed each day. In HIV, adequate adherence is when at least 95% of medication doses are taken as prescribed (Osterberg & Blaschke, 2005). Medication adherence decreases the risk of drug resistance, which in turn means the regimen will be more effective for a longer period of time. Tools for adherence include (Cichocki, 2004):

a. Integrate the regimen into daily activities.

b. Count out doses in advance using a pillbox.

c. Keep a checklist to mark off doses as they are taken to avoid double or missed doses.

d. Use an alarm on a watch or cell phone.

e. Put dosage times in a daily planner, calendar, or smartphone.

f. Call for refills a week before medications run out to avoid delays and gaps between refills.

g. Plan ahead for travel.

h. Establish and use a support network.

i. If being seen taking medications is a problem, arrange for privacy when doses are due.

j. Keep a medication diary that documents those tools and techniques that improve adherence.

k. Keep a record of medication side effects, issues with refills, etc. to share with the provider.

C. Primary/secondary/tertiary prevention.

1. Primary prevention.

a. HIV prevention also includes prevention of other sexually transmitted diseases (STDs) such as gonorrhea, syphilis, and Chlamydia. The prevention and control of STDs are based on five strategies (CDC, 2010).

b. Education and counseling of persons at risk on ways to prevent STDs through changes in sexual behavior and the use of prevention methods and services. Providers must routinely obtain a sexual history to assess for high-risk behavior.
    (1) Open-ended questions.
    (2) Understandable language.
    (3) Normalized language.
    (4) Use the 5 "Ps" of a sexual history (CDC, 2010).
        (a) Partners.
        (b) Prevention of pregnancy.
        (c) Protection from STDs.
        (d) Practices.
        (e) Past history of STDs.
c. HIV prevention methods.
    (1) Abstinence – While abstinence is the only 100% effective method of HIV prevention, maintaining abstinence is very difficult.
    (2) Reduce the number of anonymous sexual partners – Anonymous sex increases the risk of HIV exposure and infection.
    (3) Male condoms.
        (a) Use condoms for every anal, oral, and vaginal sexual encounter.
        (b) Avoid condoms with spermicides.
        (c) Lambskin condoms do not offer protection from HIV.
        (d) Use only one condom at a time; use only once and discard after using.
        (e) Withdrawal before becoming flaccid, holding onto top of condom to prevent leakage.
        (f) Apply condom before any sexual penetration occurs; precum can spread HIV and other STDs.
    (4) Female condoms.
        (a) More costly than male condoms.
        (b) Sex partners should consider using female condoms when male condoms are not available or cannot be used properly.
        (c) Empowers women with regard to safer sex.
        (d) Put in place prior to sexual contact; provides the spontaneity that male condoms do not provide.
    (5) Dental dams.
        (a) Latex squares used during oral sex; both oral-vaginal and oral-anal.
        (b) Prevents the tongue from coming in contact with bodily secretions.
        (c) Placed over the genitals during oral sex.
    (6) Avoid sharing needles.
        (a) Never share needles to inject drugs.
        (b) Get professional drug rehabilitation services to stop intravenous drug use.
        (c) If stopping drug use is not obtainable, utilize needle exchange programs to acquire clean, unused needles and syringes.
    (7) Prevent vertical transmission (transmission from mother to baby).
        (a) Enter into prenatal care and HIV care as soon as possible after conception.
        (b) HIV medications are given during pregnancy, given intravenously during delivery, and given to the newborn baby after delivery until HIV status has been determined to be negative.
        (c) HIV-positive women should not breastfeed unless commercial formula and clean water is not available.

d. Pre-exposure vaccination of persons at risk for vaccine-preventable STDs.
   (1) Human papillomavirus (HPV) vaccine (females ages 9–26).
   (2) Hepatitis A and B vaccine.

2. Secondary prevention – Identification through testing of asymptomatic HIV- or STD-infected people unlikely to seek diagnostic and treatment services.
   a. Ensure all people are treated regardless of individual circumstances (e.g., ability to pay, language spoken).
   b. People seeking testing for one STD should be tested for all common STDs, including HIV.

3. Tertiary prevention – Diagnosis, treatment, and counseling of infected persons.
   a. Identify the sexual and needle-sharing partners of infected people and arrange for testing, counseling, and treatment, if necessary.
   b. Evaluation, treatment, counseling of sex partners who are infected with an STD.
   c. Providers should encourage partner notification and urge those partners to seek medical evaluation.

D. Goals of plan of care (DHHS, 2012) – Eradication of HIV cannot be achieved with currently available medications, because the pool of latently infected CD4 T-cells are established during the earliest stages of infection and persist with a very long half-life. Therefore, the goals of HIV treatment are:
   1. Reduce HIV-associated morbidity and prolong the duration and quality of survival.
   2. Restore and preserve immunologic function.
   3. Maximally and durably suppress plasma HIV viral load.
   4. Prevent HIV transmission.

E. Education of the patient and family.
   1. Prophylaxis medication – Some patients need prophylaxis medications to protect the body from opportunistic infections while the immune system is too weak to protect the body itself. The need for prophylaxis is based on the CD4 count; people with CD4 counts less than 200 cells/mm^3 should begin prophylaxis medications of some sort. Opportunistic infections that prophylaxis will guard against include (AIDS Education & Training Centers National Resource Center, 2012):
      a. *Pneumocystis jeroveci* pneumonia (PCP).
         (1) Prophylaxis should be administered to all HIV-infected people with a CD4 count less than 200 cells/mm^3 or a CD4 percentage of less than 14% regardless of CD4 count.
         (2) Prophylaxis should be given if patient has a history of oral candidiasis (thrush) or a history of an AIDS defining illness.
         (3) Prophylaxis should be given to any patient with a history of PCP.
         (4) Identify any past sulfa allergy prior to starting prophylaxis.
         (5) Prophylaxis options:
            (a) Trimethoprim-sulfamethoxazole (TMP-SMX; Bactrim®) one double-strength tablet daily.
            (b) TMP-SMX one single-strength tablet daily.
            (c) TMP-SMX one double-strength tablet every Monday, Wednesday, and Friday.
            (d) Dapsone 100 mg once daily.
            (e) Aerosolized pentamidine 300 mg once each month.
            (f) Atovaquone 750 mg/5mL suspension; 10 mL (1500 mg) once daily.
      b. *Mycobacterium avuim* complex (MAC).
         (1) Prophylaxis should be given in patients with a CD4 count less than 50 cells/mm^3.
         (2) Rule out an active MAC or tuberculosis (TB) infection prior to starting prophylaxis.
         (3) Review current medication regimen to identify any drug that could interact with MAC prophylaxis medication.

(4) Prophylaxis options:
  (a) Azithromycin 1200 mg orally once per week.
  (b) Clarithromycin 500 mg orally twice daily (not recommended during pregnancy).
  (c) Azithromycin 600 mg twice a week.
  (d) Rifabutin 300 mg once daily.

c. Toxoplasmosis.
  (1) Caused by the organism *Toxoplasma gondii.*
  (2) Prophylaxis should be given to those patients with CD4 counts less than 100 cells/mm^3.
  (3) Prophylaxis options:
    (a) Trimethoprim-sulfamethoxazole (TMP-SMX; Bactrim®) one double-strength tablet orally three times each week.
    (b) TMP-SMX one single-strength tablet daily.
    (c) Dapsone 50 mg once daily + pyrimethamine 50 mg once weekly + folinic acid 25 mg once weekly.
    (d) Dapsone 200 mg once daily + pyrimethamine 75 mg once weekly + folinic acid 25 mg once weekly.
    (e) Atovaquone 1500 mg once daily with or without pyrimethamine 25 mg once daily + folinic acid 10 mg once daily.

d. Histoplasmosis.
  (1) Caused by the organism *Histoplasma capsulatum* found in a variety of geographical areas from the Ohio and Mississippi Valley to South America, Asia, and Africa.
  (2) Prophylaxis should be given to anyone with a CD4 count less than or equal to 150 cells/mm^3.
  (3) Prophylaxis option – Itraconazole 200 mg orally once daily (itraconazole has significant interactions with many drugs including NNR-TIs, PIs, and Maraviroc; dose adjustments may be necessary).

2. Patient education – Prophylaxis.
  a. Explain the purpose of each prophylaxis medication, explaining dosing and schedule.
  b. Discuss possible side effects and drug-drug interactions, and explain what symptoms should prompt a call to the physician.
  c. Stress the need to take the prophylaxis to prevent opportunistic infections and not to stop until instructed to do so by the provider.
  d. Stress the importance of medication adherence.
  e. For women of childbearing potential, stress the importance of effective contraception while on medication with the potential for teratogenic effects (e.g., clarithromycin).

F. Collaboration and referral.
  1. Infectious disease specialist.
  2. Home care nursing and home infusion services, as indicated.
  3. Clinical pharmacist.
  4. Nutrition counselor, as indicated.
  5. Social worker, as indicated.

G. Telehealth nursing consideration.
  1. Triage of emergent and urgent issues, described above.
  2. Sensitivity to sexual practices, and counseling for safety.
  3. Assessment for anxiety and depression.
  4. Interact with caregivers, as indicated in late stage disease.

H. Protocol/algorithm/guidelines.
  1. CDC (2010) – *Sexually Transmitted Diseases Treatment Guidelines.*
  2. CDC (Branson et al., 2006) – *Revised Recommendations for HIV Testing of Adults, Adolescents, and Pregnant Women in Health- Care Settings.*
  3. AIDS Education & Training Centers National Resource Center (2012) – *Guide for HIV/AIDS Clinical Care – Opportunistic Infection Prophylaxis, HRSA HIV/AIDS Bureau.*

4. Office of AIDS Administration (2007) – *Standards of Care: HIV Ambulatory Outpatient Medical Care Standards.*

Peptic Ulcer Disease

Patient Population: Adult

I. Overview

Approximately 14.5 million people in the United States are affected by peptic ulcer disease annually (Pleis & Lucas, 2009) with a direct cost of $3.1 billion (Sandler et al., 2002). Direct costs include physician visits, inpatient hospitalizations, outpatient hospital care, emergency visits, and pharmaceutical costs. Peptic ulcer disease is responsible for 1.4 million ambulatory care visits, 489,000 hospitalizations, and 5 million prescriptions annually (Everhart, 2008).

In 70% of patients, peptic ulcer disease occurs between the ages of 25 and 64 (Sonnenberg & Everhart, 1996). According to the Centers for Disease Control and Prevention (CDC), the hospitalization rate for peptic ulcer disease is highest for adults 65-years-old and older and is higher for men than women (Feinstein, Holman, Yorita Christensen, Steiner, & Swerdlow, 2010). The number of deaths primarily associated with peptic ulcer disease is approximately 3,000 each year (Xu, Kochanek, & Tejada-Vera, 2009).

The incidence of peptic ulcer disease and related morbidity and mortality rates have decreased over the past century. This decreased incidence is primarily related to recent discoveries of *Helicobacter pylori (H. pylori)*, a bacterium that grows in the mucous layer that lines the inside of the stomach (National Cancer Institute, 2011) and gastric acid suppressant therapies. Effective treatment modalities for peptic ulcer disease and *H. pylori* have had the greatest impact on reducing associated morbidity and mortality rates. In fact, "*H. pylori* eradication as cure of peptic ulcer received its full recognition when the Nobel Prize for Medicine and Physiology was awarded to Warren and Marshall in 2005" (Malfertheiner, Chan, & McCall, 2009, p. 1449) for their discovery of *H. pylori* and its causal relationship in peptic ulcer disease.

II. Pathophysiology

Peptic ulcer disease manifests itself within the gastrointestinal tract and can be asymptomatic depending on the location of the ulcer. Peptic ulcers can vary in location (i.e., duodenal and gastric) and are best described as breaks or damage in the protective mucosal lining of the gastrointestinal tract. Etiology is multifactorial and often the result of *H. pylori* infection, non-steroidal anti-inflammatory (NSAID) medication use, decreased blood flow to the gastric mucosa, and low-dose aspirin therapy (Malfertheiner et al., 2009). "Peptic ulcers result when there is an imbalance of aggressive gastric luminal factor acid and pepsin and defensive mucosal barrier function" (Malfertheiner et al., 2009, p. 1450). Gastric acid secretion is increased or mucosal lining is weakened as a result of one or more of the risk factors described above. Duodenal ulcers are most often associated with *H. pylori* infection and gastric ulcers with NSAID consumption (Yuan, Padol, & Hunt, 2006). *H. pylori* infection, aspirin, and NSAID use can be attributed to the majority of patients with peptic ulcer disease (Yuan et al., 2006).

III. Assessment, Screening, and Triage

A. History.
   1. Assess for signs and symptoms of uncomplicated peptic ulcers including:
      a. Dyspepsia.
      b. Epigastric pain.
      c. Fullness.
      d. Bloating.
      e. Nausea.
      f. Early satiety.
   2. Assess for signs and symptoms of duodenal ulcers including:
      a. Epigastric pain, frequently on an empty stomach, typically relieved by food intake or antacids.
      b. Heartburn.
   3. Assess for signs and symptoms of malignancy including:
      a. Loss of appetite.
      b. Unexplained weight loss.
      c. Anemia.
      d. Vomiting.

4. All patients should be queried about:
   a. Burning, dull pain in the upper abdomen after eating, and/or alleviation of symptoms after eating.
   b. Dizziness.
   c. Melena.
   d. Hematemesis.
   e. Right shoulder pain/epigastric pain.
   f. Upper gastrointestinal (UGI) bleeding.
   g. Anemia.
      (1) Observe vital signs for any indication of hypo-perfusion/bleeding.
      (2) Patients with chronic ulcers may be asymptomatic.
5. Risk factors for peptic ulcer disease:
   a. Primary and/or family history of peptic ulcers/disease.
   b. *H. pylori* infection.
   c. Medication history that includes:
      (1) NSAID therapy.
      (2) Low-dose aspirin therapy.
      (3) Glucocorticoid/corticosteroid therapy.
      (4) Anti-coagulation therapy.
   d. Cigarette smoking or tobacco chewing.
   e. Alcohol use.
   f. Substance abuse.
   g. Psychological stress factors.
B. Physical examination.
   1. Vital signs.
   2. Weight.
   3. Abdominal examination.
C. Diagnostic tests.
   1. Upper endoscopy/endoscopy with biopsy.
      a. Endoscopy to confirm diagnosis of peptic ulcer disease, associated complications, and differential diagnosis.
      b. Rapid urea test (RUT) to confirm *H. pylori* infection.
   2. Non-invasive laboratory testing for *H. pylori* infection.
      a. C-urea or C-urea breath test (UBT). Test has greater than 90% sensitivity and specificity. Use of proton pump inhibitors (PPI) within two weeks of testing may alter test results.
   b. Stool antigen test. Diagnostic for active infection and follow-up evaluation.
   c. Hematologic/serologic tests.
      (1) Presence of antibodies represents previous infection.
      (2) May not be indicative of active infection.
      (3) Compare with other diagnostic testing.
      (4) Serum gastrin levels to rule out Zollinger-Ellison syndrome.
3. Imaging studies (Ferri, 2010).
   a. Conventional upper GI barium studies identify 70–80% of peptic ulcer disease.
   b. Accuracy can be increased to approximately 90% by using double contrast.

IV. **Indications for Emergency Care or Urgent Consultation**
A. Sudden, sharp abdominal pain.
B. Development of a hard, rigid abdomen.
C. Symptoms of shock, such as fainting, diaphoresis, or confusion.
D. Hematemesis, especially dark or tarry blood.

V. **Plan of Care**
A. Pharmacotherapeutics.
   1. Treatment of *H. pylori* Infection.
      a. First-line treatment (7–14 days).
         (1) Triple therapy: Proton pump inhibitor (PPI) twice daily plus clarithromycin 500 mg twice daily.
         (2) Either amoxicillin 1 g twice daily (PPI-CA) or metronidazole 500 mg twice daily (PPI-CM) for 7–14 days.
      b. Second-line treatment (10–14 days).
      c. Re-treatment if first-line treatment fails to eradicate.
      d. Triple therapy: PPI combined with selection of combined antimicrobial medications not used in first-line treatment.
      e. Additional treatment if eradication of *H. pylori* fails; selection of antibiotic therapy and treatment should be based on microbial sensitivity to antibiotics.

f. PPI with levofloxacin or rifabutin is recommended.
2. Treatment of NSAID-induced ulcer(s) (eight weeks).
   a. Standard-dose H_2 receptor antagonists; discontinue NSAIDs.
   b. Test for *H. pylori* and treat as indicated.
   c. Antacids and sulcralfate may be used for treatment and prevention.
3. Maintenance therapy for high-risk groups may include H^2 receptor antagonists (antisecretory therapy).
   a. Ranitidine 150 mg at bedtime.
   b. Cimetidine 400 mg at bedtime.
   c. Famotidine 20 mg at bedtime.
   d. Nizatidine 150 mg at bedtime.
4. PPI (may be used).
B. Primary/secondary/tertiary prevention.
   1. Avoid NSAIDs, including aspirin.
   2. Avoid tobacco (smoking or chewing).
   3. Limit alcohol.
C. Patient and family education.
   1. Disease pathophysiology.
   2. Smoking cessation.
   3. Identification and recognition of foods that "trigger" and/or cause symptoms with associated dietary modifications.
   4. Avoidance of alcohol.
   5. Medication management including medication side effects and importance of maintenance therapy for high-risk patients.
D. Collaborations and referrals.
   1. Nutritional counseling.
   2. Smoking cessation counseling.
   3. Gastroenterology if unresponsive to treatment.
E. Community resources and advocacy – Patient and family support groups.
F. Telehealth nursing considerations.
   1. Assess severity of pain, location, onset, and characteristics.
   2. Assess for blood in emesis or stools.
   3. Rule out atypical chest pain.
G. Protocols/algorithms/guidelines.
   1. American College of Gastroenterology guideline on the management of *H. pylori* infection.

2. American College of Gastroenterology recommendations for reducing risk of peptic ulcers associated with NSAID as associated with cardiovascular and gastrointestinal risk.

Asthma

Patient Population: Pediatric

I. Overview

Asthma is a chronic inflammatory, respiratory condition that affects approximately 300 million people worldwide, and almost 25 million Americans (Centers for Disease Control and Prevention [CDC], 2011). Asthma is one of the most common chronic diseases of childhood and is found in all age groups. Children and adolescents with asthma present for care across all ambulatory health care settings, as well as in-patient for more severe symptom management. More than 7 million children under the age of 18 have been diagnosed with asthma (American Lung Association, 2011b). This is almost 10% of children in this age group, and of those diagnosed, 75% of the diagnoses are in children under the age of 5 (National Heart, Lung, and Blood Institute [NHLBI], 2007). Although asthma is being diagnosed with increasing frequency, it is still often overlooked because asthma is frequently confused with allergies, upper respiratory infections, bronchitis, and pneumonias. Both chronic and acute asthma are primarily managed in ambulatory care settings. Asthma can vary greatly from patient to patient, and its course and progression are likewise highly variable in each patient over time (NHLBI, 2007).

II. Pathophysiology
A. Asthma is defined as a chronic, inflammatory disorder of the airways that involves inflammatory cell infiltration, including neutrophils, eosinophils, lymphocytes, mast cell activation, and epithelial cell injury.
B. There are two environmental risk factors for the development, persistence, and possibly, the severity of asthma:
   1. Airborne allergens.
   2. Viral respiratory infections.

C. Asthma is characterized by airway inflammation that contributes to airway hyper-responsiveness, airflow limitation and obstruction, respiratory symptoms, and disease chronicity. Increased mucous production and tightening of muscle bands around the airways also are present (Fireman, 2003; NHLBI, 2007).

D. Recurrent episodes are usually associated with lower airway airflow obstruction that is reversible, either spontaneously or with treatment.

E. There is a distinctive pattern of interplay and interaction between airway inflammation and the clinical symptoms and pathophysiology of asthma.
1. Airway inflammation results in increased airway obstruction and hyper-reactivity to the exposure to triggers that can provoke an acute asthma exacerbation.
2. Common triggers include:
   a. Upper respiratory viral infections (URIs).
   b. Animals (feathered or furry pets).
   c. Dust.
   d. Mold or pollen.
   e. Cockroaches.
   f. Exercise.
   g. Seasonal and weather changes including heat and cold air.
   h. Emotions and stress.
   i. Environmental allergens and pollutants, such as smoke and pollution (Kirk, 2011; NHLBI, 2007).

III. Assessment and Triage
A. Key symptom indicators of asthma include:
1. Wheezing – Although a lack of wheezing does not exclude asthma.
2. Cough, which typically worsens at night.
3. Recurrent difficulty in breathing or dyspnea.
4. Recurrent chest tightness.
5. Symptoms that occur or worsen with exercise, viral infections, inhalant allergens (animals, house-dust mites, mold, pollen), irritants (tobacco or wood smoke, airborne chemicals), changes in weather, strong emotional expression (laughing or crying hard), stress, menstrual cycles.
6. Symptoms occur or worsen at night (NHLBI, 2007).

B. Triage — Identify the child's symptoms, including:
1. Appearance and color, respiratory rate, wheezing, coughing, shortness of breath (SOB), ability or difficulty with speaking, retractions, work-of-breathing. If peak-flow monitoring, compare scores to baseline and determine zone: *Green, Yellow,* or *Red* (see descriptions below).
2. Symptoms that indicate other conditions that also may require evaluation and triage, such as fever, vomiting, diarrhea, rash, pain, injury, or change in mental status.
3. Onset and duration of these symptoms.
4. Severity of the symptoms: *Mild, Moderate, Severe,* or is the child experiencing *Respiratory Distress* (see descriptions below).
5. Actions that have been taken to treat the child's symptoms.
6. Frequency of bronchodilator use during this exacerbation.
7. Compliance with controller medication, if prescribed.
8. Response to these treatments.
9. Recent emergency department visits or hospitalizations.
10. Exposure to triggers.

C. Physical assessment.
1. Full vital signs – Temperature, apical pulse, respiratory rate, and blood pressure for children age 3 or older.
2. Assessment of respiratory and circulatory function, including skin color, capillary refill and perfusion, retractions and use of accessory muscles, nasal flaring.
3. Pulse oximetry to assess oxygen saturation.
4. Observation of child's behavior and activity levels. Restlessness, apprehension, and lethargy can all be signs of respiratory distress.
5. Lung auscultation via direct skin contact (not through clothing) for adventitious breath sounds and air movement.
   a. Auscultation of all lung fields at the back and front are essential to determine even subtle wheezes, rales, rhonchi, or inadequate air movement.

b. Expiratory phase may be prolonged and wheezing may or may not be present depending on the degree of bronchospasm and obstruction of airflow due to increased airway inflammation.

D. Testing.
1. Pulmonary function testing or spirometry for children age 5 or older can be helpful in determining airway obstruction that is at least partially reversible.
2. Pulmonary function testing or spirometry is recommended for diagnosis and monitoring of asthma, and includes four key measurements:
   a. Forced expiratory volume in one second (FEV_1).
   b. Forced expiratory volume in six seconds (FEV_6).
   c. Forced vital capacity (FVC).
   d. FEV_1/FVC – Which is a more sensitive marker of impairment in children than FEV_1.

IV. Indications for Emergency Care or Urgent Consultation

If patient's asthma exacerbation, symptoms, and/or peak flow monitoring indicate:

A. *Red Zone:* Peak flow rate is < 50% of personal best baseline level.
1. Severe wheezing; severe SOB, rapid breathing; retractions; bluish lips, tongue, face, or fingernails; inability to tolerate activity; trouble walking or talking; or non-responsive.
2. Reliever medication did not help within 15–20 minutes.
3. The child sounds very sick or weak or the situation sounds life-threatening to the nurse triager.
4. This is *Respiratory Distress*, an emergent situation, and the child needs emergency care immediately.
5. The nurse triager for patients at home must instruct the parent or caregiver to call 9-1-1 and activate EMS immediately.
6. The child should be given another dose of reliever medication while EMS is activated.

B. *Yellow Zone:* Peak flow rate is 50–79% of baseline level.
1. Moderate exacerbation which requires the child to be seen immediately by the primary care provider, or if unavailable, in the emergency department.
2. Cough, wheeze, chest tightness, SOB at rest, night coughing, decreased ability to perform usual activities, after using reliever medication.
3. Asthma reliever medication is needed more frequently than every 4 hours.

C. *Green Zone:* Peak flow rate is 80–100% of baseline level.
1. A mild exacerbation is indicated by a child with no SOB at rest, mild SOB with walking, normal speaking in sentences, and wheezing that is audible by stethoscope only.
2. Most mild asthma exacerbations can be managed at home with reliever medications, along with continuation of the child's asthma action plan, including daily controller medications.
3. The nurse triager should instruct the parent or caregiver to call back to have the child seen if the symptoms persist for more than 24 hours, worsen or do not improve, or if the parent or caregiver wants the child seen.
4. *Well-controlled* asthma is indicated by being in the Green Zone every day, and may allow reduction of medications. Expirations are normal; no cough, wheeze, or SOB; no nighttime symptoms – cough or wheeze; and child has normal level of play and activity tolerance (Schmitt, 2009).

V. Plan of Care
A. Pharmacotherapeutics.
1. Medications and delivery devices need to be carefully selected to treat each patient's specific asthma condition.
2. The stepwise approach, as outlined below, is used to identify appropriate treatment options. Using the stepwise approach, the types, frequency, doses, and number of medications are increased when necessary and decreased when possible (see Figure 21-1).

3. If the patient's asthma is assessed to be not well-controlled, then the therapy should be "stepped-up." If the asthma is well-controlled, then the therapy is either continued or "stepped-down" to minimize side effects of the medications.

4. The preferred mainstays of effective long-term asthma control are the inhaled corticosteroids (ICSs), the "controller" medications.

5. Alternative controller medications include cromolyn, leukotriene receptor agonists (LTRAs), nedocromolin, and theophyline.

6. Quick-relief bronchodilator medication, often referred to as "rescue" or "reliever" medication.
   a. All patients need the short-acting beta$_2$ agonist (SABA) p.r.n. for symptoms.
   b. Use of a SABA for more than 2 days/week for symptom relief (not for prevention of exercise-induced bronchospasm) usually indicates inadequate control and the need for "step-up" treatment.

7. Medications combine a long-acting beta$_2$ agonist bronchodilator (LABA) with an ICS.

B. Primary/secondary/tertiary prevention.
   1. Primary: Prevent exposure to allergens and triggers, including secondhand smoke.
   2. Secondary: Immunize against influenza annually.
   3. Tertiary:
      a. Use controller medications routinely.
      b. Carry rescue medications for quick action when symptoms manifest.
      c. Consider allergy immunotherapy to reduce sensitivity to allergens.
      d. Identify and treat co-morbid conditions, such as obesity, obstructive sleep apnea, gastro-esophageal reflux, rhinitis, sinusitis, stress, and depression.

C. Goals of plan of care.
   1. According to the 2007 National Heart, Lung, and Blood Institute's *National Asthma Education and Prevention Program (NAEPP) Expert Panel Report 3: Guidelines for the Diagnosis and Management of Asthma*, the

goal of therapy for each patient with asthma is control. Asthma control encompasses two major criteria:
   a. Reduce impairment by preventing chronic symptoms, requiring less frequent use of SABA "rescue" medications and maintaining normal lung function and activity levels.
   b. Reduce risk by preventing exacerbations, minimizing need for emergency care or hospitalization, preventing loss of lung function, and for children, preventing reduction of lung tissue growth, and experiencing minimal or no adverse effects of therapy (NHLBI, 2007).

2. The goals of care management are to:
   a. Prevent chronic and troublesome symptoms such as cough, breathlessness (daytime, nocturnal, or after exertion).
   b. Require infrequent use (2 days/week or less) of inhaled SABA for quick relief of symptoms – Not including prevention of exercise-induced bronchospasm (EIB).
   c. Maintain (near) normal pulmonary function.
   d. Maintain normal activity levels including exercise and other physical activity, and attendance at childcare, school, or work.
   e. Prevent recurrent exacerbations of asthma.
   f. Minimize the need for emergency department visits and/or hospitalizations.
   g. Prevent loss of lung function and for children, prevent reduced lung function.
   h. Provide optimal pharmacotherapy with minimal or no adverse effects of therapy (NHLBI, 2007).

D. Education of patient and families.
   1. There are six key steps for successful management of asthma:
      a. Individualize treatment: Treatment should be tailored to the individual patient's needs and asthma control level.

Figure 21-1.

Stepwise Approach for Managing Asthma Long-Term in Children Ages 0–4 and Ages 5–11

Step up if needed (first check inhaler technique, adherence, environmental control, and comorbid conditions)

Assess control

Step down if possible (and asthma is well controlled at least 3 months)

Children 0–4 Years of Age

	Step 1	Step 2	Step 3	Step 4	Step 5	Step 6
	Intermittent Asthma	Persistent Asthma: Daily Medication				
		Consult with asthma specialist if step 3 care or higher is required. Consider consultation at step 2.				
Preferred	SABA PRN	Low-dose ICS	Medium-dose ICS	Medium-dose ICS + LABA or Montelukast	High-dose ICS + LABA or Montelukast	High-dose ICS + LABA or Montelukast + Oral corticosteroids
Alternative		Cromolyn or Montelukast				

Each Step: Patient Education and Environmental Control

- SABA as needed for symptoms. Intensity of treatment depends on severity of symptoms.
- With viral respiratory symptoms: SABA q 4–6 hours up to 24 hours (longer with physician consult). Consider short course of oral systemic corticosteroids if exacerbation is severe or patient has history of previous severe exacerbations.

Caution: Frequent use of SABA may indicate the need to step up treatment. See text for recommendations on initiating daily long-term-control therapy.

Quick-Relief Medication

Notes

- The stepwise approach is meant to assist, not replace, the clinical decisionmaking required to meet individual patient needs.
- If an alternative treatment is used and response is inadequate, discontinue it and use the preferred treatment before stepping up.
- If clear benefit is not observed within 4–6 weeks, and patient's/family's medication technique and adherence are satisfactory, consider adjusting therapy or an alternative diagnosis.
- Studies on children 0–4 years of age are limited. Step 2 preferred therapy is based on Evidence A. All other recommendations are based on expert opinion and extrapolation from studies in older children.
- Clinicians who administer immunotherapy should be prepared and equipped to identify and treat anaphylaxis that may occur.

Key: **Alphabetical listing is used when more than one treatment option is listed within either preferred or alternative therapy.** ICS, inhaled corticosteroid; LABA, inhaled long-acting beta$_2$-agonist; LTRA, leukotriene receptor antagonist; oral corticosteroids, oral systemic corticosteroids; SABA, inhaled short-acting beta$_2$-agonist.

Children 5–11 Years of Age

	Step 1	Step 2	Step 3	Step 4	Step 5	Step 6
	Intermittent Asthma	Persistent Asthma: Daily Medication				
		Consult with asthma specialist if step 4 care or higher is required. Consider consultation at step 3.				
Preferred	SABA PRN	Low-dose ICS	Low-dose ICS + LABA, LTRA, or Theophylline OR Medium-dose ICS	Medium-dose ICS + LABA	High-dose ICS + LABA	High-dose ICS + LABA + Oral corticosteroids
Alternative		Cromolyn, LTRA, Nedocromil, or Theophylline	Medium-dose ICS	Medium-dose ICS + LTRA or Theophylline	High-dose ICS + LTRA or Theophylline	High-dose ICS + LTRA or Theophylline + oral corticosteroids

Each Step: Patient Education, Environmental Control, and Management of Comorbidities

Steps 2–4: Consider subcutaneous allergen immunotherapy for patients who have persistent, allergic asthma.

Quick-Relief Medication

- SABA as needed for symptoms. Intensity of treatment depends on severity of symptoms: up to 3 treatments at 20-minute intervals as needed. Short course of oral systemic corticosteroids may be needed.

Caution: Increasing use of SABA or use >2 days a week for symptom relief (not prevention of EIB) generally indicates inadequate control and the need to step up treatment.

Notes

- The stepwise approach is meant to assist, not replace, the clinical decisionmaking required to meet individual patient needs.
- If an alternative treatment is used and response is inadequate, discontinue it and use the preferred treatment before stepping up.
- Theophylline is a less desirable alternative due to the need to monitor serum concentration levels.
- Steps 1 and 2 medications are based on Evidence A. Step 3 ICS and ICS plus adjunctive therapy are based on Evidence B for efficacy of each treatment and extrapolation from comparator trials in older children and adults—comparator trials are not available for this age group; steps 4–6 are based on expert opinion and extrapolation from studies in older children and adults.
- Immunotherapy for steps 2–4 is based on Evidence B for house-dust mites, animal danders, and pollens; evidence is weak or lacking for molds and cockroaches. Evidence is strongest for immunotherapy with single allergens. The role of allergy in asthma is greater in children than adults.
- Clinicians who administer immunotherapy should be prepared and equipped to identify and treat anaphylaxis that may occur.

Key: **Alphabetical listing is used when more than one treatment option is listed within either preferred or alternative therapy.** ICS, inhaled corticosteroid; LABA, inhaled long-acting beta$_2$-agonist; LTRA, leukotriene receptor antagonist; oral corticosteroids, oral systemic corticosteroids; SABA, inhaled short-acting beta$_2$-agonist.

Source: National Heart, Lung, and Blood Institute, 2007. Used with permission.

b. Assessment and monitoring: Utilization of multiple measures of functional impairment and risk for exacerbation.

c. Recognition of variations: Asthma is a very dynamic disease, so even patients whose symptoms are well-controlled can be at risk for severe exacerbation. The degree of control can change, sometimes quickly, over time. Patients may also experience seasonal variations in asthma symptoms.

d. Written Asthma Action Plan: Utilization of written Asthma Action Plans (or Asthma Treatment Plans) (see Figure 21-2) as fundamental to optimal asthma management. Research has shown that patients with plans manage exacerbations better than patients without plans.

e. Asthma classification and treatment options: Implementation of new treatment options.

f. Educational opportunities at multiple points-of-care: Incorporation of patient self-management skills through expanded educational opportunities (NHLBI, 2007).

2. Components of asthma care – To achieve optimal asthma control, ambulatory care nurses can assist patients in the following components of asthma care:

a. Assessment and monitoring of asthma severity and asthma control.

   (1) Asthma severity is first assessed using the asthma severity classification chart to initiate therapy (see Table 21-12).

   (2) The asthma control chart is utilized to assess both impairment and risk domains.

   (3) Asthma control is assessed and monitored periodically (and as needed) to determine if asthma therapy should be maintained or adjusted in a step-wise approach: Step-up if necessary, step-down if possible.

   (4) As asthma is highly variable from individual patient to patient, as well as over time, periodic monitoring is essential.

   (5) Follow-up care for asthma should be scheduled at 2–6 week intervals while gaining control, and can be adjusted to every 1–6 months depending on the patient's level of control.

   (6) Assessment of asthma control, controller and rescue medications used, medication technique, written asthma action plan, patient adherence, and education needs should be included in each visit.

b. Ambulatory care nurses can use a patient quality-of-life questionnaire such as the Asthma Control Test (ACT) (available at www.asthmacontrol.com) to assess the degree of asthma impairment and severity in both children and adult patients.

   (1) The ACT is completed by the patient or parent/caregiver and gives insight into frequency and intensity of symptoms, interference with normal daily activities, and SABA use.

   (2) The maximum ACT score is 25; scores between 16 and 19 indicate asthma that is not well-controlled; scores below 15 indicate very poorly controlled asthma.

c. Nursing assessment and monitoring also includes performing the nursing history at each visit for acute or chronic management. It is vitally important to assess parent/caregiver's ability to:

   (1) Recognize the child's signs and symptoms of an imminent asthma exacerbation.

   (2) Administer appropriate controller and reliever medications.

   (3) Follow the Asthma Action Plan.

Figure 21-2.
Asthma Treatment Plan – Student Form

Asthma Treatment Plan – Student

(This asthma action plan meets NJ Law N.J.S.A. 18A:40-12.8) (Physician's Orders)

 The Pediatric/Adult Asthma Coalition of New Jersey
"Your Pathway to Asthma Control"
PACNJ approved Plan available at www.pacnj.org

Sponsored by
 AMERICAN LUNG ASSOCIATION IN NEW JERSEY

 NEW JERSEY DEPARTMENT HEALTH

(Please Print)

Name	Date of Birth	Effective Date
Doctor	Parent/Guardian (if applicable)	Emergency Contact
Phone	Phone	Phone

HEALTHY (Green Zone) ⫸

Take daily control medicine(s). Some inhalers may be more effective with a "spacer" – use if directed.

You have *all* of these:
- Breathing is good
- No cough or wheeze
- Sleep through the night
- Can work, exercise, and play

And/or Peak flow above _____

MEDICINE	HOW MUCH to take and HOW OFTEN to take it
☐ Advair® HFA ☐ 45, ☐ 115, ☐ 230 _____	2 puffs twice a day
☐ Alvesco® ☐ 80, ☐ 160 _____	☐ 1, ☐ 2 puffs twice a day
☐ Dulera® ☐ 100, ☐ 200 _____	2 puffs twice a day
☐ Flovent® ☐ 44, ☐ 110, ☐ 220 _____	2 puffs twice a day
☐ Qvar® ☐ 40, ☐ 80 _____	☐ 1, ☐ 2 puffs twice a day
☐ Symbicort® ☐ 80, ☐ 160 _____	☐ 1, ☐ 2 puffs twice a day
☐ Advair Diskus® ☐ 100, ☐ 250, ☐ 500 _____	1 inhalation twice a day
☐ Asmanex® Twisthaler® ☐ 110, ☐ 220 _____	☐ 1, ☐ 2 inhalations ☐ once or ☐ twice a day
☐ Flovent® Diskus® ☐ 50 ☐ 100 ☐ 250 _____	1 inhalation twice a day
☐ Pulmicort Flexhaler® ☐ 90, ☐ 180 _____	☐ 1, ☐ 2 inhalations ☐ once or ☐ twice a day
☐ Pulmicort Respules® (Budesonide) ☐ 0.25, ☐ 0.5, ☐ 1.0 ___	1 unit nebulized ☐ once or ☐ twice a day
☐ Singulair® (Montelukast) ☐ 4, ☐ 5, ☐ 10 mg _____	1 tablet daily
☐ Other	
☐ None	

Remember to rinse your mouth after taking inhaled medicine.

If exercise triggers your asthma, take this medicine_____ ____minutes before exercise.

CAUTION (Yellow Zone) ⫸

Continue daily control medicine(s) and ADD quick-relief medicine(s).

You have *any* of these:
- Cough
- Mild wheeze
- Tight chest
- Coughing at night
- Other:_____

If quick-relief medicine does not help within 15-20 minutes or has been used more than 2 times and symptoms persist, call your doctor or go to the emergency room.

And/or Peak flow from_____ to____

MEDICINE	HOW MUCH to take and HOW OFTEN to take it
☐ Combivent® ☐ Maxair® ☐ Xopenex®_____	2 puffs every 4 hours as needed
☐ Ventolin® ☐ Pro-Air® ☐ Proventil®_____	2 puffs every 4 hours as needed
☐ Albuterol ☐ 1.25, ☐ 2.5 mg _____	1 unit nebulized every 4 hours as needed
☐ Duoneb® _____	1 unit nebulized every 4 hours as needed
☐ Xopenex® (Levalbuterol) ☐ 0.31, ☐ 0.63, ☐ 1.25 mg _	1 unit nebulized every 4 hours as needed
☐ Increase the dose of, or add:	
☐ Other	

- **If quick-relief medicine is needed more than 2 times a week, except before exercise, then call your doctor.**

EMERGENCY (Red Zone) ⫸

Take these medicines NOW and CALL 911.
Asthma can be a life-threatening illness. Do not wait!

Your asthma is getting worse fast:
- Quick-relief medicine did not help within 15-20 minutes
- Breathing is hard or fast
- Nose opens wide • Ribs show
- Trouble walking and talking
- Lips blue • Fingernails blue
- Other:_____

And/or Peak flow below _____

MEDICINE	HOW MUCH to take and HOW OFTEN to take it
☐ Combivent® ☐ Maxair® ☐ Xopenex® _____	2 puffs every 20 minutes
☐ Ventolin® ☐ Pro-Air® ☐ Proventil® _____	2 puffs every 20 minutes
☐ Albuterol ☐ 1.25, ☐ 2.5 mg _____	1 unit nebulized every 20 minutes
☐ Duoneb® _____	1 unit nebulized every 20 minutes
☐ Xopenex® (Levalbuterol) ☐ 0.31, ☐ 0.63, ☐ 1.25 mg ___	1 unit nebulized every 20 minutes
☐ Other	

Triggers
Check all items that trigger patient's asthma:

- ☐ Colds/flu
- ☐ Exercise
- ☐ Allergens
  - ○ Dust Mites, dust, stuffed animals, carpet
  - ○ Pollen - trees, grass, weeds
  - ○ Mold
  - ○ Pets - animal dander
  - ○ Pests - rodents, cockroaches
- ☐ Odors (Irritants)
  - ○ Cigarette smoke & second hand smoke
  - ○ Perfumes, cleaning products, scented products
  - ○ Smoke from burning wood, inside or outside
- ☐ Weather
  - ○ Sudden temperature change
  - ○ Extreme weather - hot and cold
  - ○ Ozone alert days
- ☐ Foods:
  - ○ _____
  - ○ _____
  - ○ _____
- ☐ Other:
  - ○ _____
  - ○ _____
  - ○ _____

This asthma treatment plan is meant to assist, not replace, the clinical decision-making required to meet individual patient needs.

Disclaimers: The use of this Website/PACNJ Asthma Treatment Plan and its content is at your own risk. The content is provided on an "as is" basis. The American Lung Association of the Mid-Atlantic (ALAM-A), the Pediatric/Adult Asthma Coalition of New Jersey and all affiliates disclaim all warranties, express or implied, statutory or otherwise, including but not limited to the implied warranties or merchantability, use or fitness for a particular purpose. ALAM-A makes no representation or warranties about the accuracy, reliability, completeness, currency, or timeliness of the content. ALAM-A makes no warranty, representation or guaranty that the information will be uninterrupted or error free or that any defects can be corrected. In no event shall ALAM-A be liable for any damages (including, without limitation, incidental and consequential damages, personal injury/wrongful death, lost profits, or damages resulting from data or business interruption) resulting from the use or inability to use the content of this Asthma Treatment Plan whether based on warranty, contract, tort or any other legal theory, and whether or not ALAM-A is advised of the possibility of such damages. ALAM-A and its affiliates are not liable for any claim, whatsoever, caused by your use or misuse of the Asthma Treatment Plan, nor of this website.

The Pediatric/Adult Asthma Coalition of New Jersey is sponsored by the American Lung Association in New Jersey. This publication was supported by a grant from the New Jersey Department of Health and Senior Services, with funds provided by the U.S. Centers for Disease Control and Prevention under Cooperative Agreement 5U58/HS00491-03. Its content are solely the responsibility of the authors and do not necessarily represent the official views of the New Jersey Department of Health and Senior Services or the U.S. Centers for Disease Control and Prevention. Although this document has been funded wholly or in part by the United States Environmental Protection Agency under Agreement XXXXXXXX-X to the American Lung Association in New Jersey, it has not gone through the Agency's publications review process and therefore, may not necessarily reflect the views of the Agency and no official endorsement should be inferred. Information in this publication is not intended to diagnose health problems or take the place of medical advice. For asthma or any medical condition, seek medical advice from your child's or your health care professional.

REVISED JULY 2012
Permission to reproduce blank form • www.pacnj.org

Permission to Self-administer Medication:
☐ This student is capable and has been instructed in the proper method of self-administering of the non-nebulized inhaled medications named above in accordance with NJ Law.
☐ This student is not approved to self-medicate.

PHYSICIAN/APN/PA SIGNATURE_____ DATE_____

PARENT/GUARDIAN SIGNATURE_____

PHYSICIAN STAMP

Make a copy for parent and for physician file, send original to school nurse or child care provider.

Source: The Pediatric/Adult Asthma Coalition of New Jersey, 2012. Used with permission. For more information, please visit www.pacnj.org.

Table 21-12.
Classifying Asthma Severity and Initiating Therapy in Children

Key: FEV₁, [in 1 second] ; ICS, inhaled ca[...] ; intensive ca[...]

Notes:

- Level of [...] both imp[...] impairm[...] recall of [...] Assign s[...] category [...] occurs.
- Frequen[...] tions ma[...] patients
- At prese[...] data to c[...] of exace[...] levels of [...] more fre[...] tions (e.[...] unsched[...] or ICU a[...] underlyi[...] treatmen[...] exacerb[...] be consi[...] who hav[...] the abse[...] consiste[...]

Components of Severity		Classifying Asthma Severity and Initiating Therapy in Children							
		Intermittent		Persistent					
				Mild		Moderate		Severe	
		Ages 0-4	Ages 5-11	Ages 0-4	Ages 5-11	Ages 0-4	Ages 5-11	Ages 0-4	Ages 5-11
Impairment	Symptoms	≤2 days/week		>2 days/week but not daily		Daily		Throughout the day	
	Nighttime awakenings	0	≤2x/month	1-2x/month	3-4x/month	3-4x/month	>1x/week but not nightly	>1x/week	Often 7x/week
	Short-acting beta₂-agonist use for symptom control	≤2 days/week		>2 days/week but not daily		Daily		Several times per day	
	Interference with normal activity	None		Minor limitation		Some limitation		Extremely limited	
	Lung Function • FEV₁ (predicted) or peak flow (personal best) • FEV₁/FVC	N/A	Normal FEV₁ between exacerbations >80% / >85%	N/A	>80% / >80%	N/A	60-80% / 75-80%	N/A	<60% / <75%
Risk	Exacerbations requiring oral systemic corticosteroids (consider severity and interval since last exacerbation)	0-1/year (see notes)		≥2 exacerbations in 6 months requiring oral systemic corticosteroids, or ≥4 wheezing episodes/1 year lasting >1 day AND risk factors for persistent asthma	≥2x/year (see notes) Relative annual risk may be related to FEV₁				
	Recommended Step for Initiating Therapy (See "Stepwise Approach for Managing Asthma" for treatment steps.)	Step 1 (for both age groups)		Step 2 (for both age groups)		Step 3 and consider short course of oral systemic corticosteroids	Step 3: medium-dose ICS option and consider short course of oral systemic corticosteroids	Step 3 and consider short course of oral systemic corticosteroids	Step 3: medium-dose ICS option OR step 4 and consider short course of oral systemic cortico[...]

The stepwise approach is meant to assist, not replace [...]

Source: National Heart, Lung, and Blood Institute, 2007. Used with permission.

d. Education on asthma self-management, and, for younger children, parent/caregiver-management, should be provided and reinforced at each asthma patient encounter. This education includes:

(1) Teaching and reinforcement of self-monitoring or parent/caregiver monitoring to assess level of asthma control and signs and symptoms of worsening asthma.

(2) For older patients, how to use peak flow monitoring for this purpose.

(3) For younger children, assess for presentation and severity of symptoms.

(4) Education also includes the patient's:

(a) Specifically written Asthma Action Plan.

(b) Correct medication administration techniques, including demonstration and return-demonstration, and use of spacer devices with metered-dose inhaler devices.

(c) Avoidance of environmental factors and triggers that worsen asthma.

(d) Instructions regarding rinsing mouth after taking inhaled medications.

(e) Specific instruction regarding prescribed medications and differences between controller medications and rescue medications.

e. Control environmental and co-morbid conditions.

(1) Assess specific trigger and symptom history and recommend measures to control exposures to allergens, pollutants, and irritants that can trigger or worsen an asthma exacerbation.

(2) Consider allergen immunotherapy for patients with persistent asthma.

(3) Inactivated influenza vaccine is recommended for all patients with asthma over 6 months of age.

(4) Identify and treat co-morbid conditions such as obesity, obstructive sleep apnea, gastroesophageal reflux, rhinitis, sinusitis, stress, and depression.

f. Context of disease management: Coordination of care includes working with the parent/caregiver to meet the goals of treatment within the context of the child's development, environment, home routines, school or child care settings, activities, and insurance coverage/payment for treatment and medications.

3. Assess for common fears and misconceptions that can lead to poor adherence and increased severity of symptoms. Educate parents, caregivers, and patients that:

a. Asthma IS NOT caused by an emotional problem.

b. Asthma involves chronic inflammation, which likely will require ongoing treatment and medications, even when there are no apparent symptoms.

c. Asthma medications ARE NOT addictive and CANNOT lose effectiveness over time. One of the most common mistakes made in asthma management is delaying the start of treatment to "wait and see" if it will get better with time or go away on its own.

d. Asthma medications and treatment require ongoing monitoring and assessment to determine effectiveness of treatment.

e. Certain asthma medications, such as metered-dose inhalers (MDIs), need to be frequently checked to ensure that the device is not empty. Most MDIs last approximately for one month if taken at prescribed daily doses.

f. Patients and parents need to be instructed regarding appropriate cleaning of asthma equipment.

g. Patients with well-controlled asthma can usually tolerate their normal activities and exercise. The goal of optimal asthma control is no restrictions on these activities.

h. When used as prescribed, inhaled corticosteroids are safe and well-tolerated and ARE NOT the same as anabolic steroids.

i. Asthma exacerbations rarely occur suddenly without any warning signs.

j. There are different but equal methods to administer asthma medications: Nebulizer medications are not superior to MDIs as long as they are used appropriately.

4. Nurse as advocate – Ambulatory care nurses can help advocate for pediatric patients and their parents/caregivers by:

a. Assessing patient's ability to pay for necessary diagnostic procedures and care, medications, equipment, and treatments.

b. Assisting with financial support and resources when necessary to assist with medication and equipment purchase.

c. Identifying community resources, including summer camps for children with asthma.

d. Advocating on the patient's behalf with the insurer and providing appropriate documentation to support medical necessity of diagnostic procedures and care, medications, equipment, and treatments.

E. Collaboration and referrals – Referral to a pulmonologist or allergist/immunologist with specialty training in asthma care is recommended if:

1. The patient has experienced a life-threatening asthma exacerbation.

2. The patient has required hospitalization or more than two bursts of oral corticosteroids in one year.

3. The pediatric patient older than the age of 5 requires Step 4 care or higher.

4. The pediatric patient 5-years-old or younger requires Step 3 care or higher.

5. Asthma is not controlled after 3–6 months of active therapy and appropriate monitoring.

6. The patient appears unresponsive to therapy.

7. The diagnosis of asthma is uncertain.

8. The patient has additional conditions which complicate management such as chronic sinusitis, nasal polyps, severe rhinitis, or vocal cord dysfunction.

9. Additional diagnostic testing is needed.

10. The patient may need allergen immunotherapy.

11. There may be non-adherence concerns (Fanta & Fletcher, 2011).

F. Telehealth nursing practice – Includes all of the components of the nursing process: The nurse triager evaluates the receipt of the triage information through the following actions:

1. Gives specific follow-up advice, including when to call back or seek emergency care:

a. Worsening symptoms despite treatment.

b. Symptoms failing to improve.

c. Onset of new symptoms.

2. Summarizes the phone call and repeats the follow-up advice.

3. Requests the caller to repeat the advice given.

4. Ends the call with a statement such as, "Please call back if there is any change, new concerns develop, or if you have any additional questions."

5. The nurse triager documents the telehealth triage call utilizing standardized documentation in accordance with the practice's policies and procedures. This documentation should include all of the previous components discussed in this section.

G. Protocols/algorithms/guidelines – Resources.

1. The National Heart, Lung, and Blood Institute (2007) – *National Asthma Education and Prevention Program (NAEPP) Expert*

Panel Report 3: Guidelines for the Diagnosis and Management of Asthma.

2. American Lung Association (2011a) – *Asthma*.
3. Asthma and Allergy Foundation of American (AAFA) (n.d.) – *AAFA Web Site*.
4. WebMD (2012) – *Allergies and Asthma*.
5. Agency for Healthcare Research and Quality (AHRQ) National Guideline Clearinghouse (n.d.) – *Asthma*.
6. American Academy of Allergy, Asthma & Immunology (AAAAI) (2012) – *Asthma Statistics*.

Sickle Cell Disease

Patient Population: Pediatric

I. Overview

Sickle cell disease is an autosomal recessive disorder of the red blood cells resulting from a single gene mutation in which glutamic acid is replaced by valine. In the United States, 1 in 10 African Americans have sickle cell trait and 1 in 325 has sickle cell disease. Sickle cell trait is not a disease. It is the carrier state and does not cause symptoms except under extreme circumstance (National Heart, Lung, and Blood Institute [NHLBI], 2004). The complications in sickle cell disease are due to vascular occlusion (also known as vaso-occlusion, a blockage of blood vessels) and chronic anemia. There are four major variants of the disease (see Table 21-13).

Newborn screening has played a significant role in decreasing mortality and morbidity by providing early identification of affected babies. This early identification provides the opportunity for early intervention. Currently, 50 states (including the District of Columbia) have mandatory newborn screening programs (National Newborn Screening and Genetics Resource Center, 2012).

The complications of sickle cell disease are episodic and the severity can be different for each individual, as well as different for one individual throughout his or her lifetime (Aliyu, Tumblin, & Kato, 2006). Individuals with sickle cell disease are now frequently surviving beyond the age of 50 (Aliyu et al., 2006). Individuals with sickle cell disease should receive the same general health care

**Table 21-13.
Nomenclature of the Four Major
Variants of Sickle Cell Disease**

Full Name	Abbreviation
Sickle cell disease-SS	SCD-SS
Sickle cell disease-SC	SCD-SC
Sickle cell disease-Sβ° thalassemia	SCD-Sβ° thal
Sickle cell disease-Sβ+ thalassemia	SCD-Sβ+ thal

Source: Adapted from National Heart, Lung, and Blood Institute, 2004.

as individuals without the disease. However, whenever possible, they should also be followed in an organized sickle cell program or in a place where the providers have knowledge and experience of the disease and its management (NHLBI, 2004).

II. Pathophysiology

Sickle cell disease is characterized by the production of abnormal hemoglobin that results in decreased red blood cell survival and polymerization of red blood cells (sickling). When the red blood cell in sickle disease loses its oxygen, it becomes deformed, hard, and sticky. This change in the red blood cells results in an increase in blood viscosity and blockage of blood vessels, leading to tissue ischemia and adherence to vessels. The red blood cell in sickle cell disease is smaller than the normal red blood cell and has a shortened lifespan, leading to a chronic anemia. The clinical manifestations of the disease are due to chronic anemia, acute anemia, and vaso-occlusion.

III. Complications
A. Fever and infection: Alteration in thermodynamics.
 1. Overview.
  a. Temperature greater than or equal to 101 °F may be indicative of life-threatening bacterial infection: A medical emergency.
  b. Increased susceptibility to bacterial infection due to decreased splenic function.

c. Leading cause of death in children with sickle cell disease under the age of 5.

d. Most common causative agents: *Streptococcus pneumoniae, Haemophilus influenzae, Neisseria meningitides, Salmonella, Staphylococcus aureus, E. coli,* and *Streptococcus pyogenes* (Pack-Mabien & Haynes, 2009).

e. Considered a medical emergency because the risk of death from overwhelming sepsis is high.

2. Pathophysiology.
   a. Sickling of red blood cells causes autoinfarction of the spleen.
   b. Spleen becomes non-functional.
   c. Spleen unable to filter bacteria from the blood stream.

3. Assessment and triage.
   a. Symptoms and history.
      (1) Fever, cough, symptoms of URI and/or UTI.
      (2) Duration of fever.
      (3) Hydration.
      (4) Baseline hemoglobin, hematocrit, O_2 saturation.
      (5) Previous admissions.
      (6) Last dose of Ceftriaxone®.
      (7) Transfusion and surgical history.
      (8) Vaccination history including pneumococcal vaccine status, including doses of pneumococcal polysaccharide vaccine (PPSV) and/or pneumococcal conjugate vaccine (both PCV7 and PCV13).
      (9) Current medications.
      (10) Allergies.
   b. Physical assessment.
      (1) Vital signs.
      (2) Chest auscultation.
      (3) Ears, throat (potential source of fever).
   c. Diagnostic tests.
      (1) Complete blood count (CBC) with differential.
      (2) Reticulocyte count.
      (3) Blood culture.
      (4) Urinalysis and urine culture for symptoms of UTI.
      (5) Chest X-ray if signs of pneumonia/ acute chest syndrome.

4. Indications for emergency care or urgent consultation.
   a. Fever of 101 °F or greater.
   b. Shortness of breath.
   c. Neurological symptoms.
   d. Severe tachypnea or tachycardia.

5. Plan of care.
   a. IV hydration.
   b. IV antibiotics.
   c. Antipyretics.
   d. Goals of plan: Patient is afebrile with negative cultures and symptoms resolved.
   e. Education of patients/family.
      (1) Emphasize that fever in a child with sickle cell disease can be indicative of a life-threatening bacterial infection.
      (2) Immediate medical attention is needed for temperature greater than or equal to 101 °F.
      (3) Do not give antipyretics unless advised by health care provider.
      (4) Penicillin prophylaxis should be given as directed. It is very important that the child does not miss a dose. Call for refills before medication runs out.
         (a) Penicillin VK 125 mg twice a day from 2 months of age until 3-years-old.
         (b) Penicillin VK 250 mg twice a day if over the age of 3.
      (5) Caregiver should demonstrate the ability to take a temperature.
      (6) Instruct caregiver to call if child has fever greater than or equal to 101 °F, diarrhea, vomiting, productive cough, irritability, or "just doesn't seem right."
      (7) Encourage good primary care follow-up and keeping immunizations up to date.
         (a) Pneumococcal vaccine.

i. Infants should receive a series of four doses of pneumococcal conjugate vaccine (PCV13).

ii. After the age of 2, children with sickle cell disease should also receive a dose of pneumococcal polysaccharide vaccine (PPSV23).

   (b) Annual influenza vaccine.

B. Vaso-occlusive painful episode: Alteration in comfort.

1. Overview.
   a. Most common type of vaso-occlusive episode.
   b. May be precipitated by extreme changes in temperature, stress, infection, dehydration, and hypoxia, but may occur without identifiable precipitating factors.
   c. Most are not life-threatening.
   d. Accounts for most hospitalizations.
   e. Onset is usually sudden, unpredictable, recurrent, and variable.
   f. Dactylitis or hand-foot syndrome.
      (1) Acute painful swelling of one or more extremities.
      (2) Usually occurs in children between 6 months and 2 years of age.
      (3) Duration is approximately one week. Can reoccur.
      (4) Can be predicative of severe disease.

2. Pathophysiology.
   a. Occurs due to the blockage of small blood vessels by sickle cells.
   b. Decreased oxygen perfusion, ischemia, infarction, and pain.

3. Assessment and triage – Usually occurs on the telephone.
   a. Symptoms and history.
      (1) Location, onset, and severity of pain. Is it typical or atypical of vaso-occlusive pain? Use appropriate pain scales to classify severity of pain as mild, moderate, or severe.
      (2) Medications taken, dose taken, time of last dose, and response to medication.
      (3) Pain medications that have worked in the past.
      (4) Effective non-pharmacologic therapies used.
      (5) Rule out possibility of trauma.
      (6) Refer for acute care management if home management unsuccessful.
   b. Physical assessment.
      (1) Vital signs.
      (2) Examination of site for swelling and erythema.
      (3) Assess spleen size if having abdominal pain.
      (4) For chest pain, attempt to determine if it is bone pain.
   c. Diagnostic tests.
      (1) CBC with differential.
      (2) Reticulocyte count.
      (3) X-ray of painful site if swelling and erythema are present.
      (4) Chest X-ray for chest pain.

4. Indications for emergency care or urgent care.
   a. Pain accompanied by fever greater than or equal to 101 °F.
   b. Severe chest pain.
   c. Left side abdominal pain and swelling.

5. Plan of care.
   a. Increase fluids.
   b. Rest and relaxation.
   c. Distraction.
   d. Massage.
   e. Warm compresses.
   f. Combination drug therapy – Opioids with NSAIDs and/or acetaminophen.
   g. If home management is unsuccessful, patient/parent should call health care provider and go to the emergency room for evaluation and IV pain management.
   h. Assess response to medication and seek change of plan as indicated.
   i. Assess respiratory status. Encourage ambulation and use of incentive spirometer.

j. Assess possible side effects to medication such as puritis, oversedation, and GI complaints. Administer stool softener, diphenhydramine, and antacids as indicated per protocol or provider order.

k. Goal of care: Alleviation of pain.

l. Education of patient and family.
   (1) Patient/family education.
      (a) FARMS (Platt & Sacerdote, 2006).
         i. **F** = Fluids and Fever – Drink plenty of fluids and seek immediate medical care for fever.
         ii. **A** = Air – Maintain adequate oxygen.
         iii. **R** = Rest – Get plenty of sleep, rest when needed, no over-exertion.
         iv. **M** = Medication – Take medication as directed.
         v. **S** = Situations – Avoid getting too hot or too cold, smoking, alcohol, and illegal drugs.
      (b) Side effects of medication, correct dosing of medication, types of non-pharmacologic treatments.
      (c) Parents should be aware that opioids can lead to severe constipation.

C. Acute exacerbation of anemia: Alteration in fluid volume; alteration in tissue perfusion.
   1. Overview (NHLBI, 2004).
      a. Usual cause – Parvovirus B19.
      b. May require hospitalization and red cell transfusion if decreasing hemoglobin results in symptoms of cardiac compromise.
      c. An outpouring of nucleated red blood cells in about 7–10 days indicates recovery.
   2. Pathophysiology.
      a. Bone marrow viral suppression of red blood cell production.
      b. Severe anemia.
   3. Assessment and triage – Usually occurs over the telephone.
      a. Symptoms and history.
         (1) Assess for fever, cough, and rash.
         (2) Determine if child has tachypnea, tachycardia, listlessness, or pallor.
         (3) Does the child have a palpable spleen?
         (4) Refer to emergency department.
      b. Physical assessment.
         (1) Vital signs.
         (2) Assess for tachypnea, tachycardia, listlessness, or pallor.
         (3) Assess spleen size.
      c. Diagnostic tests.
         (1) Complete blood count with reticulocyte count, parvovirus titer.
         (2) Type and cross for possible red blood cell transfusion.
         (3) Blood cultures if febrile.
         (4) IV hydration, IV antibiotics, if indicated.
   4. Indications for emergency care or urgent consultation.
      a. Tachypnea.
      b. Tachycardia.
      c. Listlessness.
      d. Pallor.
      e. Hypersplenism.
   5. Plan of care.
      a. Monitor hemoglobin/hematocrit, reticulocyte count.
      b. Monitor for signs of cardiovascular compromise due to decreased hemoglobin.
      c. Monitor spleen size.
      d. Isolate from others at increased risk for infection, such as pregnant women, those who are immunocompromised, and others with hemolytic anemias.
      e. Goal of plan of care.
         (1) Adequate hydration.
         (2) Resolution of acute anemia noted by outpouring of nucleated red blood cells as seen on CBC. Usually occurs in about 7–10 days.
      f. Education of patient/family.

(1) Usual cause – Parvovirus B19. Does not recur. Self-limiting.
(2) Seek medical attention if child has fever greater than or equal to 101 °F, is pale, more tired, has rapid heartbeat, or rapid breathing.
(3) May require hospitalization and red cell transfusion if decreasing hemoglobin results in symptoms of cardiac compromise.
(4) Highly contagious; siblings and other close contacts with sickle cell disease should be evaluated.

D. Acute splenic sequestration: Alteration in fluid volume.
1. Overview (NHLBI, 2004).
   a. Spleen becomes large and tender.
   b. Potentially life-threatening.
   c. Usually requires hospitalization and possibly red blood cell transfusion if decreasing hemoglobin results in symptoms of cardiac compromise.
   d. Usually occurs between the ages of 3 months and 5 years in those with SCD-SS. Recurrence is common.
2. Pathophysiology.
   a. Intrasplenic trapping of red blood cells.
   b. Precipitous fall in hemoglobin level and the potential for hypoxic shock.
3. Assessment and triage.
   a. Symptoms and history.
      (1) Onset of symptoms.
         (a) Fever.
         (b) Irritability.
         (c) Tachypnea.
         (d) Tachycardia.
         (e) Listlessness.
         (f) Pallor.
         (g) Left-sided abdominal pain and swelling.
   b. Physical assessment.
      (1) Vital signs.
      (2) Baseline hemoglobin/hematocrit, spleen size.
      (3) Assess spleen size and mark location.
      (4) Refer to emergency room.

c. Diagnostic tests.
   (1) CBC with reticulocyte count, parvovirus titer.
   (2) Type and cross for possible red blood cell transfusion.
   (3) Blood cultures if febrile.
   (4) IV hydration, IV antibiotics, if indicated.
4. Indications for emergency care or urgent consultation.
   a. Tachypnea.
   b. Tachycardia.
   c. Listlessness.
   d. Pallor.
   e. Hypersplenism.
5. Plan of care.
   a. Monitor hemoglobin/hematocrit, reticulocyte count.
   b. Monitor for signs of cardiovascular compromise due to decreased hemoglobin.
   c. IV hydration and IV antibiotics if indicated.
   d. Assess spleen size hourly and mark location.
   e. Mark level of spleen at discharge.
   f. Goal of plan of care.
      (1) Adequate hydration.
      (2) Resolution of acute anemia.
      (3) Reduction in spleen size.
   g. Patient/family education.
      (1) Seek medical attention if child has fever greater than or equal to 101 °F, is pale, more tired than usual, has rapid heartbeat, rapid breathing, complaint of left side abdominal pain.
      (2) Teach family how to palpate spleen.
      (3) Explain that splenic sequestration often recurs and child may need to be started on a chronic transfusion program. Splenectomy may be indicated, particularly if recurrence occurs while on a transfusion program.
      (4) Maintain adequate fluid intake.

E. Acute chest syndrome: Alteration in gas exchange.
   1. Overview (NHLBI, 2004).
      a. Defined as an acute illness characterized by fever and respiratory symptoms, accompanied by a new pulmonary infiltrate on a chest X-ray.
      b. Frequent cause of death in both children and adults with sickle cell disease.
      c. The second most common cause of hospitalizations in patients with sickle cell disease.
      d. Most common complication of surgery and anesthesia in these patients.
      e. May be caused by pulmonary fat embolism, pulmonary infarction, and infection.
      f. Most common organisms isolated are *Streptococcus pneumoniae, Haemophilus influenzae, Mycoplasma pneumoniae, Chlamydia pneumoniae* (Pack-Mabien & Haynes, 2009).
   2. Pathophysiology.
      a. Occlusion of the pulmonary vascular bed by sickle erythrocytes.
      b. Infection.
      c. Embolized marrow or marrow fat, and lung infarction.
   3. Assessment and triage.
      a. Symptoms and history.
         (1) Assess for fever, cough, chest pain, shortness of breath.
         (2) Assess for history of painful episodes, medications taken, decreased activity.
         (3) Refer to emergency department.
      b. Physical assessment.
         (1) Assess and monitor oxygen saturation.
         (2) Assess and monitor respiratory status.
         (3) Assess and monitor vital signs.
      c. Diagnostic tests.
         (1) Complete blood count, reticulocyte count, blood cultures type and cross, chest X-ray, monitor oxygen saturation.

   (2) Carefully monitor IV hydration.
   (3) Supplemental oxygen as needed.
   (4) IV antibiotics. Pain medication, antipyretics, and bronchodilators, as indicated.
   (5) Red blood cell transfusion, as indicated.
   4. Indications for emergency care or urgent consultation.
      a. Fever.
      b. Cough.
      c. Chest pain.
      d. Shortness of breath.
   5. Plan of care.
      a. Monitor hydration (very important to avoid over hydration). Carefully monitor intake and output.
      b. Encourage use of incentive spirometer and encourage ambulation.
      c. Monitor vital signs and laboratory values carefully.
      d. Patient/family education.
         (1) Instruct patient to complete course of antibiotics.
         (2) Use of incentive spirometer.
         (3) Importance of ambulation.
         (4) Seek medical attention if child has fever greater than or equal to 101 °F, chest pain, difficulty breathing.

F. Pulmonary arterial hypertension (PAH).
   1. Overview (Thomas, 2006).
      a. Defined as a mean pulmonary artery pressure greater than 25 mm/Hg at rest or greater than 30 mm/Hg during exercise.
      b. Can be caused by any disease that causes problems with blood flow through the lungs or that causes long periods of decreased oxygen in the blood.
      c. Increased risk for PAH in sickle cell disease due to:
         (1) Increased breakdown of red blood cells.
         (2) Decreased sensitivity to nitric oxide.
         (3) Constriction of the small arteries of the lungs.

2. Pathophysiology.
   a. Multifactorial.
   b. Prominent role for intravascular hemolysis inducing a state of vascular dysfunction.
3. Assessment and triage.
   a. Symptoms and history.
      (1) Individuals with mild disease may not show any signs or symptoms.
      (2) Assess and monitor for shortness of breath; fatigue; decreased exercise tolerance; swelling of ankles, legs, abdomen, or arms; chest discomfort or pain; light-headedness; and fainting (Pulmonary Hypertension Association, 2010).
   b. Physical.
      (1) Complete history and physical examination.
      (2) Assess and monitor oxygen saturation.
      (3) Assess and monitor respiratory status.
      (4) Assess and monitor vital signs.
   c. Diagnostic tests.
      (1) Echocardiogram.
         (a) Non-invasive.
         (b) Determines the pressure in the right ventricle.
      (2) B natriuretic peptide (BNP) level.
4. Indications for emergency care or urgent consultation.
   a. Shortness of breath.
   b. Fatigue and decreased exercise tolerance.
   c. Swelling of ankles, legs, abdomen, or arms.
   d. Chest discomfort and pain.
   e. Light-headedness and fainting.
5. Plan of care.
   a. Limited data on specific management.
   b. Control of sickle cell disease (Machado & Gladwin, 2010).
      (1) Hydroxyurea.
      (2) Red blood cell transfusion.
      (3) Hydration.
   c. Oral medications (Kato, Onyekwere, & Gladwin, 2007).

(1) Sildenafil – Reduces pulmonary pressure and improves cardiopulmonary performance.
(2) Bosentan – Endothelin receptor.
   d. Goals of plan of care.
      (1) Relief of symptoms.
      (2) Retard progression of disease.
   e. Education of patient/family.
      (1) Echocardiogram yearly starting at 10-years-old.
      (2) Seek medical attention for any signs and symptoms.
         (a) Shortness of breath.
         (b) Fatigue and decreased exercise tolerance.
         (c) Swelling of ankles, legs, abdomen, or arms.
         (d) Chest discomfort and pain.
         (e) Light-headedness and fainting.
      (3) Encourage compliance with regimen.
G. Priapism: Alteration in comfort.
   1. Overview (Field, Vemulakonda, & DeBaun, 2011).
      a. Sustained, unwanted penile erection in the absence of sexual activity or desire lasting more than 2–4 hours.
      b. High flow (arterial) priapism – Usually due to trauma.
      c. Low flow (ischemic) priapism – Type usually seen in sickle cell disease.
      d. Abnormal regulation of the nitric oxide pathway (Crane & Bennett, 2011).
      e. Risk factors:
         (1) Prolonged sexual activity.
         (2) Fever or dehydration.
         (3) Exposure to alcohol, marijuana, or cocaine.
         (4) Use of psychotropic agents, sildenafil, or testosterone.
      f. Types (NHLBI, 2004):
         (1) Prolonged priapism lasts for more than 3 hours.
         (2) Stuttering priapism lasts for less than 3 hours, but more than a few minutes. Resolves spontaneously.

g. Associated with an increased incidence of erectile dysfunction.
2. Pathophysiology.
   a. Unregulated arterial inflow to the penis.
   b. Vaso-occlusion causing obstruction of the venous drainage of the penis.
3. Assessment and triage.
   a. Symptoms and history.
      (1) Assess time of onset, presence of trauma, infection, or drug use.
      (2) Assess for fever, dysuria, and dehydration.
      (3) Assess type of home management strategies attempted.
      (4) History of prior episodes and effective treatments.
      (5) Refer to emergency room if no relief after 2 hours.
   b. Physical assessment.
      (1) Vital signs.
      (2) Assess for engorged penis, penile pain, and a soft glans.
   c. Diagnostic tests.
      (1) Complete blood count with reticulocyte count.
      (2) Urinalysis to rule out associated UTI.
4. Indications for emergency care or urgent consultation.
   a. Erection lasting more than 2 hours.
   b. Fever greater than or equal to 101 °F.
5. Plan of care.
   a. IV hydration and IV morphine.
   b. Encourage patient to empty bladder.
   c. Consult urology for possible penile aspiration if above management is unsuccessful after 2 hours.
   d. Red blood cell transfusion if indicated.
   e. Goals of plan of care: Resolution of episode.
   f. Education of patient/family.
      (1) Explain to patient that it is very important to let someone know right away when episode begins.
      (2) What to do at home: Drink plenty of fluids, attempt to empty bladder, take analgesics, and take warm shower or bath.

(3) Seek medical care if unresolved after 2 hours.
(4) Take medications as prescribed.
H. Cerebrovascular accident: Alteration in neurological status.
   1. Overview (Verduzco & Nathan, 2009).
      a. About 5–10% of children with SCD-SS are at risk for stroke (Aygun et al., 2009).
      b. Ischemic stroke accounts for 54% of stroke in the first decade and after the age of 30.
      c. Hemorrhagic strokes are seen during the 20s.
      d. 10–30% of sickle cell patients have silent strokes.
         (1) No clinical symptoms.
         (2) Associated with cognitive deficiencies.
      e. Risk factors include history of transient ischemic attack, low steady state hemoglobin concentration, sickle cerebral vasculopathy, elevated transcranial Doppler ultrasound velocity, recent or recurrent acute chest syndrome, and acute anemic events (Dowling, Quinn, Rogers, & Buchanan, 2010).
   2. Pathophysiology.
      a. Sickle red blood cell lose deformability and become sticky.
      b. Obstructive adhesion of sickle cells to each other and to vascular endothelium.
   3. Assessment and triage.
      a. Symptoms and history.
         (1) Assess for fever, headaches, syncope, altered mental status, weakness, visual changes, seizures.
         (2) History of previous neurologic events.
         (3) Refer for emergency care.
      b. Physical assessment.
         (1) Vital signs.
         (2) Complete physical with neurological examination.
      c. Diagnostic tests.
         (1) Immediate CT scan.
         (2) Brain MR studies.

      (3) Complete blood count with reticulocyte count.

      (4) Type and cross.

      (5) Hemoglobin quantitation to determine percentage of sickle hemoglobin.

4. Indications for emergency care or urgent consultation.

  a. Sudden weakness or tingling of an arm, leg, or the whole body; facial changes.

  b. Loss of vision or speech.

  c. Sudden, strong headache described as the "worst headache I've ever had."

  d. Fainting, dizziness.

5. Plan of care.

  a. Complete physical with neurological examination.

  b. ICU admission.

  c. Exchange transfusion.

  d. Consult neurology.

  e. Chronic transfusion program as secondary stroke prevention.

  f. Goals of plan of care.

    (1) Resolution of symptoms.

    (2) Prevention of further damage.

    (3) Primary stroke prevention.

      (a) Yearly transcranial Doppler.

      (b) Yearly brain MR studies.

      (c) Transfusion therapy for abnormal studies.

  g. Education of patient/family.

    (1) Seek medical attention immediately for any symptoms of stroke.

      (a) Sudden weakness or tingling of an arm, leg, or the whole body; facial changes.

      (b) Loss of vision or speech.

      (c) Sudden, strong headache described as the "worst headache I've ever had."

      (d) Fainting, dizziness.

    (2) Encourage compliance with transfusion, medications, rehabilitation.

I. Gallbladder disease (gallstones): Alteration in comfort.

1. Overview (NHLBI, 2004).

  a. Gallstones can be detected in children as young as 2-years-old.

  b. May cause blockage of common bile duct.

  c. Abdominal ultrasound is the most accurate method of detecting gallstones (Pack-Mabien & Haynes, 2009).

2. Pathophysiology.

  a. Chronic hemolysis and increased bilirubin turnover leads to a high incidence of pigmented gallstones.

  b. Biliary sludge (viscous material) may be a precursor to the development of gallstones.

3. Assessment and triage.

  a. Symptoms and history.

    (1) Onset of symptoms, may be precipitated by eating fatty or fried foods.

    (2) History of previous episodes.

    (3) Refer to emergency room if febrile or severe pain.

  b. Physical assessment.

    (1) Vital signs.

    (2) Assess for fever, increased scleral icterus, nausea, vomiting, and right upper quadrant pain.

  c. Diagnostic tests.

    (1) Complete blood count with reticulocyte count.

    (2) Hepatic panel.

    (3) Abdominal ultrasound.

4. Indications for emergency care or urgent consultation.

  a. Fever.

  b. Severe right upper quadrant pain associated with nausea or vomiting and increased jaundice.

5. Plan of care.

  a. Abdominal ultrasound.

  b. Liver function test and bilirubin profile.

  c. If recurrent episodes, cholecystectomy with pre-operative transfusion.

  d. Goals of plan of care: Resolution of problem.

  e. Education patient/family.

    (1) Seek medical attention if child has fever, right upper quadrant abdominal pain, nausea, vomiting, or increased jaundice.

(2) Dietary – Avoid fatty and fried foods.

(3) Explain need for pre-operative transfusion if surgery is indicated.

J. Renal complications.

1. Overview (NHLBI, 2004).

a. Numerous structural and functional abnormalities along the entire length of the nephron.

b. Vasa recti is susceptible to malformation due to increased sickling in this area.

c. Inability to concentrate urine leads to a high incidence of enuresis, nocturia, and polyuria.

d. Problems noted to occur involving the kidneys:

(1) Proteinuria, may be indicative of glomerulas sclerosis.

(2) Hematuria, secondary to papillar necrosis.

(3) Urinary tract infections.

(4) Renal failure.

2. Pathophysiology.

a. Sickling of erythrocytes in the vasa recta capillaries in the medulla.

b. Ischemia and infarction in the renal microcirculation.

3. Assessment and triage (Pack-Mabien & Haynes, 2009).

a. Symptoms and history.

(1) Inability to concentrate urine.

(a) Enuresis.

(b) Frequent urination.

(2) Signs of chronic renal insufficiency.

(a) Microalbuminuria.

(b) Proteinuria.

(c) Hypertension.

(d) Worsening anemia.

b. Physical assessment.

(1) Vital signs.

(2) Assess for weight change.

(3) Assess for signs of edema.

(4) Assess for supra-pubic tenderness.

(5) Assess lungs for decreased breath sounds.

c. Diagnostic tests.

(1) Yearly serum creatinine level.

(2) Routine urinalysis.

(3) Complete blood count with reticulocyte count.

(4) Chemistry profile with electrolytes.

(5) Kidney ultrasound.

4. Indications for emergency care or urgent consultation.

a. Pedal edema.

b. Hematuria.

5. Plan of care.

a. Dependent on symptoms.

b. Consult urology and nephrology as indicated.

c. Red cell transfusion as indicated.

d. Goals of plan of care: Slow progression of disease.

e. Nursing intervention/patient/family education.

(1) Encourage adequate fluid intake.

(2) Should have easy access to bathroom, particularly during school hours.

(3) Enuresis is not a cause for disciplinary action.

(4) Use of bedwetting alarm when indicated.

(5) Instruct on signs and symptoms of urinary tract infection.

K. Avascular necrosis: Alteration in comfort and mobility.

1. Overview (NHLBI, 2004).

a. Most prevalent in patients with SCD-SS.

b. Most often involves the femoral and humeral heads.

2. Pathophysiology.

a. Multifactorial.

b. Vascular occlusion (vaso-occlusion) – Interruption of the blood supply.

c. Collapse of boney structure.

d. Bone destruction, pain, and loss of joint function.

3. Assessment and triage.

a. Symptoms and history.

(1) Pain in hip or shoulder.

(2) Impaired mobility.

    b. Physical assessment.
      (1) Assess for pain in hip or shoulder.
      (2) Assess for impaired mobility.
      (3) Decreased range of motion.
    c. Diagnostic tests: X-ray and MRI of affected joints.
  4. Indications for emergency care or urgent consultation.
    a. Severe pain.
    b. Inability to ambulate.
  5. Plan of care.
    a. Consult orthopedic medicine.
    b. Treatment may include chronic transfusion to promote healing, crutches, braces.
    c. Surgery may be indicated if palliative treatment is unsuccessful.
    d. Goals of plan of care: Resolution of symptoms.
    e. Education patient/family.
      (1) Seek medical attention for pain, particularly when bearing weight or attempting to use arms.
      (2) Instruct patient to maintain follow-up with orthopedics.
      (3) Encourage patient to avoid bearing weight and to use crutches as indicated.
      (4) Explain necessity of pre-operative transfusion if surgery is indicated.
L. Retinopathy: Alteration in vision.
  1. Overview (NHLBI, 2004).
    a. Nonproliferative disease includes conjunctival vascular occlusions, iris atrophy, retinal hemorrhages, retinal pigmentary changes, and other abnormalities. High rate of spontaneous regression and lack of progression.
    b. Proliferative disease involves the growth of abnormal vascular fronds that predispose the patient to vitreous hemorrhage and retinal detachment. Increased risk of visual loss from hemorrhage and retinal detachment.
    c. Individual with SCD-SC are at higher risk.

  2. Pathophysiology.
    a. Peripheral arterial occlusions resulting in retinal hypoxia and ischemia.
    b. Neovascularization.
  3. Assessment and triage.
    a. Symptoms and history.
      (1) Complaints of visual disturbances.
      (2) Assess when patient had last ophthalmology appointment.
      (3) Assess for history of previous retinopathy.
      (4) Assess for history of trauma to the eye.
    b. Physical assessment.
      (1) Assess for signs of trauma to the eye.
      (2) Assess for signs of retinal hemorrhage.
    c. Diagnostic tests: Examination done by ophthalmologist experienced in the care of individuals with sickle cell disease.
  4. Indications for emergency care or urgent consultation.
    a. Retinal hemorrhage.
    b. Loss of sight.
  5. Plan of care.
    a. Yearly examination by ophthalmologist who specializes in diseases of the retina.
    b. Treatment reserved for disease that has progressed to the proliferative stage.
    c. Methods of treatments include laser photocoagulation and vitrectomy if retinal detachment or vitreous hemorrhage is present.
    d. Goals of plan of care.
      (1) Resolution of problem.
      (2) Slow progression of retinopathy.
    e. Education of patient/family.
      (1) Seek medical attention in the event of eye trauma, changes in vision, bleeding in the eye.
      (2) Stress importance of yearly eye examination by an ophthalmologist.

IV. Current Therapies
A. Red blood cell transfusions.
   1. Indications.
      a. Episodic transfusions for acute severe anemia, pre-operative, hypoxia/acute chest syndrome.
      b. Chronic transfusions for stroke, abnormal TCD, debilitating pain, and recurrent splenic sequestration, recurrent and severe acute chest syndrome.
   2. Goals of therapy.
      a. Episodic transfusions – Correction of anemia and increase oxygen-carrying capacity.
      b. Chronic transfusion – To reduce hemoglobin S to less than 30%.
   3. Complications.
      a. Volume overload.
      b. Iron overload.
      c. Alloimmunization and delayed transfusion reaction.
      d. Infection.
   4. Education.
      a. Explain the need for need for transfusion and the potential for transfusion reaction.
      b. Inform patient/family about the importance of maintaining the transfusion regimen.
      c. Discuss eventual need for chelation therapy due to iron overload.
B. Hydroxyurea.
   1. Chemotherapeutic agent, which increases the percent of fetal hemoglobin in the red blood cell. With a high percent of fetal hemoglobin, the formation of sickle cells can be prevented.
   2. Decreases the rate of bone marrow production of red blood cells, white blood cells, and platelets.
   3. Goals of therapy.
      a. Reduce the occurrence of acute chest syndrome, severe pain, and the need for transfusions.
      b. Increase the production of fetal hemoglobin, which reduces sickling, vaso-occlusion, and hemolysis.
      c. Raises hemoglobin level.

   4. Education.
      a. How medication should be taken.
      b. Potential side effects.
        (1) Nausea and vomiting.
        (2) Mouth sores.
        (3) Headache.
        (4) Skin rashes.
        (5) Hair loss.
      c. Need for frequent laboratory evaluations.
        (1) Complete blood count with differential/reticulocyte count.
        (2) Comprehensive metabolic panel.
C. Bone marrow transplantation.
   1. Only cure for sickle cell disease.
   2. Very risky due to possibility of graph vs. host disease.
   3. Requires matched, related donor – An unaffected sibling.
   4. Candidates usually have severe disease, which may make taking the risk of transplant worthwhile.

V. Psychosocial Management
A. Multidisciplinary team approach.
   1. Patient and family.
   2. Physician, nurse, social worker.
   3. Psychologist.
   4. Community organization.
B. School/work.
   1. Frequent absences from work or school.
   2. Families should have documentation that school or work may be interrupted due to complications of the disease.
   3. Schools should have printed materials regarding care of the child with sickle cell disease in school. Need for fluids, bathroom breaks, who to call if child should become ill.
   4. Assess need for episodic homebound education.
   5. If home management is unsuccessful, patient or caregiver should call health care provider and go to the emergency room for evaluation and IV pain management.

VI. Resources

A. Local comprehensive sickle cell center, if available.

B. Sickle Disease Association of America (National) (www.sicklecelldisease.org). Several cities have local chapters.

C. Local social service agencies.

D. General sickle cell disease information – Emory site (www.scinfo.org).

E. National Institutes of Health (NIH): National Heart, Lung, and Blood Institute (NHLBI) – Division of Blood Disorders and Resources.

Developmental Delays

Patient Population: Pediatric

I. Overview

From the moment of conception, every human being sets off on a course of growth and development that is both individualized, according to multiple internal and external factors, and somewhat predictable, according to expected norms at each stage of development. The three main domains of development (bio-physical, cognitive, and psychosocial) each involve complex systems for formation and maturation. Genetic factors, phenotype (actual physical stature and appearance), and temperament can all affect the individual's growth and development. In addition, environmental and external factors, such as parenting/caregiving, nutrition, and psychosocial influences can likewise affect these processes.

From birth through adolescence and beyond, growth and development demonstrate certain universal characteristics. Physical growth occurs in cephalocaudal (head-to-toe), proximodistal (near-to-far), general to specific, and simple to complex patterns. Pace of growth also changes during each stage of development, starting off with a rapid period from birth until age 2, slowing down until puberty, and then resuming another rapid period in later adolescence. Cognitive development includes communication, perception, thinking, memory, and language acquisition (both receptive and expressive). Psychosocial development includes emotional, psychosocial, personality, social, and interpersonal skills. Developmental milestones are typically acquired at a specific rate and in an or-

derly, sequential manner. These processes continue throughout the child's life and into adulthood. Development can be measured by assessing children for achievement of expected developmental milestones at each stage of development. Screening, assessment, early identification, and intervention for developmental delays are critical to ensure that children optimize their physical, cognitive, and psychosocial development, and reach their full potential (Centers for Disease Control and Prevention [CDC] – National Center on Birth Defects and Developmental Disabilities, 2011).

A child is considered to have a developmental delay when she or he fails to achieve skills and abilities (developmental milestones) that have been mastered by children of the same age. These delays can occur in physical, cognitive, social, language, sensory, and/or emotional development (Jones, 2009). Risk factors for developmental delays include prenatal and perinatal infection, maternal substance abuse, prematurity, parental mental illness, poverty, and child abuse and neglect (TeKolste, 2006).

Because developmental delays can be markers for future problems such as autism, cerebral palsy, hearing, vision, speech and language disorders, as well as cognitive and learning disabilities, it is imperative that screening, referral, and intervention for delays are conducted as early as possible (Sices, 2007).

In the United States, more than 17% of children have developmental or behavioral disabilities such as cognitive/intellectual disorders, autism, attention deficit/hyperactivity disorder, or speech/language delays. Less than half of these children are identified prior to starting school, by which time significant learning problems may have already taken root, and timely treatment opportunities have been missed (CDC – National Center on Birth Defects and Developmental Disabilities, 2011).

II. Assessment of Developmental Milestones

According to *Bright Futures: Guidelines for Health Supervision of Infants, Children, and Adolescents* (Hagan, Shaw, & Duncan, 2008), 50–90% of all young children are expected to have achieved the following milestones by the ages listed.

A. 2 months: Head up 45°, follows past midline, laughs, smiles spontaneously.

B. 4 months: Rolls over, follows to 180°, turns to rattling sound.

C. 6 months: Sits – No support, looks for dropped yarn, turns to voice, feeds self.

D. 9 months: Pulls to stand, takes two cubes, "dada/mama" (nonspecific), waves bye-bye.

E. 12 months: Stands alone, puts block in cup, says one word, waves bye-bye, imitates activities.

F. 15 months: Walks and can walk backwards, scribbles, says three words, drinks from cup.

G. 18 months: Walks up steps, runs, dumps raisins, tower of two cubes, points to at least one body part, says six words, removes garment.

H. 2 years: Throws ball overhand, jumps up, tower of six cubes, names one picture, combines words, puts on clothing.

I. 2.5 years: Throws ball overhand, imitates vertical line, tower of eight cubes, knows two actions, speech half understandable, washes and dries hands.

J. 3 years: Balances on each foot for one second, broad jump, thumb wiggle, imitates vertical line, tower of eight cubes, speech all understandable, names one color, knows two adjectives, names friend.

K. 4 years: Hops, draws a person with three parts, defines five words, names four colors, copies a cross (+).

III. Developmental Screening

Developmental screening is designed to assist health care professionals in the early detection of developmental and behavioral disorders, and identifying young children who should receive more intensive assessment or diagnosis for potential developmental delays.

A. Current recommendations from the American Academy of Pediatrics (AAP) and the Centers for Disease Control and Prevention (CDC) endorse universal developmental surveillance and screening of all children from birth to age 3 at preventive health care visits (AAP, 2006).

B. Standardized screening tools should be used at select age intervals (9, 18, and 24 or 30 months) and whenever developmental concerns are presented by the parent or provider (LaRosa & Glascoe, 2011).

C. Children who are identified to be at risk for developmental delays require immediate referral for developmental evaluations and early intervention services.

D. Evidence supports improved child and family outcomes when developmental disorders are identified early, and children are referred for and receive appropriate intervention (King et al., 2010).

E. The most common type of developmental screening tests used in primary care settings are parent report screening surveys.
1. Parents' Evaluations of Developmental Status (PEDS).
2. Ages and Stages Questionnaires (ASQ).
3. Infant-Toddler Checklist for Language and Communications (LaRosa & Glascoe, 2011).

F. Behavioral screening tests.
1. Eyberg Child Behavioral Inventory.
2. Pediatric Symptom Checklist.
3. Modified Checklist for Autism in Toddlers (M-CHAT) (AAP, 2006).

IV. Plan of Care

A. Developmental delays and early intervention.
1. Medical, cognitive, psychosocial, and behavioral problems require early intervention, monitoring, and treatment for a child to optimize his or her full physical, mental, and psychosocial potential (CDC, 2011).
2. Depending on the child's specific delays, infants and young children may require referrals for specialty care.
   a. Neuro-developmental pediatrician (autism, global developmental delays).
   b. Developmental-behavioral specialist (autism, cognitive, and behavioral disorders).
   c. Pediatric neurologist (autism, pervasive developmental delays).
   d. Geneticist (genetic disorders, such as Fragile X Syndrome),
   e. An early intervention program.
3. In 1986, the Infants and Toddlers with Disabilities Program (Part C) of the Individuals with Disabilities Education Act (IDEA) was enacted to do the following:

a. Enhance the development of young children with developmental disabilities.

b. Minimize adverse outcomes of developmental delays.

c. Reduce the educational costs of special education services for children who enter school with undiagnosed or untreated developmental disabilities.

4. IDEA mandates that states do the following:

a. Provide early identification and provision of services to infants and toddlers who have or are at risk for developmental delays, or who have conditions that are associated with developmental delays (U.S. Department of Education, 1997).

b. Refer children, free of charge, for a comprehensive, multidisciplinary evaluation by a team of professionals.

(1) The team works with the family to decide on which services the child needs.

(2) The result is an Individualized Family Service Plan (IFSP) that includes the implementation of early intervention (EI) services for the child with developmental problems, which are coordinated, family-centered, culturally competent, and community-based (National Early Childhood Technical Assistance Center [NECTAC], 2011).

5. The first three years of children's brain development has been the subject of much research over the past few decades, and the following evidence supports early intervention to maximize the child's fullest potential (Jones, 2009).

a. The plasticity or flexibility of the neural circuits during the first three years creates an environment for optimal learning, behavior, and health. Beyond this period, these circuits become increasingly difficult to change.

b. Stable, consistent, safe, and supportive relationships with caring and responsive adults, along with appropriate nutrition are essential for healthy brain development.

c. Early psychosocial, emotional development, and physical well-being provide the foundation for optimal development of cognitive, language, and communication skills.

6. High quality early intervention services for identified delays, and positive early experiences that enhance the child's development are crucial for future success in school, work, and community. EI services positively impact developmental outcomes across all domains:

a. General health.

b. Language.

c. Communication.

d. Cognition.

e. Social/emotional development.

f. EI services that are begun earlier in the child's life are more effective and less expensive than services that are started later (NECTAC, 2011).

B. Community resources and advocacy.

1. Nurses in ambulatory care settings have the opportunity and responsibility to ensure developmental screening and referral for appropriate early intervention services.

a. Ambulatory care nurses need to familiarize themselves with the IDEA, state and local resources, and services to assist families and meet their children's needs.

b. Nurses in primary care settings can help to implement developmental screening of children at specified preventive health care/well-child visits and when a child presents with a possible developmental concern.

c. Nurses in other ambulatory care settings, such as surgi-centers, community and public health, and additional outpatient settings can also be key in identifying and referring young children with or at risk for delays.

d. Nurses in all settings can assist parents and patients through the following activities:

   (1) Providing information to parents regarding child development, developmental milestones, and age-appropriate behavior.

   (2) Accessing appropriate early intervention and other services when indicated.

   (3) Participating in continuing education training and programs on child development, developmental screening, early intervention, resource and referral services, and billing information (CDC, 2011).

   (4) Providing emotional support, counseling, and education to parents who are concerned about the developmental progress of their children.

   (5) Helping parents who may not realize their children are at risk.

C. Guidelines and resources.

1. To integrate screening and early intervention into nursing practice, guidelines may be developed using the following resources:

   a. American Academy of Pediatrics (Hagan et al., 2008) – *Bright Futures: Guidelines for Health Supervision of Infants, Children, and Adolescents, 3rd Edition* (http://brightfutures.aap.org/).

   b. Centers for Disease Control and Prevention (CDC) (2012) – *Learn the Signs. Act Early.*

   c. Zero to Three (Jones, 2009) – *Early Intervention for Infants and Toddlers with Disabilities.*

2. Additional resources for clinicians and families are listed in Table 21-14.

Autism Spectrum Disorder

Patient Population: Pediatric

I. Overview

Autism Spectrum Disorder (ASD), also known as Pervasive Developmental Disorder (PDD), is considered a neurodevelopmental disorder. The three core deficits or characteristics of Autism Spectrum Disorder/Pervasive Developmental Disorder are impairment in socialization, impairment in communication, and stereotypic and repetitive behaviors. The term *spectrum* is used because each child will possess a different combination of characteristics and to varying degrees. There is a range of signs and symptoms, and symptoms may change with age. According to the Centers for Disease Control and Prevention (CDC, 2012), 1 in 88 children are diagnosed with ASD; boys are almost 5 times more likely to be affected than girls. The disorder occurs in all racial, ethnic, and socioeconomic groups (CDC, 2010). The number of children diagnosed with ASD has been increasing, possibly due to changes broadening the diagnostic criteria. In addition, the public is more aware, which may contribute to more parents being willing to seek this diagnosis (Peacock & Yeargin-Allsopp, 2009). Many aspects of living and overall quality of life are affected for children with ASD and for their families.

II. Pathophysiology

In a person diagnosed with this disability, the brain develops differently than the normally developing brain. People with ASD process information differently than those without the disorder. Functional MRI studies have shown that there is a disconnection between different regions of the brain that process and integrate information (Williams & Minshew, 2010). The exact cause is unknown; it is thought to be a combination of factors (Inglese & Elder, 2009). Genetics is a known contributing factor. Children with a sibling or a parent with ASD are at higher risk. Incidence in a second child is 2–18%; in identical twins, 36–95%; and in fraternal twins, 0–31% (CDC, 2012; Golnik & Maccabee-Ryaboy, 2010). Other contributing factors linked to a higher risk of ASD include thalidomide and valproic acid taken during pregnancy (CDC, 2010) and Rubella virus during early pregnancy (Vaccine Education

Table 21-14.
Resources for Clinicians and Families

- American Academy of Pediatrics – National Center of Medical Home Initiatives for Children with Special Needs (http://www.medicalhomeinfo.org/)

- *Bright Futures: Guidelines for Health Supervision of Infants, Children, and Adolescents*, 3rd Edition (http://brightfutures.aap.org/)

- Healthy Steps for Young Children (http://www.healthysteps.org)

- The Individuals with Disabilities Education Act (IDEA) (http://idea.ed.gov/)

- *Learn the Signs. Act Early* (http://www.cdc.gov/ncbddd/actearly/ccp/index.html)

- National Early Childhood Technical Assistance Center (NECTAC) (http://www.nectac.org)

- Zero to Three (http://www.zerotothree.org/)

Center at The Children's Hospital of Philadelphia, 2008). There is much ongoing research into factors contributing to this disorder (Inglese & Elder, 2009).

III. Assessment and Triage

A. Impairments in ASD include socialization, communication, and stereotypic and repetitive behaviors (CDC, 2010; National Institute of Mental Health, 2009; Trillingsgaard, Sorensen, Nemec, & Jorgensen, 2005).

1. Impairment in socialization is likely to manifest as:
   a. Limited eye contact.
   b. Poor social interaction.
   c. Lack of social reciprocity.
   d. Lack of social smile.
   e. Limited or no shared or joint attention.

2. Impairment in communication is likely to manifest as:
   a. Delayed or absent speech: About 40% of children with ASD do not talk at all. Another 25–30% of children with autism have some words at 12–18 months of age and then lose them. Others may speak, but not until later in childhood.
   b. Echolalia: The repetition of words spoken by another person.
   c. Repetitive language.
   d. Loss of language at any age.
   e. Lack of make believe or social imitative play.

   f. Deficit in receptive language skills.

3. Stereotypic and repetitive behaviors are likely to manifest as:
   a. Inflexible insistence upon routines.
   b. Limited interests.
   c. Repetitive motor movements and posturing (flaps hands, rocks, spins in circles).
   d. Sensory issues: May have unusual reactions such as hyper- or hypo-sensitivity to the way things sound, smell, taste, look, or feel.
   e. Fascination with parts of objects.

B. Screening.

1. Importance of early screening (CDC, 2010; Golnik & Maccabee-Ryaboy, 2010; Pinto-Martin, Dunkle, Earls, Fliedner & Landes, 2005; Pinto-Martin, Souders, Giarelli, & Levy, 2005; Trillingsgaard et al., 2005).
   a. Developmental screening and a thorough developmental assessment is essential to obtaining a diagnosis of ASD; there is currently no other means to diagnose the disorder, even if genetic testing reveals a higher susceptibility to ASD or an associated syndrome.
   b. Early screening and early identification of ASD are important so that individualized interventions to help the child and family can begin as soon as possible.

(1) Facilitates anticipatory guidance for parents regarding the child's development.

(2) Helps families to cope with stressors.

(3) May allow therapies early in life, especially before the child's fifth birthday, which have shown greater improvements in communication, socialization, and reduction of intensity of stereotypic behaviors.

(4) Allows services for difficulties in language and other problems before school begins, which may better prepare the child for academic and social success.

(5) Facilitates early treatment, which has been associated with better long-term outcomes for children with ASD.

(6) Enables planning by the education system for provision of services.

    (a) Children with ASD are eligible to receive special education and related services under the Individuals with Disabilities Education Act [PL 105-17].

    (b) Treating children with ASD earlier is less costly than treating them later.

2. Recommendations for screening from the American Academy of Pediatrics (CDC, 2010) (see Figure 21-3):

a. Screen all children for developmental delays and disabilities during well-child visits at 9, 18, and 24–30 months of age.

b. Screen all children specifically for ASDs at well-child visits at 18 and 24 months of age.

c. Additionally, screen in the following circumstances:

(1) High risk for developmental problems because of preterm birth or failure to meet developmental milestones. See section on *Developmental Delays* in this chapter.

(2) High risk for ASDs because of sibling or other family member with ASD, or if symptoms are present.

3. Nurses' role/involvement in screening (CDC, 2010; Pinto-Martin, Dunkle et al., 2005; Pinto-Martin, Souders et al., 2005).

a. As part of the developmental assessment, ask parents key questions and make observations (see Table 21-15).

b. Provide parents with anticipatory guidance in the form of handouts on normal developmental milestones, which may help them recognize abnormal behaviors and voice concerns.

c. Administer and score standardized screening tools.

d. Influence the timing of administration of the tool; when and where the questionnaire is given to the parent during the course of the visit has an impact on office flow and the ability of the parent to complete the questionnaire accurately.

4. Screening tools (CDC, 2010; Robins, 2008).

a. Examples of screening tools for ASD.

(1) Screening Tool for Autism in Toddlers and Young Children (STAT).

(2) Checklist for Autism in Toddlers (CHAT).

(3) Modified Checklist for Autism in Toddlers (M-CHAT) (see Table 21-16).

b. Examples of screening tools for high functioning autism or Asperger Syndrome.

(1) Autism Spectrum Screening Questionnaire (ASSQ).

(2) Australian Scale for Asperger Syndrome.

C. Diagnosis (CDC, 2010) (see Figure 21-3).

1. The clinician should refer the child to one or more of the following specialists:

a. Developmental pediatrician.

b. Child neurologist.

c. Child psychologist or psychiatrist.

2. Three main diagnoses under the umbrella of Autism Spectrum Disorder/Pervasive Developmental Disorder (see Table 21-17).

Figure 21-3.
Steps to Screening and Diagnosis of Autism Spectrum Disorder (ASD)

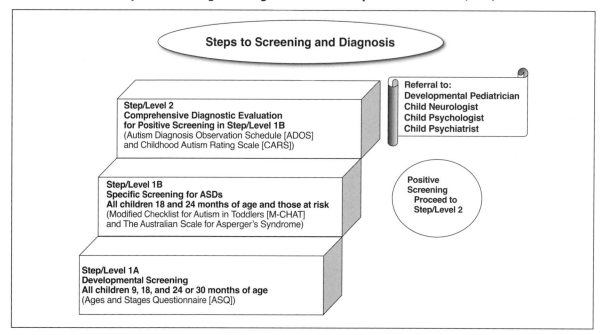

Source: Created by Deborah Byrne-Barta and Diana Anderson; adapted from CDC, 2010. Used with permission.

Table 21-15.
Nursing Developmental Assessment

Questions to ask parent:

- Does your child regularly point to show things to you?
- Does your child pretend when he or she is playing?
- Does your child seem interested in other children?
- Does your child play peek-a-boo?
- Does your child bring you things to show you?

Observations to make:

- Pay attention to how the child interacts with his or her parents.
- Does child respond to parent when called by name?
- Is language level appropriate for age?
- Allow child to explore exam room; note if child brings novel items to show others.
- How does child manipulate and play with toys (pretend play)?
- Does child make eye contact?
- Does he/she look at item when pointed at?

N.B. Developmental assessment can be performed during other procedures, such as weighing and measuring child.

Sources: Inglese, 2009; Pinto-Martin, Souders, Giarelli, & Levy, 2005.

Table 21-16.
Modified Checklist for Autism in Toddlers (M-CHAT)

- Parent-completed questionnaire designed to identify children at risk for autism in general population.
- Used for children 16–30 months of age.
- 23 questions parents fill out with follow-up interview for failed items only (5–20 minute follow-up interview).
- Failure of two critical items (items 2, 7, 9, 13, 14, 15) or any three total warrants referral to a specialist.
- Failing the follow-up interview does not diagnose ASDs; it indicates risk for ASDs.
- Sensitivity: 0.95-0.97; specificity: 0.95-0.99.

Sources: Adapted from CDC, 2010; Inglese, 2009; Robins, 2008; Robins, Fein, & Barton, 1999.

a. Autistic Disorder; "classic autism."
b. Asperger Syndrome/Disorder (AS/AD).
c. Pervasive Developmental Disorder-Not Otherwise Specified (PDD-NOS).
3. Diagnostic tools used to diagnose ASD/PDD (the CDC recommends that no single tool be used to the exclusion of another).
   a. Autism Diagnosis Interview – Revised (ADI-R).
   b. Autism Diagnostic Observation Schedule – Generic (ADOS-G).
   c. Childhood Autism Rating Scale (CARS).
   d. Gilliam Autism Rating Scale – Second Edition (GARS-2).
4. Diagnostic evaluation includes (CDC, 2010; Pinto-Martin, Souders et al., 2005):
   a. Health history.
   b. Review of child's behavior and developmental profile by one of the aforementioned specialists.
   c. The diagnosis is made based upon the criteria of the *Diagnostic and Statistical Manual-Fourth Edition-Text Revised* (DSM-IV-TR) written by the American Psychiatric Association (2000).
   d. Additional assessments may include:
      (1) Audiologic and vision screening.
      (2) Genetic testing and counseling.
      (3) Neurological assessment may include EEG (in certain circumstances).
      (4) Lead screening.
      (5) Selective metabolic testing.
D. Co-morbidities and associated genetic disorders.
1. Gastrointestinal problems/feeding issues (Golnik & Maccabee-Ryaboy, 2010; Scarpinato et al., 2010).
   a. Gastrointestinal problems may include:
      (1) Nonfunctional mealtime routines (e.g., insist that foods not touch one another on plate).
      (2) Oral aversion/sensory issues.
      (3) Selective or obsessive eating.
      (4) Chronic abdominal pain.
      (5) Constipation and diarrhea.
      (6) Food allergies or intolerances.

Table 21-17.
Three Main Types or Diagnosis Under the Umbrella of Autism Spectrum Disorder/Pervasive Developmental Disorder

Autistic Disorder ("Classic Autism")
• Usually significant social challenges. • Communication deficits; usually significant language delay. • Exhibit unusual behaviors and interests. • Many have intellectual disability; can have IQ at any level.

Asperger Syndrome/Disorder (AS/AD)
• Symptoms are usually milder than those of autistic disorder. • Experience social challenges. • Do not have language delay; may have atypical or normal language. • Have some problem with communication skills. • Exhibit unusual behaviors and interests. • Have average or above average IQ.

Pervasive Developmental Disorder-Not Otherwise Specified (PDD-NOS)
• Meet some of the criteria for Autistic Disorder or Asperger Syndrome, but not all. • Symptoms are usually fewer and milder than those of autistic disorder. • Experience social challenges. • May have difficulties with communication. • More delayed language than AS/AD. • May exhibit repetitive behaviors. • Fewer repetitive behaviors than autism and AS/AD. • Can have IQ at any level.

Sources: Adapted from CDC, 2010; Inglese & Elder, 2009.

b. Make parents aware that GI issues can compromise nutrient intake, can lead to self-injurious behavior, temper tantrums, aggression, or sleep dysfunction.
2. Sleep disturbances (American Academy of Pediatrics [AAP], 2008; Scarpinato et al., 2010).
   a. Affect one third to one half of children with ASD.

b. May cause problems with attention, irritability, and increased repetitive behaviors.

c. Etiology may be different brain wave patterns and low level of melatonin; medical issues (allergies, breathing problems, GI reflux, stomach discomfort), medications, behavior such as hyperactivity, and poor sleep routines.

d. Sleep problems include: Trouble falling asleep, night waking, early waking, nightmares, sleep terrors, and sleepwalking.

3. EEG abnormalities (Scarpinato et al., 2010).

4. Seizures (1 in 4 children with ASD develops seizures) (NIMH, 2009).

5. Psychiatric issues (Golnik & Maccabee-Ryaboy, 2010; Scarpinato et al., 2010).

   a. Aggression, self-injurious behavior (head banging, hitting, hair pulling, biting self).

   b. Anger.

   c. Anxiety.

   d. Attention-deficit/hyperactivity disorder.

   e. Bipolar disorder.

   f. Depression/major depression.

   g. Fears of physical injury.

   h. Impulsivity.

   i. Mood disorders.

   j. Obsessive compulsive disorder.

   k. Short attention span.

   l. Specific phobias.

   m. Tantrums.

6. Associated genetic disorders (CDC, 2012; Golnik & Maccabee-Ryaboy, 2010). According to the CDC, about 10% of children with ASD may have genetic and chromosomal abnormalities such as:

   a. Fragile X Syndrome.

   b. Tuberous Sclerosis.

   c. Angelman Syndrome.

   d. PTEN gene mutation.

   e. Down Syndrome.

IV. **Plan of Care**

A. Pharmacotherapeutics.

1. Commonly prescribed medications (see Table 21-18).

2. Medication safety (Elder & D'Alessandro, 2009; Inglese, 2009).

   a. Be aware of side effects, monitoring parameters, and routine laboratory work.

   b. Ask parents about complementary and alternative medicines (CAM) that they may be using for their child; biological treatment protocols may complicate management of infections, allergies, and illnesses.

B. Complementary and alternative therapies (CAM) (CDC, 2010; Golnik & Maccabee-Ryaboy, 2010).

1. Complementary and alternative therapies are controversial and may include special diets, chelation, biological- or body-based systems.

2. Prior to beginning any alternative therapies, parents should talk with their doctor.

3. Special diets: Gluten-free, casein-free; children will need vitamin and mineral supplementation (vitamin D, calcium, iron, and protein).

C. Clinic visit.

1. Children with ASD may become extremely anxious in unfamiliar surroundings and a change in their routine is stressful for them; therefore, a clinic visit may cause a great deal of anxiety (Inglese, 2009). The following are techniques and strategies nurses can use to decrease patient stress and anxiety.

   a. Preparation for clinic visit.

     (1) If possible, speak with parents prior to appointment to determine child's unique characteristics and needs.

      (a) Questions regarding communication (Golnik & Maccabee-Ryaboy, 2010; Scarpinato et al., 2010).

        i. What name does your child like to be called?

Table 21-18.
Medications Used to Treat Behavioral Symptoms in Children with Autism

Medication Class	Examples of Medication	Behaviors Addressed by Medication	Potential Side Effects	Routine Monitoring Parameters
Select Serotonin Reuptake Inhibitors (SSRIs)	Citalopram (Celexa®) Fluoxetine (Prozac®) Fluvoxamine (Luvox®) Paroxetine (Paxil®) Sertraline (Zoloft®)	Mood, problems with fixations and transitioning, impaired social skills, irritability, aggression.	Change in appetite, headache, diarrhea, racing thoughts, obsessions and compulsions, irritability, behavioral activation, sedation, tinnitus, tics.	No routine labs. Monitor for increased self-injurious behaviors, suicidal ideations.
Atypical Antipsychotics/ Neuroleptics	Risperidone (Risperdal®) Olanzapine (Zyprexa®) Quetiapine (Seroquel®) Ziprasidone (Geodon®) Aripiprazole (Abilify®)	Aggression, hyperactivity, nonverbal communication, social responsiveness, repetitive behaviors, tics, and social withdrawal.	Constipation, enuresis (bedwetting), sedation, weight gain, extrapyramidal symptoms (tremors, abnormal body movements, dystonia).	Baseline labs: Fasting lipids and glucose, liver function, electrolytes, blood count. Repeat labs 3 months after treatment begins. Monitor lipids and glucose every 6 months thereafter, as well as liver function, electrolytes, and blood count annually. Extrapyramidal symptoms assessed at three months and annually using the AIMS. Instrument. Baseline EKG for patients treated with ziprasidone, and repeated when dose of medication is increased significantly. Blood pressure, height and weight at each visit.
Stimulants	Methylphenidate (Ritalin®) Mixed salt amphetamines	Inattentive symptoms, distractibility, hyperactivity, and impulsivity.	Increased anxiety, tics and/or increase in stereotypic movements, decreased appetite, GI upset, decrease in growth velocity.	Baseline blood count and liver function, repeat annually. Blood pressure, height, and weight at each visit.
Alpha Agonists	Clonidine (Catapres®) Guanfacine (Tenex®)	Hyperactivity, impulsivity, and irritability.	Sedation, low blood pressure.	Blood pressure and heart rate.

Source: Elder & D'Alessandro, 2009.

Reprinted from *Pediatric Nursing*, 2009, Volume 35, Number 4, pp. 240-245. Used with permission of the publisher, Jannetti Publications, Inc., East Holly Avenue, Box 56, Pitman, NJ 08071-0056; (856) 256-2300; FAX (856) 589-7463; Web site: www.pediatricnursing.net. For a sample copy of the journal, please contact the publisher.

ii. What are some effective communication techniques?

iii. What is your child's developmental level?

iv. How does the child show or report pain?

(b) Questions regarding sensitivities (Scarpinato et al., 2010; Souders, Freeman, DePaul, & Levy, 2002).

   i. Does your child have hypersensitivity to touch, textures (tactile defensiveness)?

   ii. What is your child's comfort level with personal space (touch or stand back)?

   iii. Is your child hypersensitive to smells, tastes, sounds (overstimulation)?

(c) Questions regarding strategies (Golnik & Maccabee-Ryaboy, 2010; Scarpinato et al., 2010; Souders et al., 2002).

   i. What are some things that help relax and distract your child (speaking in mellow tones, counting, favorite songs)?

   ii. What things may agitate your child or trigger behaviors and what helps to calm them down?

   iii. What interventions have worked in the past for compliance with procedures and is there a need for restraints?

   iv. How are medications given at home?

(2) Preparation for tests/procedures (Inglese, 2009; Scarpinato et al., 2010; Souders et al., 2002).

(a) Ask parents: What is the best way to prepare your child for transitions, tasks, and procedures?

(b) Be aware of need for rituals or extreme fears and phobias.

(c) Inform other staff of patient's unique needs and prepare for behaviors by having extra staff on hand who are trained.

(d) If possible, allow child to manipulate instruments and materials.

(e) Prepare the environment.

   i. If possible, arrange for use of a separate waiting room.

   ii. Remove extra equipment and clutter and minimize sensory stimuli in the environment (overstimulation from noises, smells, and sounds could trigger behaviors).

   iii. Close any extra doors, especially to stairwells or nearby rooms with potential hazards because of potential for impulsive behavior.

b. During the clinic visit (Browne, 2006; Inglese, 2009; Scarpinato et al., 2010; Souders et al., 2002).

(1) Limit the number of staff and when possible, utilize staff with whom the child is familiar (many of these children have difficulty with crowds).

(2) Allow extra time for the visit; approach the child calmly, patiently, and gently.

(3) Be accepting and conscious of the child's sensitivities such as light, noise, and touch (especially to touch) before performing assessment (see Table 21-19 for various techniques and strategies that nurses can use during assessment).

Table 21-19.
Examples of Procedures and Behavioral Strategies for Nurses to Use

Measurements: Height, Weight, and Head Circumference	• Use family assistance. • Encourage child to touch, feel, and hold items. • Modeling and imitation: "My turn, your turn." • Can say, "Listen for beep," on scale. • Reward/positive reinforcement: "High five," "good job," or whatever reward parent uses.
Auscultation	• Show stethoscope and offer for child to touch it before using. • Modeling: Place stethoscope on parent or doll/toy figure, then child. • Distract with favorite toy. • Give choices when possible. • Reward/positive reinforcement.
Blood Pressure	• Child touch/hold extra BP cuff. • Modeling: Put an extra cuff on parent or doll/toy figure. • Choice of arm to use if appropriate. • High probability/low probability: Demonstrate; say, "Hold arm out straight"; praise; repeat; then put on cuff. • Distraction: ABCs, 123s, watch numbers. • Reward/positive reinforcement.

Source: Souders, Freeman, DePaul, & Levy, 2002.

Adapted from *Pediatric Nursing*, 2002, Volume 28, Number 6, pp. 555-562. Used with permission of the publisher, Jannetti Publications, Inc., East Holly Avenue, Box 56, Pitman, NJ 08071-0056; (856) 256-2300; FAX (856) 589-7463; Web site: www.pediatricnursing.net. For a sample copy of the journal, please contact the publisher.

(4) Minimize distractions to maximize chance of success.

(5) Minimize changes that could cause outbursts and know how to react appropriately to behaviors:

    (a) Recognize that behavior is a form of communication.

    (b) Say only what is essential if a child is having a tantrum; recognize how and when to redirect.

    (c) Do not verbally attend to inappropriate behaviors. Continue whatever activity was being conducted and praise the child when he or she exhibits acceptable behavior.

(6) Communicate clearly (Browne, 2006; Inglese, 2009; Scarpinato et al., 2010; Williams & Minshew, 2010).

    (a) Use the mode of communication most familiar to child, when possible.

    (b) Use visual aids if necessary; children with ASD are visual learners.

    (c) Pay attention to child's nonverbal communication.

    (d) Work with parents to interpret what child may be trying to communicate.

    (e) Speak directly to the child regardless of communication abilities, but do not insist on eye contact.

    (f) Make important information obvious or explicit by giving clear, direct, simple sentences/directions and use concrete words, not abstract.

(g) Break a procedure or task down; give one request at a time.

(h) Use the word "stop" instead of "no" to avoid tantrums and when possible, tell child *what to do* instead of what *not to do.*

(7) Use of pain assessment tools (Scarpinato et al., 2010).

    (a) If a child cannot self-report, use observational/behavior tool such as r-FLACC (Revised-Faces, Legs, Activity, Cry, Consolability). If child is able to self-report, a visual scale is most helpful; have the child place a mark on the visual scale instead of having to point or say a number.

D. Goals of plan of care.

1. Primary goals of treatment according to the American Academy of Pediatrics (Elder & D'Alessandro, 2009).

    a. Minimize deficits in order to maximize functional independence and quality of life.

    b. Promote development and learning.

    c. Promote socialization.

    d. Decrease maladaptive behaviors.

    e. Provide education and support.

2. Factors to consider when choosing a treatment program (Flippin, Reszka, & Watson, 2010; Golnik & Maccabee-Ryaboy, 2010; Inglese, 2009; Kashinath, Woods, & Goldstein, 2006).

    a. Clinical expertise of the professional.

    b. Feedback is provided; are assessment procedures specified?

    c. How closely is child's behavior observed, recorded, and measured for progress?

    d. Child's strengths match treatment modality.

    e. Individual goals: Matching child's goals and family's routines may make it feasible, acceptable, and increase use of intervention.

f. Proven safety and efficacy.

g. Integration of therapies.

h. Organization of planned activities and design of environment.

i. Promotion of generalization and embedding of interventions that parents can use at home and various settings.

j. Amount of time and attention to child.

k. Individualized tasks and rewards.

l. Intensity of program (more than 25 hours per week).

m. Will this lead to home therapy?

n. Financial factors, time commitment, and location.

E. Psychosocial considerations.

1. When choosing treatments, consider the following (Golnik & Maccabee-Ryaboy, 2010; Patterson, Smith, & Jelen, 2010):

    a. Values and needs of the family.

    b. Unique characteristics of the child.

    c. Involvement of parents.

2. Psychosocial support for families (AAP, 2008; Elder & D'Alessandro, 2009; Golnik & Maccabee-Ryaboy, 2010).

    a. Recognize that having a child with ASD can cause stress on the family (emotional, financial, and physical).

    b. Help parents recognize and work through the grieving process; it is a cycle and parents are at risk for depression.

    c. Encourage parents to ask for help, pace themselves, and utilize all resources available, such as respite care to help maintain caregiver and family well-being.

    d. High risk for abuse, peer victimization, and bullying; encourage child to report.

    e. Counseling for peer difficulties, especially for children with Asperger Syndrome (AS).

3. Adolescent issues (AAP, 2008; Frea, 2010).

    a. Explain to child that body changes at puberty are normal; educate about sexuality, appropriate social behaviors for child and others.

    b. May experience and exhibit the following: Increased fear, loneliness, confusion, anxiety, depression, anger, and sadness; higher risk of suicide. These problems may worsen as they become increasingly aware of communication and social deficits; may have regression into younger interests, repetitive activities.

c. Symptoms may change in adolescence when psychiatric disorders may appear such as Schizophrenia, Tourette Syndrome, Obsessive Compulsive Disorder, and Bipolar Disorder.

d. Teens with ASD may find electronic peer support groups helpful.

4. Sibling issues (AAP, 2008; Elder & D'Alessandro, 2009; Golnik & Maccabee-Ryaboy, 2010).

a. Monitor sibling well-being; some sibling issues include jealousy, resentment, and embarrassment.

b. Let parents know that the following are common frustrations: Inability to give siblings adequate attention, lack of "normal" family activities, and placing too many demands on the sibling; encourage setting time aside for siblings.

c. Educate siblings about diagnosis at their level of understanding.

d. Teach skills to enhance their relationship such as: Make sure they have their sibling's attention, give simple instructions, and praise good play.

e. Parents and siblings may be concerned about what role the sibling may play in the future care of the child with ASD.

f. Support groups for siblings.

F. Education of patient/family.

1. Disease process (CDC, 2010; Vaccine Education Center, 2008).

a. Provide information about the child's development.

b. Provide information about ASD.

c. Inform parents that research does not support an association between vaccines and ASD.

(1) Thimerosal (a preservative).

(a) Studies have shown there is no link between thimerosal and ASD.

(b) Thimerosal was removed from some vaccines as a precaution after 1999 recommendation.

(c) According to the CDC, the following vaccines have never contained thimerosal: MMR, Varicella (chickenpox), inactivated polio (IPV), and pneumococcal conjugate vaccines.

(2) MMR vaccine: No correlation between the MMR vaccine and autism; studies have shown prevalence of autism in children who received MMR compared to those who never received the vaccine is the same.

(3) Quantity of vaccines.

(a) New vaccines are always tested for safety and efficacy.

(b) Even though the number of vaccines has increased, the number of immunological components in them has decreased (14 vaccines contain only 150 immunological components as compared to 200 immunological components in the original smallpox).

(c) The challenge of the baby's immune system by vaccines is small in comparison to immunological challenges from the environment (babies are colonized by trillions of bacteria immediately after birth).

(d) It is estimated that babies have the capacity to respond to about 100,000 different vaccines at once.

2. Medication management and administration (Elder & D'Alessandro, 2009; Golnik & Maccabee-Ryaboy, 2010).

a. Provide information to parents about the medication their child is being prescribed.

b. Instruct parents to give Depakote® or Keppra® two hours apart from vitamin D or calcium supplement.

c. Ask about herbal, over-the-counter medications, and supplements.

d. Precaution when using Omega-3 fatty acid supplementation: Toxin contamination, excess vitamin A, and adverse effects of Omega-3 fatty acid.

e. Tell parents to withhold Omega-3 fatty acid supplementation before surgical operation.

3. Safety measures (AAP, 2008; Autism Society of America, 2008; Golnik & Maccabee-Ryaboy, 2010; National Autism Association, 2011; Patterson et al., 2010; Stull & Ladew, 2010).

a. Children with ASD are at risk for the following:

(1) Lead poisoning due to pica and mouthing objects; some symptoms of lead poisoning are similar to some symptoms for ASD, such as speech delays, inattention, aggression, and antisocial behavior.

(2) Seizures: Highest risk during preschool years and at onset of puberty; incidence is lower in Asperger Syndrome than in autism; teach seizure precautions.

(3) Self-injurious behaviors.

(4) Impulsivity; children with ASD are often impulsive and not aware of danger.

(5) Running away/elopement and wandering/getting lost: May do this to gain access to desirable items or activities (such as water), to seek attention, to avoid undesirable situations, or to seek a different level of sensory stimulation.

(a) Teach child to make a request.

(b) Teach child to swim; many children with ASD are drawn toward water; final swimming lesson should be with clothes on; vigilant supervision; remove toys from pool when not in use; fence pool; alert neighbors with pools.

(c) Teach to recall safety information; caution not to share personal information with everyone.

(d) Ensure child has proper identification: Medical ID bracelet or necklace, iron-on labels, identification card; seek out people in uniform if they get lost.

(e) Personal tracking devices worn on ankle or wrist, GPS tracking systems, perimeter systems, or service dogs.

(f) Determine cause of wandering; may need to consult a specialist.

(6) Trusting strangers; frequent family relocations make them at greater risk of getting lost and going with a stranger.

b. Restructure/modify environment (Autism Society of America, 2008; Stull & Ladew, 2010).

(1) Label everyday items and organize in see-through bins with visual labels and place on low shelves; helps the child understand the function, avoid undesirable behaviors, and prevents climbing and falling.

(2) Provide appropriate seating (arms, wrap-around style desks, corner seating) to help prevent behavioral problems and to facilitate good learning and eating behaviors.

(3) Secure eating utensils and place settings (attach utensil to string to avoid injury if thrown; secure plates, bowls, cups with adhesive Velcro®; use plastic dishes).

(4) Safeguard bath items and toys; use pump dispensers instead of open-lip bottles to avoid ingestion.

(5) Create visual signs to make expectations and limits clear (di-

viders, color-coded tape boundaries, and STOP signs).

  c. Safety devices for the home (Autism Society of America, 2008; National Autism Association, 2011; Stull & Ladew, 2010).

    (1) Consider locks and alarms for outside doors and windows, bathroom, and bedroom door and cabinets; use safety locks that you can open and not get locked in by mistake.

    (2) Plexi glass instead of plain glass if child pounds windows; boards over the window.

    (3) Electrical safety: Cover outlets, prevent access to appliances with plastic knob covers and locks, hide wires so child cannot play with them.

    (4) Obtain tot finders stickers from your local fire department for child's bedroom window.

  d. Behavioral modification techniques to teach safety (Autism Society of America, 2008; National Autism Association, 2011; Stull & Ladew, 2010).

    (1) Applied Behavioral Analysis (ABA) to teach the following of directions such as *stop, come here,* and *wait.*

    (2) Read social stories to child about fire safety; use visuals: Pair picture of oven burner or fire with STOP sign.

    (3) Activity schedules; visual rules; signs/charts.

    (4) Peer/adult modeling with positive reinforcement.

    (5) Be consistent with consequences for unsafe behaviors.

4. Exacerbations.

  a. Pain and illness (Inglese, 2009; NIMI I, 2009; Scarpinato et al., 2010).

    (1) Due to problems with sensory integration, children with ASD may lack sensitivity to pain or temperature. Conversely, they may be oversensitive to light touch and overreact to sounds or other stimuli; may cover eyes, ears.

    (2) Advise parents to seek medical attention for unusual behaviors, such as head banging, pulling hair, or biting self as they may be signs of pain and not just manifestations of their ASD.

    (3) Aggressive actions toward others such as hitting may also be an expression of pain.

  b. Adolescence (AAP, 2008; Golnik & Maccabee-Rayaboy, 2010).

    (1) May be unwilling/unable to report symptoms of new health problems; parent should be aware if child is unusually tired, has changes in appetite and behavior, or any other worrisome symptoms.

    (2) Behavior may worsen with hormonal changes at onset of puberty.

    (3) Symptoms may change in adolescence when psychiatric disorders may appear such as Schizophrenia, Tourette Syndrome, Obsessive Compulsive Disorder and Bipolar Disorder; greater use of medication may be warranted.

5. Clinical procedures and treatments (Scarpinato et al., 2010; Souders et al., 2002; Thorne, 2007).

  a. Suggest a pre-visit to a test area and allow child to manipulate instruments and materials, if possible.

  b. Ask parents to prepare child at home for visit (e.g., books about doctor visits, doctor kit).

  c. Ask parents to bring familiar/favorite toys, tokens or rewards, and communication mode normally used by the child.

  d. Consider application of analgesic for injections or blood draws if child has sensory issues.

6. Self-care of primary and secondary problems (AAP, 2008; Golnik & Maccabee-Ryaboy, 2010; Kashinath et al., 2006; Williams & Minshew, 2010).

a. Strategies to improve sleep: Develop sleep schedule and use for two weeks; ignore problem behavior; consider medications.

b. Suggest the following behavioral strategies:
   (1) ABC method for tracking behaviors; A=Antecedent: What happened before the behavior; B=Behavior; C=Consequence: What happened after the child's behavior.
   (2) Establish timeout and consequences for undesirable behaviors, such as withholding privileges.
   (3) Encourage use of positive strategies, such as rewarding child's good behavior (stickers, smiles, praise, earn privileges).
   (4) Encourage embedding intervention strategies into daily routines/daily activities to decrease parental and child stress.
   (5) Suggest keeping a behavior-monitoring log to track success of therapies.

c. Teach through visual means because visual input is important in development of language in ASD.

7. Collaboration and referrals (AAP, 2008; CDC, 2010; Chiang & Carter, 2008; Golnik & Maccabee-Ryaboy, 2010; Inglese, 2009; Kashinath et al., 2006; Williams & Minshew, 2010).

a. Early intervention services for children from birth to age 3 includes services to address communication, socialization, and motor issues. Explain to parents the importance of receiving therapies early.

b. Special preschool through the public school system over 3-years-old.

c. Some families may supplement public services with private therapies.

d. Treatment involves a multidisciplinary approach; there is no single best treatment.

e. Terms, team members, and therapies may include:

(1) Individual Education Plan (IEP); may include transportation and social work; is reviewed yearly for updating; must include present level of achievement in school, yearly goals, special education and other services, details about services and changes, transition goals and services as needs change, and measures of progress.

(2) Social workers and case managers.

(3) Behavioral therapies such as ABA, Social Skills Training.

(4) Speech therapy: Communication and feeding issues; training to achieve spontaneous communication; incorporating communication interventions such as sign language, use of augmentative devices and the Picture Exchange Communication System (PECS). PECS is a means of incorporating visual and auditory information.

(5) Occupational therapy: Self-care skills, such as using utensils and dressing; academic skills, such as writing; and sensory integration therapy.

(6) Physical therapy.

(7) Child psychologist: Social skills training, behavioral issues.

(8) Neuropsychologists, cognitive psychologist, developmental psychologist.

(9) Dietitian.

(10) Medication.

(11) Interventions in child's natural environment employed by therapist as well as parents, such as arranging environment, using positive reinforcement, using time delay, imitating contingently, modeling, and gestural/visual cueing.

f. Special considerations for adolescents (CDC, 2010; Frea, 2010; Inglese, 2009).

(1) Help them prepare for school day, events, and skills by providing detailed visual supports; allow

Table 21-20.
Informational and Support Resources

Organization	Web Site
American Academy of Pediatrics	www.aap.com
Asperger Syndrome Education Network (ASPEN)	www.aspennj.org
Association for Positive Behavior Support	www.apbs.org
Association of University Centers on Disabilities (AUCD)	www.aucd.org
Autism Society of America	www.autism-society.org
Autism Speaks	www.autismspeaks.org
Autism Wandering Awareness Alerts Response Education (AWARE)	http://awaare.org/
Center for the Study of Autism	www.autism.org
Centers for Disease Control and Prevention (CDC)	www.cdc.gov/ncbddd/autism/index.htm
CDC's Resources on Vaccines and Autism	www.cdc.gov/ncbddd/autism/vaccines.htm
ClinicalTrials.Gov	http://clinicaltrials.gov/
Cure Autism Now	www.cureautism.org
Disability	www.disability.gov
Epilepsy Foundation of America	http://www.epilepsyfoundation.org
First Signs	www.firstsigns.org
Government Benefits	www.govbenefits.gov
Interactive Autism Network	www.ianproject.org
MAPP Services for Autism, Asperger Syndrome, and PDD	www.maapservices.org
National Dissemination Center for Children with Disabilities (NICHCY)	www.nichcy.org
National Institutes of Health (NIH)	www.nih.gov
Organization for Autism Research (OAR)	www.research.autism.org
Sibling Support Project	www.siblingsupport.org
TASH	www.tash.org
The National Autistic Society	www.nas.org
The National Institute of Dental and Craniofacial Research	www.nidcr.nih.gov
The National Institute on Deafness and Other Communication Disorders	www.nidcd.nih.gov/health/voice/autism.asp
Unlocking Autism	www.unlockingautism.org
Vaccine Education at The Children's Hospital of Philadelphia	www.vaccine.chop.edu

opportunity for practicing activities/ skills in a non-threatening environment.

(2) Teen may benefit from ABA that is specifically designed to meet his or her unique needs and challenges:

    (a) Teach self-management strategies (monitor, record, and reward own behavior).

(b) Develop successful behaviors.

(c) Build an individualized plan for social skills needs and teaching conversational skills.

(d) Create social opportunities for building successful friendship.

(3) Goals:

    (a) Focus on strengths and skills.

        (b) Build confidence by setting achievable and meaningful short-term goals.

        (c) Parent and teens may want to include the following people to set long-term goals: Siblings and other family members, educators, neighbors, therapists, and others who have an understanding of the teen and with whom he or she has a meaningful relationship.

        (d) Foster independence by setting the following goals: Learning basic living skills such as cooking, cleaning, transportation, and organizational skills such as priority setting and task and time management.

    (4) Transition planning: Begin planning for transition into high school and adulthood, preferably by age 14–16; Individualized Transition Plan integrated into the IEP.

    (5) Guardianship (parents declare guardianship before age 18).

8. Community resources and advocacy.

  a. Advocate for families (Elder & D'Alessandro, 2009; Inglese, 2009).

    (1) Encourage active parent participation in development and implementation of IEP, including setting up monthly team meetings.

    (2) Negotiate/advocate/intervene for services that the child may need, including dealing with the Department of Developmental Disabilities, respite care agencies, and insurance companies.

  b. Provide parents with resources (AAP, 2008; Golnik & Maccabee-Ryaboy, 2010).

    (1) Contact information for Early Intervention administrators, and local school district for special education coordinators.

    (2) Support groups (local parent groups, Autism Society of America – local chapter).

    (3) Various services and programs; publicly funded programs such as financial, educational, medical care, job skills training, and residential services.

    (4) In most states, child will automatically become eligible for Medicaid; Supplemental Security Income (SSI) may be available to families with low-income and severely disabled child.

    (5) Home and Community-Based Waiver Services (HCBWS); funding depends upon the severity of the child's disability and how it affects the family; waiting list may be years; services may include respite care, medical equipment, and home remodeling for safety purposes.

    (6) Web sites (see Table 21-20).

  c. Planning for the future (AAP, 2008; CDC, 2010; Elder & D'Alessandro, 2009).

    (1) Transition medical home from pediatrician to adult doctor.

    (2) In preparation for independent living or group home, consider whether the child is able to live on his/her own or will require assistance upon reaching adulthood.

    (3) Consider child's future need for help managing money, cooking, cleaning, shopping, paying bills, and using public transportation.

    (4) Encourage parents to set up trusts and other financial resources.

References: Hypertension

Agency for Healthcare Research and Quality (AHRQ) National Guideline Clearinghouse. (2009). *Nursing management of hypertension*. Retrieved from http://www.guideline.gov/content.aspx?id=15610&search=nursing+management+of+hypertension

Centers for Disease Control and Prevention (CDC). (2011). *Physical activity for everyone: Guidelines: Adults.* Retrieved from http://www.cdc.gov/physicalactivity/everyone/guidelines/adults.html

Centers for Disease Control and Prevention (CDC). (2012). *High blood pressure.* Retrieved from http://www.cdc.gov/bloodpressure/index.htm

Institute for Clinical Systems Improvement. (2010). *Health care guideline: Hypertension diagnosis and treatment.* Retrieved from http://www.icsi.org/hypertension_4/hypertension_diagnosis_and_treatment_4.html

National Heart, Lung, and Blood Institute (NHLBI). (2004). *The seventh report of the Joint National Committee on Prevention, Detection, Evaluation, and Treatment of High Blood Pressure – Complete report.* Retrieved from http://www.nhlbi.nih.gov/guidelines/hypertension/jnc7full.htm

National Heart, Lung, and Blood Institute (NHLBI). (2006). *Your guide to lowering your blood pressure with DASH.* Retrieved from http://www.nhlbi.nih.gov/health/public/heart/hbp/dash/new_dash.pdf

National Institutes of Health (NIH). (2011). *Hypertension (high blood pressure).* Retrieved from http://report.nih.gov/nihfactsheets/ViewFactSheet.aspx?csid=97&key=H

U.S. Department of Health and Human Services (DHHS). (2012). *Healthy people 2020: Heart disease and stroke: Objectives.* Retrieved from http://healthypeople.gov/2020/topicsobjectives2020/objectiveslist.aspx?topicId=21

U.S. Department of Veterans Affairs. (2005). *Clinical practice guidelines: Management of hypertension (HTN) in primary care.* Retrieved from http://www.healthquality.va.gov/Hypertension_Clinical_Practice_Guideline.asp

Additional Readings: Hypertension

Centers for Disease Control and Prevention (CDC). (2012). *Hypertension.* Retrieved from http://www.cdc.gov/nchs/fastats/hyprtens.htm

Cherry, D., Lucas, C., & Decker, S.L. (2010). Population aging and the use of office-based physician services. *NCHS Data Brief, 41.* Retrieved from http://www.cdc.gov/nchs/data/databriefs/db41.pdf

Kaplan, N., & Domino, F. (2012). Overview of hypertension in adults. *UpToDate.* Retrieved from http://www.uptodate.com/contents/overview-of-hypertension-in-adults

Kaplan, N., & Rose, B. (2011). Technique of blood pressure measurement in the diagnosis of hypertension. *UpToDate.* Retrieved from http://www.uptodate.com/contents/technique-of-blood-pressure-measurement-in-the-diagnosis-of-hypertension

Papademetriou, V., Tsioufis, K., Gradman, A., & Punzi, H. (2011). Difficult-to-treat or resistant hypertension: Etiology, pathophysiology, and innovative therapies. *International Journal of Hypertension.* Retrieved from http://www.ncbi.nlm.nih.gov/pmc/articles/PMC3124360/

U.S. National Library of Medicine. (2011). *Hypertension.* Retrieved from http://www.nlm.nih.gov/medlineplus/ency/article/000468.htm

U.S. Preventive Services Task Force. (2007). *Screening for high blood pressure in adults.* Retrieved from http://www.uspreventiveservicestaskforce.org/uspstf/uspshype.htm

References: Diabetes

Agency for Healthcare Research and Quality (AHRQ). (2011). *Guide to clinical preventive services, 2010-2011.* Retrieved from http://www.ahrq.gov/clinic/pocketgd1011/gcp10s2d.htm#DiabetesT2

American Association of Diabetes Educators. (2010). *Position statement: The scope of practice, standards of practice, and standards of professional performance for diabetes educators.* Retrieved from http://www.diabeteseducator.org/DiabetesEducation/position/position_statements.html

American College of Physicians (ACP). (2007). *ACP diabetes care guide: A team based practice manual and self-assessment program.* Philadelphia: Author.

American Diabetes Association (ADA). (2011a). Clinical practice recommendations. *Diabetes Care, 34*(Suppl. 1).

American Diabetes Association (ADA). (2011b). Standards of medical care in diabetes – 2011. *Diabetes Care, 34*(Suppl. 1), 11-61.

Amylin Pharmaceuticals, Inc. (2011). *Byetta and Symlin.* Retrieved from http://amylin.com/products

Centers for Disease Control and Prevention (CDC). (2011). *National diabetes fact sheet.* Retrieved from http://www.cdc.gov/diabetes/pubs/factsheet11.htm

Segala, M. (Ed.). (2003). *Life extension disease prevention and treatment* (4th ed., pp. 709-742). Hollywood, FL: Life Extension Media.

WebMD. (2012). *Types of insulin for diabetes treatment.* Retrieved from http://diabetes.webmd.com/diabetes-types-insulin

References: Coronary Artery Disease/ Coronary Heart Disease (CAD/CHD)

Agency for Healthcare Research and Quality (AHRQ) National Guideline Clearinghouse. (2009). *Secondary prevention of coronary artery disease.* Retrieved from http://www.guideline.gov/content.aspx?id=16259&search=secondary+prevention+of+coronary+artery+disease

Agency for Healthcare Research and Quality (AHRQ) National Guideline Clearinghouse. (2011). *Effectiveness-based guidelines for the prevention of cardiovascular disease in women — 2011 update: A guideline from the American Heart Association.* Retrieved http://www.guideline.gov/content.aspx?id=33603&search=guidelines+for+the+prevention+of+cardiovascular+disease+in+women

American Heart Association (AHA). (2011). *AHA policy statement: Forecasting the future of cardiovascular disease in the U.S.* Retrieved from http://circ.ahajournals.org/content/123/8/933.full.pdf+html

American Heart Association (AHA). (2012). *Understand your risk of heart attack.* Retrieved from http://www.heart.org/HEARTORG/Conditions/HeartAttack/UnderstandYourRiskofHeartAttack/Understand-Your-Risk-of-Heart-Attack_UCM_002040_Article.jsp

Centers for Disease Control and Prevention (CDC). (2010). *Smoking and tobacco use: Heart disease and stroke.* Retrieved from http://www.cdc.gov/tobacco/basic_information/health_effects/heart_disease/index.htm

Centers for Disease Control and Prevention (CDC). (2012a). *Heart disease.* Retrieved from http://www.cdc.gov/nchs/fastats/heart.htm

Centers for Disease Control and Prevention (CDC). (2012b). *Heart disease facts.* Retrieved from http://www.cdc.gov/heartdisease/facts.htm

Centers for Disease Control and Prevention (CDC). (2012c). *Heart disease: Frequently asked questions.* Retrieved from http://www.cdc.gov/heartdisease/faqs.htm

Institute for Clinical Systems Improvement. (2011). *Health care guideline: Lipid management in adults.* Retrieved from http://www.icsi.org/lipid_management.../lipid_management_in_adults_4.html

Libby, P., & Theroux, P. (2005). Pathophysiology of coronary artery disease. *Circulation, 111,* 3481-3488.

Mohler, E. (2012). Endothelial dysfunction. *UpToDate.* Retrieved from http://www.uptodate.com/contents/endothelial-dysfunction

National Heart, Lung, and Blood Institute (NHLBI). (2012). *Classification of overweight and obesity by BMI, waist circumference, and associated disease risks.* Retrieved from http://www.nhlbi.nih.gov/health/public/heart/obesity/lose_wt/bmi_dis.htm

National Institute on Alcohol Abuse and Alcoholism (NIAAA). (n.d.). *What is a standard drink?* Retrieved from http://pubs.niaaa.nih.gov/publications/Practitioner/pocketguide/pocket_guide2.htm

National Institute on Alcohol Abuse and Alcoholism (NIAAA). (2011). *Rethinking drinking.* Retrieved from http://rethinkingdrinking.niaaa.nih.gov/WhatCountsDrink/WhatsAstandardDrink.asp

National Institute on Alcohol Abuse and Alcoholism (NIAAA). (2012). *Moderate and binge drinking.* Retrieved from http://www.niaaa.nih.gov/alcohol-health/overview-alcohol-consumption/moderate-binge-drinking

PDR Network, LLC. (2012). *Monographs and package inserts.* Retrieved from http://www.pdr.net

U.S. Department of Veterans Affairs. (2006). *Clinical practice guidelines: Management of dyslipidemia (LIPIDS).* Retrieved from http://www.healthquality.va.gov/dyslipidemia_lipids.asp

Additional Readings: Coronary Artery Disease/Coronary Heart Disease (CAD/CHD)

Agency for Healthcare Research and Quality (AHRQ). (2010). *The guide to clinical preventive services 2010-2011.* Retrieved from http://www.ahrq.gov/clinic/pocketgd.htm

American Heart Association (AHA). (2006). *AHA/ACC guidelines for secondary prevention for patients with coronary and other atherosclerotic vascular disease: 2006 update.* Retrieved from http://circ.ahajournals.org/content/113/19/2363.full

American Heart Association (AHA). (2010). *Heart disease and stroke statistics – 2010 update: A report from the American Heart Association.* Retrieved from http://circ.ahajournals.org/content/121/7/e46.full.pdf

Centers for Disease Control and Prevention (CDC). (2009). *Coronary artery disease (CAD).* Retrieved from http://www.cdc.gov/heartdisease/coronary_ad.htm

Centers for Disease Control and Prevention (CDC). (2010a). *Chronic disease prevention and health promotion. Heart disease and stroke prevention. Addressing the nation's leading killers: At a glance 2010.* Retrieved from http://www.cdc.gov/chronicdisease/resources/publications/AAG/dhdsp.htm

Centers for Disease Control and Prevention (CDC). (2010b). *Heart disease fact sheet.* Retrieved from http://www.cdc.gov/dhdsp/data_statistics/fact_sheets/docs/fs_heart_disease.pdf

National Heart, Lung, and Blood Institute. (2001). *Third report of the Expert Panel on Detection, Evaluation, and Treatment of the High Blood Cholesterol in Adults (Adult Treatment Panel III): Executive summary.* Retrieved from http://www.nhlbi.nih.gov/guidelines/cholesterol/atp_iii.htm

National Heart, Lung, and Blood Institute (NHLBI). (2011). *Coronary artery disease.* Retrieved from http://www.nhlbi.nih.gov/health/dci/Diseases/Cad/CAD_WhatIs.html

U.S. Department of Health and Human Services (DHHS). (2012). *Healthy people 2020: Heart disease and stroke: Objectives.* Retrieved from http://healthypeople.gov/2020/topicsobjectives2020/objectiveslist.aspx?topicId=21

U.S. National Library of Medicine. (2012). *Heart diseases.* Retrieved from http://www.nlm.nih.gov/medlineplus/heartdiseases.html

U.S. Preventive Services Task Force. (2009). *Aspirin for the prevention of cardiovascular disease.* Retrieved from http://www.uspreventiveservicestaskforce.org/uspstf/uspsasmi.htm

References: Chronic Heart Failure

Albert, N., Trochelman, K., Li, J., & Lin, S. (2010). Signs and symptoms of heart failure: Are you asking the right questions? *American Journal of Critical Care, 19*(5), 443-452.

American Thoracic Society (ATS). (2002). ATS statement: Guidelines for the six-minute walk test. *American Journal of Respiratory Critical Care Medicine, 166,* 111-117. doi:10.1164/rccm.166/1/111

Fonarow, G.C., Albert, N.M., Curtis, A.B., Gheorghiade, M., Heywood, J.T., Liu, Y., ... Yancy, C.W. (2011). Associations between outpatient heart failure process-of-care measures and mortality. *Circulation, 123*(15), 1601-1610.

Fonarow, G.C., Albert, N.M., Curtis, A.B., Stough, W.G., Gheorghiade, M., Heywood, J.T., ... Yancy, C.W. (2010). Improving evidence-based care for heart failure in outpatient cardiology practices: Primary results of the Registry to Improve the Use of Evidence-Based Heart Failure Therapies in the Outpatient Setting (IMPROVE HF). *Circulation, 122*(6), 585-596.

Fonarow, G.C., Yancy, C.W., Albert, N.M., Curtis, A.B., Stough, W.G., Gheorghiade, M., ... Walsh, M.N. (2007). Improving the use of evidence-based heart failure therapies in the outpatient setting: The IMPROVE HF performance improvement registry. *American Heart Journal, 154*(1), 12-38.

Goodlin, S.J. (2009). Palliative care in congestive heart failure. *Journal of the American College of Cardiology, 54*(5), 386-396.

Haglund, M. (2011). Mastering readmissions: Laying the foundation for change. Post-healthcare reform, pioneers are laying the foundation for serious readmissions-reduction work. *Healthcare Informatics, 28*(4), 10-13, 16.

Heart Failure Society of America, Lindenfeld, J., Albert, N.M., Boehmer, J.P., Collins, S.P., Ezekowitz, J. A., ... Walsh, M.N. (2010). HFSA 2010 comprehensive heart failure practice guideline. *Journal of Cardiac Failure, 16*(6), e1-194.

Heywood, J.T., Fonarow, G.C., Yancy, C.W., Albert, N.M., Curtis, A.B., Gheorghiade, M., ... Walsh, M.N. (2010). Comparison of medical therapy dosing in outpatients cared for in cardiology practices with heart failure and reduced ejection fraction with and without device therapy: Report from IMPROVE HF. *Circulation Heart Failure, 3*(5), 596-605.

Hunt, S.A., Abraham, W.T., Chin, M.H., Feldman, A.M., Francis, G.S., Ganiats, T.G., ... Yancy, C.W. (2009). 2009 focused update incorporated into the ACC/AHA 2005 Guidelines for the diagnosis and management of heart failure in adults: A report of the American College of Cardiology Foundation/American Heart Association Task Force on Practice Guidelines: Developed in collaboration with the International Society for Heart and Lung Transplantation. *Circulation, 119*(14), e391-479.

Khan, S.S., Gheorghiade, M., Dunn, J.D., Pezalla, E., & Fonarow, G.C. (2008). Managed care interventions for improving outcomes in acute heart failure syndromes. *American Journal of Managed Care, 14*(Suppl. 12), S273-286.

Roger, V.L., Go, A.S., Lloyd-Jones, D.M., Adams, R.J., Berry, J.D., Brown, T.M., ... Wylie-Rosett, J., for the American Heart Association Statistics Committee and Stroke Statistics Subcommittee. (2011). Heart disease and stroke statistics – 2011 update: A report from the American Heart Association. *Circulation, 123*(6), e240.

Setoguchi, S., Stevenson, L.W., & Schneeweiss, S. (2007). Repeated hospitalizations predict mortality in the community population with heart failure. *American Heart Journal, 154*(2), 260-266.

Silver, M.A. (2010). Depression and heart failure: An overview of what we know and don't know. *Cleveland Clinic Journal of Medicine, 77*(Suppl. 3), S7-S11.

References: Chronic Obstructive Pulmonary Disease (COPD)

Akinbami, L.J., & Liu, X. (2011). *Chronic obstructive pulmonary disease among adults aged 18 and over in the United States, 1998-2009.* Retrieved from http://www.cdc.gov/nchs/data/databriefs/db63.htm

American Thoracic Society (ATS). (2002). ATS statement: Guidelines for the six-minute walk test. *American Journal of Respiratory Critical Care Medicine, 166,* 111-117. doi:10.1164/ rccm.166/1/111

Global Initiative for Chronic Obstructive Lung Disease (GOLD). (2011). *Global strategy for the diagnosis, management, and prevention of chronic obstructive pulmonary disease (COPD).* Retrieved from http://www.goldcopd.org/guidelines-global-strategy-for-diagnosis-management.html

Mannino, D.M., & Buist, A.S. (2007). Global burden of COPD. Risk factors, prevalence, and future trends. *Lancet, 370,* 765-773.

National Heart, Lung, and Blood Institute (NHBLI). (n.d.). *Take the first step to breathing better: Learn more about COPD.* Retrieved from www.nhlbi.nih.gov/health/public/lung/copd/index.htm

Pauwels, R.A., & Rabe, K.F. (2004). Burden and clinical features of chronic obstructive pulmonary disease (COPD*). Lancet, 364,* 613-620.

Stephens, M.B., & Yew, K.S. (2008). Diagnosis of chronic obstructive pulmonary disease. *American Family Physician, 78*(1), 87-92.

World Health Organization (WHO). (2011). *Chronic obstructive pulmonary disease.* Retrieved from http://www.who.int/mediacentre/factsheets/fs315/en/index.html

References: Human Immunodeficiency Virus (HIV)

Aberg, J.A., Kaplan, J.E., Libman, H., Emmanuel, P., Anderson, J.R., Stone, V.E., ... Gallant, J.E. (2009). Primary care guidelines for the management of persons infected with human immunodeficiency virus: 2009 update. *Clinical Infectious Diseases, 49*(5), 651-681.

AIDS Education & Training Centers National Resource Center. (2012). *Guide for HIV/AIDS clinical care – Opportunistic infection prophylaxis, HRSA HIV/AIDS Bureau.* Retrieved from http://www.aids-ed.org/aidsetc?page=cg-306_oi_prophylaxis

Bebell, L.M., Pilcher, C.D., Dorsey, G., Havlir, D., Kamya, M.R., Busch, M.P., ... Charlebois, E.D. (2010). Acute HIV-1 infection is highly prevalent in Ugandan adults with suspected malaria. *AIDS, 24*(12), 1945-1952.

Branson, B.M., Handsfield, H.H., Lampe, M.A., Janssen, R.S., Taylor, A.W., Lyss, S.B., & Clark, J.E. (2006). *Morbidity and Mortality Weekly Report, 55*(RR14), 1-17. Retrieved from http://www.cdc.gov/mmwr/preview/mmwrhtml/rr5514a1.htm

Castro, K.G., Ward, J.W., Slutsker, L., Buehler, J.W., Jaffe, H.W., & Berkelman, R.L. (1992). 1993 revised classification system for HIV infection and expanded surveillance case definition for AIDS among adolescents and adults. *Morbidity and Mortality Weekly Report, 41*(RR17). Retrieved from http://www.cdc.gov/mmwr/preview/mmwrhtml/00018871.htm

Centers for Disease Control and Prevention (CDC). (2009). *Quick guide recommended adult immunization Schedule – United States, January 2009.* Retrieved from http://www.cdc.gov/mmwr/PDF/wk/mm5753-Immunization.pdf

Centers for Disease Control and Prevention (CDC). (2010). Sexually transmitted diseases treatment guidelines, 2010. *Morbidity and Mortality Weekly Report, 59*(RR-12), 2-13.

Centers for Disease Control and Prevention (CDC). (2011). *HIV in the United States: An overview.* Atlanta: Author.

Centers for Disease Control and Prevention (CDC). (2012). Recommended adult immunization schedule – United States, 2012. *Morbidity and Mortality Weekly Report, 61*(4). Retrieved from http://www.cdc.gov/vaccines/schedules/downloads/adult/mmwr-adult-schedule.pdf

Cichocki, M. (2004). *Adherence strategies that can work for you.* Retrieved from http://aids.about.com/od/adherencestrategies/a/adherestrat.htm

Cichocki, M. (2008). *Questions for a detailed sexual history: What medical professionals may ask you.* Retrieved from http://aids.about.com/od/hivprevention/a/sexualhis.htm

Cichocki, M. (2011). *Living with HIV: A patient's guide.* Jefferson, NC: McFarland Publishers.

Kane, A. (2008, September 12). CDC: Blacks, gays at high risk for HIV infections. *CNN Health.* Retrieved from http://articles.cnn.com/2008-09-12/health/hiv.blacks.gays_1_hiv-infections-young-black-gay-men-hiv-than-white-women?_s=PM:HEALTH

Marks, G., Crepaz, N., Senterfitt, J.W., & Janssen, R.S. (2005). Meta-analysis of high-risk sexual behavior in persons aware and unaware they are infected with HIV in the United States: Implications for HIV prevention programs. *Journal of Acquired Immune Deficiency, 39,* 446-453.

Office of AIDS Administration. (2007). *Standards of Care: HIV ambulatory outpatient medical care standards.* Retrieved from http://www.acphd.org/media/188326/aoa-soc-primary-care.pdf

Osterberg, L., & Blaschke, T. (2005). Adherence to medication. *The New England Journal of Medicine, 353,* 487-497.

Rotheram-Borus, M.J., & Futterman, D. (2000). Promoting early detection of human immunodeficiency virus infection among adolescents. *Archives of Pediatrics & Adolescent Medicine, 154*(5), 435-439.

Schneider, E., Whitmore, S., Glynn, M.K., Dominguez, K., Mitsch, A., & McKenna, M.T. (2008). Revised surveillance case definitions for HIV infection among adults, adolescents, and children aged <18 months and for HIV infection and AIDS among children aged 18 months to <13 years – United States, 2008. *Morbidity and Mortality Weekly Report, 55*(RR10), 1-8. Retrieved from http://www.cdc.gov/mmwr/preview/mmwrhtml/rr5710a1.htm

U.S. Department of Health and Human Services (DHHS) Panel on Antiretroviral Guidelines for Adults and Adolescents – A Working Group of the Office of AIDS Research Advisory Council (OARAC). (2012). *Guidelines for the use of antiretroviral agents in HIV-1-infected adults and adolescents.* Retrieved from http://www.aidsinfo.nih.gov/ContentFiles/AdultandAdolescentGL.pdf

University of California – San Francisco (UCSF). (2011). *What kinds of screening tests are available in the United States?* Retrieved from http://hivinsite.ucsf.edu/insite?page=basics-01-01

Additional Readings: Human Immunodeficiency Virus (HIV)

Centers for Disease Control and Prevention (CDC). (2006a). General recommendations on immunization *Morbidity and Mortality Weekly Report, 55*(RR-15). Retrieved from http://www.cdc.gov/mmwr/preview/mmwrhtml/rr5515a1.htm

Centers for Disease Control and Prevention (CDC). (2006b). HIV prevalence estimates – United States. *Morbidity and Mortality Weekly Report, 57,* 1073-1076.

Centers for Disease Control and Prevention (CDC). (2008a). HIV prevalence, unrecognized infection, and HIV testing among men who have sex with men – Five U.S. cities, June 2004 – April 2005. *Morbidity and Mortality Weekly Report, 54,* 597-601.

Centers for Disease Control and Prevention (CDC). (2008b). *HIV/AIDS surveillance in adolescents and young adults (through 2006).* Atlanta: Author.

Centers for Disease Control and Prevention (CDC). (2008c). *The HIV epidemic and United States students.* Atlanta: Author.

Centers for Disease Control and Prevention (CDC). (2008d). Youth risk behavior surveillance – United States, 2007. *Morbidity and Mortality Weekly Report, 55*(SS-5). Retrieved from http://www.cdc.gov/mmwr/pdf/ss/ss5505.pdf

Cichocki, M. (2006). *Recognizing acute HIV syndrome: When flu symptoms may not be the flu.* Retrieved from http://aids.about.com/cs/conditions/a/syndrome.htm

Cichocki, M. (2010). *Protecting yourself from HIV during oral sex: Safer sex options.* Retrieved from http://aids.about.com/cs/safesex/a/oralsex.htm

Family Practice Notebook. (n.d.). *HIV Western Blot.* Retrieved from http://www.fpnotebook.com/hiv/lab/hvwstrnblt.htm

Hall, H.I., Song, R., Rhodes, P., Prejean, J., An, Q., Lee, L.M., ... Janssen, R.S., for the HIV Incidence Surveillance Group. (2008). Estimation of HIV incidence in the United States. *Journal of the American Medical Association, 300,* 520-529.

Koko, A. (2011). *Bacillary angiomatosis.* Retrieved from http://emedicine.medscape.com/article/212737-overview

Mukherjee, J.S. (Ed.). (2006). *The community-based treatment of HIV in resource-poor settings* (2nd ed.). Retrieved from http://model.pih.org/book/export/html/190

National Institutes of Health (NIH), Office of AIDS Research. (1999). *Report of the working group to review the NIH perinatal, pediatric, and adolescent HIV research priorities.* Bethesda, MD: Author.

References: Peptic Ulcer Disease

Everhart, J.E. (2008). *The burden of digestive diseases in the United States.* Bethesda, MD: National Institute of Diabetes and Digestive and Kidney Diseases, U.S. Department of Health and Human Services.

Feinstein, L.B., Holman, R.C., Yorita Christensen, K.L., Steiner, C.A., & Swerdlow, D.L. (2010). Trends in hospitalizations for peptic ulcer disease, United States, 1998-2005. *Emerging Infectious Diseases, 16,* 1410-1418.

Ferri, F.F. (2010). *Ferri's clinical advisor* (1st ed.). St. Louis, MO: Mosby.

Malfertheiner, P., Chan, F., & McCall, K. (2009). Peptic ulcer disease. *Lancet, 374,* 1449-1461.

National Cancer Institute (NCI). (2011). *Fact sheet: Heliciobacter pylori and cancer.* Retrieved from http://www.cancer.gov/cancertopics/factsheet/Risk/h-pylori-cancer

Pleis, J.R., & Lucas, J.W. (2009). *Summary health statistics for U.S. adults: National Health Interview Survey, 2007.* Hyattsville, MD: National Center for Health Statistics.

Sandler, R.S., Everhart, J.E., Donowitz, M., Adams, E., Cronin, K., Goodman, C., ... Rubin, R. (2002). The burden of selected digestive diseases in the United States. *Gastroenterology, 122,* 1500-1511.

Sonnenberg, A., & Everhart, J.E. (1996). The prevalence of self-reported peptic ulcer in the United States. *American Journal of Public Health, 86,* 200-205.

Xu, J., Kochanek, K.D., & Tejada-Vera, B. (2009). *Deaths: Preliminary data for 2007.* Hyattsville, MD: National Center for Health Statistics.

Yuan, Y., Padol, I.T., & Hunt, R. (2006). Peptic ulcer disease today. *Journal of Gastroenterology and Hepatology, 3*(2). Retrieved from http://www.nature.com/nrgastro/journal/v3/n2/full/ncpgasthep0393.html

References: Asthma

Agency for Healthcare Research and Quality (AHRQ) National Guideline Clearinghouse. (n.d.). *Asthma.* Retrieved from http://www.guideline.gov/search/search.aspx?term=asthma

American Academy of Allergy, Asthma & Immunology (AAAAI). (2012). *Asthma statistics.* Retrieved from http://www.aaaai.org/media/statistics/asthma-statistics.asp

American Lung Association. (2011a). *Asthma.* Retrieved from http://www.lung.org/lung-disease/asthma/

American Lung Association. (2011b). *Asthma and children fact sheet.* Retrieved from http://www.lung.org/lung-disease/asthma/resources/facts-and-figures/asthma-children-fact-sheet.html

Asthma and Allergy Foundation of America (AAFA). (n.d.) *Web site.* Retrieved from http://www.aafa.org

Centers for Disease Control and Prevention (CDC). (2011). Vital signs: Asthma prevalence, disease characteristics, and self-management education – United States, 2001-2009. *Morbidity and Mortality Weekly Report, 60*(17). Retrieved from http://www.cdc.gov/mmwr/preview/mmwrhtml/mm6017a4.htm?s_cid=mm6017a4_w

Fanta, C., & Fletcher, S.W. (2011). An overview of asthma management. *UpToDate.* Retrieved from http://www.uptodate.com/contents/an-overview-of-asthma-management

Fireman, P. (2003). Understanding asthma pathophysiology. *Allergy and Asthma Proceedings, 24*(2), 79-83.

Kirk, A. (2011). Pulmonology. In *The Harriet Lane handbook* (19th ed., pp. 592-598). St. Louis, MO: Elsevier, Inc.

National Heart, Lung, and Blood Institute (NHLBI). (2007). *National Asthma Education and Prevention Program (NAEPP) Expert Panel Report 3: Guidelines for the diagnosis and management of asthma.* Retrieved from http://www.nhlbi.nih.gov/guidelines/asthma/asthgdln.htm

Pediatric/Adult Asthma Coalition of New Jersey, The. (2012). *Asthma treatment plan.* Retrieved from http://www.pacnj.org/plan.html

Schmitt, B.D. (2009). *Pediatric telephone protocols* (12th ed.). Elk Grove Village, IL: American Academy of Pediatrics.

WebMD. (2012). *Allergies and asthma.* Retrieved from http://www.webmd.com/allergies/guide/asthma-allergies

References: Sickle Cell Disease

Aliyu, Z.Y., Tumblin, A.R., & Kato, G.J. (2006). Current therapy of sickle cell disease. *Haematologica, 91*(1), 7-10.

Aygun, B., McMurray, M.A., Schultz, W.H., Kwiatkowski, J.L., Hilliard, L., Alvarez, O., … SWiTCH Trial Investigators. (2009). Chronic transfusion practice for children with sickle cell anaemia and stroke. *British Journal of Haematology, 145*(4), 524-528.

Crane, G.M., & Bennett, N.E., Jr. (2011). Priapism in sickle cell anemia: Emerging mechanistic understanding and better preventative strategies. *Anemia.* Retrieved from http://www.hindawi.com/journals/ane/2011/297364/

Dowling, M.M., Quinn, C.T., Rogers, Z.R., & Buchanan, G.R. (2010). Acute silent cerebral infarction in children with sickle cell anemia. *Pediatric Blood Cancer, 54*(3), 461-464.

Field, J.J., Vemulakonda, V.M., & DeBaun, M.R. (2011). Diagnosis and management of priapism in sickle cell disease. *UpToDate.* Retrieved from http://www.uptodate.com/contents/diagnosis-and-management-of-priapism-in-sickle-disease

Kato, G.J., Onyekwere, O.C., & Gladwin, M.T. (2007). Pulmonary hypertension in sickle cell disease: Relevance in children. *Pediatric Hematology Oncology, 24*(3), 159-170.

Machado, R.F., & Gladwin, M.T. (2010). Pulmonary hypertension in hemolytic disorders – Pulmonary vascular disease: The global perspective. *CHEST, 137*(Suppl. 6), 30-38.

National Heart, Lung, and Blood Institute (2004). *The management of sickle cell disease* (4th ed.). Bethesda, MD: National Institutes of Health.

National Newborn Screening and Genetics Resource Center. (2012). *U.S. national screening status report.* Retrieved from http://genes-r-us.uthscsa.edu/sites/genes-r-us.uthscsa.edu/files/nbsdisorders.pdf

Pack-Mabien, A., & Haynes, J., Jr. (2009). A primary care provider's guide to preventive and acute care management of adults and children with sickle cell disease. *Journal of the American Academy of Nurse Practitioners, 21,* 250-257.

Platt, A.F., & Sacerdote, A. (2006). *Hope and destiny.* Munster, IN: Hilton Publishing Company.

Pulmonary Hypertension Association. (2010). *Home page.* Retrieved from http://www.phassociation.org/

Thomas, A.V. (2006). *Pulmonary hypertension in sickle cell disease.* Retrieved from http://www.medscape.org/viewarticle/547201

Verduzco, L.A., & Nathan, D.G. (2009). Sickle cell disease and stroke. *Blood, 114*(25). Retrieved from http://bloodjournal.hematologylibrary.org/content/114/25/5117.full

References: Developmental Delays

American Academy of Pediatrics (AAP), Council on Children With Disabilities, Section on Developmental Behavioral Pediatrics, Bright Futures Steering Committee, & Medical Home Initiatives for Children With Special Needs. (2006). Identifying infants and young children with developmental disorders in the medical home: an algorithm for developmental surveillance and screening. *Pediatrics, 118*(1), 405-420. [Correction in *Pediatrics, 118*(4), 1808-1809].

Centers for Disease Control and Prevention (CDC). (2011). *Developmental monitoring and screening for health professionals.* Retrieved from http://www.cdc.gov/ncbddd/childdevelopment/screening-hcp.html

Centers for Disease Control and Prevention (CDC). (2012). *Learn the signs. Act early.* Retrieved from http://www.cdc.gov/ncbddd/actearly/ccp/index.html

Centers for Disease Control and Prevention (CDC) – National Center on Birth Defects and Developmental Disabilities. (2011). *Child development.* Retrieved from http://www.cdc.gov/ncbddd/child/development.htm

Hagan, J.F., Shaw, J.S., & Duncan, P.M. (2008). *Bright futures: Guidelines for health supervision of infants, children, and adolescents* (3rd ed.). Elk Grove Village, IL: American Academy of Pediatrics.

Jones, L. (2009). *Making hope a reality: Early intervention for infants and toddlers with disabilities.* Retrieved from http://www.zerotothree.org/public-policy/policy-toolkit/earlyintervensinglmarch5.pdf

King, T.M., Tandon, S.D., Macias, M.M., Healy, J.A., Duncan, P.M., Swigonski, N.L., … Lipkin, P.H. (2010). Implementing developmental screening and referrals: Lessons learned from a national project. *Pediatrics, 125*(2), 350-360.

LaRosa, A., & Glascoe, F. (2011). Developmental and behavioral screening tests in primary care. *UpToDate.* Retrieved from http://www.uptodate.com/contents/developmental-and-behavioral-screening-tests-in-primary-care

National Early Childhood Technical Assistance Center (NECTAC). (2011). *The importance of early intervention for infants and toddlers with disabilities and their families.* Retrieved from http://www.nectac.org/~pdfs/pubs/importanceofearlyintervention.pdf

Sices L. (2007). *Developmental screening in primary care: The effectiveness of current practice and recommendations for improvement.* Retrieved from http://www.commonwealthfund.org/usr_doc/1082_Sices_developmental_screening_primary_care.pdf?section=4039

TeKolste, K. (2006). *Developmental surveillance & screening: Monitoring to promote optimal development.* Retrieved from http://www.medicalhome.org/physicians/dev_surveillance.cfm

U.S. Department of Education. (1997). *IDEA'97: Amendments, final regulations.* Retrieved from http://www2.ed.gov/policy/speced/reg/regulations.html

References: Autism Spectrum Disorder

American Academy of Pediatrics (AAP). (2008). *Autism: Caring for children with autism spectrum disorders: A resource toolkit for clinicians.* Retrieved from http://www.aap.org/healthtopics/autism.cfm

American Psychiatric Association. (2000). *Diagnostic and statistical manual of mental disorders* (4th ed., revised). Arlington, VA: Author.

Autism Society of America. (2008). *Safety in the home.* Retrieved from http://www.autism-society.org/living-with-autism/how-we-can-help/safe-and-sound/safety-in-the-home.html

Browne, M.E. (2006). Communicating with the child who has autistic spectrum disorder: A practical introduction. *Paediatric Nursing, 18*(1), 14-17.

Centers for Disease Control and Prevention (CDC). (2010). *Autism spectrum disorders: Autism information center.* Retrieved from http://www.cdc.gov/ncbddd/autism/index.html

Centers for Disease Control and Prevention (CDC). (2012). *Autism spectrum disorder: Data and statistics.* Retrieved from http://www.cdc.gov/ncbddd/autism/data.html

Chiang, H.-M. & Carter, M., (2008). Spontaneity of communication in individuals with autism. *Journal of Autism and Developmental Disorders, 38,* 693-705.

Elder, J.H., & D'Alessandro, T. (2009). Supporting families of children with autism spectrum disorders: Questions parents ask and what nurses need to know. *Pediatric Nursing, 35*(4), 240-245, 253.

Flippin, M., Reszka, S., & Watson, L.R. (2010). Effectiveness of the picture exchange communication system (PECS) on communication and speech of children with autism spectrum disorders: A meta-analysis. *American Journal of Speech-Language Pathology, 19,* 178-195.

Frea, W.D. (2010). Preparing adolescents with autism for successful futures. *Exceptional Parent Magazine, 40*(4), 26-29.

Golnik, A., & Maccabee-Ryaboy, N. (2010). Autism: Clinical pearls for primary care. *Contemporary Pediatrics, 27*(11), 42-59.

Inglese, M.D. (2009). Caring for children with autism spectrum disorder, part II: Screening, diagnosis, and management. *Journal of Pediatric Nursing, 24*(1), 49-59.

Inglese, M.D., & Elder, J.H. (2009). Caring for children with autism spectrum disorder, part I: Prevalence, etiology, and core features. *Journal of Pediatric Nursing, 24*(1), 41-48.

Kashinath, S., Woods, J., & Goldstein, H. (2006). Enhancing generalized teaching strategy use in daily routines by parents of children with autism. *Journal of Speech, Language, and Hearing Research, 49,* 466-485.

National Autism Association. (2011). *Autism and wandering.* Retrieved from http://nationalautismassociation.org/resources/awaare-wandering/

National Institute of Mental Health (NIMH). (2009). *What are the autism spectrum disorders?* Retrieved from http://www.nimh.nih.gov/health/publications/autism/what-are-the-autism-spectrum-disorders.shtml

Patterson, S.Y., Smith, V., & Jelen, M. (2010). Behavioural intervention practices for stereotypic and repetitive behaviour in individuals with autism spectrum disorder: A systematic review. *Developmental Medicine and Child Neurology, 52,* 318-332. doi:10.1111/j.1469-8749.2009.03597.x

Peacock, G., & Yeargin-Allsopp, M. (2009). Autism spectrum disorders: Prevalence and vaccines. *Pediatric Annals, 38*(1), 22-25.

Pinto-Martin, J.A., Dunkle, M., Earls, M., Fliedner, D., & Landes, C. (2005). Developmental stages of developmental screening: Steps to implementation of a successful program. *American Journal of Public Health, 95*(11), 1928-1932.

Pinto-Martin, J.A., Souders, M.C., Giarelli, E., & Levy, S.E. (2005). The role of nurses in screening for autistic spectrum disorder in pediatric primary care. *Journal of Pediatric Nursing, 20*(3), 163-169.

Robins, D.L. (2008). Screening for autism spectrum disorders in primary care settings. *Autism, 12*(5), 537-556. doi:10.1177/1362361308094502

Robins, D.L., Fein, D., & Barton, M. (1999). *Modified checklist for autism in toddlers (M-CHAT).* Retrieved from http://www.gsu.edu/~wwwpsy/robins.html

Scarpinato, N., Bradley, J., Kurbjun, K., Bateman, X., Holtzer, B., & Ely, B. (2010). Caring for the child with an autism spectrum disorder in the acute care setting. *Journal for Specialists in Pediatric Nursing, 15*(3), 244-254. doi:10.1111/j.1744-6155.2010.00244.x

Souders, M.C., Freeman, K.G., DePaul, D., & Levy, S.E. (2002). Caring for children and adolescents with autism who require challenging procedures. *Pediatric Nursing, 28*(6), 555-562.

Stull, A., & Ladew, P. (2010, April). Safety first for children with autism spectrum disorders. *Exceptional Parent Magazine,* 54-57.

Thorne, A. (2007). Are you ready to give care to a child with autism? *Nursing2007, 37*(5), 59-61.

Trillingsgaard, A., Sorensen, E.U., Nemec, G., & Jorgensen, M. (2005). What distinguishes autism spectrum disorders from other developmental disorders before the age of four years? *European Child and Adolescent Psychiatry, 14,* 65-72. doi:10.1007/s00787-005-0433-3

Vaccine Education Center at The Children's Hospital of Philadelphia. (2008). *Q & A – Vaccines and autism: What you should know.* Retrieved from http://www.chop.edu/service/vaccine-education-center/order-educational-materials/

Williams, D.L., & Minshew, M.J. (2010, April 27). How the brain thinks in autism: Implications for language intervention. *The ASHA Leader, 8-*11.

Chapter 22

Care of the Terminally Ill Patient

Mary Elizabeth Davis, MSN, RN, CHPN, AOCNS

OBJECTIVES – *Study of the information in this chapter will enable the learner to:*

1. Describe the principles and goals of palliative care and hospice care.
2. Identify appropriate assessment and interventions to manage pain and other common symptoms in the terminally ill.
3. Recognize the impact of a culturally diverse population in caring for the terminally ill.
4. Identify the ethical and legal issues patients, families, and nurses may face when caring for the terminally ill.
5. Identify key issues for care of the patient at the time of death.
6. Apply communication principles to facilitate and enhance decision-making at the end of life.
7. Recognize the role of the nurse as an integral member of the health care team in advocating for quality of care at the end of life.

KEY POINTS – *The major points in this chapter include:*

1. Quality end-of-life care is an important but challenging goal for nurses to support patients and families in ambulatory care.
2. Pain management is complex, but nurses are key in performing individualized assessments and maintaining open dialogue with the patient, family, and health care team.
3. Nurses must work to coordinate optimal pharmacologic and non-drug treatments for end-of-life symptoms, such as anorexia and cachexia, anxiety, confusion and delirium, constipation, cough, depression, diarrhea, dyspnea, fatigue, and nausea and vomiting.
4. Issues of ethical decision-making, legal rights of patients and families, and cultural considerations are particularly important in care of the terminally ill patient.
5. Nurses facilitate the grief process by assessing grief and assisting both patients and survivors to cope with loss.
6. The nurse is often the one to facilitate a dignified, comfortable death that honors the patient's and family's choices.

Terminal illness describes an active and malignant disease that cannot be cured and is expected to eventually result in death. Americans are living longer with terminal diseases, such as AIDS, cancers, and chronic cardiac and respiratory disorders. Technologic advances have led to the medicalization of care at the end of life (EOL); this therapeutic optimism and focus on cure can overshadow the satisfaction and fulfillment of ending one's life well. Ambulatory care nurses are in a position to help patients and their families to confront the limitations of treatment, seek a balance of hope and acceptance, and recognize the reality that life is finite. Encouraging patients to live life to the fullest on their own terms while providing quality care is an important role for nurses. This can be achieved by aggressive symptom management, education, promoting patient autonomy, and fostering the establishment of personalized goals. Addressing spiritual and emotional needs, and helping patients and families cope with loss, grief, and bereavement are important aspects of nursing care at the EOL. The use of empathetic communication and a multidisciplinary team approach is essential in palliative care.

When cure is not possible, maintaining hope and promise for the living that still remains is a noble goal.

Specialized programs, such as *The End-of-Life Nursing Education Curriculum* (ELNEC), have been developed in response to a growing need to educate health care providers on EOL care. The ELNEC curriculum is a primary source for the chapter (American Association of Colleges of Nursing [AACN] & City of Hope National Medical Center, 2008).

I. **Palliative Care**
A. The World Health Organization (WHO) (2011a) describes *palliative care* as "an approach that improves the quality of life of patients and their families facing the problem associated with life-threatening illness, through the prevention and relief of suffering by means of early identification and impeccable assessment and treatment of pain and other problems, physical, psychosocial, and spiritual."
B. National Consensus Project for Quality Palliative Care (NCP): A consortium of organizations (the National Hospice and Palliative Care Organization, the American Academy of Hospice and Palliative Medicine, the Center to Advance Palliative Care, and the Hospice and Palliative Nurses Association) collaborated with the purpose of improving quality of palliative care in the United States. The "Clinical Practice Guidelines for Quality Palliative Care" was the result and serves as an educational framework and blueprint upon which to build optimal palliative care programs (NCP, 2009).
C. Philosophy of palliative care (National Comprehensive Cancer Network [NCCN], 2011b; NCP, 2009).
1. Palliative care expands traditional, disease-model, medical treatments to include the goal of enhancing quality of life by providing pain and symptom relief, and spiritual and psychosocial support according to patient and family needs, values, beliefs, and culture.
2. It is both a philosophy of care and an organized, highly structured system for the delivery of care to persons with life-debilitating or life-limiting illness.

3. It can be an integral part of disease management from diagnosis of a life-limiting disease to the end of life and bereavement. Figure 22-1 depicts the continuum of palliative care.
4. It can be delivered concurrently with life-prolonging care or as the main focus of care.
5. Palliative care affirms life and regards dying as a normal process, intending neither to hasten nor postpone death.
6. It aims to help patients and families make informed decisions and to work toward goals in whatever time they have remaining.
7. Clear, consistent, and empathetic communication with patient and family is at the core of effective palliative care.
8. Ambulatory care nurses can incorporate palliative care principles into all aspects of nursing care of the terminally ill, regardless of disease stage or need for concurrent therapies.
9. The overlap between palliative care and hospice is important to delineate: All those receiving hospice are, in a sense, receiving palliative care, but not all patients receiving palliative care are in hospice (Morrison & Morrison, 2006).
D. Hospice.
1. Hospice is a federally funded program of capitated care based on criteria initiated by Congress in 1982, known as the Medicare Hospice Benefit. Medicaid and private insurers have similarly structured benefits.
2. Eligibility criteria.
a. The patient is terminally ill with a life expectancy of 6 months or less, assuming the disease runs its normal course.
b. The patient chooses to receive hospice care rather than curative treatments for his or her illness. Some hospices have evolved a broader definition of hospice care to include treatments that improve quality and may extend life, such as blood transfusions and artificial feeding.

Figure 22-1.
Continuum of Palliative Care and Hospice Care

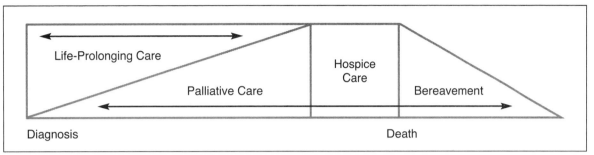

Source: Carlson, Lim, & Meier, 2011. Used with permission.

c. Patients are recertified for hospice at regular intervals and can revoke benefits at any time if goals of care change.

3. Payment for care.
   a. Medicare pays the hospice a per diem rate that is intended to cover virtually all expenses related to addressing the patient's terminal illness.
   b. There may be differing intensities of care during the course of the disease. The Medicare Benefit affords four levels of care:
      (1) Routine home care.
      (2) Continuous home care.
      (3) Inpatient respite care.
      (4) General inpatient care.

E. Common principles of hospice and palliative care.
   1. The patient and family are the unit of care; quality of life can only be viewed subjectively.
   2. Attention is given to physical, psychological, social, and spiritual needs.
   3. The multidisciplinary team approach is key to providing holistic, comprehensive care. Team typically includes physicians, nurses, social workers, chaplains, counselors, nursing assistants, therapists, and volunteers.
   4. Education about the dying process is vital, as is respect of the patient's and family's wishes regarding the dying process.

5. Bereavement support and interventions begin at admission to the program, with attention to anticipatory needs, and continue with the family following the patient's death.
6. Nurses utilize astute assessment and symptom and medication management to address the physical and emotional needs of the palliative care patient and family.

F. Benefits of early referral to palliative care services (Clayton & Kissane, 2010; Wright et al., 2008).
   1. Allows time to establish key relationships with patient and family.
   2. Emphasis can be on focusing on the present and living life to the fullest despite a life-limiting illness.
   3. Enhanced pain and symptom control during treatments, such as chemotherapy and radiation therapy, may reduce a sense of abandonment and assist in the adjustment and transition when active treatment of disease is no longer appropriate.
   4. Do not need to choose cure over care; paralleled shared care can ease transition when disease progresses.
   5. Discussion about death and dying and life goals can be a gradual process and not determined when in crises; there is time to acknowledge and define patient preferences, decreasing the decision-making burden on the family.
   6. May facilitate earlier enrollment and utilization of hospice benefit.

7. Increased likelihood of patient being cared for in his or her place of choice during terminal phase (Clayton & Kissane, 2010; Hearn & Higginson, 1998).
8. Avoidance of futile care and reduced overall health care costs.

G. Assessment of quality of life (QOL) (Egan & Labyak, 2006; Grant & Sun, 2010).
1. QOL encompasses all dimensions of a person and can only be defined by the patient based on his or her own life experience. The experience of living with terminal illness and confronting death is an individual journey involving the patient's body, mind, and spirit. As the disease progresses and there is physical decline, the psychological, spiritual, interpersonal, and social dimensions take on added meaning and purpose.
2. Physical well-being is a concern as the disease progresses, and debility, organic, and metabolic changes affect the physical health of the patient. Pain is an important concern, as well as symptoms that interfere and complicate the patient's comfort, such as shortness of breath, gastrointestinal disturbances, fatigue, and loss of appetite.
3. Psychological well-being is important because patients experience a wide range of emotional responses to illness, including anxiety, sadness, fear, depression, denial, anger, loneliness, distress, hopelessness, and guilt.
   a. Communication and support for working through unresolved issues may affect suffering.
   b. The meaning of illness, along with physical and social attributes, greatly impacts emotional responses.
   c. Coping strategies that have been helpful in the past should be explored, along with possible new strategies.
4. Social well-being problems include family distress and financial burden. The integrity of the family unit is at risk because the social structure and roles, considered normal for the family, are threatened.

   a. Becoming a burden is often a concern of the patient.
   b. Children manifest their emotional concerns in ways that may not be easily discerned.
   c. Financial concerns may arise due to lost income as well as health care expenses.
5. Spiritual well-being includes hope, inner strength, peace, dignity, a sense of faith, and a sense of connectedness to others or to God; this is often the key to transcending losses and finding meaning in life.
   a. The dying process can challenge a person's religious and/or spiritual sense of hope.
   b. Religious and/or cultural rituals are an important means of support for both patients and their families.
   c. Research indicates that both patients and families rely on spirituality and religion to help them deal with terminal illness and that they desire for their religious or spiritual concerns to be acknowledged or addressed by the health care team (National Cancer Institute [NCI], 2011c).
   d. Acknowledging the importance of the patient or family spiritual/religious concerns at diagnosis, even briefly, may facilitate better adjustment throughout the course of treatment and create a context for richer dialogue later in illness. Research has shown that support from the health care team predicted greater QOL and a greater likelihood of receiving hospice care at EOL (NCI, 2011c).
6. The focus on QOL at EOL should be not only on the patient, but also the family.
   a. The role of the caregiver has shifted in past decades from promoting convalescence to providing complex, hands-on care at EOL (Grant & Sun, 2010).
   b. Family members may have or can develop physical needs that impact their ability to care for the patient and themselves.

II. Effective Communication in the Palliative Setting

One aspect of nursing care that has been neglected in the past is how to talk to patients and families about dying. Although this has been incorporated in most curricula for nurses and physicians, it is still given very little attention. Communication involves strong collaboration between members of the multidisciplinary team, including the patient/family.

A. Communication is both verbal and non-verbal (body language, eye contact, gestures, voice intonation). Meaning of the communication is interpreted as it is perceived by the receiver of the communication.

B. Nurses as educators always need to be aware that too much information can be overwhelming and that different people absorb information through a variety of communication forms.

C. Inability to communicate effectively due to impaired cognition and sensory loss can be difficult. Capturing both verbal and non-verbal cues about pain and other symptoms is vital.

D. The palliative care plan has individualized goals based upon needs and overall condition. The patient/family must be a vital part of this planning. Clear and dynamic communication between all members of the team is imperative to excellent care.
  1. Expectations expressed by patients/families need to be addressed with respect, honesty, and guidance in exploration of realistic options.
  2. The entire team needs to have a clear understanding of these expectations and a clear plan of how to help these expectations be met.
  3. As issues of conflict arise, nurses should plan to initiate meetings with patient/family and relevant team members.

E. Health care professionals' behaviors greatly influence communication outcomes. Barriers to effective communication include:
  1. Fear of one's own mortality.
  2. Lack of personal experience with death and dying.
  3. Fear of expressing emotion; showing tears may cause avoidance of difficult topics.
  4. Fear of being blamed for causing a death when there are unrealistic expectations for cure.
  5. Fear of not knowing the answer to a question or whether to be honest when answering a question.
  6. Disagreement with patient's/family's decisions.
  7. Lack of knowledge of the patient/family's culture, end-of-life goals, wishes, and/or needs.
  8. Unresolved personal grief.
  9. Ethical concerns.
  10. Desire to keep physical and/or emotional distance from patients.

F. The value of presence: It is often enough to just be there with the patient. Presence provides compassionate confirmation and may be a nurse's greatest gift to the patient and family (Borneman & Brown-Saltzman, 2006). Touch can be a tool of presence.

G. Nurses may be concerned with not knowing exactly what to say; silence is a valuable communication tool. Compassionate listening is as important as speech.

H. Talking about death and dying: Breaking bad news or talking about death is a difficult task in our culture. While physicians generally break the bad news, nurses are in a position of reinforcing that information and providing clarification (Levin & Weiner, 2010).
  1. Clarify that disease is no longer responding to treatment and continuing other treatments may produce more side effects than benefit.
  2. Assure patient and family that full supportive care will be provided whether or not any disease-specific treatment is given.
  3. Avoid conveying that "nothing else can be done;" there is always something that can be done to reduce suffering and relieve symptoms.
  4. Be empathetic and acknowledge emotions, such as sadness, anger, and disheartenment.
  5. Ask if the patient or family is interested in learning about physical aspects of dying.

6. Encourage the patient to participate in the decision-making process according to his or her desired level of involvement. Be realistic in explaining options at EOL, such as intubation, CPR, and what "doing everything" means.

7. Elicit information about prior experience with death – What went well, what could have been done better. Previous negative experiences, such as witnessing a painful death, can be used to facilitate discussions on how the dying process can be improved and to confirm specific wishes the patient has (Levin & Weiner, 2010).

I. Techniques for responding to patient and family emotion when discussing EOL issues (Levin & Weiner, 2010).

1. 10–20 seconds of shared silence, communicating that you understand.
2. Empathy: "It really has been rough for you."
3. Validation or normalization: "What you are going through is very difficult," or "It is normal to feel sad."
4. Acknowledge emotion: "You seem angry."
5. Praise: "You are very brave."
6. Paraphrase and repeat back: "If I am hearing you correctly, you are upset because…"
7. Encourage expression: "Tell me more about how this makes you feel."
8. Apology: "I am so sorry the chemotherapy didn't work as well as planned."
9. Touch or gesture of touch. Patting bedside or chair, or offering a tissue if patients may be uncomfortable with actual touch.

J. Pediatrics (Hinds & Kelly, 2010).

1. Children usually know they have a terminal illness even if they are not directly given this information. Children can detect subtle changes in the way family and staff react to them, care for them, and talk to them.
2. A child needs to be communicated with at his or her level of understanding.
3. A child may let the nurse know he or she is finished talking by walking away, moving away to play, changing the subject, changing his or her body posture, and/or other non-verbal cues that signify withdrawal.

4. Siblings should be assessed because they may receive inadequate attention as parents focus on the dying child.
   a. Assess for acting out and either negative or "perfect child" behavior.
   b. Allow the sibling to continue his or her extracurricular activities by finding resources and support people to take the sibling to these activities.
   c. Allow siblings to verbalize feelings in a safe place without feeling as though they are making their parents feel worse.

5. Participating in EOL decision-making is understandably very difficult for parents, and inclusion of the child in these discussions will depend on a number of factors, including age, maturity, and cognition.

6. It is the nurse's responsibility to respect patients' choices and decision-making while assessing opportunities for open communication and education. The patient needs support and caring without being denied any realistic hope.

7. Parents are frequently aware of the gravity of the terminal illness of their child, but may delay EOL discussions in an attempt to maintain hope that their child will survive, which helps them maintain function and to care for the child. The team should pursue EOL discussions because they are likely to result in fewer hospitalizations, plans for the preferred location of death, and parents' feeling more prepared for the child's EOL (NCI, 2011b).

8. Factors influencing EOL decision-making for parents include:
   a. Trust of clinician.
   b. Proximity of approaching death.
   c. Information about treatment status: Have all reasonable attempts to save life been made?
   d. Parents' perceptions about being respected and trusted by health care team.
   e. Child's preference.
   f. Spirituality or religious faith.

K. Cultural communication issues at EOL include:
1. Interpreters may be needed. Family members should not be used as interpreters because they may interject their own beliefs and values. The purpose of the meeting should be explained to the interpreter. The interpreter should, ideally, meet the family in advance to gain an understanding of the situation and the family's knowledge level and beliefs, and to establish a mutual feeling of trust.
2. Conversational style is also important; patients should be asked how they should be greeted (first name, last name), and the nurse should determine whether the patient speaks for himself or if a family member will serve as a spokesperson.
3. Members of the health care team should assess and discuss the relationship of the patient to the family, and determine the key contact for information.
4. Evaluation of the patient/family view of health care professionals is also important.
5. Personal space needs can be determined by observing the patient's reactions to posturing and space. This should also be observed with eye contact and touch. Patients should always be asked for permission before they are touched.
6. People of different cultural backgrounds have different views of full disclosure of diagnosis and prognosis to the patient.

III. Pain Management in the Terminally Ill

A. *Pain* is defined by the International Association for the Study of Pain (IASP) as "an unpleasant sensory and emotional experience associated with actual or potential tissue damage, or described in terms of such damage" (1994, p. 1). McCaffery and Pasero (1999) stated that pain is "whatever the person says it is, experienced whenever they say they are experiencing it" (p. 15). This definition describes the subjectivity of pain.
B. The ambulatory nurse who has frequent contact with the patient in the community, at home, or in the outpatient setting is in a unique position to identify and appropriately assess pain,

effectiveness of management, and its impact on the patient and family.
C. Pain relief not only enhances the individual's quality of life, but may allow the patient to "let go" at the end of life.
D. Barriers to adequate pain management (Borneman et al., 2010; Fink & Gates, 2006; Jacobsen et al., 2009; Lippe, Brock, David, Crossno, & Gitlow, 2010).
1. Patient barriers:
    a. Fear of addiction.
    b. Concern that the physician may not treat the underlying disease if pain is reported; that treatment of pain will distract from treatment of underlying illness.
    c. Fatalism about the possibility of achieving relief – Not accurately reporting nature and severity because "nothing helps."
    d. Fear of becoming tolerant to effect of medications – Chronic use of pain meds will render them ineffective later.
    e. Concern over side effects – The side effects may be worse than pain (e.g., constipation, confusion, or drowsiness).
    f. Fear that increased pain indicates disease progression.
    g. Lack of access to pain management specialists.
    h. Cost prohibiting use of correct medication and dosage.
2. Health care professional barriers:
    a. Inadequate knowledge/training of principles and methodology of pain management (e.g., lack of knowledge of appropriate dosage, including conversion tables).
    b. Inability to fully evaluate or appreciate severity (inadequate pain assessment).
    c. Concerns about regulation/regulatory scrutiny (Drug Enforcement Administration [DEA], Food and Drug Administration [FDA], and Medicare).
    d. Failure to recognize and address patient barriers.

e. Inadequate management of related side effects, such as constipation prophylaxis.

f. Fear of patient addiction.

3. Health care system barriers.

a. Legal and regulatory constraints that interfere with the provision of optimal care.

b. Fragmented system with multiple specialists. Lack of continuity of care when patient is seen by multiple providers, but no one practitioner takes responsibility for overall pain management.

c. Inadequate reimbursement for pain services and for medications in some cases; lack of recognition of pain medicine as a specialty.

d. Low referrals to palliative care specialists.

e. Failure of public health agencies to make pain management and public education about pain a high priority.

4. Nurses need to recognize and reduce barriers to optimal pain management. Creating opportunity for open dialogue and education concerning patient's, family's, or caregiver's fears and concerns is critical. Knowledge or inquiry about patient's health coverage and use of pharmaceutical companies' assistance programs may be helpful.

E. Pain assessment is a continuous process and is crucial to formulate a management plan. Assessment should be ongoing, and subsequent evaluation is necessary to determine effectiveness of relief measures and to identify any new pain.

1. Assessment should include input from patient (both verbal and non-verbal). People are often unable to use the word "pain," so words such as "ache" and "hurt" may need to be interchanged. Listen carefully to the words the patient may use to describe his or her pain to evaluate the level of stoicism.

2. Input from a significant other or caretaker should also be incorporated, as well as review of medical data and feedback from other health care professionals.

3. Assessment should address type of pain, location, intensity, pattern and duration, precipitating and aggravating factors, alleviating factors, associated symptoms, cultural or psychosocial contributions, and impact on functioning and QOL.

4. Type of pain

a. Nociceptive pain:
   (1) Is related to damage to bones, tissues, or organs.
   (2) Can be visceral (originating in organs, such as stomach or intestines) or somatic (from bone, muscle, or skin).
   (3) Is usually described as aching, throbbing (somatic), squeezing, or cramping (visceral).

b. Neuropathic pain:
   (1) Is related to damage to the peripheral or central nervous system.
   (2) Tends to be chronic and less responsive to opioids.
   (3) Is usually described as burning, tingling, electrical, or shooting (e.g., diabetic neuropathy or herpes zoster [shingles]).

c. Mixed pain: Combination of both nociceptive and neuropathic pain.

5. Location of pain.

a. Patient may have pain at multiple sites: Pain in different areas or caused by different etiologies may need to be addressed separately. For example, a patient with metastatic cancer may have a tumor infiltrating a nerve, causing radiating neuropathic pain, and also have a solitary bone metastasis that presents with a localized area of pain. The use of an assessment sheet with a figure the patient can point to or record on may help provide more specific data and guide management (Fink & Gates, 2006).

b. Patient complaints of "pain all over" may be a sign of existential distress. *Existential distress* is defined as suffering that arises from a sense of meaningless, hopelessness, fear, and regret in patients who knowingly approach the EOL (Kirk & Mahon, 2010). It occurs when a person questions the meaning of his or her life. Existential distress warrants a discussion with patient and investigation into distress.

6. Intensity is a way to grade or quantify pain. Pain intensity should be monitored at present level, as well as its best, worst, and with activity. A standardized tool should be consistently used; the nurse should consider the practicality, ease, and acceptability of the tool use by the terminally ill patient. No single scale is appropriate for all patients. Examples of standardized tools are described in Chapter 14, "Nursing Process."

7. Observational tool for non-verbal or cognitively impaired patients; capturing information from verbal and non-verbal behaviors during both rest and movement, such as:
   a. Facial expressions: Frowning, grimacing, clenched teeth or jaw.
   b. Vocalizations: Moaning, groaning.
   c. Body language: Relaxed, tense, fidgeting, holding, or bracing.
   d. Physiologic indicators: Increases in blood pressure, respirations, or pulse. (Note: Elevated vital signs may occur with severe, sudden pain, but may not occur with chronic or persistent pain.)

8. Pattern of pain may be acute or chronic, constant or intermittent.
   a. Acute pain is usually associated with inflammation, tissue damage, a surgical procedure, or short-term disease process, and is of relatively brief duration – from hours to days or weeks. It is generally viewed as a time-limiting experience, has a clear cause, and disappears once the underlying cause is resolved.
   b. Chronic pain is persistent and lasts for an extended period of time – weeks to months or years. Although it can be associated with a specific injury (such as trauma, low back pain, phantom limb pain), it may be associated with a disease process, such as cancer, HIV, sickle cell disease, chronic obstructive pulmonary disease (COPD), or degenerative joint disease.
   c. Breakthrough pain (BTP) is a transient exacerbation of pain in otherwise relatively stable or adequately controlled background chronic pain (Dickman, 2011).
      (1) It can occur spontaneously or in relation to a predictable (specific) activity (like walking) or unpredictable trigger (coughing).
      (2) Generally, recurring episodes of BTP are indicative of inadequate chronic or long-term pain management.

9. Precipitating or aggravating factors: What makes the pain worse? What activities promote pain?

10. Alleviating factors: What actions have helped relieve or decreased severity of pain? What are current effective coping strategies?
    a. Medications the patient has already tried, including prescription, over-the-counter, recreational, and herbal preparations. Review schedule, dosage, and effectiveness (what they are actually taking, how often, and what is working and not working). Evaluate adverse effects, if any, and how they were managed.
    b. Other non-pharmacologic relief measures tried: Positioning, application of heat or cold, physical therapy.

11. Associated symptoms: What other things do you see or feel when you are in pain? An example is visual disturbances or nausea that accompany headache.

12. Psychosocial factors, including cultural and religious beliefs that may influence the meaning of pain, pain expression, and coping.

13. Impact of pain on functioning and QOL.

F. Physical examination contributes to determining the underlying cause of the pain.

1. Observe for non-verbal cues of pain, especially if the patient is unable to report pain; cues include signs of fatigue, grimaces, moans, irritability, holding, or bracing (see III E 7, above).
2. Examine sites for trauma, swelling, skin breakdown, changes in bony structures.
3. Palpate areas for tenderness, auscultate lungs and bowels for abnormal sounds, and percuss abdomen for gas or fluid accumulation.
4. Conduct a neurological examination to evaluate sensory and/or motor loss, as well as changes in reflexes.

G. Reassessment of the pain is critical to determine if changes are needed in the analgesic regimen.
   1. Timing of reassessment is determined by the degree to which the patient's condition and pain state is changing.
   2. Reassessment should always be done within 72 hours of change of medication.
   3. A pain diary kept by the patient or caregiver can be a very helpful tool:
      a. Times of dose of medicine with time of relief.
      b. Intensity of pain prior to and after medication.

H. Pharmacologic therapies (Freye & Levy, 2008; NCCN, 2011a; Paice & Fine, 2006).
   1. Non-opioid analgesics.
      a. Acetaminophen.
         (1) Antipyretic, may be useful as a non-specific musculoskeletal pain or as co-analgesic.
         (2) Can cause liver dysfunction with doses higher than 4,000 mg/day (caution for people with pre-existing liver disease).
      b. Aspirin.
         (1) Useful for treatment of mild to moderate pain with inflammation; reduces symptoms, such as swelling, stiffness, and joint pain.
         (2) Caution for GI bleed, impaired platelet aggregation, especially patients on chemotherapy treatment.

      c. Non-steroidal anti-inflammatory drugs (NSAIDs).
         (1) Useful for treatment of mild to moderate pain with inflammation; reduce symptoms, such as swelling, stiffness, and joint pain.
         (2) Use with caution in patients with high risk for renal, cardiac, GI, thrombocytopenia, or bleeding disorders. Side effects of cancer therapies may be increased with concomitant use (NCCN, 2011a).
         (3) Examples include ibuprofen, naproxen, and ketorolac. Topical preparations may be used for local anesthesia.
   2. Opioid analgesics.
      a. Short-acting opioids.
         (1) Onset of action in 15–20 minutes and peaking at about 45 minutes; some newer rapid onset preparations have faster onset (Fishbain, 2008).
         (2) Usually prescribed to treat acute pain; may be regularly scheduled or/and rescue dosing.
         (3) Includes codeine, oxycodone, tramadol, hydromorphone, oxymorphone, and transmucosal and buccal fentanyl.
      b. Long-acting opioids.
         (1) Slow onset of action: Pharmacokinetic profile with minimal peaks and valleys, resulting in stable blood levels.
         (2) Usually prescribed for control of persistent baseline component of chronic pain.
         (3) Includes sustained, extended, and controlled release preparations of morphine, oxycodone, oxymorphone, tramadol and hydromorphone, methadone, and transdermal fentanyl.
      c. Side effects:
         (1) Allergic reactions are rare. If a patient reports an allergy, further questioning may reveal he or she

experienced an adverse effect (such as nausea or vomiting). Opioids are contraindicated when the patient reports hypersensitivity reaction, such as wheezing or edema.

(2) Respiratory depression is rare, but greatly feared. It is usually preceded by sedation, and the greatest prevalence of this is after the first dose of a narcotic-naive patient. Morphine has been found to help patients in respiratory distress due to COPD/emphysema because it relaxes the muscles around the lungs and allows the lungs to expand.

(3) Constipation is a significant adverse effect of opioid therapy, which results from a reduction in peristalsis and increased reabsorption of water. Stool softeners and laxatives should be initiated at the first signs of constipation and then administered regularly. Newer medications, such as methylnaltrexone, may be prescribed for opioid-induced constipation.

(4) Sedation can occur, yet tolerance generally develops to this effect.

(5) Urinary retention is common in opioid-naive patients when opiate delivered intrathecally or epidurally.

(6) Nausea and vomiting may occur and are best treated with antiemetics.

3. Antidepressants are used to treat a variety of pain conditions, including neuropathic pain syndromes, and diabetic and postherpetic neuralgia. They may potentiate opioid analgesia and have an additional benefit of treating depression, anxiety, and insomnia (Mitra & Jones, 2012).
   a. Tricyclic antidepressants (TCAs).
      (1) Work by inhibiting re-uptake of serotonin and noradrenaline in spinal pain pathways.
      (2) Examples include amitriptyline and imipramine.
      (3) Side effects include sedation, akathesia (motor restlessness), and anticholinergic side effects, such as dry mouth, constipation, and urinary retention. Orthostatic hypotension, heart block, and arrhythmias can occur; cautious use in the elderly and those with cardiac disease (Bennett, 2010; Mitra & Jones, 2012).
   b. Serotonin norepinephrine reuptake inhibitors (SNRIs) are a new class of medication gaining use in the treatment of neuropathic pain.
      (1) Examples include duloxetine and venlafaxine.
      (2) Generally are well-tolerated, with nausea and somnolence as most common side effects.
      (3) Not widely studied in terminal care setting.

4. Anticonvulsants are commonly used in the management of neuropathic pain.
   a. Work by a variety of mechanisms to affect neural signals in sodium and calcium channels and release of neurotransmitters.
   b. Examples include gabapentin, pregabalin, topiramate.
   c. Common side effects include somnolence and dizziness.

5. Corticosteroids are used as analgesia for pain syndromes, including headache due to increased intracranial pressure, neuropathic pain from infiltration, or compression of neural structures, including spinal cord compression, generalized bone pain, and arthralgia (Lussier, Huskey, & Portenoy, 2004).
   a. Examples include dexamethasone, prednisone, and methylprednisolone.
   b. Usually dosed as either:
      (1) A short course of high divided daily doses followed by a scheduled taper.

(2) A long-term, low dose daily or BID schedule.

c. Side effect risk increases with dose and duration of therapy and may include hyperglycemia, fluid retention, osteoporosis, myopathy, immunosuppression, gastritis, and gastric ulceration (Mitra & Jones, 2012). Have been shown to improve appetite, nausea, malaise, and QOL in the terminal care setting (Lussier et al., 2004).

6. Bisphosphonates alleviate pain from metastatic bone disease and multiple myeloma.

   a. They inhibit osteoclast mediated bone resorption (breakdown) and reduce pathological fractures. There is some evidence they may also offer an antitumor or bone protecting role as adjuvant therapy (Hillegonds, Franklin, Shelton, Vijayakumar, & Vijayakumar, 2007).

   b. Examples include zolendronate (Zometa®, Zomera®, Aclasta®, or Reclast®) and pamidronate (Aredia®); both are given intravenously.

   c. Renal function and serum calcium levels need to be monitored; hypocalcemia can occur. (These bisphosphonate agents are also used to treat hypercalcemia of malignancy because of their calcium wasting properties.)

7. Radionuclides have been shown to help relieve pain from bone metastases and are underutilized by medical oncologists, according to some experts (Hillegonds et al., 2007; Pandit-Tasker, Batraki, & Divgi, 2004).

   a. These medications have an affinity to diseased bone. A single administration can provide significant, durable pain relief. Duration of response varies with specific radionuclide but can range from 1–15 months (Hillegonds et al., 2007). Retreatment may be an option for good responders.

   b. Examples include intravenous Strontium 89 and Samarium-153.

c. Complete blood counts need to be followed weekly for 6–8 weeks because thrombocytopenia and neutropenia are common and may occur 2–4 weeks after treatment.

d. Patients may experience a transient pain flare occurring approximately 1–5 days after administration, lasting hours to few days. This can usually be managed with additional immediate-release pain medication.

e. Patient and family must be educated about radiation safety precautions.

I. Routes of administration of pharmacologic therapies.

1. Use of a specific medication route or preparation is based on assessment of pain, patient preference and ability to administer, and response to previous preparations (efficacy and tolerance). Many patients may require more than one route of administration.

2. Oral route includes use of immediate-release tablets, long-acting tablets, and liquids, which may be swallowed or absorbed sublingually. Transmucosal patches and lozenges are used for BTP/rapid rescue. Some oral capsules may be opened into applesauce or soft foods to aid swallowing. Immediately prior to death, alternative routes may be needed.

3. Rectal route may be useful when the patient is no longer able to swallow or is having gastrointestinal issues, such as nausea or vomiting. Some long-acting opioid tablets can be absorbed via rectal mucosa; pharmacies can compound and prepare many pain preparations into suppositories. Delivery via rectal route may be difficult for family members to administer.

4. Parenteral:

   a. Advances in vascular access devices, implantable and tunneled catheters and ports, and ambulatory infusion and patient controlled analgesia (PCA) devices have eased access to continuous intravenous (IV) analgesia. Caregivers may require extensive training to manage these devices in the home setting. Visiting nursing services are valuable resources to help support catheter care and maintenance of home infusion.

    b.   Intravenous administration has a rapid onset, and can be easily titrated. Potential complications include infection, phlebitis, and thrombosis.

    c.   Subcutaneous (SC) route has a slower onset of action than IV. Continuous SC administration may be used if intravenous is not a viable option. Needle rotation, care, and assessment of site are required.

    d.   Intramuscular administration is not routinely utilized nor recommended due to wide variability in absorption, and it requires that a family member be comfortable and available to deliver.

5.   Transdermal administrations are common for long-term chronic pain control.

    a.   There is a delay in peak onset (8–12 hours), so other routes must be continued until peak is reached.

    b.   Avoid bony prominences. Place patch over non-hairy skin with good capillary flow. Fever, ascites, cachexia, and morbid obesity may impact drug absorption and distribution.

6.   Topical anesthetics (such as lidocaine, diclofenac, capsaicin) can be used as an adjuvant medication and may be helpful for isolated, neuropathic pain conditions, such as herpetic neuralgia.

7.   Epidural/spinal/intrathecal route allows targeted delivery of drugs, but it is complex and requires specialized knowledge and skills of the health care professionals and extensive teaching with caregiver.

J.   Principles regarding the use of analgesia

1.   WHO (2011b) provides a guide for medication management: A stepwise approach for selection of appropriate analgesia and dosing to manage escalating pain. Continued reassessment is necessary to modify the treatment plan based on the patient's response (see Figure 22-2).

Figure 22-2.
Pain Ladder

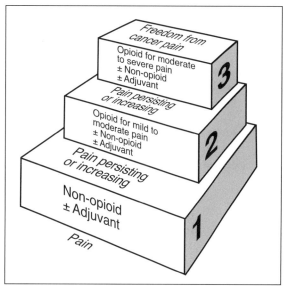

Source: Adapted from WHO, 2011b. Used with permission.

    a.   Step 1 is mild pain (1–3 on the 0–10 scale), and a non-opioid or adjuvant medication should be prescribed.

    b.   Step 2 is mild to moderate pain (4–6) and calls for the addition of weak opioids, such as codeine or hydrocodone in low doses.

    c.   Step 3 is moderate to severe pain (7–10) and indicates the need for higher doses of opioids, along with adjuvant and non-opioids.

    d.   Treatment should start at the step of the WHO analgesic ladder appropriate for the severity of the pain. Weak opioids may not be the drug of choice in moderate to severe pain; smaller doses of more potent opioids, such as morphine, are just as effective and can be titrated to relief. If the pain severity increases and is not controlled on a given step, move upwards to the next step.

2.   Begin with immediate-release formulations as needed to relieve pain. Once the patient has achieved pain relief for 24–48 hours,

calculate the 24-hour dose of opioid and convert to long-acting formulation. For example, the patient who has been taking 60 mg of liquid morphine in a 24-hour period may be converted to MS Contin® 30 mg every 12 hours or fentanyl (Duragesic®) 25 mcg every 72 hours.

3. Sustained-release formulation and around-the-clock dosing should be used for continuous pain syndromes.

4. Immediate-release (IR) formulations should be made available for BTP.
   a. The dose of IR is usually 10–20% of the total 24-hour dose of the routine opioid every 1–2 hours prn. Therefore, if the 24-hour dose of MS Contin® is 200 mg, the breakthrough dose should be 20–40 mg, starting with the lower dose and titrating, as needed.
   b. IR medication can be repeated as often as every hour; the peak effect of oral opioids is approximately 45 minutes to 1 hour.
   c. Premedication before known triggers of BTP (such as before a specific activity) is suggested.

5. Switch to a different opioid when the current one becomes ineffective after an adequate upward titration of the dose or if it produces adverse effects. If side effects or adverse events exceed the analgesic benefit, convert to an equianalgesic dose of alternative.

6. Titration should be based upon patient goals, requirements for supplemental analgesics, pain intensity, severity of undesirable or adverse drug effects, measures of functionality, sleep, emotional state, and the impact of pain on QOL.

K. Non-pharmacologic therapies.
1. Cognitive modalities, such as behavioral therapy, relaxation, guided imagery, and hypnosis.
2. Physical modalities: Supportive equipment, physical and occupational therapy, application of heat or cold, positioning instruction, trans-electrical nerve stimulation (TENS), acupuncture or acupressure, ultrasonic stimulation.

3. Interventional procedures: Kyphoplasty and vertebroplasty for painful compression fractures; neuro-ablative procedures, such as rhizotomy, or cordotomy.

4. Radiation therapy may be used to provide pain relief associated with bone metastases.
   a. Local field external beam radiotherapy is time efficient and associated with few side effects (Lutz et al., 2010).
   b. Doses may be given in single fractions or multiple fractions over a short period of time.
   c. Hemibody irradiation may also be used, but is associated with more side effects, including significant myelotoxicity (Pandit-Tasker et al., 2004).

L. Special populations.
1. Children:
   a. Are often under-treated due to misguided fears of addiction or the belief that children do not feel pain due to underdeveloped nervous systems.
   b. Unrelieved pain can produce fear, irritability, mistrust, and impaired coping, and can cause parents to feel anxiety, anger, and guilt.
   c. Pain assessment should be appropriate to child's age, developmental level, and emotional resources (Kane & Himelstein, 2007).
      (1) For children over 7 years of age, a visual analog or verbal response scale may be used.
      (2) For children ages 3–7 years, a Faces scale or pain thermometers may be more appropriate.
      (3) For children younger than 3 years of age, validated tools, such as CRIES (**c**rying, **r**equires oxygen for saturation below 95%, **i**ncreased vital signs, **e**xpression, and **s**leeplessness (Krechel & Bildner, 1995), may be utilized.
   d. Both pharmacologic and non-pharmacologic therapies should be used to manage a child's pain. Techniques incorporating play, such as deep breathing by blowing bubbles, music, or touch therapy, may be appropriate.

2. Elderly patients (Chapman, 2010; Derby & O'Mahony, 2006; Herr, Bjoro, Steffens-meier, & Rakel, 2006):
   a. Assessment may be difficult due to changes in perception of pain and cognitive abilities to report. Select appropriate pain assessment tools based on the patient's cognitive/functional abilities and adapt tools to compensate for sensory impairments. Allow sufficient time for the older adult to process information and to respond to assessment questions.
   b. Age-related physiologic changes and treatment of co-morbidities (with its associated risk of polypharmacy) impact drug absorption, metabolism, and excretion, contributing to toxicity, side effects, and drug interactions.
   c. Under-treatment of pain is a recognized problem. This may be related to barriers described above, especially fear of excessive toxicity by patients and prescribers. Elderly patients are more sensitive to the therapeutic and toxic effects of analgesia. Although it is advised to start medications at slightly lower doses and "go slow," titration should be relative to pain.

3. Patients with history of substance abuse:
   a. A thorough assessment of pain and addiction risk is critical.
   b. An interdisciplinary team approach is important.
   c. Realistic goals must be established.
   d. Co-morbid psychiatric disorders are common, particularly depression, personality disorders, and anxiety disorders. Treatment of these underlying problems may reduce aberrant behaviors and make pain control more effective.
   e. Consistency is essential.
   f. Tolerance must be considered; thus, opioid doses may require more rapid titration and may be higher than patients without a history of prior opioid use or substance abuse.

g. At the EOL, rehabilitation is not a goal, but prevention of withdrawal from opioids, benzodiazepines, and alcohol should be monitored.

4. Uninsured and socially economically disadvantaged persons.
   a. At risk for inadequate pain control at the EOL.
   b. Many analgesics, especially the newer and more sophisticated formulations, can be extremely expensive.
   c. Generic and immediate-release formulations are usually less expensive.
   d. Pharmaceutical companies have patient assistance programs that provide analgesics at reduced or no cost.

M. Pain management during the last hours of life.
   1. Decreased consciousness may make assessment complicated. If the patient is unable to report pain, non-verbal cues must be relied upon to measure pain levels (see III E 7).
   2. If the patient did not previously have pain but now appears to be in pain, first rule out other potential causes of distress (such as constipation or anxiety). A therapeutic trial of opioids may be indicated to determine if the behaviors diminish.
   3. The dosage of opioids given during the last hours of life should be based upon appropriate assessment and reassessment. The nurse should provide pain relief, and the fear of sedation or respiratory depression should not limit the use of opioids. The American Nurses Association (ANA) (1995) position statement *Promotion of Comfort and Relief of Pain in Dying Patients* supports the nurse in the role of "increasing titration of medication to achieve adequate symptom control, even at the expense of maintaining life or hastening death secondarily, is ethically justified" (p. 1).
   4. The dose of opioid needed to produce relief may be decreased during the final hours of life. Decreased renal function is one contributing factor.

5. Metabolites of opioids, particularly morphine, may accumulate due to renal dysfunction. These metabolites can produce hallucinations, myoclonus, and a hyper-irritable state. Should this occur, a change to another opioid, such as hydromorphone, may be indicated.

N. Palliative sedation therapy (Eisenchlas, 2007; Knight, Espinosa, & Bruera, 2006).
   1. Pain may become intractable at EOL, even with aggressive titration of standard opioid and other therapies. Sedation may be the only alternative to provide comfort.
   2. Palliative sedation is the use of sedative medications to relieve intolerable and refractory suffering by reducing a patient's consciousness. Along with pain, symptoms requiring palliative sedation include severe agitation or restlessness, extreme distress, delirium, dyspnea, nausea, and vomiting.
   3. Pharmacologic therapy for palliative sedation includes the use of:
      a. Anxiolytic sedatives, such as midazolam and lorazepam.
      b. Antipsychotics, such as haloperidol.
      c. Sedative antiepileptics, such as phenobarbital.
      d. General anesthetics, such as propofol.
   4. Medications are titrated by close monitoring of patients' level of distress. Use of a benzodiazepine in the presence of delirium may worsen restlessness, and in such cases, haloperidol may be helpful.
   5. Prior to administering palliative sedation to the terminally ill, the following should be established:
      a. All possible etiologies and treatments have been considered and ruled out, and the patient is suffering with intractable, unbearable symptoms.
      b. Death should be imminent (within hours to days), although confirming this is difficult; consultation with a palliative care expert is recommended.
      c. A well-planned, compassionate, and clear discussion about this therapeutic option should be held, and informed consent from patient or proxy obtained.
      d. A DNR order must be in effect.
      e. The patient or surrogate should be educated on the expected outcomes and goals of sedation. Many members of the health care team who have been involved in the case should be called upon to provide support to the patient and family.
   6. The nurse should continually assess both the patient and family for distress; promoting patient comfort is the goal.

IV. **Symptom Management**
   Multiple symptoms are common at the EOL, and symptom distress is multifactorial. Ambulatory nurses must work closely with the multidisciplinary team to coordinate an individualized treatment plan based on the extent of disease, treatment options, risks, and benefits, as well as goals and expectations of treatment. This is paralleled by an increased interest in choosing care that matches the patient's values and optimizes QOL. Patients and families require extensive teaching and support for symptom management.
A. Essential elements of symptom management:
   1. Assess the individual symptom and the complex interplay of associated and contributing physical and psychological factors.
   2. Include an evaluation of interventions utilized so far.
   3. Outline the education of plan of care for the patient and family self-care.
   4. Ensure close collaboration between nurses, physicians, and all who provide care in the home/facility. Interdisciplinary teamwork ensures that optimal care is delivered.
   5. Consider insurance coverage and other financial concerns, which may be important factors for some families.
   6. Determine criteria for ordering a diagnostic test as guided by the stage of disease, prognosis, risk/benefit ratio of proposed tests or interventions, and patient preference. If no change in management will result, tests should be questioned for appropriateness.

7. Symptoms and suffering: As with pain, other physical and psychological symptoms create suffering and distress. A multidisciplinary approach, including psychosocial intervention, is needed to complement pharmacologic strategies.

B. Anorexia and cachexia (Coss, Bohl, & Dalton, 2011; Kemp, 2006; Rosenzweig, 2006).

1. Anorexia is the loss of desire to eat, the loss of appetite, or an aversion to food.

2. Cachexia is a profound syndrome of weight loss and muscle wasting mediated, in part, by circulating cytokines released in response to stress or malignancy. The etiology of cachexia in advanced disease is rarely reversible. Cachexia can be quite distressing to the patient and family, cause a negative impact on self-concept and body image, and may serve as a constant reminder of the disease and impending death (AACN & City of Hope National Medical Center, 2008).

3. Weight loss is present in both, but anorexia and cachexia are distinct syndromes and may be difficult to differentiate in the terminally ill patient.

4. Etiology of anorexia is multifactorial.
   a. Physiological factors: Metabolic syndromes, infection, pain, nausea and delayed gastric emptying, malabsorption, vomiting, and bowel constipation and obstruction.
   b. Physical: Difficulty swallowing, changes in oral cavity (mucositis, thrush, xerostomia, ill-fitting dentures, poor dentition), constipation, and obstruction.
   c. Psychological: Depression, anxiety, and distress.
   d. Medications may directly result in anorexia or cause side effects, such as early satiety, changes in taste and smell, nausea, vomiting, mucositis, and others.
   e. Other: Patient is unable to shop, prepare, or feed oneself; social isolation (patient may not enjoy eating alone).

5. Assessment: The extent to which anorexia is investigated, and diagnostic testing ordered will depend on stage of disease, patient goals, and plan of care.
   a. Presence of symptoms described above, physical assessment: Measurements of intake, weight, body mass index (BMI), strength, and laboratory values, such as albumin, serum thyroxin-binding pre-albumin, electrolytes, iron status.
   b. Patient preferences and meal patterns, food likes and dislikes, cultural issues, meaning of food and eating.
   c. Use of validated assessment tools, such as the simplified nutritional appetite questionnaire (SNAQ), the mini nutritional assessment (MNA), or the functional assessment for anorexia cachexia therapy (FAACT) may be helpful to grade and monitor anorexia.

6. Treatment.
   a. Identify the etiology, if possible, and clarify the goal of treatment. Aggressively managing symptoms, such as nausea or mucositis, may be sufficient to increase or maintain appetite. Maintaining nutrition may help with overall tolerance of disease treatment, but eating for pleasure should be goal at EOL.
   b. Artificially provided hydration and nutrition may or may not be justified; the anticipated benefits must outweigh the anticipated burdens for any intervention to be justified. Ethical difficulties arise when it is unclear whether food and fluid are more beneficial or harmful. Outcomes, such as weight gain, increased caloric intake, or changes in laboratory test results, may not, themselves, serve as adequate justification.
   c. Dietary interventions are aimed to increase intake. Consult with a registered dietitian or swallowing expert for individualized intervention and suggestions for appropriate nutritional supplementation. Simple suggestions may include:

(1) Choose patient's favorite foods. Removing dietary restrictions may be appropriate depending on stage of disease.

(2) Offer small, frequent meals.

(3) Encourage high-calorie, high-protein snacks.

(4) Use a large plate size. Patients may be overwhelmed with a large amount of food; using a larger plate with regular portions may be helpful.

(5) Control odors and food temperature.

d. Encourage activity, as tolerated, to stimulate appetite.

e. Pharmacologic options may be helpful early in the course of treatment but may be futile in the final stages of terminal illness; weigh risks with benefits for use.

(1) Progestational agents, such as megestrol acetate, can improve appetite, promote weight gain, and increase sense of well-being. Risks include thromboembolic events, such as deep vein thrombosis, flushing, fluid retention, and suppression of testosterone in men.

(2) Corticosteroids, such as dexamethasone, increase appetite and overall well-being, and may be of particular benefit for patients who also have nausea, asthenia, and/or visceral or bone pain (Von Roenn & Paice, 2005).

(3) Cannabinoids, such as dronabinol, stimulate appetite but may cause somnolence and confusion, especially in elderly.

(4) Metoclopramide may be helpful to promote gastric emptying.

C. Anxiety.

1. A subjective feeling of apprehension, tension, insecurity, and uneasiness usually without a known specific cause. It may be associated with nervousness about the future, a preoccupation with disease, and feelings of loss of control. Anxiety may impair functioning and affect decision-making and cause repetitive questioning.

2. Etiology.

a. Disease-related: Biochemical imbalances – Endocrine or metabolic disorders, respiratory conditions causing hypoxia, treatment issues, such as unrelieved symptoms.

b. Pharmacologic effect of drugs, such as stimulants, thyroid replacement hormones, neuroleptics, corticosteroids, digitalis, antihistamines, anticholinergics, and analgesics.

c. Non-pharmacologic etiology, such as issues arising from facing uncertain futures, lifestyle changes, concern over finances, dependency, disability, and confrontation of family conflicts.

3. Assessment should be frequent, because patients with a terminal diagnosis may undergo rapid changes in lifestyle and physical well-being. Review medication history, past coping mechanisms, and the availability of support systems. Symptoms of anxiety may include:

a. Chronic apprehension.

b. Inability to sleep or relax.

c. Difficulty concentrating.

d. Persistent thoughts, ideas, or impulses.

e. Tachycardia.

f. Diaphoresis.

g. Palpitations.

h. Abdominal discomfort.

4. Treatment includes addressing and treating uncontrolled symptoms, such as dyspnea and pain, and correction of any biochemical imbalances.

a. Pharmacological treatment may include antidepressants, benzodiazepines, neuroleptics, azaspirones, and non-benzodiazepines.

b. Non-pharmacologic interventions may include:

(1) Cognitive behavioral therapy, psychotherapy, and counseling.

(2) Acknowledgment of the patient's fears.

(3) Allowing the patient to articulate anger with appropriate reassurance and support.

(4) Providing concrete information.

(5) Encouraging the use of a stress diary.

(6) Maximizing symptom management.

(7) Promoting the use of relaxation, guided imagery, and other complementary techniques.

D. Confusion/delirium/agitation.

1. *Confusion* refers to disorientation, inappropriate behavior or communication, and/or hallucinations. *Delirium* is an acute change in cognition or awareness. *Agitation* may present as a symptom accompanying delirium.

2. Etiologies include:
   a. Infection.
   b. Initiation of medications, such as opioids, hypnotics, sedatives, steroids, and anticholinergics.
   c. Rapid withdrawal of medications, such as opioids and benzodiazepines.
   d. Metabolic abnormalities.
   e. Hypoxemia.
   f. Renal or hepatic failure.
   g. Constipation.
   h. Bladder distension.
   i. Nutritional deficiencies, such as folate, thiamine, and B12.
   j. Disease processes, such as brain lesions or encephalopathy.
   k. In older adults, bladder infection should be ruled out with any sudden change in mental status.

3. Assessment should include:
   a. Physical assessment.
   b. History of onset in relation to medications or stage of disease.
   c. Identification of any spiritual distress.
   d. Cognition assessed by validated tools, such as Mini Mental Status Exam (Folstein, Folstein, & McHugh, 1975) or simply by assessing orientation to person, place, and time.
   e. Diagnostic studies, as indicated to evaluate for reversible causes, such as infections that require cultures for antibiotic selection.

4. Treatment (Dahlin, 2006).
   a. Pharmacologic.
      (1) Neuroleptics or benzodiazepines for acute agitation.
      (2) Evaluation of current medications to eliminate any non-essential drugs.
      (3) Initiation of antibiotics or correction of metabolic imbalances.
      (4) Palliative sedation for terminal delirium at EOL.
   b. Family education and support to respond to their distress due to changes in the patient. Frequent reorientation with use of clocks and calendars and reassurance to patient may be necessary.
   c. Managing the environment by reducing noise and stimuli, soft lighting, and organizing care to promote rest and sleep.
   d. Complementary therapies, such as relaxation, massage, music therapy, and acupuncture.

E. Constipation.

1. *Constipation* is defined as the infrequent passage of stool associated with symptoms of rectal pressure, straining, cramps, distension, and/or sensation of bloating. May also include feelings of inadequate evacuation and hard stools. Prevention of constipation is key.

2. Etiology includes:
   a. Obstruction, which may be partial or complete, and may be due to tumor or adhesions causing compression of the bowel.
   b. Spinal cord compression (or other condition affecting neuromuscular activity).
   c. Co-morbid conditions, such as diabetes, diverticulitis, hypercalcemia, hypokalemia, hypothyroidism, dehydration, inactivity, and pain.

d. Medications: Opiates suppress peristalsis, antidepressants slow motility, and antacids cause hardening of stool.

e. Diet: Insufficient bulk, fiber, or fluids.

3. Assessment should include:

a. Bowel history, frequency, and use of medications; should also take into account the patient's definition of constipation, with the goal being to establish what is normal for that patient.

b. Review of medications, including over-the-counter and herbal supplements.

c. Dietary habits, food and fluid intake, and amount of fiber.

d. Abdominal assessment to rule out obstruction: Examine for bowel sounds, bloating, tenderness, and rectal assessment.

e. Laboratory tests to rule out electrolyte or thyroid imbalances.

4. Treatment – If the cause cannot be eliminated, a bowel regime should be initiated. A minimum goal is for a bowel movement every 72 hours, regardless of intake. Bowel obstruction should be ruled out before any treatment is initiated.

a. Medications include stool softeners and laxatives. Suppositories and/or enemas should be considered when the patient is no longer able to tolerate oral medications.

b. Dietary and fluid interventions include encouragement of fluid intake and high-fiber foods.

c. Physical activity should be encouraged, as appropriate.

F. Cough.

1. Cough can be debilitating for the patient, causing pain, fatigue, vomiting, and insomnia.

2. Etiology of cough: Infection, bronchitis, aspiration, obstruction, medication, asthma, esophageal reflux, COPD, heart failure, sinusitis, environmental irritation, pulmonary fibrosis, pneumothorax, pulmonary embolism, or malignant involvement of lung or pleura.

3. Assessment should include a history and physical, which include information about associated precipitating and relieving factors, presence of sputum production and blood, smoking, and exposure to other environmental irritants.

4. Treatment.

a. Pharmacologic treatment may include bronchodilators, cough suppressants, opiates or local anesthetics, cough expectorants (antitussives), antibiotics, steroids, anticholinergics, and nebulized saline.

b. Non-pharmacologic techniques include adequate hydration; cool mist humidification; positioning, such as elevating the head of the bed; and avoidance of smoke, allergens, or other triggers. Radiation therapy or stent placement may relieve obstruction.

G. Depression.

1. Involves the body, mind, and thoughts; pervasive changes affect how the patient thinks, behaves, and feels about him/herself (DeLaCruz, Brown, & Passik, 2010). Persistent feelings of helplessness, hopelessness, inadequacy, depression, and suicidal ideation are not normal at the EOL and should be aggressively evaluated and treated.

2. Causes may be:

a. Disease-related: Pain, abnormal metabolic states, organic mental disorders, or drug reactions or withdrawal.

b. Medication-related: Antihypertensives, analgesics, neuroleptics, anti-Parkinson agents, steroids, chemotherapy and biologic agents, hormones, alcohol, amphetamines, sedatives, oral contraceptives, H2 blockers.

c. Psychological: Fear of death, loss of independence or control, unresolved conflict or guilt, changes in body image or social factors, such as financial and family issues, contributing to distress and exacerbating depression.

3. Assessment.
   a. Differentiating between sadness and clinical depression may be difficult. Pervasive feelings of despair, hopelessness and worthlessness, excessive guilt, and a lack of interest in usual activities likely point to depression (DeLaCruz et al., 2010).
   b. Previous psychiatric history and treatment should be assessed.
   c. Presence of risk factors should be evaluated, such as living alone, lacking a support system, uncontrollable symptoms, presence of multiple deficits (such as inability to walk, loss of bowel and bladder control, or sensory loss).
   d. Validated assessment scales may be helpful to monitor depression (see section on *Depression* in Chapter 18, "Care of the Acutely Ill Patient").
   e. The potential for suicide should be assessed by evaluating the presence of a suicidal plan, method, and resources to carry out the plan; ability to communicate intent; and intended outcome (gesture or serious attempt to die). Patients with immediate, lethal, and precise suicide plans and resources to carry out the plan should be immediately evaluated by a psychiatric professional or placed in an appropriate close supervisory state.

4. Treatment includes addressing underlying or associated factors, such as pain and infection.
   a. Pharmacologic interventions may include SSRI and tricyclic antidepressants, stimulants, non-benzodiazepines, and more rarely, monoamine oxidase (MAO) inhibitors.
   b. Non-pharmacologic interventions, such as music therapy, psychotherapy, and counseling, are suggested. The ambulatory nurse can also help by:
      (1) Using empathy: Validating and acknowledging and normalizing feelings.
      (2) Promoting and facilitating as much autonomy and control as possible.
      (3) Encouraging increasing patient and family participation in care.
      (4) Assisting the patient to do a life review to focus on accomplishments and promote closure and resolution of life events.
      (5) Grief counseling to assist in dealing with past, present, and future loss.
      (6) Maximizing symptom management to decrease physical stressors.
      (7) Assisting the patient and family to draw on previous sources of strength, such as faith and belief systems.
      (8) Educating the patient and family to understand depression, risk factors, and prescribed medications, and to develop a safety plan if suicide may be possible.

H. Diarrhea.
   1. Diarrhea, the frequent passage of loose, non-formed stool, may dramatically impact a person's quality of life. It can cause fatigue, electrolyte abnormalities, and depression, and may lead to skin breakdown and dehydration. Psychologically, it may increase anxiety and fear of appearing in public.
   2. Etiology.
      a. Disease-related: Tumors (particularly carcinoid, pancreatic, and islet cell tumors), bacterial and parasitic infection, partial bowel obstructions, malabsorption, irritable bowel syndrome, and hyperthyroidism.
      b. Treatment- or medication-related: Chemotherapy medications (particularly irinotecan, fluorouracil, and capecitabine), laxatives, antibiotics, magnesium, metoclopramide, recent bowel surgical procedures, or preparation for procedures.

c. Diet-related: Excessive dietary fiber, intolerance of certain foods, enteral feedings, and dumping syndrome.

3. Assessment requires a careful bowel history, medication history, and assessment of the nature and frequency of the stools, as well as hydration status.

   a. The onset/suddenness is important. A rapid onset may indicate fecal impaction with overflow.
   b. Watery stools in large amounts are consistent with colonic diarrhea.
   c. Foul-smelling, fatty, pale stools are associated with malabsorption.
   d. Laxative over-usage may cause cramping, urgency, or fecal leakage.
   e. Laboratory tests to evaluate for dehydration and infectious processes may be considered for blood, fat, mucous, and pus in stool.
   f. Physical assessment includes examination of abdomen, pelvis, and rectum: Auscultation of bowel sounds, palpation for masses, organomegaly, abdominal pain, tenderness, and guarding.

4. Treatment is for the underlying cause, as appropriate.

   a. Initiate a clear liquid diet; advance to low-fiber foods, solids, but avoid milk, proteins, fats, and high-gas-forming foods. "BRAT" diet: **B**ananas, **R**ice, **A**pplesauce, and white **T**oast may be helpful.
   b. Promote hydration. Sport drinks also help with electrolyte replacement.
   c. For pediatric patients with diarrhea, refer to Chapter 18, "Care of the Acutely Ill Patient," for fluid and food recommendations.
   d. Medications may be prescribed, such as antidiarrheal agents (bismuth – Kaopectate®; loperamide – Imodium®; diphenoxylate and atropine – Lomotil®), opioids, bulk-forming agents, antibiotics, and steroids. Octreotide® may be used for chemotherapy-induced diarrhea.

e. Encourage skin care – Gently wash perirectal area after bowel movements with mild soap and water, and pat dry. Sitz bath, medicated cleansing pads, and skin protectant ointments may be helpful.

I. Dyspnea (Dudgeon, 2006; Lorenz et al., 2008; Vogel, Wilson, & Melvin, 2004).

1. Dyspnea is distressing shortness of breath.
2. Etiology of dyspnea.

   a. Pulmonary compromise: Tumor, superior vena cava syndrome, aspiration, effusions, emboli, COPD, lymph infiltrates, bronchospasm, pneumothorax, fibrosis, hepatomegaly, or ascites.
   b. Cardiac-related issues: Congestive heart failure (CHF), pulmonary edema, pulmonary hypertension, pericardial effusion, or anemia.
   c. Neuromuscular disorders: Amyotrophic lateral sclerosis (ALS), myasthenia gravis, cerebrovascular disease, phrenic nerve paralysis, or trauma.
   d. Anxiety.
   e. Metabolic and paraneoplastic syndromes.
   f. Psychological or physiological distress.

3. Assessment of dyspnea is like assessment of pain: The subjective report of the patient is the only reliable indicator of this symptom. Clinical assessment determines any underlying pathophysiology and should include:

   a. Prior medical history of acute or chronic dyspnea, smoking, heart or lung disease, concurrent medical conditions, and current medications.
   b. Pattern and duration of dyspnea.
   c. Alleviating and aggravating factors.
   d. Associated symptoms, including anxiety and chest pain.
   e. Effect on functional status and QOL.
   f. Physical examination, including assessment of breath sounds, respiratory rate and depth, use of accessory muscles, and oxygenation status.

Pulse oximetry should only be used when the results will yield meaningful information, because patients and family members may focus on readings and exacerbate anxiety (Von Roenn & Paice, 2005).

4. Treatment of dyspnea would involve treating the symptom while determining whether or not to treat the underlying cause, such as antibiotics for infection or management of tumor progression. Both pharmacologic and non-pharmacologic management should be initiated.
   a. Pharmacologic: Bronchodilators, diuretics, corticosteroids, oral, subcutaneous and nebulized opioids, benzodiazepines and non-benzodiazepine anxiolytics, antibiotics for infections, anticoagulants for pulmonary embolus, and scopolamine or glycopyrolate for excessive secretions.
   b. Non-pharmacologic treatment techniques may include oxygen, pursed-lip and diaphragmatic breathing, energy conservation, rearranging environment to minimize exertion, fans and air conditioners to cool and circulate air, positioning to optimize use of accessory muscles, such as elevation of the head of the bed and support of the patient to sit in a forward and upright position. Music, relaxation, guided imagery, and other cognitive behavioral, interpersonal, and complementary therapies may also be used.
   c. Other treatments may include physical and occupational therapy, smoking cessation and avoidance of exposure to smoke and other irritants, blood transfusions to improve anemia, radiation therapy to shrink tumor or relieve airway obstruction, stent tube placement to open occluded airway, paracentesis to reduce ascites or thoracentesis to reduce effusion; catheters may be utilized for long-term drainage.

J. Fatigue.
   1. Defined as "a subjective perception and/or experience related to disease, emotional state, and/or treatment. It is multidimensional, is not easily relieved by rest, and has a profound impact on the dimensions of quality of life...is influenced by the cultural context of the individual and is associated with a reduced capacity to carry out expected or required daily activities" (Ferrell, 2000, p. 42).
   2. Etiologies include:
      a. Disease-related anemia, electrolyte imbalances, malnutrition (inadequate absorption of iron, protein or folic acid), hormonal imbalances, infection, hyperglycemia, fever, pain, organ failure, or central nervous system injury.
      b. Psychological influences include somatic symptoms associated with depression, inactivity/immobility, and spiritual distress.
      c. Treatment-related, such as side effect from chemotherapy, biotherapy, radiation, or surgery; inadequate rest; and medications, such as antihistamines, narcotics, antiepileptics, hypnotics, and antidepressants. Unrelieved side effects, such as diarrhea or vomiting, may cause or increase fatigue.
      d. Co-morbid conditions, such as cardiac disease, neuromuscular disorders, and chronic fatigue syndrome.
   3. Assessment is primarily subjective with objective evaluation playing a lesser part. Assess the timing and patterns of fatigue relative to disease and treatment.
      a. Subjective data include complaints of feeling weak and/or tired and may affect patient's functional status and ability to perform ADLs. Use of validated fatigue scales may be helpful for grading and monitoring of fatigue.
      b. Associated symptoms, such as weakness, lightheadedness, dyspnea on exertion, anxiety, difficulty concentrating, impaired memory, and changes in appetite and sleep patterns.

c. Work-up may include laboratory tests, such as complete blood count, thyroid tests, electrolytes and others, to confirm or rule out etiologic and contributing causes.

4. Treatment for fatigue involves detection and correction of reversible causes of fatigue. A multidisciplinary approach includes both pharmacological and non-pharmacological interventions, as well as patient and family education (Campos, Hassan, Riechelmann, & del Giglio, 2011).

   a. Pharmacologic treatments include low dose corticosteroids, antidepressants, psycho-stimulants, such as methylphenidate and modafinil, cholinesterase inhibitors, and erythropoietin stimulating agents for chemotherapy-related anemia.

   b. Non-pharmacologic interventions include:

      (1) Education: Provide information about common patterns of fatigue with treatments, such as cumulative fatigue during radiation therapy and cyclical fatigue with chemotherapy. This may help patient understand and interpret fatigue (as a treatment side effect rather than a symptom of progressive disease) (Cope, 2006).

      (2) Exercise: Low-intensity, progressive exercise regime matched to patient's comfort level can improve QOL. Risks and benefits should be weighed for patients with anemia, bone metastases, neutropenia, thrombocytopenia, and fever (Barsevick, Newhall, & Brown, 2008). Physical and occupational therapists may help identify helpful assistive devices.

      (3) Energy conserving techniques and provision of assistance can help the patient maintain independence and functional abilities as long as possible. Balance activities with periods of rest. Assist patient to plan and prioritize activities.

      (4) Encourage good sleep hygiene: Set and maintain regular sleep and wake times, avoid caffeine, alcohol, and nicotine within several hours of bedtime.

K. Nausea and vomiting.

1. Nausea and vomiting are multifactorial and have extremely complex pathophysiology. They may be acute, anticipatory, or delayed. Etiology includes:

   a. Disease process: Gastric irritation and stasis, constipation, intestinal obstruction, pancreatitis, ascites, liver failure, intractable cough, electrolyte imbalances, hypercalcemia, uremia, infection, increased intracranial pressure, and pain.

   b. Psychological: Emotional factors can be a result of stimulation of emetic receptors in the brain.

   c. Treatment-related: Recent surgery, radiation therapy, chemotherapy, and other drugs that stimulate the chemoreceptor zone.

   d. Vestibular disturbances: Toxic action of drugs (such as ASA and opiates) and local tumors within the brain stimulate the vestibular apparatus.

2. Clinical assessment should include:

   a. Pattern, onset, duration, and severity of nausea and vomiting.

   b. History of consistency, frequency, and volume of emesis.

   c. Identification of activities that may precipitate nausea and vomiting, such as odors, position changes and medications, and other contributing factors, such as pain, constipation, or anxiety.

   d. Past history and effectiveness of treatment.

3. Treatment is dictated by the presumed cause. Treat underlying cause and try any interventions that have worked in the past.

   a. Pharmacologic:

(1) Routine antiemetics, including prochlorperazine (Compazine®), are used for mild nausea, or metoclopramide (Reglan®), which is also used to treat gastric stasis or ileus.

(2) 5HT3 medications, such as ondansetron and granisetron, are appropriate for chemotherapy-induced nausea and vomiting.

(3) Corticosteroids, such as dexamethasone, may be used as an adjuvant antiemetic.

(4) Anticholinergics, such as meclizine or scopolamine, treat motion sickness, intractable vomiting, or small bowel obstruction.

(5) Antihistamines are used for increased intracranial pressure, peritoneal irritation, or vestibular cause.

(6) Lorazepam (Ativan®) is most effective in treating anxiety-induced nausea, including anticipatory nausea with cancer chemotherapy.

(7) Haloperidol (Haldol®) may be used to treat opioid and chemically or mechanically induced nausea.

b. Non-pharmacologic techniques include dietary interventions, such as serving small, frequent meals at room temperature; avoiding strong odors; and other complementary therapies, such as distraction, relaxation, acupuncture, music therapy, hypnosis, and herbs, such as ginger.

V. Ethical Issues in EOL

A. Advances in medical technology, changes in family and social systems, managed care, and multiple health care choices have added to the complexity of EOL care and ethical decision-making.

B. EOL care raises questions about the meaning of life, QOL, dependency on others, and the meaning of pain and suffering, illness, and death.

C. The nurse's role in addressing ethical issues is complex, understanding that each member of the care team, including the patient and family, comes with his or her own values, morals, and life experiences.

D. Issues of decision-making and communication at EOL are complex and often provide challenges. Chapter 6, "Legal Aspects of Ambulatory Care Nursing," and Chapter 12, "Ethics," provide information about ethical principles and legal regulation of patients' and families' rights that are particularly important to consider with a terminally ill patient.

1. Discussions centered on issues, such as understanding prognosis and current health status, advance directives, Do Not Resuscitate (DNR) orders, assisted suicide, and withholding and withdrawing treatment, increasingly involve the nurse (Stanley & Zoloth-Dorfman, 2006).

2. Nurses have the responsibility to understand and articulate ethical rationale for health care decisions. Open and sensitive communication, educating, and enabling the patient and family to make fully informed decisions about EOL care is paramount.

3. The ANA position statement *Registered Nurses' Responsibility in Providing Expert Care and Counseling at End of Life* supports nurses facilitating informed decision-making at EOL. It is meant to provide information to guide the nurse in vigilant advocacy for patients throughout their lifespan as they consider EOL choices and includes discussion of personal ethical dilemmas that can occur when caring for the dying patient (ANA, 2010a).

4. The fundamental principle of ethical decision-making is respect for the inherent worth, dignity, and human rights of each individual.

5. Truth telling: Dealing with family requests not to have specific discussions with the adult patient may be difficult for the nurse. Although cultural values may dictate how the family filters information for the patient, it is equally important for the nurse to elicit

what the patient wants to know. Requests to withhold truth should prompt a discussion or meeting to address family fears and concerns.

6. After discussion with parent and assessment of the ability of the child to participate in EOL, EOL discussions with children must be age-appropriate.

7. Ethical dilemmas arise when patients are unable to ascertain their own rights, such as children, those incarcerated, patients in critical care units or psychiatric care centers, or others with a diminished capacity for decision-making (ANA, 2010b).

E. Advance care planning is a process of decision-making and communication of those decisions between the person and his or her family, friends, physicians, and other health care providers who ensure that the patient's choices are known, preferably long before a crisis situation, or when wishes can no longer be communicated. If these discussions are considered or introduced as routine care when providing information about treatment, it may reduce anxiety.

1. Do Not Resuscitate/No Code orders confirm that if a cardiopulmonary arrest occurs, no resuscitative measures are initiated. This requires a written physician order. It is not required by standard or law for admission to hospice.

2. Designating a health care proxy involves the patients deciding and designating whom they would like to make health care decisions for them in the event they cannot make them for themselves. A growing number of states include some type of provision for surrogate consent if a patient does not complete proxy designation. See *Advance Directives* discussion in Chapter 6, "Legal Aspects of Ambulatory Care Nursing."

3. New laws regarding discussion at EOL are being adopted by some states. In New York, the "Palliative Information Act" went into effect in 2011, mandating that health care practitioners provide information regarding the patient's options of palliative and EOL care. The goal of these new laws is to empower the dying patient and ensure his or her right to receive information and counseling at EOL.

4. Several states now provide a shortened form of the living will that is signed by the physician, so it then becomes a physician's order for life-sustaining treatment. Patients with a terminal illness should keep these documents in plain sight in their homes so that emergency personnel and caregivers have information of the patient's wishes readily available.

5. Decision-making near EOL is an ongoing, dynamic process; the patient and/or proxy have the right to change their decisions at any time.

6. Decisions communicated ahead of time decrease the chances of conflict in future decision, decrease the potential for ethical dilemmas, and take the burden off the family and health care team.

F. Nurses must advocate and contribute to effective pain and symptom management. Nurses may be reluctant to administer adequate analgesia for fear of respiratory depression and that they will "cause" the patient death. The increasing titration of medication to achieve adequate symptom control, even if hastening death secondarily, is ethically justified (ANA, 1995). Those who work with patients at the end of life often report that patients who are in pain often pass when their pain is under control because the body is relaxed and suffering is assuaged.

G. Withholding or withdrawing of potentially life-sustaining treatment is usually done because of patient choice, undesirable QOL, burdens outweighing benefits, or prolongation of the dying process. Common situations include withdrawal of medically provided hydration or nutrition, ventilation, CPR, and/or dialysis. The courts have upheld the validity of advance directives drawing a distinction between allowing a patient to die and purposely causing a patient's death. There is, however, no legal or moral distinction between withholding and removing life-prolonging measures (Ackermann, 2007).

1. The decision to withdraw or withhold is a decision that allows the disease to progress on its natural course. It is not a decision or action intended to cause death.
2. Nurses need to clarify with patient and family that withdrawing or withholding life-sustaining measures does NOT equate with withdrawal of care. Regardless of the decision made, nurses and the health care team will still be present to provide high-quality EOL care. For example, if the decision is made not to utilize or to remove artificial nutrition, the nurse will continue to minimize patient discomfort by offering ice chips and providing mouth and skin care.

H. Physician-assisted suicide (PAS):
1. Specific states, such as Oregon, Washington, and Montana, have passed laws allowing terminally ill patients to end their lives through the voluntary self-administration of lethal medications expressly prescribed by a physician for that purpose. Several other states are considering similar legislation.
2. ANA has based its position on PAS from the philosophical stance of respect for patients that is extensively explicated in the *Code of Ethics for Nurses*; the position clearly states that "nurses may not act with the sole intent of ending a patient's life, even though such action might be motivated by compassion, respect for autonomy, and QOL consideration" (ANA, 2001, p. 8).
3. Nurses have the right to conscientiously object to participating in situations they may find morally objectionable.

I. Dealing with statements or requests to die (Coyle & Sculco, 2004; Hudson, Kristjanson et al., 2006; Hudson, Schofield et al., 2006).
1. Nurses have the responsibility to respond to requests in a way that supports the needs and expectations of the patient while offering care that is both ethical and legal.
2. The desire to die statement may be an expression of anger, despair, hopelessness, or existential distress. It may be a way for the patient to communicate distress and to seek help, and a reaction to current circumstances or unrelieved symptoms. Common factors associated with a desire for a hastened death include:
   a. Being a burden on family and friends.
   b. Loss of autonomy or loss of self.
   c. Unrelieved physical symptoms.
   d. Loss of future, hopelessness, depression.
   e. Existential concerns.
3. The initial nursing response should never be a "yes" or "no" reply, but rather, an invitation for discussion. Encourage the patient to express feelings and explore issues behind request. Listen.
4. Be aware of one's own verbal and nonverbal response to the patient statement. Responses such as shock, impatience, or anger can have a negative impact/effect on the conversation and may limit future conversations.
5. Assess possible contributing factors, such as lack of social support, depression, unrelieved symptoms, and interpersonal factors.
6. Address potentially reversible causes, such as unrelieved symptoms. Develop a management plan with patient and evaluate effectiveness.
7. Inform the health care team of patient disclosure and offer multidisciplinary support to the patient, such as chaplaincy and social services.
8. Patient's views may fluctuate over time, which reinforces the need for ongoing assessment, discussion, and review.

J. Nurses strive to remain committed to the delivery of patient care and non-abandonment. There may be situations in which nurses need to remove themselves from the care of a particular patient based on an ethical objection. Nurses are obligated to provide for the patient's safety and seek alternative sources of care (Matzo & Sherman, 2001).

K. Issues of justice impact EOL care.
1. Quality EOL care is not consistently available to all people.

2. Health care systems are beginning to identify and understand the need for the incorporation of quality palliative and hospice care. However, rural hospitals that are struggling to maintain financial solvency may be having difficulty justifying the expense of these programs and are likely to cut them from their budgets.

3. After the death of the patient, there is a responsibility to support the family through bereavement. This is mandated by Medicare in the hospice benefit; however, most hospices provide bereavement services in their community to families whether the patient was on the hospice service or not.

4. Families may shoulder the financial burden of caregiving in the home and/or need for placement of patients in nursing homes. Families are often drained of future financial stability.

L. Each state's nurse practice act and other public health regulations provide essential information related to EOL care, such as the pronouncement of death, prescriptive practices, and laws governing controlled substances and disposition of opioids in the home after death.

M. When ethical dilemmas occur, the nurse's role is as advocate, with the responsibility to assure that the patient and family fully understand the options available so they can make informed decisions, and to facilitate that the patient's and family's wishes are clarified and communicated to the interdisciplinary team of caregivers.

N. Cultural considerations at EOL.
1. Cultural practices are defined as a system of shared symbols, serving as guides for interactions. Cultural and spiritual issues may be best addressed through collaboration with clergy, pastoral care counselors, and representatives from the patient's cultural community.
2. Beliefs regarding death and dying, the afterlife, and bereavement vary within different cultural frameworks. Cultural and religious beliefs and practices around time of death should be anticipated and carefully managed (NCCN, 2011b).

VI. Grief, Loss, and Bereavement

As a death-denying society, Americans often suppress the need to express grief and feel the pain that accompanies a loss; however, both are beneficial to healing. The nurse's role includes facilitating the grief process by assessing grief and assisting the survivor to feel the loss, express the loss, and complete the tasks of the grief process. Grief affects survivors physically, psychologically, socially, and spiritually.

A. Grief is a process, unique to each person, a constellation of responses to a significant loss, real, perceived, or anticipated.

B. Grief can express itself in unexpected times and places. No one can predict when the grief work will be complete because there will always be times when a memory, object, anniversary, or feelings of loss will occur.

C. Grief can be a very isolating experience and most especially for the patient who is dying (Loomis, 2009).

D. Normal or uncomplicated grief reactions.
1. Can be physical, emotional, cognitive, and/or behavioral.
2. May include reactions, such as shock, anxiety, emotional numbness, denial, disbelief, and symptoms of depression with eventual recovery.
3. Are marked by a gradual acceptance of loss, and although difficult, continuation of basic daily activities.

E. Anticipatory grief.
1. Begins before death for the patient and survivors as they anticipate and experience loss.
2. May begin at diagnosis of a life-limiting or life-debilitating disease.
3. Examples include grief reactions to actual or fear of potential loss of health, independence, body part, financial stability, choice, or mental function.
4. Anticipatory grief provides the family members time to absorb the reality of the loss; they have time to complete unfinished business, such as saying, "I love you," or "goodbye" (NCI, 2011a).

F. Complicated grief.
1. Complicated grief can be described as:

a. Prolonged or chronic, characterized by normal grief reactions that do not subside and continue over long periods of time.

b. Delayed, characterized by normal grief reactions that are suppressed or postponed, and the survivor consciously or unconsciously avoids the pain of the loss.

c. Exaggerated or distorted, characterized by extremely intense or atypical symptoms, such as self-destructive behaviors (e.g., suicide).

d. Masked or absent, with little evidence of normal grief. Survivor may not be aware that behaviors that interfere with normal functioning are the result of the loss.

2. Reactions include:

a. Difficulty acknowledging the death.

b. Preoccupation with distressing thoughts of loved one and his or her death.

c. Bitterness and sense of disbelief.

d. Severe isolation and avoidance behavior.

e. Persistent pangs of emotional pain and yearning for the deceased.

f. Violent or workaholic behavior or suicidal ideation.

g. Replacing loss of relationship quickly.

h. Excessive loneliness.

3. Risk factors for complicated grief include sudden or traumatic death, death of a child, multiple losses, and unresolved grief from prior losses, concurrent stressors, active or history of depression, pessimistic thinking, and lack of support system or faith system.

4. Complicated grief causes significant functional impairment of social, occupational, and other areas, and an inability to resume normal routine.

G. Disenfranchised grief occurs when a loss is experienced and cannot be openly acknowledged, socially sanctioned, or publicly shared. This may occur with ex-spouses, lovers, co-workers, children experiencing the death of a step-parent, women with a terminated pregnancy, or partners of patients with HIV/AIDS.

H. Children's grief (NCI, 2011a).

1. Children's grief is often not recognized by adults who are dealing with their own sense of grief and loss and have not realized the impact on the children involved.

2. Adults often try to hide their own feelings of loss to protect children.

3. Symptoms of unresolved grief in younger children include anxiety; nervousness; uncontrollable rages; frequent sickness; disturbances in eating, sleeping, and bowel and bladder function; accident proneness; hyperactivity; nightmares; compulsive behavior; and dependency on remaining adults.

4. Symptoms of unresolved grief in older children include difficulty concentrating, forgetfulness, poor school work, insomnia or sleeping too much, reclusiveness, antisocial behavior, resentment of authority, overdependence, talk of or attempted suicide, nightmares, frequent sickness, eating disorders, or experimentation with drugs, alcohol, or sex.

5. Though highly individualized, a child's grief may appear brief, but it may last a lifetime and can be revisited during significant life events, such as graduations, marriages, and births.

6. Factors that influence grief in a child include:

a. Age and developmental level.

b. Relationship with the deceased.

c. Previous experience with death.

d. Availability of support systems.

e. Opportunity to express feelings and memories.

f. Stability of the child's life after the loss.

7. Interventions for grieving children include:

a. Discussing death with simple, direct, and truthful explanations.

b. Using correct language such as "death" and "died," rather than "gone to sleep," "we lost him," or "he passed on."

c. Reassuring security of child.

d. Encouraging participation of child in mourning rituals as they feel comfortable, such as allowing a younger child to carry flowers, or an older child to say a prepared reading in funeral service.

   e. Explaining what the child should expect at mourning ritual: What they will see or hear, such as the casket and crying or wailing.

I. Grief assessment includes the patient, family, and significant others. It is ongoing throughout the course of an illness and for the bereavement period after the death for the survivors. Nurses should assess:

1. Type of grief, reactions, stages and tasks, and factors that may affect the grief process.
   a. Personality of the individual and his or her previous coping skills/experience of losses.
   b. History of substance abuse, mental illness, or suicidal tendencies.
   c. Relationship to the deceased and age.
   d. Religious/spiritual belief system and cultural traditions.
   e. Type of death and preparation for the death.
   f. Concurrent stressors, support systems.

2. Many caregiver survivors do not care for themselves while caring for the patient. Nurses may want to suggest a thorough physical examination and psychosocial and spiritual evaluation.

J. Mourning.

1. The outward, social expression of loss; a public display of grief. It is often dictated by cultural norms, customs, practices (including rituals), and traditions. It is influenced by the individual's personality, beliefs, religion, and life experiences (Corless, 2006).

2. An important part of mourning for survivors is learning how to live in the world without their loved one physically present; they need to learn how to adjust the relationship and move forward (Loomis, 2009).

K. Bereavement.

1. The length of time it takes to mourn, though grief may persist, and the acuity usually softens.

2. Bereavement includes grief and mourning: The inner feelings and outward reactions of the survivor.

L. It is the nurse's responsibility to be aware of the cultural characteristics of grief and mourning for patients and family members.

M. Bereavement interventions may come from a variety of resources and should include an interdisciplinary approach based upon the plan of care that has been developed after the assessment. Interventions may include:

1. Presence, active listening, touch, silence.
2. Identification of support systems.
3. Use of bereavement specialists, bereavement resources (hospice is a primary source to use).
4. Normalizing the grief process and individual differences.
5. Actualizing the loss and facilitating living without the deceased.
6. Public funerals, memorial services, rites, rituals, and traditions.
7. Spiritual care.

N. Bereavement interventions for children and parents are often available through community hospices and schools. Parents may be encouraged to attend support groups in the community.

O. Nurses, as all professionals, must recognize and respond to their own grief to provide quality palliative and bereavement care.

P. The nurse will, at one time or another, experience death anxiety and/or a sense of cumulative loss and grief.

1. Working with dying patients can trigger the nurse's awareness of his or her personal losses or fears about death or mortality.
2. Death anxiety occurs when the nurse is confronted with fears about death and has few resources or support systems to explore and express thoughts and emotions about dying/death.
3. When overwhelmed by death anxieties, nurses may use defenses to allay fears, including focusing only on physical care needs or evading emotionally sensitive conversations. This may result in emotional distancing at a time when patients and families need intensive interpersonal care.

4. Personal death awareness allows the nurse to come to a sense of comfort to explore, experience, and express his or her personal feelings regarding death (Vachon, 2006).

5. Cumulative loss is a succession of losses experienced by nurses who work with patients with life-threatening illnesses, often on a daily basis. When the nurse is exposed to death frequently, he or she may not have the time to resolve grief issues.

Q. Nurses new to working with dying patients may need to emotionally and spiritually adapt to caring for the terminally ill. Factors that influence the nurse's adaptation process include:

1. Professional training and ability to verbalize feelings and emotions.

2. Personal death history – Experiences on a personal and/or professional level.

3. Life changes and how the nurse has coped with those changes.

4. Support systems – Presence or absence of people who can provide emotional support.

R. Systems that are available for nurse support.

1. The nurse possesses the ability to provide compassionate, quality care to dying patients and their families, balanced with finding personal satisfaction in work as a professional.

2. The support system should be evaluated to determine if it inhibits or supports professional growth, adaptation, and development in caring for dying patients and families.

3. Formal support systems can include preplanned gatherings where team members can express feelings in a safe environment, post-clinical debriefings, and ceremonies or programs to acknowledge and express grief (memorial services).

4. Informal support is derived from co-workers, peers, or other team members.

5. Spiritual support may be provided by pastoral care workers or the nurse's personal spiritual aid.

VII. Preparation and Nursing Care at the Time of Death

A. The final days to hours before a patient dies may be the most significant moments for a patient and his or her family while preparing for death, saying goodbyes, and completing EOL closure tasks.

B. The nurse is often the one to facilitate a dignified, comfortable death that honors patient/family choices. The nurse may take on many roles as advocate, companion on the journey, professional caregiver, educator, and facilitator of resources. The nurse's challenge is to gain knowledge and skills to promote competence and provide dignified EOL care in any practice setting.

C. Individuals specializing in the care of the dying (nurses in hospice, spiritual counselors, social workers, volunteers, nursing aides) should be utilized as a resource. The team can help assess individual situations and identify problems, issues, and opportunities specific to the patient/family.

D. Dying is a unique experience. There is no typical death. Each person dies in his or her own way, own time, with his or her own culture, belief system, values, and unique relationships with others.

E. Dying is a physical, psychological, social, and spiritual event with the patient and family together as the unit of care.

F. Patients who are aware they are dying usually know where and with whom they want to die.

1. Nurses need to advocate for these patient/family choices no matter what the setting (hospital, home, nursing facility, group home, prison, or hospice).

2. Each setting should provide a supportive physical environment.

3. The nurse should avoid a change of setting in the final stages of life. The setting should be changed only if all options have failed and preferably only if the patient and family request the change.

4. The nurse should provide options in care, education about care, and/or increased support as early as possible so the patient can die where he or she chooses, and the

patient and family are not making rash decisions.

G. The team must be open and engage in honest communication to promote trust and informed decision-making.
   1. Information should be conveyed in simple, uncomplicated terms.
   2. Avoid overloading, overwhelming the patient/family by providing simple answers to questions in accordance with the patient/family understanding and readiness for responses.
   3. Family members may be tired, have difficulty concentrating, and focus on the present and not the future. The nurse may need to answer the same questions and provide the same information repeatedly because the family may be in crisis, and the ability to retain information may be greatly diminished.
   4. Patients often have a greater awareness that they are dying than those around them. If the patient asks if he or she is dying, be honest, and explore the patient's fears and concerns.
   5. If the family is fearful of the patient knowing he or she is dying, address these concerns by educating the family that the patient may already know he or she is dying, and encourage open, honest communication while respecting patient/family requests.
   6. The family may need education about the signs and symptoms of the dying process, such as what may happen, what they can expect regarding physical changes, and psychosocial and spiritual needs. Most hospice and palliative care programs have educational booklets that help explain these changes and guide them through the process of the body shutting down.
   7. Maintaining presence is the most important role nurses have; providing companionship, active listening, and reassurance that someone will be available during the dying process.

H. The death vigil occurs when death is imminent. Family will often want to be constantly at the bedside during the hours to days before death. In some situations, however, they may be uncomfortable due to their own fears. Education and support to the family is important at this time.
   1. Common fears include:
      a. Fear of being alone with the patient.
      b. Fear that the patient will have a painful death and/or they will have to watch the patient suffer.
      c. Fear of being alone with the patient when he or she dies and that they will not know what to do.
      d. Fear they will not know if the patient has died.
      e. Fear of giving the last dose of pain medication and hastening death.
   2. Nursing interventions include:
      a. Calming family fears, reassuring the family the patient will be kept as comfortable as possible.
      b. Educating the family about the signs and symptoms of the dying process, death, what they should do if they suspect the patient has died, and that they should call the nurse for any questions they may have at any time.
      c. Providing intensive physical comfort care, including mouth care, turning and positioning, and pain and symptom management.
      d. Offering spiritual comfort through presence, prayer, rites, and rituals.
      e. Honoring cultural beliefs, traditions, rites, and rituals.

I. The imminently dying patient.
   1. The dying process is a natural slowing down of physical and mental processes, and may occur weeks, days, or only hours prior to death.
   2. Signs and symptoms of the dying process only serve as a guideline. Not all patients experience all symptoms, and the signs and symptoms do not necessarily occur in sequence.
   3. Psychological and spiritual symptoms include fear of dying; abandonment or fear of the unknown; withdrawal from family, friends, and caregivers; and/or increased focus on spiritual issues.

4. Physical symptoms include:
   a. Extreme weakness and fatigue, periods of drowsiness or difficulty concentrating, confusion, and disorientation. One may also see surges of energy, restlessness, agitation, or delirium.
   b. Decreased oral intake, decreased or lack of swallow reflex, fever, and changes in bowel and bladder elimination (incontinence or retention/constipation) may occur.
   c. Imminent death signs include cold and mottled extremities, breathing pattern changes, dyspnea, noisy, bubbly, or moist breathing.
5. The nurse should clarify with family members their desires at time of death. Individuals have unique needs, and the nurse has an opportunity to help make the death easier for them (Berry & Griffie, 2006). Do they wish to be present? Are there other loved ones who would be supportive or that they would want present?

J. Telling the family the patient has died should be done with sensitivity. Provide small amounts of information at the family's level of understanding. Information about the death may need to be repeated due to the family feeling overwhelmed or shocked by the actual death.

K. Signs of death include absence of heartbeat or respirations, release of stool and urine, eyes remain open with fixed pupils, pale body color, body temperature drops, and jaw may fall open.

L. To pronounce the death, the nurse should know guidelines and procedure for the practice setting and state or county. If the patient is an organ donor, follow the procedure as planned.

M. Time with the body, post-mortem care, and removal of the body should be appropriate to the family's need to say goodbye and to religious or cultural rituals and traditions. The nurse may invite family to participate in cleaning and dressing, if they are comfortable. Parents may be encouraged to hold or cuddle their child after death. Allow siblings to participate in rituals and traditions according to their desires and developmental level (Berry & Griffie, 2006).

N. Preparing the body after death:
   1. Unless autopsy is planned, remove all tubes, IVs, and medical supplies to help provide a personal closure experience for the family, leaving the family with memories of the deceased as a loved one rather than a patient.
   2. Bathe and dress the body, placing dressings on leaking wounds and diaper for incontinence. Ask the family to assist if they want and to provide clothing if they prefer.
   3. Rigor mortis occurs 2–4 hours after death. Positioning or aligning of the body and limbs for viewing post-mortem may be important, such as placing dentures in place and a rolled washcloth under the chin to keep jaws closed. After the body is positioned, air may escape lungs and those present may hear a sighing sound similar to breathing. Alert the family to this possibility.
   4. Be aware of cultural practices with preparing the body. At the time of removal of the body, ask the family if they have preferences to covering or uncovering the face and whether or not they want to be in the room when the body is actually removed.

O. The nurse may want to assist the family with phone calls. The nurse should be the one to contact physicians, co-workers, or other health care agencies involved.

P. In a home setting, refer to local/state laws regarding destruction of patient medications. If the family asks the nurse to leave medications for them, the nurse should assess reasons/issues for the request. Offer to call the physician, as indicated, for an assessment of the survivor's issue/problem and/or to obtain a prescription unique to his or her needs.

Q. Funeral arrangements are best completed prior to death, but that option is not always available. If the family requests, provide options to promote family choice.

R. Following the death, the nurse should initiate bereavement support by providing compassion, active listening, and presence. In addition, the nurse should assess grief reactions and assess risk factors. For survivors who may need continued bereavement support, refer to community resources, such as hospice and support groups.

Table 22-1.
Valuable Resources for Palliative Care

Resource	Web Site
End-of-Life Nursing Education Curriculum (ELNEC). Washington, DC: American Association of Colleages of Nursing (AACN) & City of Hope National Medical Center.	www.aacn.nche.edu/elnec
Textbook of Palliative Nursing (2nd ed). B.R. Ferrell & N. Coyle (Eds.). New York: Oxford University Press.	Bookstores
National Hospice and Palliative Care Organization (NHPCO) is an organization representing hospice and palliative care programs and professionals in the United States. Web site includes directory of organizations and hospices in the U.S.	www.nhpco.org
National Cancer Institute (NCI) is a government-run Web site with a multitude of resources for specific cancers, as well as Web pages devoted to supportive and palliative care.	http://www.cancer.gov/cancertopics/coping
Education in Palliative and End-of-Life Care for Oncology (EPEC™-O) is a comprehensive multimedia curriculum available in CD-ROM format for health professionals caring for persons with cancer.	http://www.cancer.gov/cancertopics/cancerlibrary/epeco
Palliative.info is a Web site that offers an organized, up-to-date collection of links to palliative care resources on the Internet, as well as locally developed palliative care material.	http://palliative.info
The Center to Advance Palliative Care (CAPC) is a national organization dedicated to increasing the availability of quality palliative care services for people facing serious illness. It provides health care professionals with the tools, training, and technical assistance necessary to start and sustain successful palliative care programs.	http://www.getpalliativecare.org/resources
American Academy of Hospice and Palliative Medicine (AAHPM) is an organization of physicians and other medical professionals dedicated to excellence in palliative medicine and the prevention and relief of suffering among patients and families by providing education and clinical practice standards, fostering research, facilitating personal and professional development of its members, and by public policy advocacy.	http://www.aahpm.org/
Americans for Better Care of the Dying (ABCD) is an organization with the goal to improve EOL care by learning which social and political changes will lead to enduring, efficient, and effective programs. It works with the public, clinicians, policymakers, and other EOL organizations to institute change.	http://www.abcd-caring.org/
Bioethics Resources is a government-sponsored Web site that provides a compilation of links with the aim of helping individuals and groups explore the vast array of issues in bioethics at EOL.	http://bioethics.od.nih.gov/endoflife.html

S. The nurse may experience feelings of anxiety when caring for a dying patient, caring for a dead body, or supporting the family. Nurses grieve the loss of their patients and should not work in isolation while providing care for an imminently dying patient. Post-clinical debriefings can assist the nurse in exploration and expression of feelings of loss and grief.

VIII. Advocating for Quality Palliative Care

Nurses, individually and collectively as a profession, play a vital role in improving care at the EOL, promoting ethical quality care, respecting patient and family wishes, and helping patients to "die a good death."

A. Clarify the misconception that palliative care is solely for those who are actively dying or associated with imminent death (Clayton & Kissane, 2010). Nurses can incorporate palliative care principles (effective communication, pain and symptom management) within their own practice regardless of the setting/disease continuum.

B. Encourage, contribute to, and lobby for efforts to educate and promote autonomy and ethical decision-making at EOL. Stay knowledgeable of current issues and for health care reforms and trends.

C. Nurses can advance and implement evidence-based management to improve control of pain and other distressing symptoms of the terminally ill.

D. Nurses must be conscious of financial costs as well as the burden of treatments and therapies on the patient/family.

E. The death of the patient has typically not been seen as a positive outcome of care. Improving care at the EOL can be determined by measuring outcomes that reflect the positive outcomes of quality EOL closure. Some examples are length of stay in hospice program, the number of hospice services utilized by the patient and family, and patient/family satisfaction with symptom management.

F. Interdisciplinary teamwork extends to community resources. Early access of needed resources can significantly decrease stress and the perception of burden, especially for patients/families that do not have extended family to assist the primary caregiver.

G. There are many resources available about palliative and hospice care. Table 22-1 contains some valuable resources for nurses caring for the terminally ill.

References

Ackermann, R.J. (2007). Withholding and withdrawing potentially life – Sustaining treatment. In A. Berger, J. Shuster, & J. Von Roenn (Eds.), *Principles and practice of palliative care & supportive oncology* (3rd ed.). Philadelphia: Lippincott, Williams & Wilkins.

American Association of Colleges of Nursing (AACN) & City of Hope National Medical Center. (2008). The end-of-life nursing education curriculum (ELNEC). Washington, DC: Author.

American Nurses Association (ANA). (1995). *Position statement: Promotion of comfort and relief of pain in dying patients.* Kansas City, MO: Author.

American Nurses Association (ANA). (2001). *Code of ethics for nurses with interpretive statements.* Silver Spring, MD: Author.

American Nurses Association (ANA). (2010a). *Position statement: Registered nurses' responsibility in providing expert care and counseling at end of life.* Washington, DC: Author.

American Nurses Association (ANA). (2010b). *Position statement: The nurse's role in ethics and human rights: Protecting and promoting individual worth, dignity, and human rights in practice settings.* Washington, DC: Author.

Barsevick, A.M., Newhall, T., & Brown, S. (2008). Management of cancer related fatigue. *Clinical Journal of Oncology Nursing, 12S*(5), 21-25.

Bennett, M.I. (2010). Effectiveness of antiepileptic or antidepressant drugs when added to opioids for cancer pain: Systematic review. *Palliative Medicine, 25*(5), 553-559.

Berry, P., & Griffie, J. (2006). Planning for the actual death. In B.R. Ferrell & N. Coyle (Eds.), *Textbook of palliative nursing* (2nd ed., pp. 561-580). New York: Oxford University Press.

Borneman, T., & Brown-Saltzman, M. (2006). Meaning in illness. In B.R. Ferrell & N. Coyle (Eds.), *Textbook of palliative nursing* (2nd ed., pp. 605-616). New York: Oxford University Press.

Borneman, T., Koczywas, M., Sun, V.C., Piper, B.F., Uman,G., & Ferrell, B. (2010). Reducing patient barriers to pain and fatigue management. *Journal of Pain and Symptom Management, 39*(3), 486-501.

Campos, M.P., Hassan, B.J., Riechelmann, R., & del Giglio, A. (2011). Cancer-related fatigue: A review. *Revista da Associação Médica Brasileir, 57*(2), 206-214.

Carlson, M.D., Lim, B., & Meier, D.E. (2011). Strategies and innovative models for delivering palliative care in nursing homes. *Journal of the American Medical Directors Association, 12*(2), 91-98.

Chapman, S. (2010). Managing pain in the older person. *Nursing Standard, 25*(11), 35-39.

Clayton, J.M., & Kissane, D.W. (2010). Communication about transitioning patients to palliative care. In D.W. Kissane, B.D. Bultz, P.M. Butow, & I.G. Finlay (Eds.), *Handbook of communication in oncology and palliative care* (pp. 203-214). New York: Oxford University Press.

Cope, D. (2006). Fatigue. In D. Camp-Sorrell & R.A. Hawkins (Eds.), *Clinical manual for the oncology advanced practice nurse* (pp. 1127-1132). Pittsburgh: Oncology Nursing Society.

Corless, I.B. (2006). Bereavement. In B.R. Ferrell & N. Coyle (Eds.), *Textbook of palliative nursing* (2nd ed., pp. 531-544). New York: Oxford University Press.

Coss, C.C., Bohl, C.E., & Dalton, J.T. (2011). Cancer cachexia therapy: A key weapon in the fight against cancer. *Current Opinions in Clinical Nutrition and Metabolic Care, 14,* 268-273.

Coyle, N., & Sculco, L. (2004). Expressed desire for hastened death in seven patients living with advanced cancer: A phenomenologic inquiry. *Oncology Nursing Forum, 31*(4), 699-706.

Dahlin, C. (2006). Confusion/delirium. In D. Camp-Sorrell & R.A Hawkins (Eds.), *Clinical manual for the oncology advanced practice nurse* (pp. 877-883). Pittsburgh: Oncology Nursing Society.

DeLaCruz, A., Brown, R., & Passik, S. (2010). Ambulatory care nurses responding to depression. In D.W. Kissane, B.D. Bultz, P.M. Butow, & I.G. Finlay (Eds.), *Handbook of communication in oncology and palliative care* (pp. 439-448). New York: Oxford University Press.

Derby, S., & O'Mahony, S. (2006). Elderly patients. In B.R. Ferrell & N. Coyle (Eds.), *Textbook of palliative nursing* (2nd ed., pp. 635-660). New York: Oxford University Press.

Dickman, A. (2011). Integrated strategies for the successful management of breakthrough cancer pain. *Current Opinion in Supportive and Palliative Care, 5,* 8-14. doi:10.1097/SPC. 013e3283434515

Dudgeon, D. (2006). Dyspnea, death rattle and cough. In B.R. Ferrell & N. Coyle (Eds.), *Textbook of palliative nursing* (2nd ed., pp. 249-264). New York: Oxford University Press.

Egan, K.A., & Labyak, M.J. (2006) Hospice care: A model for quality end-of-life care. In B.R. Ferrell & N. Coyle (Eds.), *Textbook of palliative nursing* (2nd ed., pp. 7-26). New York: Oxford University Press.

Eisenchlas, J.H. (2007). Palliative sedation. *Current Opinion in Supportive and Palliative Care, 1,* 207-212.

Ferrell, B.R. (2000). Analysis of palliative care. *Journal of Palliative Care, 16*(1), 39-47.

Fink, R., & Gates, R. (2006). Pain assessment. In B.R. Ferrell & N. Coyle (Eds.), *Textbook of palliative nursing* (2nd ed., pp. 97-130). New York: Oxford University Press.

Fishbain, D.A. (2008). Pharmacotherapeutic management of breakthrough pain in patients with chronic persistent pain. *The American Journal of Managed Care, 14*(5), S123-S128.

Folstein, M., Folstein, S., & McHugh, P. (1975). "Mini mental state": A practical method for grading the cognitive state of patients for the clinician. *Journal of Psychiatric Research, 12,* 189-198.

Freye, E., & Levy, J.V. (2008). *Opioids in medicine: A comprehensive review on the mode of action and the use of analgesics in different clinical pain states.* Dordrecht, The Netherlands: Springer Science + Business Media B.V.

Grant, M., & Sun, V. (2010). Advances in quality of life at the end of life. *Seminars in Oncology Nursing, 26*(1), 26-35.

Hearn, J., & Higginson, I. (1998). Do specialist palliative care teams improve outcomes for cancer patients? A systematic review of the literature. *Palliative Medicine, 12,* 317-332.

Herr, K., Bjoro, K., Steffensmeier, J., & Rakel, B. (2006). *Evidence-based practice guideline: Acute pain management in older adults.* Iowa City: University of Iowa, Research Dissemination Core.

Hillegonds, D.J., Franklin, S., Shelton, D., Vijayakumar, S., & Vijayakumar, V. (2007). The management of painful bone metastases with an emphasis on radionuclide therapy *Journal of the National Medical Association, 99*(7), 785-794.

Hinds, P.S., & Kelly, K.P. (2010). Helping parents make and survive end of life decisions for their seriously ill child. *Nursing Clinics of North America, 45,* 465-474.

Hudson, P.L., Kristjanson, L.J., Ashby, M., Kelly, B., Schofield P., Hudson, R., ... Street, A. (2006). Desire for hastened death in patients with advanced disease and the evidence base of clinical guidelines: A systematic review. *Palliative Medicine, 20,* 693-701. doi:10.1177/0269216306071799

Hudson, P.L., Schofield, P., Kelly, B., Hudson, R., Street, A., O'-Connor, M., ... Aranda, S. (2006). Responding to desire to die statements from patients with advanced disease: Recommendations for health professionals. *Palliative Medicine, 20,* 703-710.

International Association for the Study of Pain (IASP). (1994). *IASP taxonomy.* Retrieved from http://www.iasp-pain.org/AM/Template.cfm?Section=Pain_Definitions

Jacobsen, R., Liubarskien, Z., Møldrup, C., Christup, L., Sjøgren, P., & Samsanavicient, J. (2009). Barriers to cancer pain management: A review of empirical research. *Medicina, 45*(6), 427-433.

Kane, J.A., & Himelstein, B.P. (2007). Palliative care in pediatrics. In A. Berger, J. Shuster, & J. Von Roenn (Eds.), *Principles and practice of palliative care & supportive oncology* (pp. 813-824). Philadelphia: Lippincott, Williams & Wilkins.

Kemp, C. (2006). Anorexia and cachexia. In B.R. Ferrell & N. Coyle (Eds.), *Textbook of palliative nursing* (2nd ed., pp. 169-176). New York: Oxford University Press.

Kirk, T.W., & Mahon, M.M. (2010). National Hospice and Palliative Care Organization position statement and commentary on the use of palliative sedation in imminently dying terminally ill patients. *Journal of Pain and Symptom Management, 39*(5), 914-923.

Knight, P., Espinosa, L.A., & Bruera, E. (2006). Sedation of refractory symptoms and terminal weaning. In B.R. Ferrell & N. Coyle (Eds.), *Textbook of palliative nursing* (2nd ed., pp. 131-153). New York: Oxford University Press.

Krechel, S.W., & Bildner, J. (1995). CRIES: A new neonatal postoperative pain measurement score: Initial testing of validity and reliability. *Paediatric Anaesthesia, 5*(1), 53-61.

Levin, T., & Weiner, J.S. (2010). End of life communication training. In D.W. Kissane, B.D. Bultz, P.M. Butow, & I.G. Finlay (Eds.), *Handbook of communication in oncology and palliative care* (pp. 216-227). New York: Oxford University Press.

Lippe, P.M., Brock, C., David, J., Crossno, R., & Gitlow, S. (2010). The First National Pain Medicine Summit – Final summary report: The AMA pain and palliative medicine specialty section council. *Pain Medicine, 11,* 1447-1468.

Loomis, B. (2009). End-of-life issues: Difficult decisions and dealing with grief. *Nursing Clinics of North America, 44,* 223-231.

Lorenz, K.A., Lynn, J., Dy, S.M., Shugarman, L.R., Wilkinson, A., Mularski, R.A., ... Shekelle, P.G. (2008). Evidence for improving palliative care at the end of life: A systematic review. *Annals of Internal Medicine 148*, 147-159.

Lussier, D., Huskey, A.G., & Portenoy, R.K. (2004). Adjuvant analgesics in cancer pain management. *The Oncologist, 9*, 571-591.

Lutz, S., Berk, L., Chang, E., Chow, E., Hahn, C., Hoskin, P., ... Hartsell, W. (2010). Palliative radiotherapy for bone metastases: An ASTRO evidence-based guideline. *International Journal of Radiation Oncology & Physics, 79*(4), 965-976.

Matzo, M.L., & Sherman, D.W. (Eds.). (2001). *Palliative care nursing: Quality care to the end of life*. New York: Springer Publishing Company.

McCaffery, M., & Pasero, C. (1999). *Pain: Clinical manual* (2nd ed.). St. Louis, MO: Mosby.

Mitra, R., & Jones, S. (2012). Adjuvant analgesics in cancer pain: A review. *American Journal of Hospice and Palliative Care, 29*(1), 70-79.

Morrison, L.J., & Morrison, R.S. (2006). Palliative care and pain management. *Medical Clinics of North America, 90*, 988-1004.

National Cancer Institute (NCI). (2011a). *Grief bereavement and loss.* Retrieved from http://www.cancer.gov/cancertopics/pdq/supportivecare/bereavement/Healthprofessionals

National Cancer Institute (NCI). (2011b). *Last days of life: Health professionals' version.* Retrieved from http://www.cancer.gov/cancertopics/pdq/supportivecare/lasthours/healthprofessional

National Cancer Institute (NCI). (2011c). *Spirituality in cancer care: Health professionals' version.* Retrieved from http://www.cancer.gov/cancertopics/pdq/supportivecare/spirituality/HealthProfesional

National Comprehensive Cancer Network (NCCN). (2011a). *Adult pain guidelines* [version 1.2011]. Fort Washington, PA: Author.

National Comprehensive Cancer Network (NCCN). (2011b). *Palliative care guidelines* [version 1.2011]. Fort Washington, PA: Author.

National Consensus Project for Quality Palliative Care (NCP). (2009). *Clinical practice guidelines for quality palliative care* (2nd ed.). Retrieved from http://www.nationalconsensusproject.org

Paice, J.A., & Fine, P.G. (2006). Pain at the end of life. In B.R. Ferrell & N. Coyle (Eds.), *Textbook of palliative nursing* (2nd ed., pp. 131-153). New York: Oxford University Press.

Pandit-Tasker, N., Batraki, M., & Divgi, C.R. (2004). Radiopharmaceutical therapy for palliation of bone pain from osseous metastases. *The Journal of Nuclear Medicine, 45*(8), 1358-1365.

Rosenzweig, M.Q. (2006). Anorexia/cachexia. In D. Camp-Sorrell & R.A Hawkins (Eds.), *Clinical manual for the oncology advanced practice nurse* (pp. 485-490). Pittsburgh: Oncology Nursing Society.

Stanley, K.J., & Zoloth-Dorfman, L. (2006). Ethical considerations. In B.R. Ferrell & N. Coyle (Eds.), *Textbook of palliative nursing* (2nd ed., 1031-1053). New York: Oxford University Press.

Vachon, M.L.S. (2006). The experience of the nurse in end of life in the 21st century. In B.R. Ferrell & N. Coyle (Eds.), *Textbook of palliative nursing* (2nd ed., pp. 1011-1030). New York: Oxford University Press.

Vogel, W.H., Wilson, M.A., & Melvin, M.S. (Eds.). (2004). Dypsnea. In *Advanced practice oncology and palliative care guidelines*. Philadelphia: Lippincott, Williams & Wilkins.

Von Roenn, J.H., & Paice, J.A. (2005). Control of common, non-pain cancer symptoms *Seminars in Oncology, 32*, 200-210.

World Health Organization (WHO). (2011a). *Definition of palliative care.* Retrieved from http://www.who.int/cancer/palliative/definition/en/

World Health Organization (WHO). (2011b). *WHO's pain ladder.* Retrieved from http://www.who.int/cancer/palliative/painladder/en/index.html

Wright, A.A., Zhang, B., Ray, A., Mack, J.W., Trice, E., Balboni, T., ... Progerson, H.G. (2008). Associations between end of life discussions, patient mental health, medical care near death and caregiver bereavement adjustment. *Journal of the American Medical Association, 300*(14), 1665-1673.

Glossary

Glossary

Abandonment – Relationship between patient and health care provider is terminated abruptly; provider disregards legal and ethical obligations to facilitate continuity of care and to avoid harm caused by prematurely terminating the relationship.

Absence (Petit Mal) Seizure – Resulting in brief loss of consciousness, usually 10 seconds or less, with the absence of hypertonicity or muscular contracture.

Accessibility of Care – Refers to the ease with which consumers can initiate interaction with a clinician about health problems; includes activities to eliminate barriers raised by geography, financing, culture, race, language, etc.

Accreditation Association for Ambulatory Health Care (AAAHC) – A private, non-profit agency that offers voluntary, peer-based review of the quality of health care services of ambulatory health organizations, including ambulatory and office-based surgery centers, managed care organizations, as well as Indian and student health centers, among others.

Advance Directives – Allow competent adults to make certain kinds of health care decisions in advance of an acute (such as a car accident) or chronic (such as Alzheimer's or cancer) incapacity, thus ensuring that their wishes are respected even if they are unable to communicate them directly; three types are: living wills, durable power of attorney for health care, and DNR ("Do Not Resuscitate") order.

Advanced Cardiac Life Support (ACLS) – Protocols and algorithms created through the American Heart Association to provide guidelines for medical management of cardiac arrest and/or arrhythmia, respiratory arrest and/or respiratory support, and stroke.

Advocacy – Act or process of advocating or supporting (a cause or proposal) on behalf of another.

Ambulatory Care – Outpatient care in which patients stay less than 24 hours and are discharged to their normal residential situation after care.

Ambulatory Care Nursing – A specialty practice area that is characterized by nurses responding rapidly to high volumes of patients in a short span of time while dealing with issues that are not always predictable.

Ambulatory Patient Classifications (APCs) – Used by the Centers for Medicare and Medicaid Services for prospective payment in hospital outpatient departments and ambulatory surgery centers; based on procedures and adjusted for severity.

Ambulatory Patient Groups (APGs) – Patient classification system designed to explain amount and type of resource used in ambulatory care visit.

Americans with Disabilities Act (ADA) – Prohibits discrimination on the basis of disability in employment, state and local government, public accommodations, commercial facilities, transportation, and telecommunications.

Anaphylactoid Reaction – An allergic reaction induced by drug infusion; anaphylactoid reactions are not caused by immunoglobulins (IgE).

Anaphylaxis – An allergic reaction caused by immunoglobulins (IgE) that affects whole body systems; can be fatal if not immediately treated.

Assisted Suicide – A practice whereby a person other than the patient provides a means to him or her with the knowledge that the patient will use the means to commit suicide.

Asthma – Chronic inflammatory disorder of the airways; chronically inflamed airways are hyperresponsive to triggers, which can lead to acute asthma exacerbation; exposure to triggers contributes to an increased level of airway inflammation with edema, acute bronchoconstriction, and mucus plug production.

Asthma Action Plan – A written, individualized asthma management/action plan that includes routine treatment, pre-exercise treatment, and a plan for emergency exacerbation.

Attention Deficit Hyperactivity Disorder (ADHD) – A persistent pattern of inattention and/or hyper-activity-impulsivity that is more frequently displayed and more severe than is typically observed in individuals at a comparable level of development.

Atypical (Psychotic) Depression – Depression that is accompanied by unusual symptoms, such as hallucinations or delusions.

Aura – Subjective indication of oncoming seizure; patients may describe a change in vision, taste, or smell pursuant to the onset of seizure activity.

Automated External Defibrillator (AED) – Device delivering electrical joules in response to shockable cardiac arrhythmias utilizing ACLS protocol.

Autonomy – Self-determination; the freedom to choose one's course of action.

Balanced Scorecard – Graphic or pictorial display of the organization's indicators chosen to support the strategic plan and vision of the organization; allows for examination of relationships among the separate indicators (care, quality, financial, operational, etc.).

Basic Life Support (BLS) – Process of providing circulation and respiration through artificial means (e.g., chest compressions and rescue breathing) in an organized, scientifically proven way in an effort to sustain life until advanced care can be provided.

Benchmarking – A continuous measurement of a process, product, or service in comparison to those of the toughest competitor, to those considered industry leaders, or to similar activities in the organization and using the information to change/improve practices, resulting in superior performance as determined by measured outcomes.

Beneficence – Doing good; requires defining what is meant by "good" in the situation.

Bereavement – Includes grief and mourning; the inner feelings and outward reactions of the survivor.

Body Mass Index (BMI) – Weight (kilograms) ÷ Height (meters)^2; or Weight (pounds) X 703 X Height (inches)^2.

Capitation – Method for funding expenses of enrollees in prepaid health plans; pays providers a fixed fee per member regardless of whether or not the service is provided. For example, a plan pays a per member per month (PMPM) amount to a physician group to provide primary care services for each enrollee in the plan.

Care Coordination – A process that seeks to achieve the optimal cost-effective use of scarce resources by helping individuals obtain health and appropriate social and life support services that meet their unique needs at a given point in time or across the lifespan.

Case Management – A collaborative process of assessment, planning, facilitation, and advocacy for options and services to meet an individual's health needs through communication and available resources to promote quality cost-effective outcomes; a method for managing the provision of health care to members/patients with catastrophic or high-cost medical conditions.

Centers for Medicare and Medicaid Services (CMS) – Formerly Health Care Financing Administration (HCFA); division within the U.S. Department of Health and Human Services that determines the standard rules and reporting mechanisms for health care services.

Certification – Process that uses predetermined standards to validate and recognize an individual's knowledge, skills, and abilities in a defined functional and clinical area of specialty practice.

Certified Diabetes Educators – Registered nurses, registered dietitians, and other professionals with diabetes education and experience who have passed the CDE examination.

Chronic Bronchitis – The presence of a productive cough for three months in each of two successive years in an individual for whom other causes of chronic cough have been excluded.

Chronic Obstructive Pulmonary Disease (COPD) – Disease state characterized by airflow limitation that is not fully reversible; airflow limitation is usually progressive and associated with an abnormal inflammatory response of the lungs to noxious particles or gases.

Clinical Care Classification (CCC) – Formerly Home Health Care Classification (HHCC); Saba's Georgetown System for Patient Problems, Interventions, and Outcomes.

Clinical Practice Guidelines – Statements that have been systematically developed to assist practitioners and patients in making decisions about appropriate health care for specific clinical circumstances.

Cluster Headaches – Sharp, extremely painful headaches that tend to occur several times a day for months, then go away for a similar period of time; can occur after patient has fallen asleep, located near or above the eye, and associated with nasal congestion.

Collaboration – Working together toward a common goal; to pursue a common purpose and a sharing of knowledge to resolve problems, decide issues, and set goals within a structure of collegiality.

Commercial Indemnity Plans – A type of insurance contract in which the insurer pays for care received up to a fixed amount per encounter or episode of illness.

Competence – Having the ability to demonstrate the technical, critical thinking, and interpersonal skills necessary to perform one's job responsibilities.

Complementary, Alternative, and Integrative Therapies (CAM) – Care that includes non-traditional therapies either in place of or together with conventional medicine.

Confidentiality – To protect the patient's and family's right to privacy regarding information that the nurse or institution holds about the patient.

Confusion – Disorientation, inappropriate behavior or communication, and/or hallucinations.

Co-Payment – Out-of-pocket expense paid by an individual for a specific service defined in the insurance plan.

Cost Benefit Analysis – A formal financial analysis completed by organizations to determine the cost of a program, projected revenues, and to identify and quantify program benefits; includes assumptions about specific expenses and potential revenue based on projected volumes.

CPT – *The Physicians' Current Procedural Terminology,* published by the American Medical Association; the internationally recognized coding system for reporting medical services and procedures.

Credentialing – Review and verification of credentials (i.e., education, training, licensure, certification, experience). In some cases (such as in most nursing homes and an increasing number of other health care facilities), this includes performing criminal background checks.

Cultural Competence – Requires developing cultural awareness (conscious learning process through which one becomes appreciative and sensitive to the cultures of other people), cultural knowledge (process of understanding the key aspects of a group's culture), cultural skills (ability to collect relevant data regarding health histories and perform culturally specific assessments), and cultural encounters (process that encourages one to engage directly in cross-cultural interactions with people from culturally diverse backgrounds).

Decision Support System – Automated tool that enhances the nurse's ability to make decisions in semi-structured, uncertain situations by bringing necessary information, evidence, expertise, and resources to the point of care.

Deductible – Amount an insured individual is responsible to pay before insurance pays. For example, an individual may have to pay a $200 deductible for hospitalization before the remainder of the hospital stay is covered by insurance.

Delegation – The transfer of responsibility for the performance of a task from one person to another.

Delirium – An acute change in cognition or awareness, with agitation presenting as an accompanying symptom.

Deontology – Also known as duty-based ethics; based on the belief that there are duties to which one must be faithful and which one is obligated to carry out because these duties are owed to all human beings and because of the expectations implied by one's professional role.

Depression (Major) – Possessing five or more symptoms of depression (e.g., insomnia, fatigue, weight loss or gain, low self-esteem, sudden bursts of anger, excessive sleeping).

Diabetes – See *Type 1 Diabetes* and *Type 2 Diabetes*.

Diagnosis-Related Groups (DRGs) – A system for classifying hospital inpatients into groups requiring similar quantities of resources according to characteristics such as diagnosis, age, procedure, complications, and co-morbidities.

Dietary Approaches to Stop Hypertension (DASH) – Evidence-based eating plan that is low in saturated fat, cholesterol, and total fat; reduced consumption of red meats, sweets, and sugar-containing beverages; concomitant emphasis on fruits, vegetables, and low-fat dairy products; rich in magnesium, calcium, protein, and fiber; sodium consumption is limited from 1,500–2,400 mg/day.

Disinfection – Process that destroys many or all pathogenic microorganisms (except bacterial spores) on inanimate objects, usually by use of liquid chemical or wet pasteurization.

Distance Learning – Provides access to learning modalities initially designed to reach/include persons in rural/isolated areas, providing educational opportunities/resources.

Domain of Ambulatory Nursing Practice – The overall scope of nursing practice in the ambulatory arena; it includes attributes of the environment in which practice occurs, patient requirements for care, and specific nursing role dimensions.

Dyslipidemia – See *Hyperlipidemia*.

Dysthymia – Depression that is chronic in nature; milder than major depression, lasting up to two years.

Education Process – Systematic planned course of action consisting of two major interdependent operations: teaching and learning.

Emergency Medical Treatment and Active Labor Act (EMTALA) – Federal law passed in 1986 to ensure patient access to emergency services regardless of ability to pay.

Emotional Intelligence – Ability to accurately perceive one's own and others' emotions, to understand the signals that emotions send about the relationship, and to manage one's own and others' emotions.

Emphysema – The abnormal enlargement of airspaces distal to the terminal bronchioles with destruction of their walls without obvious fibrosis.

Environmental Management – The assurance of appropriate management plans to provide a safe, accessible, effective, and functional environment of care.

Epilepsy – Diagnosis for congenital or acquired brain disease, resulting in seizure activity.

Equal Employment Opportunity Commission (EEOC) – A federal agency that enforces regulations concerning equal opportunity.

Ethics – A branch of philosophy dealing with the values related to human conduct, with respect to the rightness or wrongness of certain actions; and to the goodness and badness of the motives and ends of such actions; a set of moral principles or values, the principles of conduct governing an individual or a group.

Ethnopharmacology – Emerging field of research that is increasingly focusing on the effect of genetic and cultural factors on absorption, metabolism, distribution, and eliminations and the mechanism of action and effects of drugs.

Evidence-Based Practice – The conscientious, explicit, and judicious use of current best evidence in making decisions about the care of individual patients; combines research and clinical expertise.

Existential Distress – Occurs at a time when a person is questioning the meaning of his or her life. This response encompasses the physical, psychosocial, and spiritual angst that may occur at the end of life.

Fee for Service – Reimbursement method in which payment is made for each service or item.

Fidelity – Faithfulness; involves duty owed to patients, families, and colleagues to do what one says.

Fixed Costs – Costs do not change with volume of service units or activity, such as patient visits.

Focal Seizure – Seizure activity initiating from one side of the brain; presentation of seizure activity is seen on the opposite side of the body; may or may not generalize to include both sides of the body.

Food Guide Pyramid (United States Department of Agriculture) – Provides a visual key to the proper dietary balance of the five food groups.

Grand Mal Seizure – See *Tonic-Clonic Seizure.*

Grief – The individualized feelings and responses that a person makes to real, perceived, or anticipated loss.

Health Care Financing Administration (HCFA) – See *Centers for Medicare and Medicaid Services (CMS).*

Health Care Financing Administration (HCFA) Common Procedure Coding System (HCPCS) – A uniform method for health care providers and medical suppliers to report professional services, procedures, and supplies to health care plans.

Health Care Team – Includes the patient, family, and other members of the health care system who are involved in the development and implementation of the care plan.

Health Insurance Portability and Accountability Act (HIPAA) – Federal law that establishes a "floor" for privacy protection and implementing privacy and security regulations; applies to all health plans, health care clearinghouses, and those health care providers (including nurses) who bill electronically for their services; basically provides that patients have a right to control their information and must "authorize" use or disclosure of their health information.

Health Literacy – Degree to which individuals have the capacity to obtain, process, and understand basic health information and services needed to make appropriate health decisions.

Health Maintenance Organization (HMO) – A health plan that uses physicians as gatekeepers. In this model, the patient chooses a primary care provider (PCP) who is responsible for all aspects of care management and who must authorize (gatekeeper) or give permission for referral to other providers; another model of HMO places risk on the providers for medical expenses. In this instance, providers are encouraged to provide appropriate medical services, but not medically unnecessary services, in exchange for larger premiums.

Healthy People 2020 – Federal government's health care improvement priorities managed by federal agencies; provides measurable objectives applicable at national, state, and local levels; increases public awareness and understanding of determinants of health.

Heart Failure – A complex clinical syndrome in which the cardiac myocytes or contractile apparatus of the heart does not pump enough blood to meet the needs of the tissues; peripheral perfusion is altered, leading to subsequent mechanical, neuroendocrine, and inflammatory responses in an attempt to improve systemic organ flow; compensatory mechanisms fail to improve contractility over time and lead to a maladaptive state characterized by "ventricular remodeling."

HEDIS® – A set of standardized performance measures designed to assure that purchasers and consumers have the information they need to reliably compare the performance of health plans; sponsored and maintained by NCQA.

Hospice – Comprehensive, non-curative services are provided to a terminally ill patient and his or her family by an interdisciplinary team (including physicians, nurses, social workers, chaplains, counselors, certified nursing assistants, therapists, and volunteers) wherever the patient is.

Hyperlipidemia – An elevation of any lipid in blood plasma; increased levels of low-density lipoprotein (LDL) incorporate themselves into fatty plaque development on the intima wall of the blood vessel causing atherosclerotic changes, stiffening of the arteries, and reducing blood flow to vital organs.

Hypertensive Emergency – Severe elevation of blood pressure (BP) (>180/120 mm Hg) complicated by evidence of impending or progressive target organ dysfunction.

ICD-9-CM (*International Classification of Diseases,* 9th revision, Clinical Modification) – Published by the U.S. National Center for Health Statistics; the internationally recognized system for the purposes of international morbidity and mortality reporting; in the United States, used for coding and billing purposes.

ICD-10-CM (*International Classification of Diseases,* 10th edition, Clinical Modification Procedure Coding System) – New classification system that captures more detailed clinical information to reflect advances in clinical medicine; uses 3–7 alpha or numeric digits.

Independent Practice Association (IPA) – A legal entity whose members are independent physicians who contract with the IPA for the purpose of having the IPA contract with one or more HMOs.

Informed Consent – Process by which a patient is provided relevant information about a proposed procedure, test, or course of treatment; given an opportunity to ask questions; and asked to voluntarily agree.

Institute of Medicine (IOM) – An independent, non-profit organization that works to provide unbiased and authoritative advice to decision-makers and the public to improve health.

Interstate Compacts – Allow that nurses may practice across state lines, physically or electronically, unless under discipline or a monitoring agreement that restricts interstate practice. Nurses are licensed where they live (the "home state").

The Joint Commission (TJC) (Formerly The Joint Commission on Accreditation of Healthcare Organizations [JCAHO]) – An independent, non-profit organization that evaluates and accredits more than 15,000 health care programs in the United States.

Justice – Fair, equitable distribution of resources.

Magnet Recognition Program® – American Nurses Credentialing Center's program to recognize health care organizations that provide the very best in nursing care and uphold the tradition within professional nursing practice.

Major Depression – See *Depression.*

Managed Care – A system that combines financing and care delivery through comprehensive benefits delivered by selected providers and financial incentives for enrolled members to use these providers; goals of managed care are quality, cost-effectiveness, and accessible health care. It is a coordinated system of health care, which achieves outcomes (reduced utilization and improved population health) through preventive care, case management, and the provision of medically necessary and appropriate care.

Medicaid – A plan jointly funded by federal and state governments, introduced in 1966 to cover poor individuals; it is managed by each state.

Migraine Headache – Severe, recurrent headache with other symptoms, including visual changes, nausea and vomiting, and photophobia; starts on one side of the head and may spread to both sides; some may have an aura before onset; pain is described as throbbing, pounding, or pulsating.

Moderate Sedation – Use of medication resulting in amnesia and/or analgesia to sufficiently blunt, but not remove, a patient's protective reflexes in order to allow the performance of a procedure or test; patient should exhibit a state of reduced consciousness that allows the patient to tolerate unpleasant procedures while retaining the ability to independently and continuously maintain cardiorespiratory function and appropriately respond to physical stimulation and/or verbal commands.

Motivational Interviewing (MI) – Method of guiding patients to explore their own health behaviors and to strengthen their motivation to change.

Mourning – The outward, social expression of loss; often dictated by cultural norms, customs, and practices, including rituals and traditions; is also influenced by the individual's personality and life experiences.

National Committee for Quality Assurance (NCQA) – An independent, non-profit organization that assesses, evaluates, and publicly reports on the quality of health plans, health care provider groups, and individual physicians.

National Patient Safety Goals (NPSGs) – The Joint Commission's series of specific actions that accredited organizations are required to meet with the purpose of preventing medical errors and improving processes for patient safety.

Negligence – A duty of care owed to the patient is breached, with a reasonable direct relationship to the patient suffering damages.

Nonmaleficence – Acting in such a way that avoids harm, either intentional harm or harm as an unintended outcome.

North American Nursing Diagnosis Association (NANDA) Nomenclature –Terminology used by nurses to document diagnoses in all settings where nursing care is delivered.

Nursing Informatics – A specialty that integrates nursing science, computer science, and information science to manage and communicate data, information, and knowledge in nursing practice.

Nursing Interventions Classification (NIC) – Taxonomy for classifying nursing interventions; used in all settings where care is delivered to document nursing interventions; developed by a team at University of Iowa, led by McCloskey and Bulechek.

Nursing Minimum Data Set (NMDS) – A concept developed to ensure that all data important to nursing was collected in a standardized manner in every encounter, across all settings; includes 16 data elements; not widely implemented in practice.

Nursing-Sensitive Outcomes – Changes in the actual or potential health status, behavior, or perceptions of individuals, families, or populations that can be attributed to nursing interventions provided.

Nursing Services – Organized services delivered to groups of patients by nursing staff; includes nursing care as well as services to support or facilitate direct care, such as referral and coordination of care.

Obesity – Body weight 120% of ideal; body mass index (BMI) equal to or greater than 30; or adipose deposition patterns.

Occupational Safety and Health Administration (OSHA) – Branch of the U.S. Department of Labor responsible for enforcing laws and regulations on workplace safety.

Omaha VNA System– A system for problems, interventions, and outcomes; used by nurses to describe and document care in community settings; contains 40 nursing problems (diagnoses) and a number of associated nursing interventions and outcomes (composed of knowledge, behavior, and status subscales).

Orientation – A structured plan created by the organization to "on-board" new staff to provide smooth assimilation into a new position; key components include a general organizational overview, department specifics, and individualized job duties.

Osteoarthritis – Disease manifested by progressive degeneration of cartilage in joints; as cartilage becomes thin, bone ends come closer together, bone spurs develop at tendon and ligament attachment sites, synovial fluid may leak, and cysts may develop on the bone; also known as degenerative joint disease (DJD).

Otitis Externa – Infection of the ear canal.

Otitis Media – Infection occurring just behind the eardrum; presents as collection of fluid, bloody or purulent, visible by otoscope.

Out-of-Pocket Expense – Refers to the portion of health care cost for which the individual is responsible.

Ozbolt's Patient Care Data Set (PCDS) – Taxonomy used by nurses to document care in all settings, but primarily developed for the acute care setting; comprises nursing diagnoses, patient care actions, and nursing outcomes.

Pain – An unpleasant sensory and emotional experience associated with actual or potential tissue damage, or described in terms of such damage.

Palliative Care – Both a philosophy of care and an organized, highly structured system for delivery of care; its goal is to prevent and relieve suffering and to support the best possible quality of life for patients and their families, regardless of the stage of the disease or the need for other therapies.

Patient-Centered Medical Home (PCMH) – A care delivery model that facilitates partnerships between individual patients, their health care team, and, when appropriate, the patient's family; attributes include patient-centeredness, continuous improvement, and care that is comprehensive, coordinated, and accessible.

Patient Education – Process of assisting people to learn health-related behaviors (knowledge, skills, attitudes, and values) so they can incorporate them into their everyday lives.

Patient Protection and Affordable Care Act (PPACA) – U.S. law passed in 2010 to reform health care, focused on health promotion, disease prevention, and increased access through insurance reform.

Pay for Performance – Government and other third-party payer programs to incentivize adherence to suggested evidence-based guidelines that lead to improved patient outcomes.

Pediatric Advanced Life Support (PALS) – Protocols and algorithms created through the American Heart Association to provide guidelines for medical management of potentially fatal health conditions in the pediatric population, and to provide guidelines for medical management of cardiac arrest and/or arrhythmia and respiratory arrest and/or respiratory support.

Peer Review – Process of reviewing and assessing the clinical competence and conduct of health professionals on an ongoing basis; an integral part of quality assessment and improvement processes.

Performance Improvement – Systematic analysis of the structure, processes, and outcomes within systems for the purpose of improving the delivery of care.

Perfusion – Tissues in the body exchanging metabolic waste (carbon dioxide) and receiving oxygen through arterial/venous circulation.

Perioperative Nursing Data Set (PNDS) – Developed by the Association of periOperative Registered Nurses (AORN); used by perioperative registered nurses and surgical service managers in a variety of perioperative settings.

Petit Mal Seizure – See *Absence Seizure.*

Physician Hospital Organization (PHO) – Legal organization often developed for purposes of contracting with managed care plans; links physicians to specific hospitals for hospitalization care.

Point of Service (POS) – A plan that defines service providers in the service area outside of the usual preferred provider network.

Polypharmacy – Involves clients with one or more conditions who are using multiple medications, some of which are not clinically indicated.

Post-Ictal Period – Time after a seizure during which the client may present with confusion and lethargy.

Postpartum Depression – Feeling of sadness or "blue mood" after delivery; usually induced by hormonal changes.

Precertification – Process of obtaining authorization or certification from a health plan for hospital admissions, referrals, procedures, or tests.

Preferred Provider Organization (PPO) – Program in which contracts exist between the health plan and care providers at a discount for services; typically, the plan provides incentives for patients to use in-network providers as opposed to nonparticipating providers (independent/noncontracted) through decreased co-payments.

Premenstrual Dysphoric Disorder (PMDD) – Feeling of depression with onset one week prior to menses; after onset of menstruation, symptoms resolve.

Presence – Effective listening; occurs at five different levels: hearing, understanding, retaining information, analyzing and evaluating information, and helping/active empathizing.

Priapism – Sustained, unwanted, and painful penile erection usually unrelated to sexual activity, due to vaso-occlusion, causing obstruction of the venous drainage of the penis.

Primary Care – The provision of integrated, accessible health care services by clinicians who are accountable for addressing a large majority of personal health care needs, developing a sustained partnership with patients, and practicing in the context of family and community.

Primary Prevention – Includes health promotion (HP) interventions and specific protections (SP); may be directed at individuals, groups, or populations; targeted at well populations or those already ill (e.g., HP = nutrition education; SP = use of seatbelts, avoidance of allergens, or importance of inoculations).

Productivity – Measure of the efficiency with which labor and materials are converted into service or care; volume of output related to amount of resources consumed/used to produce a specified output/service.

Rebound Headache – Occurs after medication for pain relief of headaches has been taken away; reintroducing the pain reliever does not decrease pain.

Relative Value Unit (RVU) – Established by HCFA/CMS to approximate the work, practice expense, and malpractice expense for delivery of physician services.

Report Cards – Identify performance measures that include quality indicators (immunization, Pap smear, and mammogram rates), utilization indicators (membership, access, finances, hospital, and ER admission), and satisfaction levels; consumers use report card data to compare the performance of different organizations against a predetermined standard/best practice.

Research Utilization – A process of using research findings as a basis for practice; typically based on a single study.

Resource-Based Relative Value Scale (RBRVS) – A classification system that attempts to assign the resource requirements within a defined setting based on weights, according to relative cost of each service.

Respiratory Arrest – Lung tissue is not able to receive carbon dioxide or give oxygen to circulating blood.

Revenue – Total amount of income received or that is entitled to be received based on services rendered or goods provided.

Risk Management – An organization-wide program to identify risks, control occurrences, prevent damage, and control legal liability; a process whereby risks to an institution are evaluated and controlled.

Root Cause Analysis – A method to determine the fundamental reason that causes variation in performance.

Seasonal Affective Disorder (SAD) – Feeling of depression that ensues during the autumn and winter months due to decreased length of daylight.

Secondary Prevention – Involves early diagnosis and prompt treatment to avoid disability (e.g., screening, biopsies, medication, surgery).

Seizure – Increased neuronal activity in the brain caused by disease process or trauma, leading to hypertonicity and muscular contracture.

Sickle Cell Disease – An autosomal recessive disorder characterized by the production of abnormal hemoglobin, causing a decrease in red blood cell survival and polymerization of red blood cells (sickling).

SNOMED-CT® – Systematic Nomenclature for Medicine-Reference Terminology (College of American Pathologists) comprehensive, multiaxial nomenclature classification system created for the indexing of the entire medical and health care vocabulary.

Splenic Sequestration – Intrasplenic trapping of red blood cells, which causes a precipitous fall in hemoglobin level and the potential for hypoxic shock.

Standard – An authoritative statement developed and disseminated by a professional organization or governmental or regulatory agency by which the quality of practice, services, research, or education can be judged.

State Practice Acts – A combination of laws and regulations that define and regulate the practice of medicine, nursing, and other health professions.

Status Epilepticus – Increased neuronal activity in the brain, resulting in seizure activity that continues for more than 10 minutes; considered a medical emergency.

Sterilization – Process that destroys or eliminates all forms of microbial life that is carried out in health care facilities by physical or chemical methods; required to be carried out on critical items and those that enter sterile tissue or the vascular system.

Strategic Planning – The continuous process of systematically evaluating the nature of the ambulatory care organization, defining its long-term objectives, identifying quantifiable goals, developing strategies to reach these objectives and goals, and allocating resources to carry out these strategies.

Supervision – The direction and oversight of the performance of others.

Telehealth – Delivery, management, and coordination of health services that integrate electronic information and telecommunications technologies to increase access, improve outcomes, and contain or reduce costs of health care.

Telehealth Nursing – Delivery, management, and coordination of care and services provided via telecommunications technology within the domain of nursing; encompassing practices that incorporate a vast array of telecommunications technologies (telephone, fax, electronic mail, Internet, video monitoring, and interactive video) to remove time and distance barriers for the delivery of nursing care.

Telephone Nursing – All care and services within the scope of nursing practice that are delivered over the telephone; component of telehealth nursing practice restricted to the telephone.

Telephone Triage – An interactive process between the nurse and patient that occurs over the telephone; involves identifying the nature and urgency of client health care needs and determining the appropriate disposition; a component of telephone nursing practice that focuses on assessment and prioritization and referral to the appropriate level of care.

Tension Headache – Caused by tight, contracted muscles in shoulders, neck, scalp, and jaw; brought on by stress, depression, anxiety, overwork, lack of sleep, not eating properly, and/or alcohol or drug use.

Tertiary Prevention – Involves rehabilitation to return to maximum use of remaining capacities (such as maximizing functional status of the COPD patient with pulmonary toilet and oxygen administration).

Tonic-Clonic (Grand Mal) Seizure – Increased neuronal activity in the brain with presenting loss of consciousness, muscle rigidity, involuntary muscular twitching, and incontinence.

Transitional Care – Directed at making a smooth transition between levels of care and/or settings.

TriCare – A federal program providing coverage to families of active duty military personnel, military retirees, spouses, and dependents, which replaced CHAMPUS (Civilian Health and Medical Program of the United States).

Type 1 Diabetes – Onset is usually acute with pronounced symptoms; autoimmune disease characterized by loss of pancreatic beta cell function; insulin required in a regimen designed for the individual in a way that imitates non-diabetes insulin production.

Type 2 Diabetes – Onset is usually gradual, with or without symptoms in those with family history of Type 2 diabetes and other risk factors; insulin production at onset may be normal or elevated, but insulin resistance, elevated liver production of glucose, and other factors may prevent insulin from functioning normally; treatment includes healthy eating, exercise, oral medications, and/or insulin to control blood glucose levels.

U.S. Preventive Services Task Force (USPSTF) – Non-governmental expert panel of primary care, evidence-based medicine experts who review current preventive services and make practice recommendations.

Usual, Customary, and Reasonable (UCR) – A method used to determine if a fee is usual, customary, and reasonable; *customary* is based on a percentile of aggregated fees charged in the geographic area for the same service; *usual* refers to fees normally charged by a doctor or health care provider for a service.

Utilitarianism – Also known as consequence-based ethics; the theory that seeks to choose the thing that will offer the most good to the greatest number of people, increase pleasure, and avoid pain.

Utilization Management – The second process of care coordination across the continuum of care; the management and evaluation of the medical necessity, appropriateness, and efficiency of the use of health care services, procedures, and facilities under the auspices of the applicable health benefit plan.

Variable Costs – Costs that vary with changes in volumes of service units, such as patient visits.

Ventilation – Mechanism by which the blood gives off carbon dioxide and takes on oxygen in the lungs.

Ventricular Fibrillation – Fatal heart arrhythmia that results in pulselessness; ventricles contract in an unorganized manner resembling a quiver and produce no cardiac output.

Ventricular Tachycardia – Fatal heart arrhythmia with wide QRS complexes; not necessarily resulting in pulselessness initially; rapid rate of ventricular contraction inhibits adequate blood filling and decreased cardiac output.

Veracity – Truth telling.

Definitions taken from text.

Index

Index

A

Bolded page numbers indicate location of glossary definitions.

t = table
f = figure

Bolded page numbers indicate location of glossary definitions.	*t* = table *f* = figure

Bolded page numbers indicate location of glossary definitions.
t = table
f = figure

Bolded page numbers indicate location of glossary definitions.

t = table
f = figure

Bolded page numbers in-
dicate location of glossary
definitions.

t = table
f = figure

N

Bolded page numbers indicate location of glossary definitions.

t = table
f = figure

Bolded page numbers indicate location of glossary definitions.

t = table
f = figure

R

Race, cultural diversity of population and, 218–219, 218*t*, 219*t*
Radionuclides, for pain management, 482
Ramsey scale, 339
REALM, 235
Rebound headache, **519**
Records, retention, requirements for, 94
Red blood transfusions, for sickle cell disease, 445
Referrals, kickbacks, 98
Refusal of assignment, 90
Registered nurses
    delegation and, 38–39
    role in ambulatory care nursing practice, 6–7, 12, 16
    scope of ambulatory nursing practice, 38
Regulations, in nursing practice, 78–82
Regulatory standards, 101–111, 127–128
Rehydration therapy, 322*t*
Relative value unit (RVU), **519**
Renin, 362
Renin inhibitors, for coronary artery disease, 384*t*
Report cards, 163, **519**
Reporting
    of incompetent/inappropriate behavior, 83
    mandates, 97
Research utilization, **519**
Resource-based relative value scale (RBRVS), 56, **519**
Resource management, 57–58
Resources, for cultural competence, 228*f*–229*f*
Respirations, 204
Respiratory arrest, 292–295, **519**
Retinopathy, with sickle cell disease, 444
Revenue, 51–52, **519**
Risk management
    definition of, **519**
    linkage with advocacy and ethics, 116
    for telehealth nursing practice, 133–136
Root-cause analysis, 162, **519**
Rotovirus vaccine, 285
RVU (relative value unit), **519**

S

SAD (seasonal affective disorder), 303, **519**
Safe Medical Device act, 46
Safety
    counseling, 251–252
    cultural, 222–223
    definition of, 22
    patient *(See Patient safety)*
    of staff, 42–43
Safety culture, evolution of, 101–102
SBAR, 82
SBIR, 82
Scope of practice, 38, 85*t*
Screenings. *See also specific screening tests*
    adolescents/children, 283–285
    adult, 265–276
    infant, 283
SCT (Social Cognitive Theory), 237–238
Seasonal affective disorder (SAD), 303, **519**
Secondary prevention, 245, 264, **519**
Security issues, for office practice, 43
Sedation
    for ambulatory surgical practice, 332–333
    pharmacological agents used during, 339
Sedation scale, 339
Seizure, 295–297, **520**
Select serotonin reuptake inhibitors (SSRIs), 455*t*
Self-efficacy, 242
Self-management, 242, 244*t*, 351–352
Self-monitoring, of blood glucose, 377–378
Serotonin norepinephrne reuptake inhibitors (SNRIs), 481
Settings. *See Practice settings*
Sexually transmitted diseases (STDs)
    adult/adolescent, 313–315
    counseling, 252, 257–258
    HIV/AIDS *(See HIV/AIDS)*
    screenings, 280–283
Shock
    anaphylactic, 298–300
    hypoglycemic, 297–298
Sickle cell disease, 434–446
    complications, care plans for, 434–444

Bolded page numbers indicate location of glossary definitions. *t* = table, *f* = figure.

Bolded page numbers in-dicate location of glossary definitions.	*t* = table *f* = figure

Violence
    adolescent, counseling for, 253–254
    domestic, 305–307
Vision screening, 270–272, 284
Visual acuity, 210–211
Vital signs, 200–201
Vomiting, pediatric, 320–322, 322*f*

W

Waist-hip ratio (WHR), 274–275
Wellness, 264
Whistle blowing, 97
WHO analgesic ladder, 483, 483*f*
WHR (waist-hip ratio), 274–275
Workload variability/intensity, in ambulatory *vs.*
    inpatient setting, 24*t,* 26